The Diabetic Foot

CONTEMPORARY DIABETES

ARISTIDIS VEVES, MD, DSc
SERIES EDITOR

The Diabetic Foot, Second Edition, edited by *Aristidis Veves*, MD, DSC, *John M. Giurini*, DPM, *and Frank W. LoGerfo*, MD, *2006*

The Diabetic Kidney, edited by PEDRO CORTES, MD AND CARL ERIK MOGENSEN, MD, *2006*

Obesity and Diabetes, edited by *Christos S. Mantzoros*, MD, *2006*

THE DIABETIC FOOT
Second Edition

Edited by

ARISTIDIS VEVES, MD, DSc

JOHN M. GIURINI, DPM

FRANK W. LOGERFO, MD

Beth Israel Deaconess Medical Center
Harvard Medical School
Boston, MA

To Joe,

Thank you for all your help advice and guidance over the years

TanTi grazie,

John

HUMANA PRESS
TOTOWA, NEW JERSEY

© 2006 Humana Press Inc.
999 Riverview Drive, Suite 208
Totowa, New Jersey 07512

www.humanapress.com

Production Editor: Tracy Catanese

Cover design by Patricia F. Cleary

Cover Illustration: Figure 4 from Chapter 12, "Imaging of the Diabetic Foot," by Mary G. Hochman, Yvonne Cheung, David P. Brophy, and J. Anthony Parker.

For additional copies, pricing for bulk purchases, and/or information about other Humana titles, contact Humana at the above address or at any of the following numbers: Tel.: 973-256-1699; Fax: 973-256-8341, E-mail: orders@ humanapr.com; or visit our Website: www.humanapress.com

This publication is printed on acid-free paper.∞

ANSI Z39.48-1984 (American National Standards Institute) Permanence of Paper for Printed Library Materials.

Printed in the United States of America.   10 9 8 7 6 5 4 3 2 1

Library of Congress Cataloging-in-Publication Data

e-ISBN 1-59745-075-8

The diabetic foot / edited by Aristidis Veves, John M. Giurini, Frank W. LoGerfo. -- 2nd ed.
      p. ; cm. -- (Contemporary diabetes)
   Prev. ed. has subtitle: medical and surgical management.
   Includes bibliographical references and index.
   ISBN 1-58829-610-5 (alk. paper)
   1. Foot--Diseases. 2. Diabetes--Complications.   I. Veves, Aristidis. II. Giurini, John M. III. LoGerfo, Frank W.
IV. Series.
   [DNLM: 1. Diabetic Foot--therapy.   WK 835 D53518 2006]
   RD563.D495 2006
   617.5'85--dc22

                                                                                                2005034356

PREFACE

It has been more than 4 years since the first edition of *The Diabetic Foot* was published. Over this period of time, it has become absolutely clear that diabetes is becoming a pandemic that challenges the health care resources of all societies, from the developing ones to the most advanced. It is therefore not surprising that diabetic foot disease is still a major problem and, if anything, is growing in size rather than coming under control.

One positive development is that our knowledge of the pathophysiology of foot problems in diabetes has considerably expanded. Furthermore, it has been realized that impairment in wound healing is associated with pathways that are related to the development of cardiovascular disease, both in the micro- and macrocirculation.

In *The Diabetic Foot: Second Edition*, we have tried to keep the spirit of the first edition, which is to give the interested reader a full view of diabetic foot disease and to emphasize the need for a multidisciplinary approach in its management. As with the first edition, we have relied on the long tradition of the Joslin-Beth Israel Deconess Foot Center, one of the oldest and most experienced diabetic foot centers. We have also tried to emphasize new developments in basic and clinical research that we hope will be translated to clinical practice in the future. It is our hope that *The Diabetic Foot: Second Edition* will be helpful not only to clinicians but also to the research community with an interest in this field.

Aristidis Veves, MD, DSc
John M. Giurini, DPM
Frank W. LoGerfo, MD

CONTENTS

CONTRIBUTORS

OSCAR M. ALVAREZ, PhD • *Center for Palliative Wound Care, Calvary Hospital, Bronx and Department of Medicine, New York Medical College, Valhala, NY*

DAVID G. ARMSTRONG, DPM, PhD • *Chair of Research and Assistant Dean, Dr. William M. Scholl College of Podiatric Medicine and Director, Center for Lower Extremity Ambulatory Research, Rosalind Franklin University of Medicine and Science, North Chicago, IL*

CHRISTOPHER E. ATTINGER, MD • *Director, Wound Healing Center, Georgetown University Hospital and Professor of Plastic and Orthopedic Surgery, Georgetown University School of Medicine, Washington, DC*

DAVID P. BROPHY, MD, FRCSI, FRCR, MSCVIR • *St. James's Hospital, Trinity College Dublin, Dublin, Ireland*

A. J. M. BOULTON, MD, FRCP • *Professor of Medicine, University Department of Medicine, Manchester Royal Infirmary, Oxford Road, Manchester, UK*

DAVID CAMPBELL, MD • *Division of Vascular Surgery, Beth Israel Deaconess Medical Center, Harvard Medical School, Boston, MA*

YVONNE CHEUNG, MD • *Assistant Professor of Radiology and Orthopedics, Dartmouth Medical School, Hanover, NH*

I. KELMAN COHEN, MD • *Emeritus Professor of Surgery, Virginia Commonwealth University, and President and CEO, Tissue Technologies LLC, Richmond VA*

JEFFREY M. DAVIDSON, PhD • *Department of Pathology, Vanderbilt University School of Medicine and Veterans Affairs Medical Center, Nashville, TN*

THANH DINH, DPM • *Clinical Instructor in Surgery, Beth Israel Deaconess Medical Center, Harvard Medical School, Boston, MA*

LUISA DiPIETRO, DDS, PhD • *Burn and Shock Trauma Center, Department of Surgery, Loyola University Medical Center, Maywood, IL*

VINCENT FALANGA, MD, FACP • *Professor of Dermatology and Biochemistry, and Chairman, Department of Dermatology, Roger Williams Medical Center, Providence, RI*

ROBERT G. FRYKBERG, DPM, MPH • *Chief, Podiatry Section, Carl T. Hayden VA Medical Center, Phoenix, AZ*

JOHN M. GIURINI, DPM • *Chief, Division of Podiatry, Beth Israel Deaconess Medical Center and Associate Professor in Surgery, Harvard Medical School, Boston, MA*

ALLEN HAMDAN, MD • *Division of Vascular Surgery, Department of Surgery, Beth Israel Deaconess Medical Center, Harvard Medical School, Boston, MA*

LAWRENCE B. HARKLESS, DPM • *Louis B. Bogy Professor of Podiatric Medicine and Surgery, Department of Orthopedics, University of Texas Health Science Center at San Antonio, San Antonio, TX*

CHANTEL HILE, MD • *Division of Vascular Surgery, Department of Surgery, Beth Israel Deaconess Medical Center, Harvard Medical School, Boston, MA*

MARY G. HOCHMAN, MD • *Chief, Musculoskeletal Imaging Section, Beth Israel Deaconess Medical Center and Instructor in Radiology, Harvard Medical School, Boston, MA*

KAKRA HUGHES, MD • *Division of Vascular Surgery, Beth Israel Deaconess Medical Center, Harvard Medical School, Boston, MA*

NIKHIL KANSAL, MD • *Division of Vascular Surgery, Department of Surgery, Beth Israel Deaconess Medical Center, Harvard Medical School, Boston, MA*

ADOLF W. KARCHMER, MD • *Chief, Division of Infectious Diseases, Beth Israel Deaconess Medical Center, and Professor of Medicine, Harvard Medical School, Boston, MA*

LAWRENCE A. LAVERY, DPM, MPH • *Associate Professor, Department of Surgery, Scott & White Memorial Hospital, Texas A & M University College of Medicine, Temple, TX*

FRANK W. LOGERFO, MD • *Division of Vascular Surgery, Department of Surgery, Beth Israel Deaconess Medical Center, Harvard Medical School, Boston, MA*

THOMAS E. LYONS, DPM • *Clinical Instructor in Surgery, Harvard Medical School, Beth Israel Deaconess Medical Center, Harvard Medical School, Boston, MA*

LEE MARKOWITZ, DPM • *Center for Palliative Wound Care, Calvary Hospital, Bronx, NY*

LYNNE V. MCFARLAND, MS, PhD • *VA Research Health Science Specialist and Affiliate Associate Professor, Department of Medicinal Chemistry, University of Washington, Seattle, WA*

COLEEN NAPOLITANO, DPM • *Assistant Professor, Department of Orthopedic Surgery and Rehabilitation, Loyola University Stritch School of Medicine, Maywood, IL*

J. ANTHONY PARKER, MD • *Associate Professor of Radiology and Staff Radiologist, Nuclear Medicine, Beth Israel Deaconess Medical Center, Harvard Medical School, Boston, MA*

MICHAEL PINZUR, MD • *Professor, Department of Orthopedic Surgery and Rehabilitation, Loyola University Stritch School of Medicine, Maywood, IL*

FRANK B. POMPOSELLI, JR., MD • *Division of Vascular Surgery, Beth Israel Deaconess Medical Center, Harvard Medical School, Boston, MA*

GAYLE E. REIBER, MPH, PhD • *VA Career Scientist and Professor, Departments of Health Services and Epidemiology, University of Washington, Seattle, WA*

BARRY I. ROSENBLUM, DPM • *Division of Vascular Surgery, Department of Surgery, Beth Israel Deaconess Medical Center, Harvard Medical School, Boston, MA*

RONALD A. SAGE, DPM • *Professor, Department of Orthopedic Surgery and Rehabilitation, Loyola University Stritch School of Medicine, Maywood, IL*

SHERRY D. SCOVELL, MD • *Director, Endovascular Surgery, Division of Vascular Surgery, Beth Israel Deaconess Medical Center, Harvard Medical School, Boston, MA*

PETER SHEEHAN, MD • *Associate Professor of Medicine (Clinical), New York University School of Medicine, and Director, Diabetes Foot and Ankle Center, New York, NY*

ARLENE SMALDONE, DNSc, CPNP, CDE • *Assistant Professor of Nursing, Columbia University, New York, NY*

ERIC SOLLER, MSME • *Department of Mechanical Engineering, Massachusetts Institute of Technology, Cambridge, MA*

DAVID L. STEED, MD • *Professor of Surgery, Division of Vascular Surgery, University of Pittsburgh School of Medicine, Pittsburgh, PA*

RODNEY STUCK, DPM • *Associate Professor, Department of Orthopedic Surgery and Rehabilitation, Loyola University Stritch School of Medicine, Maywood, IL*

SOLOMON TESFAYE, MD, FRCP • *Consultant Physician and Senior Lecturer, Royal Hallamshire Hospital, Sheffield, UK*

LUIGI UCCIOLI, MD • *Department of Internal Medicine, University of Rome Tor Vergata, Rome, Italy*

C. H. M. VAN SCHIE, MSc, PhD • *Department of Rehabilitation, Academic Medical Center, University of Amsterdam, Amsterdam, The Netherlands*

ARISTIDIS VEVES, MD, DSc • *Research Director, Microcirculation Lab and Joslin-Beth Israel Deaconess Foot Center, and Associate Professor, Harvard Medical School, Boston, MA*

KATIE WEINGER, EdD, RN • *Investigator, Joslin Diabetes Center and Assistant Professor of Psychiatry, Harvard Medical School, Boston, MA*

MARTIN WENDELKEN, DPM, RN • *Center for Palliative Wound Care, Calvary Hospital, Bronx, NY*

STEPHANIE WU, DPM, MSc • *Assistant Professor, Department of Surgery, Dr. William M. Scholl College of Podiatric Medicine and Fellow, Center for Lower Extremity Ambulatory Research, Rosalind Franklin University of Medicine and Science, North Chicago, IL*

IOANNIS V. YANNAS, PhD • *Departments of Biological and Mechanical Engineering, Massachusetts Institute of Technology, Cambridge, MA*

Introduction to Diabetes
Principles of Care in the Surgical Patient With Diabetes

Peter Sheehan, MD

INTRODUCTION

The medical and surgical management of foot disorders in the patient with diabetes should have as its basis a thorough understanding of the complications and metabolic consequences of diabetes mellitus. This is especially true in the patient who is undergoing a surgical procedure. Diabetes is rapidly increasing in prevalence worldwide and surgery in patients with diabetes is more common. Foot complications are already a major cause of admissions for diabetes, and comprise a disproportionately high number of hospital days because of increased surgical procedures and prolonged length of stay.

With advances in surgical techniques and anesthesia, surgery has become safer for patients with diabetes; nonetheless, patients with diabetes are high-risk group for perioperative complications, such as infection and myocardial infarction (MI). These may be avoided or minimized with proper anticipation and awareness of the patient's medical condition. Despite the increase in morbidity and mortality that has been observed in the surgical patient with diabetes, there are no widely accepted guidelines for the many clinical issues that are present in the perioperative period. The objective of this chapter is to present current concepts in the assessment and management of the surgical patient with diabetes, as well as the pathophysiological basis on which these concepts rest. To this end, an overview of diabetes mellitus and its complications also will be presented, with the understanding that more thorough reviews exist elsewhere, which are beyond the scope of this chapter.

OVERVIEW OF DIABETES AND ITS COMPLICATIONS

Epidemiology

In the past few decades, there has been an alarming rise in the prevalence of diabetes, particularly type 2 diabetes. In the well-studied town of Framingham, Massachusetts, the prevalence has risen from 0.9% in 1958 to 3% in 1995 *(1)*. Recently, the Centers for Disease Control estimated the US prevalence of diagnosed diabetes at 7.3% in 2001, in comparison with a similar study in 1990 reporting 4.9%, representing nearly a 48% increase over the decade *(2)*. Most disturbing was a 76% increase in the prevalence among

From: *The Diabetic Foot, Second Edition*
Edited by: A. Veves, J. M. Giurini, and F. W. LoGerfo © Humana Press Inc., Totowa, NJ

the 30–39 year age group. Furthermore, there exists a nearly as large group in the population who are undiagnosed. This estimate comes from the National Health and Nutrition Examination Survey (NHANES) II and III studies of large-scale population screening, in which only 50% of people found to have diabetes were previously diagnosed *(3)*.

The increased prevalence of diabetes in the United States is correlated with the rising rates of obesity, which now afflicts more than 20% of adult Americans. The prevalence of diagnosed diabetes also increases with age, affecting more than 10% of those over 65 years of age in the United States. It is also slightly over-represented in women in comparison with men. Some ethnic populations have a two- to fivefold increase in risk of developing diabetes. The highest incidence is seen in Native Americans, followed by Hispanics, African Americans, Asians, and Pacific Islanders. The risk of diabetes in all groups is associated with higher rates of obesity and, more specifically, with an increase in the waist–hip ratio, a measure of central adiposity.

Worldwide, the rates of diagnosed diabetes are rising, especially in developing nations. Indigenous peoples of the Americas and Polynesia are those with the highest risk. The Pima tribe in Arizona has the highest prevalence of type 2 diabetes in the world, affecting nearly 50% of all adult members. Asians and Africans are of intermediate risk. People of European descent are actually among those with the lowest risk of developing diabetes *(4)*. Most epidemiological studies suggest that lifestyle changes introduced with increasing industrialization and economic development may be responsible. Higher prevalence of diabetes can also be seen in urban dwellers *vis-a-vis* their rural counterparts. The obvious contributing factors are a more abundant and richer diet, a sedentary lifestyle, and higher rates of obesity.

One cohesive theory tying the genetic predisposition of type 2 diabetes seen in certain ethnic groups to a higher prevalence of obesity is one of the "thrifty phenotype" *(5)*. According to this hypothesis first proposed by Neel in 1962, these high-risk ethnic groups, primarily indigenous peoples, have been adapted over the millennia to survive conditions of scarcity and episodic "feast or famine." As a consequence of natural selection, they have developed a degree of metabolic efficiency, or "thriftiness," that allows storage of ingested calories as fat with less energy expenditure or waste. This predisposes therefore to higher tendency to obesity, especially of the central type, when placed in an environment of surfeit, rich foodstuffs. With the development of obesity, there is in turn insulin resistance and a greater risk of type 2 diabetes.

At this time, approx 1% of the population of China has diabetes, but the prevalence is rising, especially in urban areas. Indeed, the prevalence of diabetes is approx 4% in Beijing. It is estimated that if that country assumes a more industrial, Western lifestyle, the prevalence would rise to 8–10%. This alone would cause nearly a doubling of the world's population with diabetes. Similar projections are proposed for South Asians as well. It is clear that we are presently in a pandemic of diabetes that will pose an even greater and more frequently encountered medical issue. The decade of incident diabetes has now given way to a time of prevalent diabetes. This portends a new wave of chronic diabetic complications presenting in the coming decade.

Diagnosis

An expert committee of the American Diabetes Association (ADA) amended the diagnostic criteria for diabetes mellitus in 1997 *(6)*. Previously, the diagnosis was made with the Fajans–Conn criteria as the standard. By that definition, a person was diagnosed with diabetes when: (1) signs and symptoms of diabetes (polyuria, polydipsia, and so on) with glycosuria or a random blood glucose >200 mg%; (2) fasting blood glucose greater than 140 mg% on two separate occasions; or (3) after an oral 75 g glucose load, a 2-hour blood glucose and an interval blood glucose greater than 200 mg%. The problem with the use of these criteria was the lack of sensitivity in the fasting blood glucose value in diagnosing diabetes in comparison with the 2-hour glucose tolerance test. Furthermore, the Wisconsin epidemiological study of diabetic retinopathy and NHANES III data suggested that retinopathy was associated with fasting blood glucose as low as 120 mg% *(7)*. It was concluded that using a lower diagnostic value would improve correlation with the incidence and prevalence of microvascular complications, i.e., retinopathy, and would increase the sensitivity correlating similar to the oral glucose tolerance results. Therefore, the ADA expert consensus criteria for the diagnosis of diabetes are as follow:

1. Symptoms and a casual blood glucose greater than 200 mg%.
2. Fasting blood glucose greater than 126 mg% (7 mmol/dL) on two separate occasions.
3. Two-hour blood glucose greater than 200 mg% after a 75 g oral glucose load.

The new criteria thus encourage the use of the fasting blood glucose as an efficient and reliable measure in the diagnosis of diabetes.

Most recently, the ADA defined a "normal" blood glucose as less than 100 mg%. Persons with fasting values between normal (<100 mg%) and diabetes (>126 mg%) would be classified as having "prediabetes." Formerly called impaired glucose tolerance (IGT), the term "prediabetes" underscores the progressive nature of this metabolic condition and the high conversion rate to type 2 diabetes and its complications.

CLASSIFICATION

The classification of diabetes also has revised nomenclature. Type 1 diabetes refers to β-cell destruction and absolute insulin deficiency, previously called "juvenile" or "insulin dependent" diabetes. It is a chronic autoimmune disease affecting pancreatic β-cells. The typical patient is a 12-year-old child presenting with diabetic ketoacidosis (DKA). Clearly, however, it can be seen in older persons with less dramatic, insidious presentation. In the United Kingdom Prospective Diabetes Study (UKPDS), many adult patients had evidence of islet cell autoimmunity, especially the younger, less obese subgroups *(8)*.

More than 90% of people with diabetes have type 2 diabetes, which typically affects an older population, and is associated with a family history of diabetes, as well as obesity and sedentary lifestyle. In the past, type 2 diabetes was referred to as "adult-onset" and "noninsulin dependent" diabetes. This nomenclature is less accurate in that many of these patients are treated with insulin, and there is presently a rising incidence in the younger population, even in childhood ages. As will be discussed, type 2 diabetes is characterized by insulin resistance and an absolute or relative impairment in insulin secretion. It is now reaching epidemic occurrence rates worldwide.

Secondary causes of diabetes are uncommon, but should be considered, especially if management of the patient is unusual or problematic. Pancreatic disease leads to insulin deficiency and diabetes, but is also associated with marked insulin sensitivity because of exocrine insufficiency, malabsorption, and glucagon deficiency. Endocrine disorders may cause hyperglycemia that may be reversible, and are usually recognized by their own stigmata. These include Cushing's disease, acromegaly, and hyperthyroidism. There are also rare hereditary and acquired disorders of extreme insulin resistance. These are often associated with an intertriginous dermopathy and acanthosis nigricans.

Finally, an increasingly more common presentation is diabetes during pregnancy, or gestational diabetes mellitus. Often occurring in the third trimester, it can lead to fetal wastage, macrosomia, and fetal malformation, especially neural crest and heart defects. The hyperglycemia typically resolves after delivery, implicating some placental factor as central to the pathogenesis. Nonetheless, these women are phenotypically insulin resistant and are at high risk for future development of diabetes, with a 10-year postpartum incidence of more than 30%.

Pathogenesis of Diabetes

Type 1 Diabetes

Many studies over the past two decades have validated the characterization of type 1 diabetes as a chronic autoimmune disease *(9)*. The familiar pathological finding of "insulitis" demonstrating lymphocytic infiltration of the pancreatic islets with loss of insulin-containing β cells suggests cell-mediated immune activation. In addition, 90% of individuals at presentation with type 1 diabetes have autoantibodies against islet cells and insulin. These include islet cell antibodies, insulin auto antibodies, and glutamic acid decarboxylase antibodies. Whether these antibodies are cause or result of β-cell destruction is not certain, but they serve as ancillary evidence of the autoimmune nature of this disorder.

Importantly, the presence of autoantibodies can be demonstrated years before the diagnosis of type 1 diabetes, underscoring the chronic, silent nature of its development. This belies the familiar, often-dramatic clinical presentation of acute diabetic ketoacidosis in a young person. It is important to note that some older patients felt to have type 2 diabetes may in fact have type 1 diabetes, as suggested by the demonstration of circulating islet cell antibodies and glutamic acid decarboxylase antibodies. These patients tend to be leaner and younger at presentation, and progress rapidly to requiring insulin treatment over 2 or 3 years *(8)*. The smoldering autoimmune destruction of the β cells may also be arrested. These same autoantibodies also are highly predictive of future development of type 1 diabetes, and serve as a screening mechanism in studies designed to prevent the onset of hyperglycemia with immune modulation *(10)*.

Type 1 diabetes follows ethnic and geographical variation. The highest incidence in contrast to type 2 diabetes is found in Scandinavian and Northern European populations. Early-onset type 1 diabetes is associated with specific human leukocyte antigen (HLA) phenotypes on chromosome 6 responsible for class-II histocompatability complexes, namely DR3, DR4, and DR3/DR4. Other genes in the closely located DQ locus may confer increased risk or protection from clinical type 1 diabetes *(11)*. Because concordance rates in HLA-identical twins are less than 50%, and fewer than 15% of newly diagnosed patients have an affected first degree relative, environmental factors are implicated in the pathogenesis of type 1 diabetes. Possible environmental triggers include viruses (mumps, Coxsackie's B, and rubella) and dietary substances (bovine milk albumin and gluten) *(12)*.

The current model of the pathogenesis is that an environmental factor triggers an autoimmune response against the pancreas, leading chronically over years to progressive

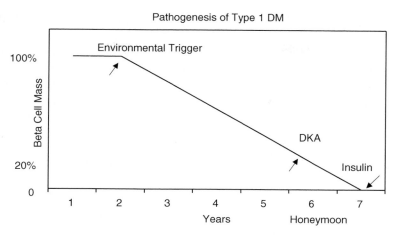

Fig. 1. Schema of the development of type 1 diabetes in a model individual. After activation by environmental trigger, the autoimmune attack against pancreatic β cells results in progressive loss of β-cell mass over several years. Clinical presentation often occurs with DKA when the β-cell mass is approx 20% of its original content. Over the next 1 or 2 years, the autoimmune attack persists resulting in complete loss of β-cell mass and true insulin-dependence. The honeymoon period is the term for this temporary time when use of little or no insulin is required. (From ref. 9.)

loss of β-cell mass, and impairment of insulin secretion (Fig.1). When there is loss of 80–90% of β-cell mass, fasting hyperglycemia may develop. If there is also severe coincident or intercurrent illness, typically a viral infection, the initial presentation may be fulminant diabetic ketoacidosis. Indeed 20% of type 1 patients present with DKA. After stabilization, β-cell function may improve, and for a time the patient then requires little or no exogenous insulin. This is known as the "honeymoon period" of type 1 diabetes. However, months or years later, autoimmune β-cell destruction is complete. There is no endogenous insulin secretion extant and the patient is rendered "insulin-dependent."

Type 2 Diabetes

The pathogenesis of type 2 diabetes can be best understood as heterogeneous, having both genetic and environmental causes. Although type 2 diabetes typically presents in later life than type 1 diabetes, there has been an increasing incidence in younger individuals. This is best explained by the association of type 2 diabetes with obesity, which is now more prevalent in the same population under 30 years of age. The recently reported increase in the prevalence of diabetes in the United States is highly correlated with a contemporaneous increase in the prevalence of obesity. Indeed, almost 90% of patients who present with type 2 diabetes are overweight. As will be discussed, increasing obesity leads to increasing insulin resistance in these individuals, causing insulin requirements that exceed the secretory capacity of the pancreas. A common clinical observation is that the presentation of type 2 diabetes is often at the time of the individual's lifetime maximum weight.

The strong genetic basis in the etiology of type 2 diabetes is substantiated by several observations. There is usually a family history of diabetes in affected individuals, typically involving a first-degree relative. Indeed, the concordance rates in identical twins approaches 100%. The clustering of diabetes in certain ethnic and racial groups, particularly Native Americans and other indigenous peoples, underscores its hereditary nature.

One disturbing observation is the new increased incidence of type 2 diabetes in childhood in the United States. This is seen when strong expression of both primary risk factors, genetic predisposition and obesity, affect a young individual. Presently, type 2 diabetes in childhood is more common in members of high-risk ethnic populations in the United States, namely, Native Americans, Hispanics, and African Americans *(14)*. Therefore, young age no longer distinguishes type 1 from type 2 diabetes. In fact, it is estimated that 50% of children with diabetes have type 2, and a new public health problem must now be addressed.

Insulin Resistance

Although type 2 diabetes in unequivocally a genetic disorder, the exact nature of the inherited defect is not clear, and may likely be complex and polygenic. Insulin resistance is the most likely inherited factor. First, it is seen is almost all newly diagnosed individuals with type 2 diabetes. Furthermore, it is only partially reversible with treatment. Finally, studies in lean, nondiabetic, first-degree relatives of patients with type 2 diabetes, and in patients with impaired glucose tolerance, have documented a state of insulin resistance in these "prediabetic" conditions *(14)*.

Insulin resistance has been most accurately quantified with the use of the euglycemic hyperinsulinemic clamp study *(15)*. In this procedure, a subject is infused with insulin in high concentrations, resulting in plasma levels of approx 100 microIU/mL. To defend against hypoglycemia, the subject is also given a variable glucose infusion at a rate that preserves euglycemia. The amount of glucose infused is a quantitative reflection of the subject's insulin sensitivity: the lower the infusion, the more insulin-sensitive; the higher the infusion, the more insulin-resistant. Studies in subjects with type 2 diabetes have confirmed the presence of insulin resistance in comparison with normal control subjects. Insulin resistance is also found in those with IGT, suggesting that it precedes the development of type 2 diabetes. Studies of subjects with diabetes using glucose extraction studies over various organ beds have placed the site of insulin resistance overwhelmingly at the level of skeletal muscle uptake. This is important conceptually when considering the importance of exercise in the prevention and treatment of type 2 diabetes. Thus, insulin resistance is fundamental in the pathogenesis of type 2 diabetes, and may be the primary inherited defect.

Insulin Secretion

It is important to note that not all insulin resistant states result in hyperglycemia. This suggests that a loss of β-cell function, either relative or absolute, is also a requisite for the development of type 2 diabetes. Much of the impairment of insulin secretion is probably acquired, as β-cell loss in type 2 diabetes is approx 20–40%. Some of the defect can be explained by the concept of "glucose toxicity," whereby hyperglycemia *per se* can impair insulin secretion and insulin action, thus becoming cause and consequence of decompensated diabetes. The insulin secretory defect is partially reversible, and may improve considerably with correction of the hyperglycemia. This also underscores the concept that functional, rather than intrinsic cellular, abnormalities of the β cells explain the impaired insulin secretion associated with type 2 diabetes.

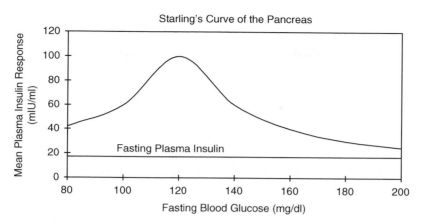

Fig. 2. Cross-sectional data from oral glucose tolerance testing in four different groups: normal fasting blood glucose, impaired glucose tolerance (IGT), type 2 diabetes, and uncontrolled type 2 diabetes. Curve is best fit to emphasize the compensatory increase and subsequent decrease in insulin secretion seen in IGT and diabetes. It is a model for the progression to type 2 diabetes observed in longitudinal studies. (From ref. *16.*)

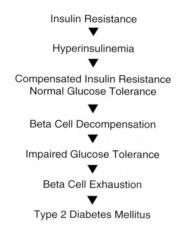

Fig. 3. Progression to type 2 diabetes. (From ref. *17.*)

The defects in insulin secretion are best conceptualized by the "Starling curve" proposed by DeFronzo *(16)* (Fig. 2). This model was drawn from a meta-analysis of cross-sectional studies of insulin secretion in response to an oral glucose load in four different clinical groups: normal fasting glucose, IGT, diabetes, and uncontrolled diabetes. The compensatory increase in insulin secretion seen in patients with IGT disappeared in the group with diabetes. In those with uncontrolled diabetes, insulin secretion was significantly impaired. Though taken from cross-sectional data, this model proposes a mechanism the observation of conversion of people with IGT to type 2 diabetes. Indeed, in the Pima tribe, a longitudinal study of "progressors" from IGT to type 2 diabetes revealed that the lack of compensatory increase in insulin secretion in insulin resistant subjects was predictive of the development of diabetes *(17)* (Fig. 3).

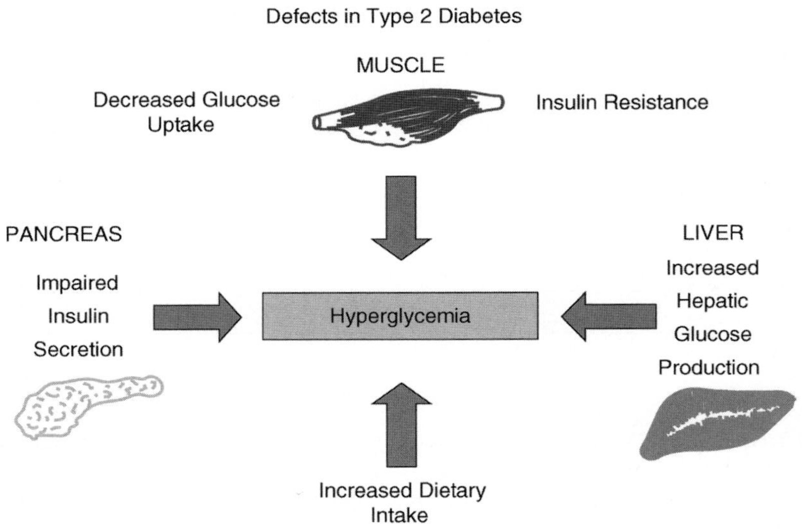

Defects in Type 2 Diabetes

Fig. 4. Defects in type 2 diabetes.

A simplified model of the pathogenesis of type 2 diabetes is offered *(18)*. Insulin resistance has primacy in the development of type 2 diabetes, and is inherited in identifiable families and ethnic groups. This results in a compensatory increase in endogenous insulin secretion. Environmental factors, such as obesity and sedentary lifestyle add to the insulin resistance, causing increased metabolic stresses. Through a compensatory increase in insulin secretion, the individual may maintain normal blood glucose levels or progress to a state of impaired glucose tolerance, prediabetes. Over a period of time, however, the β-cell compensation fails. Defective insulin secretion can result from genetically determined limits, from aging, from senescent "β-cell exhaustion," or from the "glucose toxicity" of intermittent hyperglycemia. A marked decrease in β-cell function then leads to a conversion to fasting hyperglycemia and overt type 2 diabetes, as seen in the "progressors" in the Pima tribe.

Metabolic Abnormalities of Type 2 Diabetes Mellitus

The appropriate management of diabetes mellitus requires a basic understanding of the pathophysiolic mechanisms contributing to the development of hyperglycemia. For the sake of brevity the discussion will focus on type 2 diabetes, because type 1 diabetes has a relatively less complex pathophysiology, and is less commonly encountered. As defined by DeFronzo and Ferranini, three metabolic abnormalities (Fig. 4) that have been identified in patients with type 2 diabetes, which lead to the development and persistence of hyperglycemia:

1. Insulin resistance;
2. Impaired insulin secretion; and
3. Increased hepatic glucose production.

In the fasting state, normal blood glucose is supported by the endogenous production of glucose, primarily by the liver with some contribution from the kidneys. The

Table 1
Clinical Features

	Type 1	Type 2
Age <30 years	Yes	No
Ketosis	Yes	No
Obesity	No	Yes (90%)
Family history	Possible	Usual
Ethnic groups	European	Indigenous peoples
Concordance twins	40%	90%
HLA type	DR3/4	None
Autoantibodies	90%	10%
Complications	Micro	Macro
Primary defect	↓Insulin secretion	↑Insulin resistance
Pathogenesis	Autoimmune	Heterogenous

rate of hepatic glucose production is approx 2 mg/kg per minute, or 125 g daily in an average individual. The purpose of this endogenous glucose production is to provide fuel to the brain and central nervous system. This hepatic production constitutes for the most part the fasting blood glucose that is commonly measured clinically.

With the ingestion of an oral glucose load, specific events must occur in concert to ensure the maintenance of normal glucose tolerance. First, insulin secretion is stimulated. The increased insulin secretion then prevents hyperglycemia by suppressing endogenous glucose production (primarily in the liver), and stimulating glucose uptake and disposal in the peripheral tissues (primarily in muscle).

In the fasting state, there is increased hepatic glucose production.

Several defects in the normal physiological regulation of blood glucose exist in type 2 diabetes. In patients with type 2 diabetes, despite increased ambient concentrations of plasma insulin. The increased glucose production rate is evidence of insulin resistance at the level of the liver, and is suppressible only with higher concentrations of insulin. Second, the insulin secretory response to oral glucose is impaired initially in early type 2 diabetes with a loss of the rapid or "first-phase" release of insulin, and subsequently with a relative or absolute deficiency in the total secretion, as discussed in the "Starling Curve" model of insulin secretion. Third, muscle glucose uptake in response to oral glucose or exogenous insulin is reduced, and is indeed the primary site of insulin resistance in type 2 diabetes. The earliest defect is in the nonoxidative muscle glucose uptake and storage as glycogen.

These events interplay to result in worsened hyperglycemia. According to the concept of "glucose toxicity," hyperglycemia then in turn worsens insulin resistance and further impairs insulin secretion. The initiation of the vicious circle of glucose toxicity contributes to the progressive decline in insulin secretion and insulin action that characterize type 2 diabetes, and provides a model to explain the "progressors," the individuals who convert from impaired glucose tolerance to type 2 diabetes *(19)*. In the management of uncontrolled diabetes, treating hyperglycemia may interrupt the vicious cycle of glucose toxicity and result in improved insulin secretion and insulin action.

The clinical characteristics of type 1 and type 2 diabetes are summarized in Table 1.

COMPLICATIONS OF DIABETES

Acute Complications

Diabetic Ketoacidosis

DKA is a medical emergency in patients with diabetes, with an incidence of 4–8 per 1000 patient-years *(21)*. It affects type 1 patients almost exclusively, with approx 25% manifesting clinical DKA at the time of onset of diabetes, but may also occur in type 2 patients with severe intercurrent illness. Patients often require hospitalization; mortality rates are 2–5%.

The pathogenesis of DKA is absolute insulin deficiency in the face of abnormally high concentrations of counter-regulatory hormones, usually in the setting of an intercurrent illness. The hormones involved are related to sympathoadrenal activation, specifically cortisol and epinephrine, as well as glucagon, growth hormone, and thyroxin. The underlying illness is usually infection, typically of viral etiology. Other provocative events include surgery, MI, cerebrovascular accident, pulmonary embolus, pregnancy, and omission of insulin treatment.

The metabolic condition of increased counter regulatory hormones in the state of deficient or absent insulin results in a marked increase in glucose production primarily by the liver. This results in polyuria, free water loss, and eventual dehydration. Glucose uptake in muscle is impaired, and alterations in mitochondrial fatty acid oxidation result in excessive production of ketones—potent organic acids. Systemic acidosis results in anorexia, abdominal pain, nausea, and vomiting, further contributing to dehydration. Respiratory compensation to metabolic acidosis is often characteristic deep, labored Kussmaul respirations. Treatment is urgent and consists of vigorous fluid and electrolyte replacement as well as high doses of insulin (0.1 U/kg/hour) to inhibit ketone production. DKA is preventable with early recognition: it is most important to treat dehydration and to adjust—but not omit—insulin treatment during illness or surgery.

Hyperosmolar Hyperglycemic Nonketotic Syndrome

Hyperosmolar Hyperglycemic Nonketotic Syndrome (HHNK) is an acute complication usually seen in older patients with type 2 diabetes. It results in more severe hyperglycemia and dehydration than in DKA, and with lesser or absent ketosis *(21)*. Unlike a viral infection causing DKA, it is usually a smoldering bacterial infection, typically of the respiratory or urinary tracts, which precipitates HHNK. The hyperglycemia causes polyuria and increased fluid losses. Patients affected often have underlying renal disease or are taking diuretics, further limiting urinary concentrating ability to prevent free water loss. The presence of a finite concentration of insulin in the patient with type 2 diabetes prevents the development of ketoacidosis, but allows the progression of hyperglycemia and increasing dehydration. Patients may present with marked hyperglycemia, often >700 mg%, after being ill for days to weeks. Neurological manifestations, such as seizures or coma, are common. Fluid deficits are often 6–10 L, and potassium losses may approach 400 meq. Mortality rates range from 10% to 50%, usually as a consequence of neurological sequelae or concurrent bacterial infection and sepsis.

In contrast to DKA, treatment of HHNK should emphasize fluid replacement rather than insulin administration. Patients require gradual rehydration (approx 50% of estimated fluid deficit replaced in first 24 hours) to avoid induction of cerebral edema. Potassium replacement should be concomitant with administration of insulin, as uptake of glucose and potassium in muscle may precipitate hypokalemia and cardiac arrhythmias. A thorough search for the presence of a bacterial infection as well as empiric systemic therapy with antibiotics may decrease the mortality of HHNK from related sepsis. With the advent of home glucose monitoring and patient education, HHNK should be largely preventable, and incidence should be reduced from the current rate of 0.6 per 1000 patient years *(22)*. Indeed, it is usually now seen only in patients who were not previously diagnosed with diabetes without awareness for recognition of the symptoms.

Hypoglycemia

Though it is rarely life threatening, hypoglycemia is an acute complication of the pharmacological treatments of diabetes. It can result in mental status change, seizures, and coma if sustained and prolonged. Most episodes are mild-to-moderate. The causes are related to insulin excess that is absolute (from exogenous insulin or oral secreta-gogue) or relative (from exercise, alcohol, or lack of food). The earliest symptoms are a result of glucose counterregulation and sympathoadrenal activation—specifically epinephrine—that occur at a glycemic concentration of 55–70 mg%. Epinephrine is responsible for the characteristic symptoms, such as shakiness, palpitations, sweating, hunger, and irritability, which are accompanied with signs of pallor and diaphoresis. Neuroglycopenia usually occurs at glycemic concentrations <55 mg%. This often results in confusion and altered mental status. A severe episode of hypoglycemia is one that requires the assistance of another individual for correction. Of clinical importance is the observation that patients with frequent episodes of hypoglycemia may lose the early counterregulatory "warning" symptoms, and sporadically develop severe episodes with neuroglycopenia and mental changes. This "hypoglycemic unawareness" is often seen in patients receiving intensive insulin therapy. Strict avoidance of hypoglycemic episodes can result in the restoration of the early counterregulatory response *(23)*.

The treatment of hypoglycemia should be prompt but not excessive, as over treatment may result in marked hyperglycemia. The elevation of the ambient counter-regulatory hormones may cause a rebound with treatment from a low blood sugar to an excessively high blood sugar. The "rule of 15" is a treatment neumonic: 15 g of glucose orally and retest in 15 minutes. This translates into three glucose tablets or 4 ounces of soda or juice. For a severe episode in which the patient's consciousness is impaired, glucagon (1 mg) should be administered parenterally, rather than risk aspiration with forced oral treatment.

Chronic Complications

Pathogenesis of Microvascular Complications

A consensus for the pathogenesis of the microvascular complications of diabetes has not yet been reached, and a review of the possible candidate mechanisms is beyond the scope of this chapter. Epidemiological studies, particularly of retinopathy, have strongly implicated hyperglycemia as a factor in the causal pathway. Retinopathy can be traced to the duration and the degree of hyperglycemia, which suggests a dose–response relationship. It is more prevalent in patients with poorly controlled diabetes, and in those with diabetes of longer duration. Conversely, achieving tight glycemic control and near-normalization of blood glucose may prevent or postpone the development of complications *(24)*. Theories that incorporate hyperglycemia in their paradigm for the microvascular complications of diabetes include the hyperfiltration hypothesis *(25)*, increased polyol-sorbitol pathway activity *(26)*, accumulation of advanced glycosylation end products *(27)*, activation of cytokines through the receptor for accumulation of advanced glycosylation end products *(28)*, and activation of protein kinase C *(29)*. These are presently areas of intense scientific investigation. Recently, a "unifying hypothesis" has been proposed by Brownlee *(30)*, incorporating several of these hypotheses with a common initiating mechanism of hyperglycemia and increased mitochondrial oxidative stress. The discussion of microvascular complications will be limited to retinopathy and nephropathy. Diabetic neuropathy, which includes elements of both microvascular and macrovascular etiologies, is the subject of a more comprehensive discussion (*see* Chapter 6).

Retinopathy

Although nearly 80% of patients with diabetes will have some retinopathy in their lifetime, most will be limited to background disease that carries little risk of loss of vision and blindness. Findings on fundoscopic exam include micro aneurysms, small "dot and blot" hemorrhages, retinal ischemic lesions (cotton wool spots), and exudates that consist of lipid (hard) and plasma proteins (soft). Background retinopathy is a manifestation of retinal ischemia owing to capillary loss and dropout, and increased capillary permeability to macromolecules. Visual disturbance and blurriness result from macula edema. This may occur if the central vision area of the macula is affected by excessive capillary leak. Macula edema may require treatment with laser photocoagulation to decrease local edema, which results in improvement in acuity over the ensuing months.

After 20 years of type 1 diabetes, the prevalence of proliferative retinopathy is approx 20% *(31)*. It is hypothesized that in response to retinal ischemia and capillary dropout there is an increased production of angiogenic factors. These result in neovascularization of the retina, particularly around the more proximal vessels emerging from the optic disk. A likely candidate angiogenic factor is vascular endothelial growth factor (VEGF), which has been shown to be in high concentrations in the vitreous humor of patients with retinopathy *(32)*. The neovascularization progresses in a dysregulated manner, creating abhorrent fronds and vessels growing out of the plane of the retina into the vitreous, characteristic of proliferative retinopathy. These frail vessels can spontaneously bleed, initially causing vitreal hemorrhage and acute blurring of vision. With time, there is clot organization and retraction that may result in retinal detachment and loss of vision. As a proof of concept of the importance of VEGF in the progression of diabetic retinopathy, early data using either an antibody or an aptamer inhibitor of VEGF have shown some early clinical success in stabilizing disease *(33)*.

For more than 30 years, proliferative retinopathy has been successfully treated with pan-retinal laser photocoagulation. In this procedure, multiple laser burns are induced in the peripheral, ischemic areas of the retina. After treatment, there is regression of the more proximal neovascular vessels, presumably as a result of eliminating the production of angiogenic factors by now infarcted, photocoagulated cells. Until there is active retinal hemorrhage, most patients are asymptomatic, making screening and prevention paramount. Patients generally should begin yearly dilated eye examinations within 3–5 years of diagnosis; type 2 patients should be examined at the time of diagnosis *(34)*. Prevention and lack of progression may be achieved by tight glucose control as reported in the diabetes control and complication trial (DCCT) *(35)*. The DCCT also showed elegantly that the risk of retinopathy increases with each incremental rise in the glycosylated hemoglobin (HbA1C). In addition, aggressive blood pressure control, particularly with angiotensin-converting enzyme (ACE) inhibitors, has been shown to have some effectiveness.

Nephropathy

Nephropathy remains an all too common complication of diabetes, with a lifetime incidence of 30–50%. Approximately 40% of cases of end-stage renal disease in the United States are owing to diabetic nephropathy. Fortunately, better understanding of the pathophysiology has lead to improved screening for and detection of early nephropathy, whereas interventional treatment with ACE inhibitors has improved the outlook for the individual and for the entire population with diabetes.

The pathogenesis of nephropathy is best understood by hemodynamic hypothesis as advanced by Brenner *(36)*. At the time of onset of hyperglycemia, the glomerular filtration rate (GFR) increases to more than 140 mL per minute in the average-sized individual. With this hyperfiltration of the nephrons, there is the development of compensatory renal hypertrophy. Over several years, alterations in the renal vasculature occur, with loss of negatively charged heparan sulfate binding sites and increased capillary permeability. This allows for leak of macromolecules that deposit in the mesangium, causing expansion of the mesangial matrix and proliferation of cellular elements. Subsequent capillary and glomerular sclerosis causes loss of functioning nephrons. This further stresses remaining individual units with more hyperfiltration and intraglomerular hypertension. Thus, a vicious cycle is established. Inexorable and progressive loss of functioning nephrons leads to single nephron hyperfiltration and further nephron injury, whereas the hemodynamic hypothesis is the paradigm that best explains the clinical progression of diabetic nephropathy. In addition, excessive production of the inflammatory growth factor, transforming growth factor β_1, has been under intense study and may play a role in the progressive renal injury *(37)*.

Microalbuminuria is the first clinical manifestation of incipient nephropathy, preceding renal insufficiency and azotemia by 8–10 years. Systemic hypertension may also occur in incipient nephropathy and, in turn, accelerate its progression. Ultimately, clinical diabetic nephropathy may develop, characterized by decreasing GFR, rising serum creatinine, and overt proteinuria of >300 mg per 24 hours. It should be emphasized that serum creatinine is often reduced in early nephropathy because of the supranormal GFR; accordingly, a minimal elevation in serum creatinine in a patient with diabetes may indicate the development of significant nephropathy.

Along with hyperglycemia, hypertension has a significant causal role in the development of diabetic nephropathy. Unlike retinopathy, nephropathy is only partly related to disease duration: after 15 years of diabetes, the incidence may actually start to decline *(32)*. This may be related to the requisite covariable of hypertension. Quite simply, systemic hypertension may exacerbate the established intraglomerular hypertension seen in diabetic nephropathy. The observed higher prevalence in certain ethnic groups, for example, African Americans, can be explained by the clinical link of diabetes with the tendency to hypertension in these populations *(38)*.

The management of nephropathy relies on early detection by screening for microalbuminuria. This should be performed yearly with acceptable ranges of <30 mg per 24 hours, <30 μm/mg creatinine, or <20 μm per minute (timed) *(39)*. Aggressive treatment of hypertension to <130/80 has a renal sparing effect, as demonstrated in the UKPDS *(40)*. This benefit has also been shown with tightly controlling blood glucose. Perhaps the most significant population-based intervention in altering the course of nephropathy has been the use of ACE inhibitors, which, in addition to lowering blood pressure, specifically reduce hyperfiltration and intraglomerular hypertension. If instituted in a timely period, ACE inhibition may forestall the development of overt nephropathy by more than a decade *(41)*. The ADA recommends use of an ACE inhibitor in all patients with diabetes and microalbuminuria, or an angiotensin receptor blocker in those with type 2 diabetes and microalbuminuria *(42)*.

Pathogenesis of Macrovascular Complications

Diabetes is a major factor for the development of cardiovascular disease (CVD), and by itself, is considered a CVD "equivalent," increasing the relative risk by three- to four-fold over normal. The leading cause of death in patients with diabetes is coronary artery disease. Other clinical manifestations of macrovascular complications are congestive heart failure, peripheral arterial disease (PAD) of the lower extremities, and stroke. The relative risk of these complications is greater in women, resulting in a more equal male/female distribution than is found in the nondiabetic population in which CVD is predominant in men.

Many patients with type 2 diabetes will exhibit significant macrovascular disease at the time of diagnosis. Moreover, impaired glucose tolerance, *per se*, is an identifiable risk factor for CVD, implicating the prediabetic state in conferring part of the risk. These observations have lead to the conceptual model of the "metabolic syndrome" as the basis for most CVD seen in the population with type 2 diabetes *(43)*. The cornerstone of this paradigm is the presence of insulin resistance. Indeed, it has long been observed that the major cardiovascular risk factors—diabetes, obesity, and hypertension—are all conditions of insulin resistance. Insulin resistance is also associated with the clinical constellation of glucose intolerance, central adiposity, dyslipidemia, hyperuricemia, and a procoagulant state—the so-called syndrome X as defined by Reaven *(44)*. This clinical syndrome has proven to be responsible for a large portion of CVD-related complications in developed nations. It is now clear that the macrovascular complications of diabetes have their origins in metabolic abnormalities that precede the onset of clinical diabetes by years, even decades. Insulin resistance appears to have a pivotal role. Recently, this "metabolic syndrome" has been defined by the presence of three of five clinical findings of increased waist circumference, hypertension, hyperglycemia, low high-density lipoprotein (HDL), and hypertriglyceridemia *(45)*.

One plausible explanation is the clustering of known cardiovascular risk factors within this patient population, the so-called fertile field. Glucose intolerance, hypertension, dyslipidemia, central obesity, and a sedentary lifestyle often occur coincidently in the same individuals. In addition, the same individuals have higher circulating levels of plasminogen activator inhibitor-1, resulting in a procoagulant state *(46)*. The importance of insulin resistance in the pathogenesis of CVD is supported by the recent observation that insulin-resistant IGT is associated with coronary risk factors, but not IGT with normal insulin sensitivity *(47)*.

Perhaps the most intriguing observation in the pathogenesis of CVD in diabetes is the endothelial dysfunction and impaired vascular reactivity associated with insulin resistance. These abnormalities are ultimately associated with deranged activity of nitric oxide pathways of endothelial-mediated vasodilatation, and can be seen in individuals with diabetes, as well as in other insulin resistant states such as IGT and first-degree relatives of type 2 diabetes *(48)*.

The conceptual model of the multiple metabolic syndrome gives primacy to insulin resistance. What is provocative is the concept that diabetes may be only one manifestation of this central metabolic disturbance that may also express itself clinically as hypertension, obesity, dyslipidemia, endothelial dysfunction, and/or a procoagulant state. Individuals may present with some, many, or none of these clinical findings, but nonetheless share a common metabolic disorder responsible for the development of atherosclerosis.

Cardiovascular Disease and Diabetes

The macrovascular disease in diabetes has unique clinical characteristics. The atherosclerosis tends to be diffuse and more distal in location, affecting smaller sized vessels such as the coronary, the tibial trifurcation, and the internal carotid arteries. Patients may present with symptoms such as angina pectoris, claudication, or transient ischemic neurological attacks. Unfortunately, many patients with vascular complications are relatively asymptomatic, often attributed to the coexistence of sensory neuropathy, which prevents full appreciation of pain and symptoms of ischemia. This is especially true for those individuals with coronary artery disease (CAD) and "silent ischema" of the myocardium. People with diabetes have a high prevalence of CAD. Haffner and colleagues *(49)* have strikingly observed that the risk of MI in patients with diabetes alone is equal to that of nondiabetic patients with known CAD, thus constituting a CVD equivalent (Fig. 5). This makes screening and surveillance, especially for CAD, crucial in the long-term management of patients with diabetes.

Treatment of CVD in patients with diabetes is often surgical owing to the late presentation of patients and the significance of their underlying disease. Carotid endarterectomy, coronary artery bypass vein-graft (CABG), and infrapopliteal bypass with saphenous vein are more frequently encountered in this population. Interventional procedures such as percutaneous balloon angioplasties of the coronary and iliofemoral arteries are performed, but have an excessively high rate of restenosis, making them less durable than surgery for the long-term management of CAD and CVD in diabetes. It has been unequivocally shown that CABG results in better long-term outcomes for patients with diabetes in comparison with percutaneous coronary angioplasty *(50)*. Presently, the use of endovascular stents is increasing as a means of preventing restenosis, but evidence-based recommendations the indications for patients with diabetes are still evolving.

With or without surgery, medical management and risk factor reduction are essential in the prevention of progression of vascular disease. Weight loss, moderate exercise, and smoking cessation should be emphasized at the onset of diabetes, and reinforced frequently throughout the course of long-term management. Although it is important to control

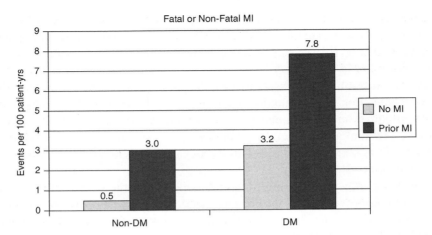

Fig. 5. Results of epidemiological study comparing coronary event rates in diabetic (DM) and nondiabetic (non-DM) cohorts. The striking observation is that the fatal and nonfatal occurrence rate of myocardial infarction (MI) for subjects with diabetes and no known history of MI is almost equal to the MI occurrence rate for nondiabetic individuals with a confirmed history of MI. This demonstrates the excess coronary risk imposed on individuals with diabetes. For patients with both diabetes and prior MI the rate increases sharply to an even higher degree. (From ref. *51*.)

blood glucose to reduce the microvascular complications of diabetes, the impact of glycemic control in type 2 diabetes on macrovascular complications may be outweighed by that of control of hyperlipidemia and hypertension *(51)*. The lipid abnormalities in diabetes include increased triglyceride levels, decreased HDL cholesterol, and increased low-density lipoprotein (LDL) cholesterol. Many long-term studies have shown the benefit of treatment of dyslipidemia in the reduction of CVD death, MI, and stroke. It appears from subgroup analysis that the benefits of treatment of hyperlipidemia are even greater for those patients with coexisting diabetes *(52)*. Because of the potential of prevention of cardiovascular events, optimal goals of treatment as recommended by the ADA are fairly stringent *(53)*. The ADA recommended lipid levels for people with diabetes are:

1. LDL <100 mg%;
2. HDL >50 mg%; and
3. Triglycerides <150 mg%.

Therapy should always include diet and lifestyle changes, but owing to the degree of difficulty for most patients to achieve these goals, pharmacological management with statins is usually required. Statins should be initiated promptly in any patient with known CVD. Hypertriglyceridemia can be managed with improved glycemic control, and if necessary, high-dose statins or fibrates *(54)*. The publication of the recent PROVE IT *(55)* and CARDS *(56)* studies has provoked a paradigm shift for goals of lipid reduction in patients with diabetes and high cardiovascular risk *(57)*. Presently, the ADA recommends pharmacological treatment for a person with diabetes and total cholesterol >135 mg%. If there is known CVD, the target LDL is <70 mg%.

The beneficial impact of tight blood pressure control was demonstrated in the UKPDS *(58)*. A modest lowering of blood pressure (10 mmHg systolic) translated into a significant reduction in deaths, congestive heart failure, and stroke. Patients were managed with either a β-blocker or an ACE inhibitor with equal efficacy. The results of the heart outcomes prevention evaluation study showed a 24% risk reduction in CVD endpoints in patients with diabetes receiving ramipril *(59)*. Because of these findings, as well as the known renal sparing effects of ACE inhibitors, they are often recommended for treating hypertension. It is the recommendation of the ADA to achieve a blood pressure of <130/80 mmHg *(60)*. ACE inhibitors or angiotensin receptor blockers are recommended if microalbuminuria is present.

Because of the high prevalence of CAD in patients with diabetes, screening recommendations are evolving to reduced thresholds to proceed to exercise tolerance testing (ETT) or "stress test." These recommendations were derived at a consensus conference of the ADA on the evaluation of CAD in patients with diabetes *(61)*. Any typical or atypical symptom should serve as an indication for ETT. For asymptomatic patients, the presence of any other risk factors, an abnormal electrocardiogram, or any evidence of PAD or carotid disease warrants an evaluation. Those patients with a high probability of significant CAD by ETT should proceed to coronary angiography. Those with low probability should be followed every 1–2 years. Intermediate or moderate risk patients may be better assessed with nuclear perfusion imaging with thallium for better specificity and risk stratification.

For those patients with diabetes who present with acute MI, the use of β-blockers as an acute intervention to reduce mortality has been recommended. A long-term benefit has also been seen in use as a secondary intervention *(62)*. In addition, strict glycemic control may also be important. Interestingly, the Diabetes Mellitus, Insulin Glucose Infusion in Acute Myocardial Infarction (DIGAMI) study showed a marked and significant reduction in deaths from MI with the use of a glucose/insulin infusion to maintain glycemia between 126 and 196 mg% *(63)*. The initial infusion was followed by four subcutaneous insulin injections daily for 4 months. The benefit was seen over 5-year follow-up observation. It is speculative but also possible that insulin *per se* has a cardio protective effect through its action on endothelial-mediated vasodilatation and vascular inflammation (reducing elevated C-reactive protein [CRP]) *(64)*.

Of note, the current understanding of an acute ischemic syndrome is that there is thrombus formation in an area of disruption of inflamed, vulnerable plaque, mediated by platelet aggregation. There is an affirmation among clinicians of a shift to a medical model in the approach to CAD, especially in patients with diabetes. Studies utilizing intravascular ultrasound have confirmed plaque rupture as the cause of the thrombosis in acute MI, moreover, multiple areas of plaque rupture have been demonstrated in 80% of episodes *(65)*. Invasive procedures may correct symptoms of coronary artery stenoses, but may not be as meaningful in preventing events. In fact, in 4% stent deployment procedures are complicated by MI. Therefore, a treatment strategy of maximal medical risk intervention addressing hypertension, dyslipidemia, and antiplatelet therapy is gaining a foothold, especially in asymptomatic patients. A large prospective study comparing medical and surgical management of coronary artery disease in patients with diabetes, Bypass Angioplasty Revascularization Investigation (BARI)-2, is presently being conducted.

Diabetes may be viewed as a hypercoaguable state, part of the multiple metabolic syndrome. The benefits of daily intake of aspirin in reducing mortality in patients with diabetes and CAD has been observed, and in fact exceed that seen in patients without diabetes *(66)*. Therefore, all patients with any risk should be placed on daily aspirin. For patients with CVD who fail or are intolerant of aspirin, antiplatelet treatment with ticlopidine or clopidrogrel should be considered. Recently, an ADA consensus statement on PAD added that patients with diabetes and PAD may benefit more from clopidogrel than aspirin *(67)*.

MANAGEMENT OF DIABETES: GLYCEMIC CONTROL

Rationale and Goals of Treatment of Diabetes

Diabetes is a chronic metabolic disorder requiring long-term management and patient education to achieve with the objectives to an improved quality of life, to prevent acute complications, and to reduce the risk of chronic complications. The benefits of improved glycemic control are many. Correction of hyperglycemia reduces the likelihood of acute complications and decompensation into DKA or HHNK, as well as relieves symptoms polyuria, polydipsia, blurry vision and weight loss. The risks of developing microvascular complications (retinopathy, nephropathy, and neuropathy) are also reduced with improved glycemic control. For individuals with type 1 diabetes, this was established by the DCCT, in which the overall microvascular risk reduction was 50–75% *(68)*. There was no glycemic threshold for the development of microvascular complications, with benefit even at the lowest HbA1c. Severe hypoglycemia limited the intensity of control. The UKPDS offers insight into treatment strategies for type 2 diabetes *(69)*. In this trial, 3867 patients with new-onset type 2 diabetes were randomized into intensive or standard treatment and followed for a median time of 10 years. In brief, the study showed a reduction of microvascular complications in the intensively treated group, with a 35% risk reduction with each 1% drop in the HbA1c. A trend for a decrease in macrovascular complications was seen, but reached significance only in the subgroup treated with metformin. As discussed previously, intensive treatment of hypertension significantly reduced macrovascular complications, as well as microvascular end points. Thus, it is clear that good glycemic control not only reduces acute complications of diabetes and improves the day-to-day life of the patient, but also prevents the onset and progression of certain chronic complications. Because of these observations, the ADA presently recommends treatment goals of near-normalization of blood glucose, with fasting glucose <120 mg% and HbA1c <7%, and the addition of pharmacological treatment (after diet and exercise) if HbA1c exceeds 8% *(70)* (Table 2). Some patients may be individualized to less stringent goals, such as the elderly, children, and those with comorbid conditions. For the prevention of macrovascular complications in type 2 diabetes, additional risk factor reduction with treatment of hypertension, dyslipidemia, and antiplatelet therapy should be instituted as previously discussed.

Pharmacological Treatment of Diabetes

Diet, exercise, and patient education are fundamentals in the management of diabetes and should be emphasized in any and all treatment regimens. In the interest of parsimony, this discussion will be restricted to the pharmacological management of diabetes. This

Table 2
Glycemic Guidelines of the American Diabetes Association

Biochemical index	Normal	Goal	Action suggested
Fasting blood glucose	<100 mg/dL	80–120 mg/dL	<80 or >140 mg/dL
Bedtime glucose	<120 mg/dL	100–140 mg/dL	<100 or >160 mg/dL
Hemoglobin A1c	<6%	<7%	>8%

Source ref. *62.*

Table 3
Pharmakokinetics of Insulin Preparations

Insulin preparation	Onset of action	Peak action	Duration of action
Rapid-acting analog (Lispro)	5 minutes	45 minutes	4 hours
Short-acting (Regular)	30 minutes	2 hours	5–8 hours
Intermediate-acting (NPH or Lente)	1–3 hours	6–12 hours	16–24 hours
Long-acting (Ultralente)	4–6 hours	8–20 hours	24–28 hours
Long-acting analog (Glargine)	4–6 hours	8–20 hours	24–28 hours
Mixtures (70/30 or 50/50)	30 minutes	6–12 hours	16–24 hours

should not be interpreted to mean that other therapies are subservient to pharmacology. In contrast, successful pharmacological therapy depends on a foundation of a healthy lifestyle of diet and exercise in a patient with good self-management skills.

Type 1 Diabetes

In type 1 diabetes, loss of β-cell mass renders the patient completely insulin-dependent. There is no question regarding whether to treat with insulin, but only one of the choice insulin preparations and regimen. To achieve tight glycemic control, patients are generally required to use multidose regimens of intermediate and short-acting insulin preparations in an attempt mimic the basal and postprandial blood insulin excursions seen in normal individuals (Table 3).

The fundamental principle of insulin therapy is to attempt to recapitulate physiological insulin secretion by providing a finite basal amount of insulin supplemented with mealtime bolus injections. Basal insulin is provided with long-acting insulin once daily (Ultralente, Glargine), or with twice daily injections intermediate acting insulin (NPH, Lente). When using twice-daily intermediate-acting insulin, generally two-thirds of the total dose is given in the morning, and one-third in the evening. Meal requirements are satisfied by short-acting insulin injections (Regular, Lispro, Aspart). Inhaled insulin may also provide rapid insulin coverage with meals. In general, with any insulin regimen used in type 1 diabetes, the average daily insulin requirement totals 0.6 U/kg (42 units for a 70-kg man). This should provide a benchmark to guide the clinician in initiating and adjusting the dose of insulin. Many patients benefit from the continuous subcutaneous insulin infusion (CSII) made possible with an insulin pump. CSII provides continuous basal insulin, and allows for bolus amounts at mealtime. It predictably reduces insulin daily use by 25% because of its efficiency, and may reduce episodes of subclinical hypoglycemia (hypoglycemia unaware) seen with multistick regimens *(71).*

Type 2 Diabetes

The principles of pharmacological management of type 2 diabetes have been the subject of many reviews *(72)*, and change with time as new concepts of treatment as well as new agents are introduced. Pharmacological intervention is indicated when diet and exercise fail to attain desired goals of therapy, i.e., Hgb A1C >8%. Current treatment philosophy embraces polypharmacy to improve efficacy and reduce adverse effects of medications. The management should be flexible, realizing that correction of "glucose toxicity" results in a feed-forward, positive feedback of improved insulin secretion and insulin action. Therefore, initial treatment is not binding, and adding and withdrawing treatments is typical.

The selection of pharmacological agents is presently expanding. For reasons of parsimony, the specific agents will not be addressed in detail, rather, the medications will be reviewed by class in terms of their clinical use. To be clear, the observations of the UKPDS show benefits from intensive control of hyperglycemia, but support no single pharmaceutical agent or class as superior to others, with the exception of the decrease in macrovascular end points seen in patients intensively treated with metformin *(73)*. Treatment regimens then should be individualized, and may not apply to all patients with type 2 diabetes.

Insulin

Insulin therapy is required in 10–30% of type 2 diabetes. The natural history of type 2 diabetes is one of progressive loss of β-cell function and eventual failure of oral agents, making insulin treatment necessary over many years. In addition, there is heterogeneity in type 2 diabetes, with some patients actually demonstrating autoantibodies suggesting type 1 β-cell destruction *(74)*. These patients are insulinopenic and have been shown to progress rapidly to insulin therapy.

Insulin can be used as monotherapy, or in combination therapy with oral agents. Most commonly, nocturnal intermediate or long-acting insulin is used in combination with day time oral agents. Insulin regimens are also used to achieve tight glycemic control in type 2 diabetes similar to regimens used in type 1. Another regimen for tight control would utilize rapid acting insulin analogs solely to minimize postprandial hyperglycemia. Finally, in symptomatic patients in which glycemia exceeds 300 mg% and glucose toxicity is present, temporary intervention with exogenous insulin may be necessary. This may reverse the defect in endogenous insulin secretion and action, restoring euglycemia. Afterward, the patient may be safely withdrawn from therapy and placed on an oral agent. Concerns over the issue of glucose toxicity has lead some clinicians to advocate early insulin treatment of type 2 diabetes, with the objectives of improved glycemic control and a possible β-cell-sparing effect.

Oral Agents

Oral agents have become the most common treatment modality for type 2 diabetes, and are often used in combination. From the UKPDS we have learned that monotherapy for type 2 diabetes is unlikely to achieve tight control after a few years of treatment *(75)*. Therefore, combination regimens are necessary as well as desirable for many patients. When a two-drug regimen fails, often a third drug or insulin will be added. Combinations should capitalize on the synergy of using drugs with different mechanisms of action (Table 4). The three basic mechanisms are stimulation of insulin secretion,

Table 4

	Sulfonylureas	Meglitinides	Metformin	Thiazolidinediones	Acarbose
Mechanism of action	Increase in insulin secretion	Increase in insulin secretion	Decrease in hepatic glucose production; increase in muscle insulin sensitivity	Increase in muscle insulin sensitivity; decrease in hepatic glucose production	Delayed absorption of dietary carbohydrates
Decrease in FPG (mg/dL)	60–70	60–70	60–70	35–40	20–30
Decrease in HgbA1c	1.5–2%	1.5–2%	1.5–2%	1–1.2%	0.7–1%
LDL level	No effect	No effect	Decrease	Increase	No effect
HDL level	No effect	No effect	Increase	Increase	No effect
Triglycerides	No effect	No effect	Decrease	Decrease	No effect
Body weight	Increase	Increase	Decrease	Increase	No effect
Plasma insulin	Increase	Increase	Decrease	Decrease	No effect
Adverse events	Hypoglycemia	Hypoglycemia	GI disturbances; lactic acidosis	Anemia; hepatic toxicity	GI disturbances

Table 5

Oral agent	Starting dose (mg)	Maximum dose (mg)	Duration of action
Sulfonylureas			
Chlorpropamide	250 qd	500 qd	60 hours
Tolbutamide	250 bid	1000 tid	6–12 hours
Tolazamide	100 qd	500 bid	12–24 hours
Glyburide	2.5–5 qd	10 bid	16–24 hours
Glipizide	5 qd	20 bid	12–24 hours
Glimeperide	1–2 qd	8 qd	24 hours
Thiazolidinediones			
Rosiglitazone	2 qd	8 qd	3–4 weeks
Pioglitazone	15 qd	45 qd	3–4 weeks
Meglitinides			
Repaglinide	1.5 tid	4 tid	4–6 hours
Nateglinide	30 tid	180 tid	4 hours
Metformin	500 bid	850 tid	3–4 weeks
Acarbose	25 tid	100 tid	4 hours

inhibition of hepatic glucose production, and improvement in insulin sensitivity. A list of oral agents and appropriate doses is also presented (Table 5).

Sulfonylureas

As a class, sulfonylureas have been in use for decades and remain the most potent oral hypoglycemics. The mechanism of action is stimulation of insulin secretion, which in turn inhibits hepatic glucose production and increases muscle glucose uptake. Earlier findings of improved insulin sensitivity were likely an indirect result of the improved glycemia and correction of glucose toxicity. Sulfonylureas are well tolerated, but carry a risk of hypoglycemia, especially in elderly patients and with renal disease.

Metformin

A second-generation biguanide, metformin has significantly less reported lactic acidosis than its predecessor, phenformin. Metformin lowers glycemia primarily by inhibiting hepatic glucose production, and to a lesser extent by increasing insulin sensitivity in muscle (76). This causes some decrease in plasma insulin. It has some beneficial effects on lipids, and may cause weight loss, making it the preferable agent for use in obese patients. As mentioned, the UKPDS suggested that metformin monotherapy may have added benefits in prevention of macrovascular end-points. The major side effects are gastrointestinal disturbances, which are generally selflimited and transient.

Thiazolidinediones: Rosiglitazone and Pioglitazone

Because troglitazone was withdrawn from the marketplace for hepatotoxic events, two thiazolidinediones have been introduced in the United States: rosiglitazone and pioglitazone. The mechanism of action is improvement of insulin sensitivity through the stimulation of peroxisome proliferator-activated receptor (PPAR)-γ, resulting in increased expression of glucose transporters (77). These "insulin sensitizers" also have some effect in reducing hepatic glucose production. They are used in combination with other agents or as monotherapy. Thiazolidinediones are particularly useful in reducing insulin dose in poorly controlled patients. They are probably not as potent as monotherapy as are sulfonylureas or metformin. Adverse effects on hepatic function are of potential concern. Because of their salutary effect on the insulin resistance seen in diabetes and prediabetes, the thiazolidinediones are under study as cardiovascular protective agents.

Meglitinides: Repaglinide and Nateglinide

A nonsulfonylurea, repaglinide is a rapid acting insulin secretagogue that can be complimentary when used in combination with metformin and thiazolidinediones. It is particularly helpful in reducing postprandial hyperglycemia. It has more hypoglycemic potential when used in combination with metformin *(78)*. Nateglinide is a phenylalanine analog that stimulates insulin secretion, but only in the presence of glucose *(79)*. It thus has little hypoglycemic potential. It is also short acting. Meglitinides are used increasingly as more attention is being directed toward the importance of postpradial hyperglycerimia in glycemic control and chronic complications.

Acarbose

The use of acarbose, an α-glycosidase inhibitor that delays the absorption of dietary carbohydrate, is limited by the frequency of the gastrointestinal side effects of diarrhea and flatulence. Its effect is primarily on postprandial hyperglycemia and dampening the swings in daytime glycemia. It has been used successfully in combination with other agents and insulin, but has received Food and Drug Administration (FDA) approval only as monotherapy.

Exenatide and the Incretins

The "incretins" are a new class of parenteral pharmaceuticals, which have a hypoglycemic effect through specific binding with the glucagan-like peptide (GLP)-1 receptor. By acting as "gut factors," the incretins potentiate meal-stimulated endogenous insulin secretion. The first compound to be FDA approved is exenatide. Originally isolated in the saliva of a southwestern US reptile, the Gila Monster, the peptide is a potent GLP-1 receptor agonist. In the pivotal trial of patients treated with metformin, the addition of exenatide lowered HbA1c approx 0.8%, with 46% of patients attaining a HbA1c less than 7%. Because of its effects on gastric motility, exenatide also allowed a mean weight loss of 2.8 kg over the 30-week trial *(80)*.

Approach to the Surgical Patient with Diabetes

The patient with diabetes poses a complex management problem when hospitalized, especially in the event of surgery and anesthesia. Not only are there associated morbidities and complications of diabetes that require evaluation, there is also the unpredictable effect of the stress of surgery and intercurrent illness on glycemic control. The only treatment guideline that is universally accepted is that the management of diabetes allows for flexibility and feedback. After general considerations are reviewed, the focus of the remaining discussion will be on the unique issues of surgical patients with diabetes, in particular those with foot complications and peripheral arterial disease.

Preoperative Assessment

The evaluation of the patient with diabetes in anticipation of surgery should include the same principles of preoperative assessment used in all patients, with the expectation of frequent associated comorbidities. In the patients with neuropathy and foot disease, there are usually attendant microvascular and macrovascular complications. Although an attempt should be made to optimize the medical condition before surgery, this is often not feasible owing to the extent of the comorbidities and the urgency of the procedure. Indeed, if the patient is medically unstable with infection and altered hemodynamics, this is more often an indication rather than a contraindication for necessary surgery.

Microvascular Complications

Although most concern is directed toward macrovascular complications as will be discussed, microvascular disease should be evaluated for its impact on the perioperative course. Nephropathy may result in abnormal fluid retention and electrolyte disturbances, especially hyperkalemia from type IV renal tubular acidosis (hyporeninemic hypoaldosteronism). Renal disease causes a prolonged clearance of anesthetic drugs. Anemia is commonly encountered as a consequence of poor erythropoetin secretion. Proteinuria and sub clinical nephropathy incur a risk of acute tubular necrosis after contrast angiography; patients should be well hydrated and volume replete before any angiography *(81)*. Patients with end-stage renal disease have impaired wound healing and are at high risk for limb amputation. They also pose difficulty for vascular surgery because of generalized arterial and soft tissue calcification from an increased calcium–phosphorous product.

In patients with neuropathy, autonomic neuropathy contributes to more frequent cardiac arrhythmias and is associated with silent myocardial ischemia. It also confers a risk of aspiration in those with gastroparesis. Sensory neuropathy is the primary cause of most foot ulcers and infections, but may fortuitously permit less anesthesia, allowing more use spinal, regional, and local methods. Patients with retinopathy should be assumed to have significant microvascular abnormalities ubiquitously. In addition, microalbuminuria has been found to be an independent cardiovascular risk factor, and may be a marker of impaired vascular reactivity and endothelial dysfunction *(82)*. This has implications of impaired cutaneous microcirculation and impaired healing.

Cardiovascular Risk: Assessment and Management

Perhaps the single most important preoperative assessment in the patient with diabetes is that for CAD. Diabetes confers by itself an odds ratio of 3–4 in comparison with the nondiabetic population. As mentioned, the risk of fatal and nonfatal MI in the general population with diabetes is equal to that of the nondiabetic population that has had a prior MI, thus constituting a CVD equivalent *(85)*. In the surgical group of patients with diabetes and peripheral vascular disease, the majority will have significant CAD that should be addressed.

There have been several clinical guidelines and position papers drafted to assist in the assessment and perioperative management of patients with CAD *(86)*. Although none specifically addresses the issues of the patient with diabetes, certain common features can be gleaned that may be generalized. The noncardiac procedures that pose the greatest risk to the patient with CAD are emergency procedures and peripheral vascular surgery. For patients with diabetes, lower extremity vascular surgery has an associated death and cardiac complication rate of as high as 10%; for aortic procedures the rate increases to as high as 25% *(85)*.

In addition to the risk of the procedure, the preoperative assessment should include identification of potentially serious heart disease such as prior MI or angina, prior coronary revascularization, congestive heart failure, and significant arrhythmia. Each of these conditions confers added risk of cardiac end-points postoperatively. Advanced age (>70 years) is *per se* an added risk factor. When these historical features are considered, along with the general history of comorbid conditions (e.g., renal disease and chronic obstructive pulmonary disease), the physical exam, functional capacity, and the resting electrocardiogram, a fairly accurate assessment of low vs high risk can be made (86). This Bayesian approach to the probability of CAD has been advocated simple and reliable method of risk stratification.

In patients of indeterminant or intermediate risk, further preoperative testing may be necessary as a "tie-breaker." Echocardiography may identify patients with left ventricular dysfunction. A low ejection fraction (<35%) increases the risk of noncardiac surgery (87). Exercise stress testing and pharmacological stress testing may assist in the evaluation, especially in stratifying patients of indeterminate or moderate risk. The most useful noninvasive evaluation is perfusion nuclear imaging with thallium. Patients increase their risk stratification if there are more than two reversible perfusion defects on thallium imaging. For patients with diabetes, the most important independent predictors of postoperative death are advanced age, resting EKG abnormalities, and thallium abnormalities (88). It should be understood that in patients with diabetes who are undergoing peripheral vascular surgery the prevalence of thallium imaging abnormalities is high. In a study of patients with diabetes undergoing vascular surgery at the Deaconess Hospital in Boston, over 90% of patients with clinical evidence of cardiac disease had abnormal dipyridimole thallium scans, whereas more than 50% of those without clinical disease had abnormalities (89). The clinical caveat is that all patients with diabetes undergoing vascular surgery should be managed with a high index of suspicion for significant CAD, whether or not noninvasive testing is performed.

THE HIGH-RISK PATIENT

A more complex decision tree is present when a patient is identified as high risk. The consideration of proceeding to invasive testing and coronary angiography rests on the decision to commit the patient to CABG or percutaneous transluminal coronary angioplasty (PTCA). This decision generally is based on three probabilities: the prior Bayesian probability of CAD, the risks of the revascularization procedure, and the risks of the proposed surgery. It is generally felt that with close monitoring, the high-risk patient going directly to vascular surgery will fare better in terms of all outcomes than the same patient subjected to the potential morbidity and mortality of presurgical coronary angiography and revascularization (90). This is even truer for less risky surgical procedures. Therefore, the short-term benefit of preoperative coronary revascularization usually is outweighed by the combined risks of both coronary revascularization and the intended operative procedure. Patients should not have coronary surgery solely in preparation for another noncardiac procedure (91).

It should be remembered, however, that coronary revascularization has evidence-based proof of benefit for long-term survival in selected patients. The American College of Cardiology/American Heart Association includes in their recommendations patients with unstable angina, triple-vessel or left main CAD, and double-vessel with left anterior descending disease *(92)*. Patients should be evaluated for coronary revascularization by the clinical criteria for long-term prognosis independent of the preoperative evaluation. This also holds true for PTCA, which is less commonly advocated for patients with diabetes because of the high restenosis rate and less favorable outcomes in comparison with CABG *(93)*. The use of coronary stents is increasingly added to PTCA, but prospective data for short-term benefits of perioperative stent placement are lacking.

β-*Blockers*

For the high-risk patient, use of β-blockers is becoming more routine. A landmark study on perioperative β-blockade in high-risk patients undergoing vascular surgery showed a striking reduction of MI and death *(94)*. In this prospective randomized trial, patients with abnormal thallium reperfusion imaging were randomized to bisoprolol or placebo before peripheral vascular surgery. There was a significant reduction of perioperative and in-hospital mortality, which persisted throughout the treatment period of 6 months. A similar though less dramatic effect was previously reported with the use of atenolol *(95)*. Most observers consider the beneficial results are class effects of β-blockers rather than specific drug effects.

If these clinical results are substantiated with more general use, the preoperative management of the high-risk patient, especially with diabetes, will be more simplified and focus on vigilant perioperative monitoring and routine use of β-blockers. This philosophy of care has already been adopted at many centers with busy vascular surgery sections *(96)*. The preoperative evaluation of coronary disease has evolved to a Bayesian evaluation of clinical risk and prior probability of disease, with or without noninvasive studies such as pharmacological nuclear perfusion imaging or echocardiography *(97)*. The high-risk patient could then be initiated on β-blockade, and followed closely during and after surgery. For low-risk patients or for those undergoing low-risk procedures, good medical support and vigilance should be sufficient. These simple clinical approaches require little ancillary testing, eliminate most invasive angiography, and should result in a substantial decrease in postoperative coronary events. One should realize, however, that even in the best circumstances, the mortality rates of vascular surgery in the high-risk patients with diabetes would most likely remain a finite quantity of 1–2%.

Glycemic Control in the Surgical Patient: Rationale

The most important point in the rationale for glycemic control in the perioperative period is to avoid the acute dangers of hypoglycemia, hyperglycemia, and ketoacidosis. After providing sound medical management, there remains a question of how tight the glycemic control should be. Although the benefits of tight control have been documented in the prevention of long-term complications of diabetes by the DCCT and the UKPDS, the short-term benefits of near normal glycemia are not as clear in the perioperative period. It becomes an individual assessment of potential benefits vs demands of the increased resource utilization and risks of hypoglycemia with tight control.

Infection

One concern is the increased risk of perioperative infection in patients with diabetes; however, this may be multifactorial and only partly a result of hyperglycemia. Many in vitro studies have demonstrated impaired chemotaxis of neutrophils, generally at glucose concentrations above 240 mg%. This concentration has thus been used as the high water mark for perioperative control. The clinical translation of an observed decrease in infection rates with tight glycemic control following surgery has been lacking. Hyperglycemia in the postoperative patient with diabetes has been associated with an increased risk of infection, and suggests that hyperglycemia *per se* is an independent risk factor for infection *(98)*. However, in a study in cardiacthoracic surgery patients tighter control of hyperglycemia resulted only in a "trend" to fewer infections *(99)*.

The issue may be of less priority in patients hospitalized for foot disease, who are often already receiving systemic antibiotic therapy for infections and in which surgery often treats infection rather than its causes. It should be underscored that hyperglycemia may also be a clinical sign of concurrent infection. Therefore, hyperglycemia should be considered as a factor associated with infection, and may prove variably to be either a cause or a consequence.

Wound Healing

The effects of glycemic control on wound healing are even less well documented. Diabetes clearly contributes to faulty wound healing, but this may be attributed to associated factors such as infection, macrovascular disease and microvascular disease *(100)*. Acute corrections in glycemia are likely to be of minor consequence in changing these impairments to healing. Animal models have shown impaired healing of acute wounds in diabetes, but these findings may not be generalized as these animals are more moribund and catabolic than their human counterparts.

Of interest and perhaps of more importance in impaired healing is the contribution of the low tissue oxygen tension that may be observed in the wounds of some patients with diabetes. This can be explained by poor oxygen delivery because of macrovascular and microvascular diseases. Low oxygen tension has also been found to be a predictor of subsequent surgical wound infection *(101)*. A study assessing the use of supplemental perioperative oxygen has demonstrated a decrease in abdominal surgical wound infections. In this study, patients who were breathing 80% oxygen during surgery and for 2 hours afterward had nearly 60% less infections than those randomized to receiving 30% oxygen *(102)*. Supplemental oxygen may prove to be an useful adjunct in postoperative wound healing and prevention of infection. It is premature to recommend routine use as no similar prospective data are yet available for surgical patients with diabetes.

INSULIN INFUSION

There is growing interest in the effects of insulin *per se* on operative outcomes independent of glycemic control. As mentioned previously, the DIGAMI study demonstrated a beneficial effect on cardiac events and death in diabetic patient with acute MI who received glucose and insulin infusion acutely, followed by intensive insulin therapy for several months *(103)*. Furthermore, a study of intensive care patients treated with insulin infusion showed a significant reduction in morbidity and mortality *(104)*. One hypothesis posed by observers is that insulin *per se* may account for some of this beneficial effect independent of the improved glycemia. Insulin has vasodilatory actions mediated through endothelial nitric oxide synthase *(105)*, and it is postulated that insulin infusion may have salutary effects on tissue hypoxia. In one study in patients with diabetes undergoing coronary bypass, insulin infusion resulted in better glycemic control and less deep infections than in patients given subcutaneous insulin *(106)*. Insulin infusion may also have beneficial effects on neutrophil function *(107)*. Insulin is also a potent stimulator of pyruvate dehydrogenase, and, as such, may help to clear the accumulation of lactic acid often seen in critically ill patients. A prospective study is needed to determine if insulin infusion is beneficial in surgical patients with diabetes who are at high risk for infection and poor wound healing.

In summary, the benefits of tight glycemic control in the perioperative period of infection and wound healing are only partly evidence based, and must be considered in the light of the risks of hypoglycemia and the costs of resource utilization and personnel to deliver the care. For most clinicians, it is acceptable to maintain the glucose level during surgery between 150 and 200 mg% to avoid hypoglycemia, and continue this into the postoperative period. For those desiring tight glycemic control of 90–130 mg%, those targets are probably best achieved by intravenous insulin infusion in the perioperative period.

THE GLUCOSE BALANCING ACT

In approaching the preoperative patient with diabetes, the attention is often initially directed to the issue of hypoglycemia owing to the restriction of oral intake to prevent emesis and aspiration. Usually, the first intervention is the reduction of the dose of insulin and pharmacological treatment for diabetes to avoid hypoglycemia during and after surgery. It should be emphasized, however, the stress and metabolic consequences of surgery often result in an increased insulin requirement *(108)*. In patients undergoing surgery, marked and significant increases in the levels of counterregulatory hormones are seen. These include growth hormone, glucagons, cortisol, epinephrine and norepinephrine. In addition, gluconeogenic precursors such as lactate, amino acids, and free fatty acids are increased. In patients without diabetes, this is accompanied by marked increases in insulin and c-peptide levels, reflecting an increased secretion of insulin to compensate for the metabolic changes. The increased insulin secretion also prevents associated protein breakdown and catabolism, and promotes protein synthesis. These metabolic changes are generally resolved and near normal by the day following surgery, provided no subsequent physiological stress is superimposed.

In the patient with diabetes, the challenge of this metabolic stress may not be met adequately with increased insulin secretion. The most predictable consequence of the elevation in counterregulatory hormones is an increase in hepatic glucose output from both increased gluconeogenesis and release of stored glycogen. Gluconeogenesis is fueled by the increases in plasma lactate, amino acids and free fatty acids, and can result in hyperglycemia—despite the restricted oral intake in the surgical patient. Furthermore, the acute worsening of insulin resistance impairs glucose uptake and utilization by muscle. In the patient with type 1, these metabolic demands in the setting of little or absent insulin secretion can result in increased ketogenesis and ketoacidosis.

Thus, it is not surprising that the most common error in the management of the patient with diabetes undergoing surgery is an excessive reduction of insulin dose for fear of hypoglycemia from food restriction. The endogenous glucose and ketone production during the stress of surgery may actually increase insulin requirements and acutely decompensate glycemic control. The net glycemic outcome is a balancing act between the counterregulatory hormones and stress driving the glucose up, and the caloric restriction and medications driving it down. Whatever treatment regimen is chosen, the lack of predictability makes the feedback of frequent glucose monitoring essential for glycemic control.

TREATMENT REGIMENS FOR GLYCEMIC CONTROL DURING SURGERY

Intravenous Insulin Infusion

In the past, insulin infusion was generally reserved for insulin-requiring patients who were undergoing surgical procedures of long duration, or for patients who were unstable with poor glycemic control *(109)*. However, in the light of the recent studies showing improved outcomes in critically ill patients, insulin infusion algorithms are increasingly utilized for operative patients. In patients in whom tight glycemic control is desired, intravenous insulin infusion is usually preferable to subcutaneous insulin injection in that better glycemic control is achieved, usually with lesser insulin dosage *(110)*. Insulin infusion permits a more adjustable and dynamic treatment method.

The different infusion regimens have their advocates, but none has clearly been shown to be superior. The two most commonly utilized are combined glucose–potassium–insulin infusion, and separate glucose and insulin infusion. The former is based on a 500 cc mixture of 10% dextrose, 10 mM potassium, and 15 U of crystalline zinc insulin. The infusion is initiated at 50 cc (1.5 U) hourly, and then titrated to the blood glucose. Mean dosage is 3.2 U per hour. Increased doses are required in infected patients, obese patients, and those on corticosteroids *(111)*. Glucose–potassium–insulin protocols are favored for their predictability and ease of use.

Separate glucose and insulin infusions are used to more accurately regulate each variable. Insulin is infused from 0.5 to 5 U each hour. It is useful and reassuring to recall from pathophysiology that the usual hepatic glucose production rate in the fasting state is 2 mg/kg per minute, and that peripheral glucose uptake is maximized at an insulin infusion of 0.1 U/kg per hour. In a 70 kg individual, one can be confident that a glucose infusion rate >8.4 g per hour (84 cc of D10 W/hour) will prevent most hypoglycemia. The insulin dose in the same individual should not exceed 7 U per hour. One practical issue is the nonspecific binding of insulin to the intravenous plastic tubing, so precise dosing is not feasible, and adaptability and responsiveness to frequent glucose monitoring are required.

Finally, there are advocates of intermittent insulin bolus of 10 U every 2 hours and adjustment according to glycemic response *(112)*. This is simpler but less precise in achieving control. Much depends on the goals of therapy: to achieve a glycemic level between 90 and 130 mg% during surgery, bolus therapy should be sufficient.

Subcutaneous Insulin Regimens

All patients with type 1 and many patients with type 2 are insulin requiring, and subcutaneous insulin regimens for these patients are appropriate in the setting of brief, less complicated procedures. This is especially true of a morning procedure with a prompt recovery time to allow the patient to resume meals. Generally, patients are given one-half to two-thirds of their usual morning dose in the form of intermediate acting insulin (NPH or Lente). Before surgery, patients should not receive short-acting insulin (Regular, Lispro, os Aspart) unless they are unstable with hyperglycemia.

As previously stated, insulin requirements usually increase with the stress of surgery despite the absence of oral intake. Thus, patients are usually undertreated with insulin so as to avoid hypoglycemia, and often require supplemental insulin immediately after surgery. Traditional "sliding scale" insulin regimens, relying solely on short-acting insulin, are not recommended because of more frequent episodes of hyperglycemia and hyperglycemia. The use of intermediate or long-acting insulin with standing or corrective dosing of short-acting insulin with meals is the present recommendation *(113)*. If the procedure is delayed more than a few hours, intravenous glucose at 5–10 g per hour (2 mg/kg/minute) should prevent hypoglycemia. Patients who are receiving CSII "pump" therapy should be maintained on their usual basal infusion rate, with an anticipation of increasing the rate postoperatively to compensate for the metabolic stress of surgery.

For the patient with type 2 who is on nonpharmacological (diet and exercise) or pharmacological therapy, insulin treatment during or after surgery may be required to correct hyperglycemia, and the management should allow for that possibility. Usually, patients are maintained on their usual regimens. Oral agents used to control glycemia have been reviewed previously. Generally, oral hypoglycemic drugs are not given the morning of surgery, and are safely resumed postoperatively. It should be noted that the hypoglycemic effect of sulfonylureas might persist after the drug is eliminated, and there is some hypoglycemic risk despite holding the dose. If medication is taken on the day of surgery, close monitoring with or without glucose infusion is appropriate. Much effort has been made to avoid the use of metformin within 48 hours of surgery or contrast injection because of concerns of precipitating lactic acidosis. Recently, an estimate of the incidence of lactic acidosis in metformin users placed at 9 per 100,000 patient-years suggests that this concern is overstated *(114)*, and that surgery should not be postponed or delayed if a patient has been inadvertently given metformin.

The maintenance of satisfactory glycemic control is highly individualized and is dependent on the rapidity of recovery, the stress of surgery and/or infection, and the ability to consume dietary regimens. The recommended goals are a premeal blood glucose of 90–130 mg%, and a postprandial blood glucose of <180 mg% *(115)*. These targets are difficult to achieve when relying on oral agents, which allow little flexibility and titration in an acute setting. If supplemental insulin is required, it is best to give intermediate-acting insulins that work physiologically to control endogenous glucose production. Bedtime dosing is especially useful in patients with type 2 to normalize the fasting blood glucose. Use of short-acting insulins may be necessary, but should not be used solely in "sliding scale" coverage schedules. Without the "reservoir" of longer-acting insulin, the patient may be unprotected for 4–6 hours with short-acting insulin regimens, allowing time for hyperglycemia and ketosis to develop. There is evidence that sliding-scale insulin regimens when utilized solely frequently result in more episodes of hyperglycemia *(116)*. Standing or corrective dosing of short-acting insulin regimens should be used on a "base" of long or intermediate-acting insulin, or in combination with oral agents. The metabolic consequences of uncomplicated surgery should be normalized within 48 hours, allowing a rapid return to the patient's preoperative regimen.

CONCLUSION

In conclusion, the management of the surgical patient with diabetes should be based on a knowledge of the pathophysiology of diabetes and on an assessment of its chronic complications. Of most importance in achieving satisfactory outcomes is an awareness of the presence of cardiovascular disease and avoidance of perioperative MI. In patients undergoing high-risk procedures, a clinical Bayesian approach of establishing prior probability of CAD, with or without ancillary noninvasive testing, can accurately assess risk. High-risk patients should be treated with β-blockers. All patients should be managed with a high index of suspicion for coronary disease and appropriate monitoring. Good glycemic control will prevent acute complications such as DKA and hypoglycemia, and is associated with better outcomes in hospitalized patients. Recent guidelines for glycemic management in the perioperative period have urged stricter glycemic control, preferably with intravenous or subcutaneous insulin therapy, and treatment regimens that are flexible and adaptable to the "feedback" of frequent glucose monitoring. The benefits of tight glycemic control should be viewed with respect for the utilization of resources required to deliver the care. With proper awareness of expected consequences of surgery and with heightened vigilance for postoperative complications, surgical outcomes for patients with diabetes should continue to improve.

REFERENCES

1. Kenny SJ, Aubert RE, Geiss LS. Prevalence and incidence of non-insulin-dependent diabetes, in *Diabetes in America* (Harris MI, ed.). National Institute of Health, Washington, DC, 1995, pp. 37–46.
2. Mokdad AH, Ford ES, Bowman BA, et al. Prevalence of obesity, diabetes, and obesity-related health risk factors, 2001. *JAMA* 2003;289(1):76–79.
3. Harris MI, Flegal KM, Cowie CC, et al. Prevalence of diabetes, impaired glucose tolerance in US adults. The third National Health and Nutrition Examination Survey, 1988–1994, *Diabetes Care* 1998;21:518–524.
4. Zimmet PZ. Kelly West Lecture 1991. Challenges in diabetes epidemiology—from the west to the rest. *Diabetes Care* 1992;15:232–252.
5. Neel JV. Diabetes Mellitus: a "thrifty" genotype rendered detrimental by "progress"? *Am J Hum Genet* 1962;14:353–362.
6. Expert Committee for the Diagnosis and Classification of Diabetes Mellitus. *Diabetes Care* 1997;20:1183–1197.
7. Harris MI. Prevalence of retinopathy since time of diagnosis of type 2 diabetes: WESDR study, 1980–1988, *Consultant* 1997;37(Suppl):S9–S14.
8. Turner R, Stratton I, Horton V, et al. UKPDS25: autoantibodies to islet-cell cytoplasm and glutamic acid decarboxylase for prediction of insulin requirement in type 2 diabetes. UK Prospective Diabetes Study Group. *Lancet* 1997;350:1288–1293.
9. Eisenbarth GS. Type I diabetes mellitus—a chronic autoimmune disease. *N Engl J Med* 1986;314:1360–1368.
10. Coutant R, Carel JC, Timsit J, Boitard C, Bougneres P. Insulin and the prevention of insulin-dependent diabetes mellitus. *Diabetes Metab* 1997;23(Suppl 3):25–28.

11. Eisenbarth GS. Lilly lecture 1986, genes, generator of diversity, glycoconjugates and autoimmune beta-cell insufficiency in type I diabetes. *Diabetes* 1987;36:355–364.

12. Dalhquist GG. Primary and secondary prevention strategies of pre-type 1 diabetes. Potentials and pitfalls. *Diabetes Care* 1999;22(Suppl 2):B4–B6.

13. Rosenbloom AL, Joe JR, Young RS, Winter WE. Emerging epidemic of type 2 diabetes in youth *Diabetes Care* 1999;22:345–354.

14. Gulli G, Ferrannini E, Stern M, Haffner S, DeFonzo RA. The metabolic profile of NIDDM is fully established in glucose-tolerant offspring of two Mexican-American NIDDM parents. *Diabetes* 1992;41:1575–1586.

15. DeFronzo RA, Tobin JD, Andres R. Glucose clamp technique: a method for quantifying insulin secretion and resistance. *Am J Physiol* 1979;237:E214–E223.

16. DeFronzo RA. Lilly Lecture 1987, the triumvirate: beta-cell, muscle, liver. A collusion responsible for NIDDM. *Diabetes* 1988;37:667–687.

17. Weyer C, Bogardus C, Mott DM, Pratley RE. The natural history of insulin secretory dysfunction and insulin resistance in the pathogenesis of type 2 diabetes mellitus. *J Clin Invest* 1999;104:787–794.

18. DeFronzo RA, Bonadonna RC, Ferrannini E. Pathogenesis of NIDDM. A balanced overview. *Diabetes Care* 1992;15:318–368.

19. Rossetti L. Glucose toxicity: the implications of hyperglycemia in the pathophysiology of diabetes mellitus. *Clin Invest Med* 1995;18:225–260.

20. Buse JB, Polonsky KS. Diabetic ketoacidosis, hyperglycemic hyperosmolar nonketotic coma, and hypoglycemia, in *Principles of Critical Care Medicine* (Hall JBM, Schmidt GA, Woods LDH, eds). 2nd ed., McGraw Hill, New York, 1998, pp. 1183–1193.

21. Arieff AI, Carroll HJ. Nonketotic hyperosmolar coma with hyperglycemia: clinical features, pathophysiology, renal function, acid–base balance, plasma-cerebrospinal fluid equilibria and the effects of therapy in 37 cases, *Medicine* 1972;51:73–94.

22. Buse JB. The patient with Diabetes, in *Management of Office Emergencies* (Barton CW, ed.) McGraw Hill, New York, 1999, pp. 73–95.

23. Cranston I, Lomas J, Maran A, MacDonald I, Amiel SA. Restoration of hypoglycaemia awareness in patients with long-duration insulin-dependent diabetes. *Lancet* 1994;344:283–287.

24. The Diabetes Control and Complications Trial Research Group. The effect of intensive treatment of diabetes on the development and progression of long-term complications in insulin-dependent diabetes mellitus. *N Engl J Med* 1993;329:977–986.

25. Zatz R, Brenner BM. Pathogenesis of diabetic microangiopathy. The hemodynamic view. *Am J Med* 1986;80:443–453.

26. Greene DA, Lattimer SA, Sima AA. Sorbitol, phosphoinositides, and sodium-potassium-ATPase in the pathogenesis of diabetic complications. *N Engl J Med* 1987;316:599–606.

27. Brownlee M. The pathological implications of protein glycation. *Clin Invest Med* 1995;18:275–281.

28. Schmidt AM, Yan SD, Wautier JL, Stern D. Activation of receptor for advanced glycation end products: a mechanism for chronic vascular dysfunction in diabetic vasculopathy and atherosclerosis. *Circ Res* 1999;84:489–497.

29. Koya D, King GL. Protein kinase C activation and the development of diabetic complications. *Diabetes* 1998;47:859–866.

30. Brownlee M. The pathobiology of diabetic complications: a unifying mechanism. *Diabetes* 2005;54(6):1615–1625.

31. Krolewski AS, Warram JH, Rand Li, Kahn CR. Epidemiologic approach to the etiology of type I diabetes mellitus and its complications. *N Engl J Med* 1987;317:1390–1398.

32. Aiello LP, Avery RL, Arrigg PG, et al. Vascular endothelial growth factor in ocular fluid of patients with diabetic retinopathy and other retinal disorders. *N Engl J Med* 1994;331:1480–1487.

33. Adamis AP, Shima DT. The role of vascular endothelial growth factor in ocular health and disease. *Retina* 2005;25(2):111–118.
34. Fong DS, Aiello L, Gardner TW, et al. Retinopathy in diabetes. *Diabetes Care* 2004;27(Suppl 1):S84–S87.
35. The Diabetes Control and Complications Trial Research Group. The effect of intensive treatment of diabetes on the development and progression of long-term complications in insulin-dependent diabetes mellitus. *N Engl J Med* 1993;329:977–986.
36. Zatz R, Brenner BM. Pathogenesis of diabetic microangiopathy. The hemodynamic view. *Am J Med* 1986;80:443–453.
37. Border WA, Noble NA. Evidence that TGF-beta should be a therapeutic target in diabetic nephropathy. *Kidney Int* 1998;54:1390–1391.
38. Cowie CC, Port FK, Wolfe RA, Savage PJ, Moll PP, Hawthorne VM. Disparities in incidence of diabetic end-stage renal disease according to race and diabetes. *N Engl J Med* 1989;321:1074–1079.
39. Diabetic nephropathy, ADA position statement. *Diabetes Care* 2000;23(Suppl 1):S69–S72.
40. UK Prospective Diabetes Study. Tight blood pressure control and risk of macrovascular and microvascular complications in Type 2 diabetes: UKPDS 38. *BMJ* 1998;317:703–713.
41. Viberti G, Mogensen CE, Groop LC, Pauls JF. Effect of captopril on progression to clinical proteinuria in patients with insulin diabetes mellitus and microalbuminuria. European Microalbuminuria Captopril Study. *J Am Med Assoc* 1994;271:275–279.
42. American Diabetes Association, Standards of medical care in diabetes. *Diabetes Care* 2005;28:S4–S36.
43. Zimmet P, Boyko EJ, Collier GR, de Courten M. Etiology of the metabolic syndrome: potential role of insulin resistance, leptin resistance, and other players. 1999;892:25–44.
44. Reaven GM. Pathophysiology of insulin resistance in human disease. *Physiol Rev* 1995;75:473–486.
45. Third Report of the Expert Panel on Detection, Evaluation, and Treatment of High Blood Cholesterol in Adults (Adult Treatment Panel III) Executive Summary, NIH Publication No. 01-3670, May 2001.
46. Meigs JB, Mittleman MA, Nathan DM, et al. Hyperinsulinemia, hyperglycemia, and impaired hemostasis: the Framingham Offspring Study. *JAMA* 2000;283:221–228.
47. Haffner SM, Mykkanen L, Festa A, Burke JP, Stern MP. Insulin-resistant prediabetic subjects have more atherogenic risk factors than insulin-sensitive prediabetic subjects: implications for preventing coronary heart disease during the prediabetic state. *Circulation* 2000;101:975–980.
48. Steinberg HO, Chaker H, Leaming R, Johnson A, Brechtel G, Baron AD. Obesity/insulin resistance is associated with endothelial dysfunction. Implications for the syndrome of insulin resistance. *J Clin Invest* 1996;97:2601–2610.
49. Haffner SM, Lehto S, Ronnemaa T, Pyorala K, Laakso M. Mortality from coronary heart disease in subjects with type 2 diabetes and in nondiabetic subjects with and without prior MI. *N Engl J Med* 1998;339:229–234.
50. The bypass angioplasty revascularization investigation (BARI) investigators. Comparison of coronary bypass surgery with angioplasty in patients with multivessel disease. *N Engl J Med* 1996;335:217–225.
51. Turner RC. The U.K. Prospective Diabetes Study. A review. *Diabetes Care* 1998;21(Suppl):C35–C38.
52. Haffner SM. Management of dyslipidemia in adults with diabetes (technical review). *Diabetes Care* 1998;21:160–178.
53. American Diabetes Association. Dyslipidemia management in adults with diabetes, position statement. *Diabetes Care* 2004;27(Suppl 1):S68–S71.

54. Haffner SM. Management of dyslipidemia in adults with diabetes. *Diabetes Care* 1998;21: 160–178.

55. Cannon CP, Braunwald E, McCabe CH, et al. Pravastatin or atorvastatin evaluation and infection therapy—thrombolysis in MI 22 investigators. Intensive versus moderate lipid lowering with statins after acute coronary syndromes. *N Engl J Med* 2004;350(15): 1495–1504.

56. Colhoun HM, Betteridge DJ, Durrington PN, et al. CARDS Investigators. Primary prevention of cardiovascular disease with atorvastatin in type 2 diabetes in the Collaborative Atorvastatin Diabetes Study (CARDS): multicentre randomised placebo-controlled trial. *Lancet* 2004;364(9435):685–696.

57. Grundy SM, Cleeman JI, Merz CN, et al. National Heart, Lung, and Blood Institute. American College of Cardiology Foundation; American Heart Association. Implications of recent clinical trials for the National Cholesterol Education Program Adult Treatment Panel III guidelines. *Circulation* 2004;110(2):227–239.

58. UK Prospective Diabetes Study Group. Efficacy of atenolol and captopril in reducing risk of macrovascular complications in type 2 diabetes, UKPDS39. *BMJ* 1998;317: 713–720.

59. Heart Outcomes Prevention Evaluation Study Investigators. Effects of ramipril on cardiovascular and microvascular outcomes in people with diabetes mellitus: results of the HOPE study and MICRO-HOPE substudy. *Lancet* 2000;355:253–259.

60. American Diabetes Association, Hypertension management in adults with diabetes. *Diabetes Care* 2004;27(Suppl 1):S65–S67.

61. Consensus Development Conference on the Diagnosis of Coronary Heart Disease and Diabetes, 10–11 February 1998, Miami, Florida, American Diabetes Association. *Diabetes Care* 1998;21:1551–1559 (review).

62. Tse WY, Kendall M. Is there a role for beta-blockers in hypertensive diabetic patients? *Diabetic Medicine* 1994;11:137–144 (review).

63. Malmberg K. Prospective randomised study of intensive insulin treatment on long term survival MI in patients with diabetes mellitus. DIGAMI (Diabetes Mellitus Glucose Infusion in Acute MI) Study Group. *BMJ* 1997;314:1512–1515.

64. Dandona P, Aljada A, Chaudhuri A, Mohanty P. Endothelial dysfunction, inflammation and diabetes. *Rev Endocr Metab Disord* 2004;5(3):189–197.

65. Nissen SE. Application of intravascular ultrasound to characterize coronary artery disease and assess the progression or regression of atherosclerosis. *Am J Cardiol* 2002;89(4A):24B–31B.

66. Harpaz D, Gottlieb S, Graff E, Boyko V, Kishon Y, Behar S. Effects of aspirin treatment on survival in non-insulin-dependent diabetic patients with coronary artery disease. Israeli Bezafibrate Infarction Prevention Study Group. *Am J Med* 1998;105:494–499.

67. American Diabetes Association Consensus Statement: peripheral arterial disease in people with diabetes. *Diabetes Care* 2003;36:3333–3341.

68. The absence of a glycemic threshold for the development of long-term complications: the perspective of the diabetes control and complications trial. *Diabetes* 1996;45: 1289–1298.

69. UK Prospective Diabetes Study Group. Intensive blood-glucose control with sulphonylureas or insulin compared with conventional treatment and risk of complications in patients with type 2 diabetes (UKPDS 33). *Lancet* 1998;352:857–853.

70. American Diabetes Association. Standards of medical care for patients with diabetes mellitus, position statement. *Diabetes Care* 2005;28:S4–S36.

71. Bode BW, Steed RD, Davidson PC. Reduction in severe hypoglycemia with long-term continuous subcutaneous insulin infusion in type I diabetes. *Diabetes Care* 1996;19: 324–327.

72. DeFronzo RA. Pharmacologic therapy for type 2 diabetes mellitus. *Ann Intern Med* 1999;31:281–303.
73. UK Prospective Diabetes Study. Effect of intensive blood-glucose control with metformin on complications in overweight patient with type 2 diabetes (UKPDS 34). *Lancet* 1998; 352:854–865.
74. Turner R. Stratton I, Horton V, et al. UKPDS25: autoantibodies to islet-cell cytoplasm and glutamic acid decarboxylase for prediction of insulin requirement in type 2 diabetes. UK Prospective Diabetes Study Group. *Lancet* 1997;350:1288–1293.
75. Turner RC, Cull CA, Frighi V, Holman RR. Glycemic control with diet, sulfonylurea, metformin, or insulin in patients with type 2 diabetes mellitus: progressive requirement for multiple therapies (UKPDS 49), UK Prospective Diabetes Study (UKPDS) Group. *J Am Med Assoc* 1999;281:2005–2012.
76. DeFronzo RA, Barzilai N, Simonson DC. Mechanism of metformin action in obese and lean non-insulin-dependent diabetic subjects. *J Clin Endocrinol Metab* 1991;73:1294–1301.
77. Spiegelman BM. PPAR-[gamma]: adipogenic regulator and thiazolizinedione receptor. *Diabetes* 1998;47:507–514.
78. Moses R, Slobodniuk R, Boyages S, et al. Effect of repaglinide addition to metformin monotherapy on glycemic control in patients with type 2 diabetes. *Diabetes Care* 1999;22: 119–124.
79. Dunn CJ, Faulds D. Nateglinide. *Drugs* 2000;60:607–615.
80. DeFronzo RA, Ratner RE, Han J, Kim DD, Fineman MS, Baron AD. Effects of exenatide (exendin-4) on glycemic control and weight over 30 weeks in metformin-treated patients with type 2 diabetes. *Diabetes Care* 2005;28(5):10, 92–100.
81. Manske CL, Spraka JM, Strony JT, Wang Y. Contrast nephropathy in azotemic diabetic patients undergoing coronary angiography. *Am J Med* 1990;89:615–620.
82. Tooke JE. Microvascular function in human diabetes: a physiological perspective. *Diabetes* 1995;44:721–726.
83. Haffner SM, Lehto S, Ronnemaa T, Pyorala K, Laakso M. Mortality from coronary heart disease in subjects with type 2 diabetes and in nondiabetic subjects with and without prior MI. *N Engl J Med* 1998;339:229–234.
84. Palda VA, Detsky AS. Perioperative assessment and management of risk from coronary artery disease. *Ann Intern Med* 1997;127:313–328.
85. Hood DB, Weaver FA, Papnicolaou G, Wadhawani A, Yellin AE. Cardiac evaluation of the diabetic patient prior to peripheral vascular surgery. *Ann Vasc Surg* 1996;10:330–335.
86. Fleisher LA, Eagle KA. Screening for cardiac disease in patients having noncardiac surgery, *Ann Intern Med* 1996;124:767–772.
87. Eagle KA, Brundage BH, Chaitman BR, et al. Guidelines for perioperative cardiovascular evaluation for noncardiac surgery: an abridged version of the report of the American College of Cardiology/American Heart Association Task Force on Practice Guidelines. *Mayo Clin Proc* 1997;72:524–531.
88. Cohen MC, Curran PJ, L'Italien GJ, Mittleman MA, Zarich SW. Long-term prognostic value of preoperative dipyridamole thallium imaging and clinical indexes in patients with diabetes mellitus undergoing peripheral vascular surgery. *Am J Cardiol* 1999;83:1038–1042.
89. Zarich SW, Cohen MC, Lane SE, et al. Routine perioperative dipyridamole 201T1 imaging in diabetic patients undergoing vascular surgery. *Diabetes Care* 1996;19:355–360.
90. Mangano DT. Assessment of the patient with cardiac disease: an anesthesiologist's paradigm. *Anesthesiology* 1999;91:1521.
91. McFalls EO, Ward HB, Moritz TE, et al. Coronary—artery revascularization before elective major vascular surgery. *N Engl J Med* 2004;351:2795–2804.
92. Guidelines and indicators for coronary artery bypass graft surgery: a report of the American College of Cardiology/American Heart Association Task Force or Assessment of

Diagnostic and Therapeutic Cardiovascular Procedures (Subcommittee on Coronary Artery Bypass Graft Surgery). *J Am Coll Cardiol* 1991;17:543–589.

93. Comparison of coronary bypass surgery with angioplasty in patients with multivessel disease. The bypass angioplasty revascularization investigation (BARI) investigators. *N Engl J Med* 1996;335:217–225.

94. Poldermans D, Boersma E, Bax JJ, et al. The effect of bisoprolol on perioperative mortality and MI in high-risk patients undergoing vascular surgery. Dutch echocardiographic cardiac risk evaluation applying stress echocardiography study group. *N Engl J Med* 1999;341:1789–1794.

95. Mangano DT, Layug EL, Wallace A, Tateo I. Effect of atenolol on mortality and cardiovascular morbidity after non cardiac surgery. *N Engl J Med* 1996;335:1713–1720.

96. Monahan TS, Shrikhande GV, Pomposelli FB, et al. Preoperative cardiac evaluation does not improve or predict perioperative or late survival in asymptomatic diabetic patients undergoing elective infrainguinal arterial reconstruction. *J Vasc Surg* 2005;41(1):38–45.

97. Mehat RH, Bossone E, Eagle KA. Perioperative cardiac risk assessment for noncardiac surgery. *Cardiologia* 1999;44:409–418.

98. Pomposelli JJ, Baxter JK 3rd, Babineau TJ, et al. Early postoperative glucose control predicts nosocomial infection rate in diabetic patients. *JPEN J Parenter Enteral Nutr* 1998;22:77–81.

99. Golden SH, Peart-Vigilance C, Kao L, Brancati FL. Perioperative glycemic control and the risk of infectious complications in a cohort of adults with diabetes. *Diabetes Care* 1999;22:1408–1414.

100. Diabetic Foot Wound Care, consensus statement, American Diabetes Association. *Diabetes Care* 1999;22:1354–1360.

101. Hopf JW, Hunt TK, West JM, et al. Wound tissue oxygen tension predicts the risk of wound infection in surgical patients. *Arch Surg* 1997;132:997–1004.

102. Greif R, Akca O, Horn HP, Kurtz A, Sessler DI. Supplemental perioperative oxygen to reduce the incidence of surgical-wound infection. *N Engl J Med* 2000;342:161–167.

103. Malmberg K. Prospective randomised study of intensive insulin treatment on long term survival MI in patients with diabetes mellitus. DIGAMI (Diabetes Mellitus Glucose Infusion in Acute MI) Study Group. *BMJ* 1997;314:1512–1515.

104. Van den Berghe G, Wilmer A, Hermans G, et al. Intensive insulin therapy in the medical ICU. *N Engl J Med* 2006;354(5):449–461.

105. Zeng G, Quon MJ. Insulin-stimulated production of nitric oxide is inhibited by wortmannin. Direct measurement in vascular endothelial cells. *J Clin Invest* 1996;98:894–898.

106. Furnary AP, Zerr KJ, Grunkemeier GL, Starr A. Continuous intravenous insulin infusion reduces the incidence of deep sternal wound infection in diabetic patients after cardiac surgical procedures. *Ann Thorac Surg* 1999;67:353–360.

107. Rassias AJ, Marrin CA, Arruda J, Whalen PK, Beach M, Yeager MP. Insulin infusion improves neutrophil function in diabetic cardiac surgery patients. *Anesth Analg* 1999;88:1011–1016.

108. Rümelin A, Nietgen M, Pirlich PT, et al. Postoperative pattern of various hormonal and metabolic variables. *Curr Med Res Opin* 1999;15:339–348.

109. Jacober SJ, Sowers JR. An update on perioperative management of diabetes. *Arch Intern Med* 1999;159:2405–2411.

110. Kaufman FR, Devgan S, Roe TF, Costin G. Perioperative management with prolonged intravenous insulin infusion versus subcutaneous insulin in children with type I diabetes mellitus. *J Diabetes Complications* 1996;10:6–11.

111. Husban DJ, Thai AC, Alberti KGMM. Management of diabetes during surgery with glucose–insulin–potassium infusion. *Diabet Med* 1986;3:69–74.

112. Alberti KG, Gill GV, Elliott MJ. Insulin delivery during surgery in the diabetic patient. *Diabetes Care* 1982;5(Suppl 1):65–77.

113. Clement S, Braithwaite SS, Magee MF, et al. American Diabetes Association Diabetes in Hospitals Writing Committee. Management of diabetes and hyperglycemia in hospitals. *Diabetes Care* 2004;27(2):553–591.
114. Stang M, Wysowski DK, Butler-Jones D. Incidence of lactic acidosis in metformin users. *Diabetes Care* 1999;22:925–927.
115. Garber AJ, Moghissi ES, Bransome ED Jr, et al. American College of Endocrinology Task Force on Inpatient Diabetes Metabolic Control. American College of Endocrinology position statement on inpatient diabetes and metabolic control. *Endocr Pract* 2004;10(1):77–82.
116. Queale WS, Seidler AJ, Brancati FL. Glycemic control and sliding scale insulin use in medical inpatients with diabetes mellitus. *Arch Intern Med* 1997;157:545–552.

2

Epidemiology and Health Care Costs for Diabetic Foot Problems

Gayle E. Reiber, MPH, PhD and Lynne V. McFarland, MS, PhD

INTRODUCTION

The global prevalence of diabetes is predicted to double by the year 2030 from 2.8% to 4.4% *(1)*. Of individuals with diabetes, a substantial number will develop lower extremity disease including peripheral neuropathy, foot ulcers, and peripheral arterial disease (PAD). In this chapter, the current epidemiology of lower extremity disease in individuals with diabetes is reviewed with a focus on foot ulcers. Population-based and hospital discharge survey data from several sources illustrate the magnitude of the problem in the United States. Analytic and experimental studies conducted in several countries, which used robust multivariable modeling techniques, are discussed to describe foot ulcer risk factors. The chapter concludes with information on the economic impact of lower extremity disease, primarily diabetic foot ulcers.

LOWER EXTREMITY DISEASE IN DIABETES

The majority of lower extremity disease in people with diabetes is treated in outpatient, clinic, or office settings. Surveillance of lower extremity disease is uncommon in these health care settings. Therefore, to estimate the extent of this problem, the 1999–2000 population-based US Health and Nutrition Survey conducted interviews and lower limb examinations in a sample of the population. These data provide an accurate estimate of the frequency of lower extremity disease, specifically diabetic foot ulcers, peripheral neuropathy, and PAD in individuals ages ≥40. The prevalence (history) of peripheral neuropathy (≥1 insensate area) in people with diabetes was 28.5% and the prevalence of PAD (defined as an ankle brachial index of <0.9) was 9.5%. The prevalence for both conditions was double that observed in individuals without diabetes. In people with diabetes, 7.7% met the criteria for a history of foot ulcer which was three times higher than that observed in persons without diabetes *(2)*.

HOSPITAL DISCHARGE FREQUENCY AND RATES

Hospital discharge data from several national surveys are available to describe the magnitude of lower extremity disease in hospitalized individuals. Trends in lower extremity conditions were tracked over a 10-year interval, 1993–2002, using data

From: *The Diabetic Foot, Second Edition*
Edited by: A. Veves, J. M. Giurini, and F. W. LoGerfo © Humana Press Inc., Totowa, NJ

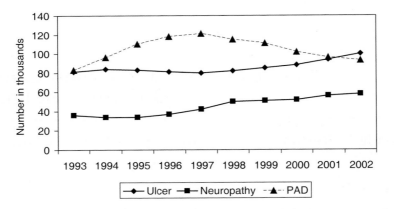

Fig. 1. Frequency of lower extremity conditions in the US population with diabetes/1000. Hospital discharge data for ulcer/inflammation/infection (ulcer), peripheral neuropathy, and peripheral arterial disease, 1993–2002. (Source: Centers for Disease Control *[4]*).

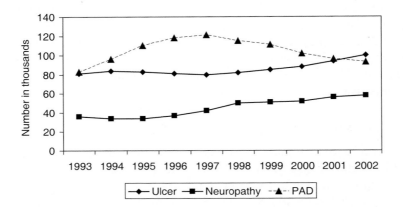

Fig. 2. Age-adjusted hospital discharge rates for lower extremity disease in the US population with diabetes/1000. Ulcer/inflammation/infection (ulcer), peripheral neuropathy, and peripheral arterial disease, 1993–2002. (Source: Centers for Disease Control *[4]*).

from the US National Hospital Discharge Survey, in order to determine the number of hospital discharges in people with diabetes and lower extremity disease. The International Classification of Disease CM-9 codes used were: diabetes ICD-9-CM 250; foot ulcer/infection (454, 707.1, 680.6–680.7, 681.1, 682.6–682.7, 711.05–711.07, 730.05–730.07, 730.15–730.17, 730.25–730.27, 730.35–730.37, 730.85–730.87, 730.95–730.97, 785.4); peripheral neuropathy (337.1, 357.2, 355, 358.1, 713.5, 094.0, 250.6); and peripheral arterial disease (250.7, 440.2, 442.3, 443.8, 443.9, 444.22) *(3,4)*.

Figure 1 shows that the frequency of lower extremity conditions requiring hospitalization for people with diabetes and foot ulcers increased from 81/1000 to 100/1000 between 1993 and 2002. Hospitalizations for peripheral neuropathy increased from 36/1000 to 58/1000 whereas hospitalizations for peripheral arterial disease were 85/1000 in 1993, increased to a high in 1997 of 121/1000 and declined to 93/1000 by 2002. Figure 2 shows the age-adjusted hospital discharge rates for foot ulcers, peripheral neuropathy,

Table 1
Frequency of US Hospitalization for Ulcer-Related Conditions in Individuals With Diabetes by Diagnosis, 2001–2002

Type of ulcer	ICD-CM codes	Estimated frequency	
		2001	2002
Cellulitis, abscess, or infected ulcer	681.1	26,685	29,347
Other cellulitis and abscess, foot except toes	682.7	81,367	83,954
Ulcer of lower limbs, except decubitus	707.1	209,088	216,785
Osteomyelitis	730.07	60,989	66,591
	730.17		
	730.27		
	730.37		
	730.87		
	730.97		
Chronic nonhealing ulcers	707.0	129,466	134,274
	707.9		
Atherosclerosis of lower limb with ulcer or gangrene	440.23	83,546	78,983
	440.24		

Source: Nationwide Inpatient Sample, 2001, 2002 *(6).*

and PAD from 1993 to 2002 using US hospital discharge survey data as the numerator and the US diabetes prevalence from the National Health Interview Survey applied to census population estimates as the denominator. Important methodological changes were made to the denominator used in the survey in 1997 when the diagnosis of diabetes was lowered from 145 mg/dL to 127 mg/dL and other denominator computations influenced by Census data. Age-adjusted hospital discharge rates for foot ulcers declined from 8.5/1000 in 1993 to 6.2/1000 in 2002. Age- and gender-specific foot ulcer rates for individuals with diabetes hospitalized with foot ulcers show the hospitalization rates increased steadily with age, from 5.5/1000 for ages 0–44; 6.4/1000 for ages 45–64; 8.8/1000 for ages 65–75; and finally 11.2/1000 for those aged 75+. The age-adjusted ulcer rates were 6.5/1000 in males and 6.1/1000 in females. Extensive missing hospital discharge data on racial and ethnic categories preclude an accurate estimate of these variables. The age-adjusted trend in peripheral neuropathy hospitalizations showed a slight increase between 1993 and 2002 from 5/1000 to 5.7/1000. The age-adjusted hospital discharge rate for PAD peaked in 1996 at 7.8/1000, then declined by over half to 3.6/1000 in 2002. These estimates exclude long-term care facility and federal hospital patients from the numerator.

FOCUS ON FOOT ULCERS

Foot ulcers are defined as a cutaneous erosion extending through the dermis to deeper tissue, resulting from various etiological factors and are characterized by an inability to self-repair in a timely and orderly manner *(5).* Table 1 shows the frequency of specific foot ulcer-related conditions in people with diabetes based on the Nationwide Inpatient Sample for 2001 and 2002 *(6).* Estimates for the three most frequent conditions reported in 2002 were 216,785 discharges for lower limb ulcer, except decubitus; 134,274 discharges for

Table 2
Population-Based Diabetic Foot Ulcer Incidence and Prevalence from Selected Studies

First author (reference)	Population studied	Foot ulcer annual incidence/100	Foot ulcer prevalence/100
Abbott *(17)*	Cohort of 6613 patients in 6 district clinics in NW England followed for 2 years, type 1,2 diabetes	2.2	4.7
Borssen *(32)*	375 patients Umea County Sweden, age 15–50, type 1 = 298, type 2 = 77	2	10.0 IDDM 9.0 NIDDM
Kumar *(12)*	Cross-sectional study of 811 type 2 patients from three UK cities	1	5.3
Lavery *(33)*	Cohort of 1666 patients, San Antonio, TX, 51% Mexican Americans, followed for 2 years	3.4	—
Malgrane *(34)*	664 patients from 16 French diabetes centers	—	15.8%
MMWR *(35)*	2000–2002 BRFSS US survey of adults >18 years	—	11.8%
Moss *(15)*	Cohort of 2990 patients with late and early onset diabetes	2.4 younger 2.6 older	9.5 younger 10.5 older
Ramsey *(28)*	Nested case–control study in HMO, 8905 type 1, type 2	1.9	
Walters *(14)*	Cross-sectional study of 1077 type 1, 2 patients in 10 UK general medicine practices	4.1	7.4

chronic nonhealing ulcer; and 83,954 discharges for cellulitis and abscess of the foot, excluding toes. Long-term care facility and federal hospital patients are also excluded from these estimates.

Selected geographic population-based incidence and prevalence data are available from nine studies (Table 2) and show the annual ulcer incidence (new onset) ranges from 1% to 4.1% depending on the risk profile of the population. Prevalence (history) of foot ulcer in these diabetic populations ranges from 4.7% to 15.8%. The lifetime risk of a foot ulcer in people with diabetes has been estimated at 15% *(7)*.

In a study of causal pathways leading to foot ulcers involving patients in a US and British setting, 77% of the causal pathway included minor trauma as the initiating event. The most common components in development of foot ulcers in these settings were peripheral neuropathy (78%), minor trauma (77%), and deformity (63%) *(8)*. A study of 669 patients with diabetic foot ulcers reported the three most common ulcer-initiating events were trauma owing to ill-fitting footwear (21%), falls (11%), and self-inflicted foot care injuries such as trimming the nails (4%) *(9)*.

Table 3
Anatomic Site and Outcome of Diabetic Foot Lesions in Two Prospective Studies

	All lesions $N = 314$; Apelqvist (36)[a]	Most severe lesion $N = 302$; Reiber (11)[b]
Lesion site, %		
Toes (dorsal and plantar surface)	51	52
Plantar metatarsal heads, midfoot, and heel	28	37
Dorsum of foot	14	11
Multiple ulcers	7	NA
Total	100	100
Lesion outcomes		
Re-epithelialization/primary healing	63	81
Amputation at any level	24	14
Death	13[c]	5
Total	100	100

[a]Study included consecutive patients whose lesions were characterized according to Wagner Criteria from superficial nonnecrotic to major gangrene.
[b]Study patients were enrolled with a lesion through the dermis that could extend to deeper tissue.
[c]Includes eight amputees who had not yet met the 6-month healing criteria.

The anatomic location of a foot lesion has both etiological and treatment implications. Table 3 presents data from two large prospective studies showing the most common ulcer sites were the toes (dorsal or plantar surface), followed by the plantar metatarsal heads *(10,11)*. The authors caution that ulcer severity is more important than ulcer site in determining the final outcome *(10)*.

RISK FACTORS FOR FOOT ULCERS

Independent risk factors for diabetic foot ulcers were identified from 10 selected analytic or experimental studies that used multivariate modeling techniques to control confounders. Results summarized in Table 4 show the most consistent independent risk factors for foot ulcers were measures of peripheral neuropathy, measures of peripheral vascular disease, and prior foot ulcer. Several other independent risk factors also were identified. Long duration of diabetes, even after controlling for age, was a statistically significant finding in three studies *(12–14)*. In the study by Rith-Najarian *(13)*, long duration of diabetes increased the risk of foot ulcers over sixfold comparing persons with a diabetes duration ≤9 years to those with a duration of ≥20 + years.

Peripheral neuropathy was assessed using several semiquantitative and quantitative measures, and neurological summary scores. Nine studies found an association between peripheral neuropathy and foot ulcers, and one study not showing an association had no lower limb peripheral neuropathy measures *(15)*. In randomized clinical trials using vibration perception threshold (VPT) ≥25 as an entry criteria, Abbott and colleagues *(16)* identified both baseline VPT and a combined score of reflexes and muscle strength as significant predictors of incident foot ulcers. In Abbott's cohort study, VPT was not a significant predictor in the final model, whereas abnormal neuropathy disability score, insensitivity to the 10-g monofilament, and abnormal ankle reflexes were significantly

Table 4
Risk Factors for Foot Ulcers in Patients With Diabetes Mellitus From the Final Analysis Models of Select Studies

Author (reference) and type of analysis	Study design, diabetes type	Age	Long DM duration	Male gender	Peripheral neuropathy (monofilament, reflex, vibration, or neurological summary score)	Peripheral arterial disease (low AAI, TcPO$_2$ or absent pulses)	High HbA1c	Foot deformity	History Smoking	History Ulcer
Abbott (16), Cox regression analysis	RCT, patients with VPT ≥25; (US, UK, Canada), type 1 = 255, type 2 = 780		0		0 Monofilament, + VPT + MI DPN score	Exclusion criteria				Exclusion criteria
Abbott (17), Cox regression analysis	Cohort, 6613 type 1 or 2, patient followed 2 years, NW UK	+	0	0	0 VPT; + reflex + monofilament + neuropathy disability score	+ AAI + pulses		+	0	+
Boyko (19), Cox regression analysis	Cohort, veterans; type 1 = 48, type 2 = 701; followed mean 3.7 years		0		+ Monofilament	+ AAI + TcPO2	0	+ Charcot	0	+
Carrington (18), Cox proportional hazards	Cohort, 169 patients with diabetes, 22 nondiabetic controls		0		+ Motor nerve conduction velocity	0	0			Control factor

44

Study, statistical method	Population						
Kumar (12), logistic regression	Cross-sectional 811 type 2 from UK general practices	+	+ NDS	+		0	0
Litzelman (22,23,24), GEE	RTC 352 type 0, 2 patients, followed 1 year	0	0	+ Monofilament + thermal sensitivity	0	0	+
Moss (15), Logistic regression	Cohort, 1878 patients with early and late onset diabetes, followed 4 years	+ in older onset		+	+ older onset		+ older onset onset
Pham (20), Logistic regression	Cohort, 248 patients at three sites, followed 30 months	0	0	+ NDS + VPT + monofilament			
Rith-Najarian (13), Chi-square analysis	Cohort, 358 type 2 Chippewa Indians, followed 32 months	+		+ Monofilament		0	
Walters (14), Logistic regression	Cohort, 10 UK general practices 1077 type 1, 2	+	+ Absent light touch + impaired pain, perception 0 VPT	+ Absent pulses, 0 doppler	0		

+, significant positive association; 0, no association; blank, not addressed; GEE, generalized estimating equations; AAI, ankle arm index; DM, diabetes; HbA1c, hemoglobin A1c; MI DPN score, Michigan diabetic peripheral neuropathy score; NDS, neuropathy disability score; RCT, randomized controlled trial; TcPo2, VPT = vibration perception threshold transcutaneous oxygen tension.

associated with a subsequent foot ulcer *(17)*. Carrington reported motor nerve conduction velocity as the best predictor of new ulcer after removing prior ulcer history from the model. Over the 6-year follow-up interval, 37% of these study participants developed at least one foot ulcer *(18)*. Several studies identified increased ulcer risk in patients unable to detect the 5.07 monofilament, a semiquantitative measure of light touch *(13,17,19–23)*. There was no statistically significant association between monofilament findings and foot ulcer risk in two other studies *(14,16)*.

Peripheral arterial disease was measured as absent pulses, decreased transcutaneous oxygen tension (TcPO$_2$), and a low ankle arm index (AAI). These variables were significant in the final ulcer prediction model in four studies. Low TcPO$_2$ indicating diminished skin oxygenation, and low ankle arm index, suggesting impaired large vessel perfusion, were both independent predictors of foot ulcers in the study by Boyko *(19)*. In this study, laser Doppler flowmetry did not predict foot ulcer. Kumar *(12)* defined peripheral vascular involvement as the absence of two or more foot pulses or a history of previous peripheral revascularization. He found this variable was a significant predictor of foot ulcers. Walters *(14)* found that an absent dorsalis pedis pulse was associated with a 6.3-fold increased risk of foot ulcer (95% CI 5.57–7.0). Abbott found that reduced number of pedal pulses (0–2) was associated with a 1.57 increased risk of new foot ulceration *(17)*.

Glycated hemoglobin was measured in four studies; only one reported an independent association between elevated HbA1$_c$ or blood glucose levels and foot ulcers in the final model. In a cohort study by Moss, the odds ratio was 1.6 (95% CI 1.3–2.0) showing the significant association between high levels of HbA1$_c$ and subsequent foot ulcers *(15)*.

Five of the studies reported in Table 4 address the relationship between foot deformity and subsequent foot ulcer. Abbott found an abnormal foot deformity score of 3–6 increased the relative risk to 1.57 (95% CI 1.22–2.02). The foot deformity score includes muscle wasting, hammer toes, bony prominences, Charcot arthropathy, and limited joint mobility *(17)*. The study by Boyko *(19)* found an independent association between Charcot deformity and foot ulcer, but other foot deformities were not independent ulcer predictors. Foot deformity did not enter the final analytic model in the studies by Rith-Najarian, Litzelman, or Walters *(13,14,24)*.

The relationship between smoking and foot ulcers was assessed in four studies reported in Table 4. Smoking was only of borderline significance in the older population in the Wisconsin study *(15)*. The risk associated with a prior history of ulcers and amputations was assessed in four studies. Boyko, Abbott, and Litzelman *(17,19,24)* reported a prior history of ulcers significantly increased the likelihood of a subsequent ulcer. Kumar *(12)* reported a relationship between prior amputation and subsequent ulcer. Boyko's *(19)* cohort study also identified higher body weight, insulin use, and history of poor vision as three additional independent predictors of foot ulcer.

Health care access and availability of diabetes education has been reported to influence development of foot ulcers. In a randomized trial conducted by Litzelman *(24)* in a county hospital population, patients were randomized to education, behavioral contracts, and reminders as concurrently their providers received special education and chart prompts. The control population in this study received usual care and education. After 1 year, patients in the intervention group reported more appropriate foot self-care behaviors, including inspection of feet and shoes, washing of feet, and drying between toes.

Table 5
Direct Cost for Foot Ulcers in Persons With Diabetes From Two Studies

Author (reference)	No. of patients/study type	Outcome	Average episode cost (US $)	Inpatient cost (%)	Outpatient cost (%)
Apelqvist (27)	Prospective 314 general internal medicine patients	Primary healing = 63%, healed after amputation = 24%	$6664[*], $44,790[**]	61	39
Ramsey (28)	Nested case-control study in HMO of 8905 type 1,2	Primary healing = 84%, amputation = 16%	$27,987 total attributable cost	18	82

*No surgery
**Including amputation

Patients in the intervention group developed fewer serious foot lesions including ulcers than did those in the control group *(24)*.

Foot ulcers recur in many patients with diabetes *(25)*. Abbott *(17)* reported prior podiatry clinic attendance as a risk factor for foot ulcer. This variable is likely intermediary in the pathway and a proxy for other conditions. Risk factors for foot ulcer recurrences were addressed in a UK study by Mantey and colleagues *(26)*. Diabetic patients with an initial foot ulcer and two ulcer recurrences were compared with patients with diabetes who had only one ulcer and no recurrences over a 2-year interval. The authors reported greater peripheral sensory neuropathy and poor diabetes control in the ulcer recurrence group. Members of the ulcer recurrence group waited longer from observing a serious foot problem until seeking care and consumed more alcohol than did the group without ulcer recurrences *(26)*.

HEALTH CARE COSTS

Optimally, the estimation of diabetic foot ulcer costs spans an entire ulcer episode from lesion onset to final resolution. Two studies provided direct costs associated with the entire diabetic foot ulcer history (Table 5). This methodology captures the many inpatient and outpatient costs/charges associated with foot ulcers and is preferable to reporting only charge for a single hospitalization or limited time interval *(27,28)*.

The study by Apelqvist *(27)* followed 314 patients across an entire ulcer episode, from ulcer presentation until final resolution. Healing was achieved in ≤2 months in 54% of patients, in 3–4 months in 19% of patients, and in ≥5 months in 27% of patients. There were 63% of patients who healed without surgery at an average cost of $6664. Lower limb amputation was required for 24% of patients at an average cost of $44,790. The 13% of patients who died before final ulcer resolution were excluded from this analysis. The proportion of all costs that were related to hospitalization was 39% among ulcer patients and 82% among amputees *(27)*. Ramsey's nested case–control study was conducted in a large HMO involving 8905 patients with diabetes. In this group, 514 individuals with diabetes developed one or more foot ulcers and 11% of these patients required amputation. Costs were computed for the year before the ulcer and

Table 6
Ulcer Reimbursement to Hospitals for Patients With and Without Diabetes, 2002

DRG	Condition	Medstat (private)[a]		Medicare[b]	
		Length of stay	Average $ Reimbursement	Length of stay	Average $ reimbursement
18	Peripheral neuropathy with complications	5.6	9036	5.5	4782
19	Peripheral neuropathy without complications	4.8	6061	3.6	3034
277	Cellulitis >age 17 with complications	4.8	6823	5.7	4000
278	Cellulitis >age 17 without complications	3.4	4426	4.2	2192
271	Skin ulcers	11	11,638	7.3	5227
238	Osteomyelitis	5.9	9913	8.7	7376
130	Peripheral arterial disease with complications	5.1	7743	5.6	4554
131	Peripheral arterial disease without complications	4.3	5768	4.1	2375

DRG, diagnostic-related group.
Source: [a]Medstat Group, Thompson Corporation, 2005; and
[b]Centers for Medicare and Medicaid Services, 2005.

the 2 years following the ulcer for both cases and controls. The excess costs attributed to foot ulcers and their consequences were $27,987 per patient for the 2-year period following ulcer presentation *(28)*.

A Markov model was developed to estimate lifetime health and economic effects of optimal metabolic and foot prevention and treatment strategies for patients with type 2 diabetes in the Netherlands. Modeling allocated patients to management according to guidelines or standard care. The authors reported guideline-based care improved quality-adjusted life years, decreased foot complications, and cost *(29)*.

In the United States, hospital care for lower extremity disease includes both a hospital and a physician component. Table 6 provides the hospital length of stay and reimbursement for lower extremity conditions described earlier in the chapter. Physician, outpatient, and other follow-up care costs would be added across the ulcer episode to these figures for a complete estimate of direct costs. Length of stay and reimbursement by diagnostic-related group (DRG) codes is shown for patients receiving private hospital care (Medstat) and Medicare. For example, under DRG 271, skin ulcer hospitalizations were longer for private patients (11 days) than Medicare patients (7.3 days). The average reimbursement to the private hospital was $11,638 whereas the reimbursement for the shorter Medicare hospitalization was $5227. Table 6 also has DRG codes for peripheral neuropathy with and without complications, cellulitis with and without complications, osteomyelitis and peripheral arterial disease with and without complications *(30,31)*. Payment for the health care provider is not included in these figures.

SUMMARY

Persons with diabetes who develop foot ulcers are at high risk for subsequent foot ulcers and amputations. The hospital discharge rate for foot ulcers has decreased in the United States in recent years; however methodological differences may be partially responsible. The major independent risk factors for foot ulcers identified from population-based, analytic and experimental studies include measures of peripheral neuropathy, peripheral vascular disease, and a history of a prior ulcer. Specific evidence is available demonstrating the benefit of better blood glucose control, and self-care strategies learned through patient education to prevent lesions in high-risk patients.

The average private hospital reimbursement for a foot ulcer was $11,638 for 11 days, whereas Medicare reimbursement for foot ulcer conditions was $5227 for 7.3 days. The direct economic cost attributable to foot ulcers from onset for 2 years approaches $28,000. Guideline-based care is reported to improve outcomes and provide cost savings in comparison with standard care.

REFERENCES

1. Wild S, Roglic G, Green A, Sicree R, King H. Global prevalence of diabetes: estimates for the year 2000 and projections for 2030. *Diabetes Care* 2004;27(5):1047–1053.
2. Gregg EW, Sorlie P, Paulose-Ram R, et al. Prevalence of lower-extremity disease in the U.S. adult population >40 years of age with and without diabetes. *Diabetes Care* 2004;27(7):1591–1597.
3. ICD-9-CM Professional for Hospitals, (2004,), *International Classification of Diseases.* (Hart AC, Hopkins CA, eds.), Volumes 1–3, 6th ed., St. Anthony Publishing/Medicode, Ingenix, 2003.
4. CDC. Data & Trends—Diabetes Surveillance System—Hospitalizations for Lower Extremity Conditions: Methodology. National Center for Chronic Disease Prevention and Health Promotion, Diabetes Public Health Resource, Available at: http://www.cdc.gov/diabetes/statistics/hosplea/methods.htm [accessed 7/05]; 2005.
5. Lazarus GS, Cooper DM, Knighton DR, et al. Definitions and guidelines for assessment of wounds and evaluation of healing. *Arch Dermatol* 1994;130:489–493.
6. AHRQ. Healthcare Cost and Utilization Project (HCUP), Nationwide Inpatient Sample, 2001, 2002. Available at: http://www.hcup-us.ahrq.gov (accessed 7/05).
7. Palumbo P, Melton L. *Peripheral Vascular Disease and Diabetes.* US Government Printing Office, Washington, DC, 1985.
8. Reiber G, Vileikyte L, Boyko E, et al. Causal pathways for incident lower-extremity ulcers in patients with diabetes from two settings. *Diabetes Care* 1999;22(1):157–162.
9. Macfarlane RM, Jeffcoate WJ. Factors contributing to the presentation of diabetic foot ulcers. *Diabet Med* 1997;14(10):867–870.
10. Apelqvist J, Castenfors J, Larsson J. Wound classification is more important than site of ulceration in the outcome of diabetic foot ulcers. *Diabet Med* 1989;6:526–530.
11. Reiber GE, Lipsky BA, Gibbons GW. The burden of diabetic foot ulcers. *Am J Surg* 1998;176(2A):5S–10S.
12. Kumar S, Ashe HA, Fernando DJS, et al. The prevalence of foot ulceration and its correlates in type 2 diabetic patients: a population-based study. *Diabet Med* 1994;11:480–484.
13. Rith-Najarian SJ, Stolusky T, Gohdes DM. Identifying diabetic patients at high risk for lower-extremity amputation in a primary health care setting. *Diabetes Care* 1992;15(10):1386–1389.
14. Walters DP, Gatling W, Mullee MA, Hill RD. The distribution and severity of diabetic foot disease: a community study with comparison to a non-diabetic group. *Diabet Med* 1992;9:354–358.

15. Moss SE, Klein R, Klein BEK. The prevalence and incidence of lower extremity amputation in a diabetic population. *Arch Intern Med* 1992;152:610–616.
16. Abbott CA, Vileikyte L, Williamson S, Carrington AL, Boulton AJM. Multicenter study of the incidence of and predictive risk factors for diabetic neuropathic foot ulceration. *Diabetes Care* 1998;21:1071–1075.
17. Abbott CA, Carrington AL, Ashe H, et al. The North-West Diabetes Foot Care Study: incidence of, and risk factors for, new diabetic foot ulceration in a community-based patient cohort. *Diabet Med* 2002;19:377–384.
18. Carrington AL, Shaw JE, Van Schie CHM, Abbott CA, Vileikyte L, Boulton AJM. Can motor nerve conduction velocity predict foot problems in diabetic subjects over a 6-year outcome period? *Diabetes Care* 2002;25(11):2010–2015.
19. Boyko E, Ahroni JH, Stensel V, Forsberg RC, Davignon DR, Smith DG. A prospective study of risk factors for diabetic foot ulcer: the Seattle Diabetic Foot Study. *Diabetes Care* 1999;22:1036–1042.
20. Pham H, Armstrong DG, Harvey C, Harkless LB, Giurini J, Veves A. Screening techniques to identify people at high risk for diabetic foot ulceration: a prospective multicenter trial. *Diabetes Care* 2000;23:606–611.
21. Frykberg RG, Lavery LA, Pham HT, Harvey C, Harkless L, Veves A. Role of neuropathy and high foot pressures in diabetic foot ulceration. *Diabetes Care* 1998;21(10):1714–1719.
22. Litzelman DK, Marriott RJ, Vinicor F. The role of footwear in the prevention of foot lesions in patients with NIDDM. *Diabetes Care* 1997;20(2):156–162.
23. Litzelman DK, Marriott DJ, Vinicor F. Independent physiological predictors of foot lesions in patients with NIDDM. *Diabetes Care* 1997;20(8):1273–1278.
24. Litzelman DK, Slemenda CW, Langefeld CD, et al. Reduction of lower extremity clinical abnormalities in patients with non-insulin-dependent diabetes mellitus. A randomized, controlled trial. *Ann Intern Med* 1993;119(1):36–41.
25. Maciejewski ML, Reiber GE, Smith DG, Wallace C, Hayes S, Boyko EJ. The effectiveness of diabetic therapeutic footwear in preventing reulceration. *Diabetes Care* 2004;27:1774–1782.
26. Mantey I, Foster AVM, Spencer S, Edmonds ME. Why do foot ulcers recur in diabetic patients. *Diabet Med* 1999;16:245–249.
27. Apelqvist J, Ragnarson-Tennvall G, Persson U, Larson J. Diabetic foot ulcers in a multidisciplinary setting: an economic analysis of primary healing and healing with amputation. *J Intern Med* 1994;235:463–471.
28. Ramsey SD, Newton K, Blough D, et al. Incidence, outcomes, and cost of foot ulcers in patients with diabetes. *Diabetes Care* 1999;22(3):382–387.
29. Ortegon MM, Redkop WK, Niessen LW. Cost-effectiveness of prevention and treatment of the diabetic foot. *Diabetes Care* 2004;27:901–907.
30. HCFA. DRG Inpatient Billing Data, 2002: Health Care Finance Administration, Bureau of Data Strategy and Management, 2005.
31. MEDSTAT. DRG Guide Descriptions and Normative Values. Ann Arbor, MI, 2005.
32. Borssen B, Bergenheim T, Lithner F. The epidemiology of foot lesions in diabetic patients aged 15–50 years. *Diabet Med* 1990;7:438–444.
33. Lavery LA, Armstrong DG, Wunderlich RP, Tredwell J, Boulton AJM. Predictive value of foot pressure assessment as part of a population-based diabetes disease management program. *Diabetes Care* 2003;26(4):1069–1073.
34. Malgrange D, Richard JL, Leymarie F. Screening diabetic patients at risk for foot ulceration. A multi-centre hospital-based study in France. *Diabetes Metab* 2003;29(3):261–268.
35. MMWR. History of foot ulcer among persons with diabetes—United States 2000–2002. *Morb Mortal Wkly Rep* 2003;52(45):1098–1102.
36. Apelqvist J, Larsson J, Agard C. Long term prognosis for diabetic patients with foot ulcers. *J Int Med* 1993;233:485–491.

3

The Evolution of Wound Healing

From Art to Science

I. Kelman Cohen, MD

INTRODUCTION

Man's struggle to heal wounds is as old as history itself. As life forms evolved from single cell life to amphibian and finally mammal, the pristine ability to heal by regeneration was lost and thus repairs by inflammation and subsequent deposition of matrix protein (scar) evolved as the method of mammalian healing. This evolutionary change leading to scar (the deposition of collagen) seems to be the key to preventing regeneration. It is well known that when the point is reached on the ladder where regeneration on longer occurs, inflammation and collagen deposition are the difference. In fact, if one takes a form of life, which seems the first link between regeneration and scar formation and a collagen cross-linking inhibitor is fed to the animal, then regeneration will once again occur! If we could only bridge this gap, imagine how successful we could become in the management of diabetic wounds. Although uncertain regarding why this occurred in the evolutionary process, it is hypothesized that as mammals became sophisticated, they needed rapid healing to protect themselves from other predators and to eke out a physical survival in a very hostile environment. In early-recorded history, the Egyptians repaired wounds with primitive suture materials (such as insect claws) and used clean sheets on surgical fields to prevent "suppuration." The Greeks, led by Hippocrates, devised methods of treatment for primary wounds and chronic wounds. They used various gauze materials empirically which included wine, milk, honey, and other substances in open wounds similar to our treatment today. Today, one can assign scientific rationale to some of these ancient empirical choices. For example, the complex sugars of honey are known to suppress the growth of Gram-positive bacteria. Wine will suppress pseudomonas proliferation. Milk products may contain cytokines or serve as buffers to control wound pH. Although the ancients had no idea that pus was actually is made up of proteins and dead leukocytes, they understood that drainage of localized products of infection was a good sign (laudable pus). They understood that when signs opf inflammation could not be localized that death would inevitably follow. During the early Roman era, Celsius, unaware of the existence of bacteria, did recognize and describe the cardinal signs of clinical infection being (1) *rubor*—erythema, (2) *tumor*—swelling, (3) *dolor*—pain, and (4) *calor*—heat.

From: *The Diabetic Foot, Second Edition*
Edited by: A. Veves, J. M. Giurini, and F. W. LoGerfo © Humana Press Inc., Totowa, NJ

THE ORIGINS OF SCIENTIFIC STUDYING OF THE WOUND

Even the ancients took a scientific approach to wound healing by their observations, rationale, and conclusions. However, during the Dark Ages the domination of the church over thought processes overran the free thinkers in the arts and the sciences. Regardless, each generation brought forth new tools for the scientific mind to utilize for discovery and progress in wound healing. For example, Pare, the young French surgeon in the 16th century (1510–1590) made the following observations on the battlefield, which allowed him to "think out of the box" and radically change principles of wound management. "I had not yet seen wounds made by gun shot … it is true I had read in John de Vigo that wounds made by weapons of fire for their cure commands to cauterize them with oyle of Elders scalding hot…I was willing to know first, before I applied it, how the other Chirurgions did which was to apply the sayd oyle the hottest that was possible in the wounds insomuch as I took courage to doe as they did. At last I wanted oyle, and was constrained in steed therefore, to apply a digestive of yolks of eggs, oyle of Roses, and Turpentine. In the night I could not sleep in quiet, fearing some default in not cauterizing, that I should find those to whom I had not used the burning oyle dead impoysoned; which made me rise very early to visit them, where beyond my expectation I found those to whom I had applied my digestive medicine, to feel little pain, and their wounds without inflammation or tumor, having rested reasonably well in the night: the others to whom was used the sayd burnign oyle, I found them feverish, with great pain and tumor about the edges of their wounds." Therefore, Pare concluded, "And I resolved with myself never so cruelly, to burne poore men wounded with gunshot."

In the 17th century, great minds such as John Hunter (…) interested in science, anatomy and evolution could not be suppressed. Just one of his accomplishments was the first description of angiogenesis (one of the hot buttons at the moment for diabetic healing research). Hunter hypothesized that obliteration of blood flow would impede growth. Therefore, he ligated the carotid artery of a young deer and then observed antler growth on the ligated compared with the normal side. To his surprise, antler growth was retarded for a short period of time but then growth began again until the antler reached normal size. He hypothesized that the ligature had come off the carotid. When he sacrificed the animal, he was surprised to find that the ligature was intact but there was extensive growth of new vessels in the area, which compensated for the ablated blood flow from carotid ligation. Therefore, he concluded that hypoxia had stimulated new blood vessel growth and although he did not know the factor involved, he coined the phrase angiogenesis to brand his observation. This occurred over 200 years before the seminal work of Judah Folkman. Think of the impact today on cancer and wound research and treatment. It is quite possible that the poor blood flow in diabetes is not only related to nitric oxide vascular changes but also to a lack of angiogenesis in diabetic wounds related to wound proteases, which destroy the angiogenic growth factors.

In the 18th and 19th centuries came the recognition that a factor passed from care givers to patients would kill. These observations were made by Holmes, Semmelweiss, and many others. All were rejected by the leading professors of the day. The failure to support new ideas is still a major flaw in the scientific system. New ideas are often rejected for lack of validation of the very idea the investigator wishes to explore. Those in academic power continue to suppress the new. Yet the observations of Semmelweiss and others promoted the discovery of bacteria by Pasteur and the concept of antisepsis by Lister. All were in part made possible by the 17th century fervor for anatomical studies, the age of the scientific method, the discovery of the microscope and bacterial culture. Similarly, in the 21st century, new ideas that are worthwhile often break through the prejudices and judgment of "peers."

It is Claude Bernard (1813–1878) who really played a major role in development of laboratory methods for the advancement of clinical medicine and hence the advancements that would occur in wound healing in general and the diabetic wounds in particular. "I consider the hospital the antechamber of medicine, it is the first place where the physician makes his observations. But the laboratory is the temple of the science of medicine." Such pronouncement was justified in his day as the practice of medicine had no scientific basis beyond observation. In contrast, Bernard's laboratory findings would lead to scientific facts, which would alter patient care. This philosophy would change drastically in the 20th century when it became obvious that work in animals and cell culture could not supplant the data, which can be derived from human studies.

The late 19th to mid-20th century saw the advent of antibiotics, which has had both positive and negative effects on wound care; mainly, the effects have been positive. Perhaps one of the most interesting observations of discovery in this area again is the fortuitous observation. Yes, Fleming discovered penicillin but as an annoying mold which was hampering his studies of bacteria. It was his associates Chain and Florey who recognized that they should be studying the mold rather than the bacteria and hence penicillin. One must learn from these lessons. Keen and simple observation can change the course of medical history for the better. Failure to look objectively at new ideas can cripple the growth and development of health-related science.

THE EVOLUTION OF WOUND HEALING STUDY

In the 1940s wound healing studies evolved in cell culture, animal models and eventually in man. Alexis Carrel was really the father of modern day wound healing studies for in the first part of the 20th century. He grew fibroblasts in culture, studied wound contraction in World War I combat injuries, and did the first microsurgery (for which he was awarded the Nobel Prize). By the end of War II, many exposed to the devastating injuries of this struggle were stimulated to study wound healing on a more formal basis. These included John Schilling at the University of Oklahoma who created a stainless steel wire mesh chamber, which he implanted subcutaneously in rats. Schilling then measured histological and biochemical events which occurred over time in the chambers. Moreover, the chambers could be injected with various materials to see the effects of these materials on the healing process. About the same time, Egbert Dumphy, at Harvard, started a series of experiments in various animals and humans examining a number of factors which might effect healing including nutrition, oxygen, shock, and so on. Stan Levinson started his medial career in Boston where he witnessed the care of burn victims after the Cocoanut Grove Fire. This early experience led him to his career in burns, wounds, shock, and metabolism. These two surgical leaders published the first texts and symposium on the subject and either trained or inspired such future leaders in wound healing research such as Tom Hunt who trained with Dumphy and picked up on the Schilling chamber. In parallel, were those spawned from a more traditional academic investigative career. For example, Jerry Gross graduated from Harvard Medical School and went straight into research of developmental biology and tissue repair. Gross actually discovered Gross collaborated with his surgical colleague, Hermes Grillo. Therefore, the basic data of Gross led to Grillo's classic work on the biology of tracheal scarring and contraction. These laboratory experiences led Grillo to the operating room armed with the basic biological principles of healing he had learned working with Gross. In the operating room, he was then able to develop biologically based operations, which were of major importance in the restoring the lives of those with congenital and acquired tracheal injuries.

Working in relative isolation in Chapel Hill North Carolina, a young Erle E. Peacock Jr., stimulated by those mentioned earlier and knowing that collagen was the predominant protein in tissue matrix, performed wound healing experiments involving wound contraction and prevention of scarring using collagen crosslink inhibitors. Like Dumphy, Schilling, and Gross, he mentored many of today's leaders in the wound-healing field.

All of these advances took more than inquisitive ambitious minds. Since the 1970s there has been a logarithmic growth in the laboratory tools available to seek answers to the problems of wound healing pathogenesis in general and diabetic wounds in particular. Wound healing researchers have taken advantage of each new "laboratory toy" which has come along to discover how the "toy" could be used to unlock a wound healing problem crying for solution. Tissue culture, electron microscopy, protein analysis, Western blot, Northern blot, PCR, and now gene array. The list of tools seems endless and increases daily.

Perhaps the greatest discovery for all was the defining structure and means for analysis of DNA and RNA. Without Rosalind Franklin, Watson and Crick, Linus Pauling, and a whole host of scientists of the day, these phenomena and spin off analytical methods would not be available to us. Technology has led to our ability to identify rapidly protein structure, map genes, and characterize materials with great speed accuracy. The explosion of new biological information for those interested in correcting wound-healing abnormalities is dramatic and great strides in our knowledge and therapies is predictable in the near future.

One cannot forget the humanistic areas of science, which has helped in wound care. The pharmacological treatment of depression, education of patients, and caregivers are all part of the advancing science of wound healing. One of the greatest needs along these lines is the education of caregivers, which remains appallingly poor. Perhaps the most important "science of education" to be explored is how to get new valid information to caregivers and see that they learn to separate scientific fact from marketing propaganda.

MAJOR STEPS IN OUR UNDERSTANDING OF WOUND HEALING PROCESS (GROWTH FACTORS, MMPS, AND SO ON)

To treat a clinical wound today without having a basic understanding of the biological principles of wound repair is like trying to sail across the ocean without a compass. (Some of the newer tools being developed will add the equivalent of GPS to the armamentarium of the clinician.) Several classical wound-healing texts will provide the basics of repair (…) along with Chapter 4 in this text.

WOUND HEALING TODAY: HOW MUCH OF ART AND HOW MUCH OF SCIENCE

In the 45 years that this author has had a focused interest in the biology of wound healing and wound care, there have been few changes in care that make a difference. However, there has been a great deal of exciting science, which has defined some of the basic pathophysiology of chronic wounds. Now it is a matter of increasing the scientific base and translation into clinical care. The science is described in the Chapter by Davison. Moreover, there is a great deal of new science, which relates directly or indirectly to wound healing which increases daily. Many of these advances have been resulting from Federal Government support via the National Institutes of Health (NIH). Unfortunately, most industrial support for wound healing research has been with specific product orientation. However, there are a few significant exceptions to this as some responsible manufacturers have given funds for basic wound healing research.

Perhaps the most interesting phenomena I have observed of wound care product manufacturers is the discovery that wound care is a market worth billions of dollars. Therefore, over the past 25 years, there has been a tremendous drive to dazzle the wound care consumers with virtually thousands of new products each claiming to have an important role in wound management. They have been able to convince third party payers and the federal government that their products should be on the market without much evidence to support their claims. They are driven by profit and not by scientific, clinical truths. They have found spokesmen for their products among "brand name" wound healing nurses and physicians who have sold their endorsements of these therapies for a price rather than take a real objective view of the product. There are some nurses and doctors who have totally lost touch with patient care who market themselves as wound healing experts and travel around the country teaching "wound healing" and often endorsing products of questionable merits. They have created a self-serving business for themselves. Clearly many of the manufacturers and their health care advocates have abused the taxpayer. They have been allowed by the government to add their oft times expensive products of questionable clinical value to the armamentarium used daily for wound care. Moreover, as large populations of wound care givers are nurses, they have fallen for the pseudoscience often offered up by the marketing forces of industry. They are indeed successful and those who actually use the products are won over by marketing rather than scientific data. Unfortunately, the same is true for a number of treating physicians!! Somehow, a strong ethical branch of the wound care industry must ban together with an untainted group of true wound healing experts to develop products, which will actually accelerate the healing of chronic wounds and control the healing aberrations of fibrosis. A leading driver for such reform will come from the federal agencies, which control health care costs and are beginning to look at wound care costs in particular.

AN OUTLOOK OF THE FUTURE

Several events will improve wound care in the next few decades. They can be divided into scientific and care related.

Scientific

1. *Proteases:* why are wounds stuck in an early inflammatory phase and making excessive proteases. Although attaching the protease issue is relevant, it is only the tip of the iceberg. The protease issue looms big. For example, sections in this text will focus on angiogenesis, yet a key to effective angiogenesis will be protease control so angiogenic factors are not destroyed. One possible form of new therapy would be enhancement of endogenous antiproteases. Can one develop gene therapy to enhance the activity of antiproteases and thereby enhance healing? Another would be better understanding and control of free radical production by polymorphonuclear leukocytes (PMNs) as free radicals stimulate inflammation and hence proteases. What are the role of nitric oxide and especially the role of inducible nitric oxide synthase (iNOS) in the induction of inflammation?

2. *Gene Therapy:* we are still wandering in this area and the "scientific tricks," although interesting, are flawed when it comes to clinical application and the health care expenses associated with it. Yet, I expect that we will see cost-effective gene therapy in the future—it will not be soon. Much has been made of stimulating growth factor production with gene therapy. It would seem more appropriate to direct attention at gene therapy to inhibit proteases as growth factors will never be effective in the presence of high levels of proteases.

3. Modulation of temperature to control pressure necrosis leads to cell death and ulcer formation in the patient with diabetes. Cooling as well as pressure relief will be important in the management of diabetic foot wounds. Cooling to prevent the inflammatory changes with pressure and the flow–reflow phenomena may provide a very simple form of low-cost improvement in our prevention of diabetic wounds and pressure sores. After all, pressure is a major cause of both chronic wounds.

4. New drugs to treat diabetes itself: the better one can keep blood sugar in a normal range, the less glycosylation there is of all sorts of tissues in the body; hence the fewer diabetic complications.

Care-Related Issues

1. Industry must "clean house" and listen to the science rather than the marketing genius who will simply push product rather than the scientific basis of the product.

2. Education: many of the "courses" on wound healing simply propagate bad ideas and practice. There are even national meetings, which are contaminated by bad data given by bad speakers.

3. The concept of wound healing centers is excellent, but often the execution is lacking. There must be more formal education for the health care gives in these centers and frequent reviews and updates.

4. We live in an era in which computerized communication is superb, yet we in wound healing have not taken advantage of this for the benefit or our patients. Google and PubMed are a big help for those willing to dig out data. However, the busy practitioner needs to be fed information in a simple and easily accessed fashion. More can be done

5. The federal government should be more involved in evaluation of products for their scientific merit and having some control over what is and what is not paid for by government agencies.

6. Every wound is attached to the patient and the patient must be treated emotionally as well as physically. Every wound is associated with an underlying pathological process and all of these phenomena must be examined in great detail. How often I am referred a wound rather than being referred a patient. How often I discover that the patient has not had an adequate evaluation. Once the emotional aspects are clear and the patient becomes part of the wound care team and once the underlying disease is properly treated, it is amazing how well the patient will do and the wound will heal without expensive or esoteric therapies.

7. Finally, I urge basic scientists, clinicians and even government regulators to get involved in wound healing. The problem is enormous worldwide and needs major attention. The incidence of diabetes and morbidity and mortality from the diabetic wound continues out of

control. Not enough attention is being paid to the problem and all must fight this dreaded disease and its complications.

SUGGESTED READING

1. Claude IB. *An Introduction to the Study of Experimental Medicine, 1927*, Reprint, Dover Publications, New York, 1957.
2. Nuland SB. *The Doctors' Plague*, WW Norton, New York, 2003.
3. Majno G. *The Healing Hand. Man and Wound in the Ancient World*, Harvard University Press, Cambridge, MA, 1975.
4. Kobler J. *The Reluctant Surgeon: A Life of John Hunter*, Heinemann, London, 1960.

The Wound-Healing Process

Jeffrey M. Davidson, PhD and Luisa DiPietro, DDS, PhD

INTRODUCTION

Diabetes is on the rise in the United States and the rest of the world, and its complications are even more evident in the aging population. Among the most severe complications of diabetes are impaired circulation and wound healing. The former condition, together with peripheral neuropathy, contributes to an insensate, poorly vascularized lower extremity that is prone to the development of chronic wounds. Lack of sensation leads to aggravation of the injury, which can frequently lead to the spread of infection and the loss of all or part of the lower limb. The circulatory defects occur in both conducting vessels—which are prone to atherosclerosis—and the microcirculation, which shows signs of basement membrane thickening and diminished reparative capacity. Surgical intervention can sometimes alleviate the macrovascular defects, but grafting procedures cannot guarantee that tissue perfusion can be restored. With the exception of the retina, the poor growth of new capillary vessels in diabetes broadly diminishes the capacity to repair.

WORKING DEFINITIONS

For the purposes of this discussion, we define wound repair as the effort of adult tissues to restore normal tissue function and architecture after one of a variety of physical, mechanical, biological, or chemical insults. The primary demands of a system that is undergoing wound repair are the restoration of normal blood and lymphatic circulatory patterns, the formation of a surface barrier to fluid loss and further infection, the suppression and elimination of foreign organisms and material from the injury site, and reestablishment of mechanical integrity. Often these events occur with great urgency; thus, perfect reorganization is sacrificed in the name of adequate function. On the other hand, regeneration implies the complete restoration of pre-existing tissue architecture and all cellular elements in the absence of scar formation. Although regeneration is an ideal in the wound-healing world, it is typically only found in embryonic development, lower organisms, or in restricted tissue compartments such as bone. Angiogenesis is a crucial element of wound repair. In its broadest sense, it is defined as the formation of new blood vessels from a pre-existing, surrounding blood supply. In the healing wound, new blood vessel formation is a rapid and

From: *The Diabetic Foot, Second Edition*
Edited by: A. Veves, J. M. Giurini, and F. W. LoGerfo © Humana Press Inc., Totowa, NJ

transient phenomenon, which occurs during the proliferation of granulation tissue. Fibrosis refers to the excess formation of extracellular connective tissue that often accompanies wound repair processes. Excess of connective tissue accumulation may go beyond the function of restoring mechanical integrity and act to impede the normal architecture and physiological function of the injured tissue. Fibrosis in the skin can result in mild disfigurement or severe loss of mobility.

HISTORY

The record of wound-healing analysis and therapy goes back many centuries. Works by Majno *(1)* and Needham *(2)* give very nice accounts of the earliest efforts in wound repair up to and including the modern era. Wound healing has always been a major interest of the surgeon, and, with the discovery of antiseptic procedures and antibiotics, the extent to which surgical solutions to wound-healing problems can be applied has grown enormously. Nevertheless, there are a wide range of wound-healing complications which do not respond to simple, surgical treatment: nonhealing wounds, wounds that heal excessively, and wounds that become locked in uncontrolled growth (tumors). With the advent of modern biochemical and molecular techniques, a new perspective of the process has been opened before us *(3,4)*. These discoveries have, in turn, created a new prospect for our understanding and treatment of the problem wound *(5)*.

TERMINOLOGY

There are a few general terms that should be described before dealing with specific issues of wound repair. The term cytokines is used to describe a collection of small protein molecules that are used to provide communication between cells of the inflammatory system. Perhaps the best known of this group are the interleukins, leukocyte intercellular signaling molecules; however, there are also a wide variety of other secreted gene products which act on specific receptors to induce responses such as cell movement, cell growth, or even cell death. In contrast to cytokines, which are frequently involved in regulating inflammation, a distinct group of proteins crucial to the repair process are the cellular growth factors. As implied by their name, the principal function of these proteins molecules is thought to be the promotion of cell and tissue growth; in addition, these molecules can also act to stimulate cell movement and cell migration. Some of the growth factors also stimulate cells to produce more connective tissues. All these molecules can be thought of as hormones that act at the local tissue level to bring about specific tissue responses. As such, they act in autocrine (on like cells), paracrine (on unlike cells), or juxtacrine (on nearby cells) fashion depending on the nature of the target cell.

A crucial class of proteins involved in tissue repair is the proteinases. These are protein-degrading enzymes that can be released by both inflammatory and connective tissue cells. When proteinases act outside the cell, they are crucial for degradation of foreign material, for promoting cell movement through tissue spaces, and for tight regulation of the abundance and distribution of various molecules in the extracellular space. Some proteinases are also important catalysts for further enzymatic reactions.

COMPONENTS AND MEDIATORS IN THE SKIN

Extracellular Matrix

The integrity and mechanical properties of every tissue are governed by its extracellular matrix. This consists of a complex mixture of fibrous and adhesive macromolecules that determine such physical characters as tensile strength, elasticity, hydration, and compressibility *(6)*. The best known and most abundant component in this class is collagen, which is a family of fiber-forming proteins characterized by a rope-like arrangement of three individual polypeptide chains, which confers to every collagen molecule a high degree of stiffness, resistance to proteolytic degradation, and highly defined, rigid structure. Collagen molecules characteristically assemble into higher-order fibrils and fibers whose organization is stabilized by covalent chemical cross-links between individual molecules to produce the predominant material of tendons, ligaments, blood vessels, and skin. Some members of the collagen family of proteins serve more specialized functions, such as determining overall fibril diameter or promoting interactions with other components in the extracellular matrix. In addition, several of the collagen types (presently types I–XXVII) have very restricted distributions in either the basement membrane underlying epithelial surfaces or in structures that attach epithelium to underlying connective tissue.

Under physiological conditions, fibrous collagen is only degraded by highly specialized proteolytic enzymes known as collagenases. The collagenases are in turn members of a much larger class of proteinases, the matrix metalloproteinases (MMPs).

Elastin is, as the name implies, a rubber-like protein, which is often found in association with collagen in skin, blood vessels, and other elastic tissues. Unlike collagen, elastin does not form highly organized fibers, perhaps because this would interfere with its function as a rubbery, cross-linked network *(7)*. The principal role of elastin appears to be the development of elastic properties in tissues. Elastin is noteworthy in wound healing because, at least in the skin, it is one of the last components to be replaced during the repair sequence.

Proteoglycans are composite molecules as the name implies. They consist of a core protein to which are attached acidic sugar chains distinctively built up from the addition of disaccharide subunits. These highly charged molecules play an important role in maintaining hydration of tissue spaces, and they also interact strongly with many other components in the extracellular space, including connective tissue proteins and growth factors. Proteoglycans that contain heparan sulfate side chains are particularly significant because they can bind many other molecules.

Because the diabetic state invariably involves hyperglycemia, nonenzymatic glycation of collagen, and other proteins can be extensive. The relatively long half-life of matrix proteins in combination with this modification can lead to the formation of undesirable cross-links among molecules, which reduces solubility of the matrix. In addition to stiffening of blood vessels, hyperglycemia may contribute to atherosclerosis and other vascular complications *(8–12)*. Further investigation is needed to determine if strategies that reduce the formation of these byproducts can reduce the wound-healing deficit in diabetes.

ADHESIVE PROTEINS

Cells, whether they are moving about in tissue or fixed in place, require adhesive interactions with their surroundings. This is accomplished by the interaction of specific cell surface receptors with molecules in the extracellular environment. The classic example of this system and cell–matrix interactions is the family of integrin molecules. These matrix receptors consist of two subunits that are mainly external to the cell but which transverse the cell membrane and may be closely associated with many elements of the cytoskeleton on the cell interior. On the cell surface, these integrins interact with specific sites in extracellular matrix components to provide adhesion and even some recognition functions. Although integrins can bind to a number of different matrix macromolecules, they are importantly associated with a group of molecules known as cellular attachment factors, most of which are glycoproteins that have branched sugar chains attached to the protein backbone *(3)*. The best known of these adhesive glycoproteins is the molecule fibronectin, a component of plasma, which is also produced in a variant form by cells during wound repair. This molecule has many different interactive regions. Fibronectin can form a bridging link from cells (via integrins) to collagen, to heparin or heparan-containing proteoglycans, and to fibrin. Thus, this glycoprotein is a prototype for the intercellular cement that links many of the elements of the matrix together with its constituent cells. Another prominent plasma attachment factor is the protein vitronectin. Cells themselves produce many attachment and migration factors including osteopontin, osteonectin/SPARC, tenascin, and thrombospondin. In some cases these latter three molecules, depending on the cell type and circumstances, may have anti-adhesive properties.

BASEMENT MEMBRANES

There is highly specialized extracellular matrix organization found in the basement membrane underlying all epithelial cells *(13)*. These structures surround the endothelial lining of all blood vessels and underlie epidermal surfaces. Although they are often very thin and evanescent, basement membranes serve an important function in maintaining the polar organization of the epithelium assuring its appropriate attachment to underlying connective tissue and acting as a physical barrier to large molecular complexes and cells. Basement membranes characteristically contain some unique members of each of the extracellular matrix classes we have already discussed: type-IV collagen, which tends to form lattices rather than extended fibers; laminin—a large, multifunctional, cross-shaped attachment factor, and perlecan—a proteoglycan that is particularly rich in heparan sulfate side chains. Basement membrane collagens do not have a continuous triple helical structure, so they are susceptible to degradation by a wider range of proteinases.

CELL POPULATIONS

A variety of cell populations play a role in wound healing. In the epidermis, the upper layer of the skin, the predominant cells are the keratinocytes. This is a self-renewing cell population in which the basal cells remain closely associated with the basement membrane whereas their daughter cells differentiate and move upward through the epidermis to produce the cornified layers that protect the skin. Other epidermal cells include the Langerhans cell and the dendritic cell, which are involved in host defense and antigen presentation. Lymphocytes can also appear in the epidermis under pathological conditions. Melanocytes produce pigment that is transferred to the keratinocyte. In the deeper layer of the skin, the dermis, the predominant cell type is the fibroblast, which is embedded in a dense meshwork of extracellular matrix molecules. Blood is brought to the skin by vascular channels lined with endothelial cells. The pericyte is a smooth muscle cell-like component, which is closely associated with capillary endothelial cells. The larger vessels, both arteries and veins, will have surrounding vascular smooth cells. A number of cells of the inflammatory system also reside in the dermis. The mast cell is a key participant in any immunological and allergic reactions, and resident tissue macrophages are also critical to immune surveillance. During injury, many new cell types move from the circulation into connective tissue space. These include leukocytes: macrophages, lymphocytes and neutrophils, and platelets.

CYTOKINES, GROWTH FACTORS, AND THEIR RECEPTORS

Growth factors have powerful, positive actions during the wound-healing process. The prototypical growth factor is epidermal growth factor (EGF). It was originally identified as a small protein produced in the salivary gland of male mice by Stanley Cohen, and it was noted for stimulating the premature opening of eyelids of the fetal mouse. EGF is actually a part of a family of related proteins, which include EGF, transforming growth factor (TGF)-α, betacellulin, heparin-binding EGF, epiregulin, neuregulin, and amphiregulin *(14)*. As true of all the growth factors, these proteins bind to very specific and selective cellular receptors that transmit a set of signals within the cell to stimulate cell growth and division. An unusual feature of the EGF family is that many members actually are synthesized as much larger cell surface proteins with "tails" penetrating into the cell interior. The active forms are then cleaved from the exterior of the cell surface by specific enzymatic activities. EGF has been shown in a number of studies to stimulate wound repair both in fibroblasts and epithelial cells. It has not achieved much clinical success, although it is presently used in some formulations for corneal lubrication.

A second important class of growth stimulating molecules is the platelet-derived growth factors (PDGFs) *(15)*. These molecules are contained in platelet granules, and the release of PDGF at sites of injury during clot formation is certainly an important aspect of the repair process. Commercial preparations of platelet lysates have shown success in clinical application, most likely because of the presence of PDGF and other growth factors. This molecule has been widely implicated in the pathological growth of vascular smooth muscle cells during atherosclerosis, and one of the two peptide chains of PDGF is closely related to a viral (v-*sis*) oncogene. Thus, growth factor-like molecules are involved in growth control of transformed cells. As with EGF, the response to this stimulus is dictated by the presence of specific PDGF receptors. PDGF is produced in two isoforms (A and B) and PDGF molecules exist as AA, AB, or BB forms which are selectively recognized by two different kinds of PDGF receptors.

Two growth factor types are significant for their ability to stimulate angiogenesis. Fibroblast growth factor (FGF) refers to a family of proteins that interact with one or more of four related receptors on a variety of cell types *(16)*. FGF-1 and -2 (acidic and basic FGF) are particularly noteworthy for their ability to stimulate endothelial cell growth and capillary cell invasion in a variety of models. Most forms of FGF have growth effects on many cell populations, but endothelial cells appear to have a greater sensitivity; however, there are two novel forms of FGF (FGF-7 and -10 or keratinocyte growth factors-1 and -2) that specifically stimulate the proliferation and differentiation of epithelial cells because of unique receptors present on these cells *(17)*. These two growth factors have a classical paracrine mode of action because they are produced in the dermis and act on the epidermis. Vascular endothelial growth factor (VEGF) or vascular permeability factor is the most selective of the growth factors for endothelial action. As first name implies, VEGF acts to stimulate endothelial cell growth and recruitment *(18,19)*. The latter name, vascular permeability factor, refers to an important property of VEGF, the ability to increase capillary permeability and leakage of plasma into tissue space. VEGF has received very recent notoriety for its ability to stimulate the revascularization of ischemic limbs and cardiac muscle *(20)*. It is very likely that this molecule is going to assume an important role in the therapy of wound repair particularly in which blood supply is compromised. VEGF-C is exclusively responsible for the process of lymphangiogenesis, the growth of new lymphatic structures.

Connective tissue growth factor (CTGF) is another, newer growth factor *(21)*. Although this molecule appeared to have some antigenic similarity to PDGF, it is chemically a very different structure. It appears to be highly specific for connective tissue cells such as fibroblasts and chondrocytes. Its expression is associated with sites of tissue repair. CTGF has been reported to stimulate connective tissue formation as well *(21)*. Perhaps more significant is the observation that CTGF is strongly induced by treatment of cells and tissues with another growth factor, transforming growth factor (TGF)-β. Recent findings suggest that CTGF may be the downstream signal molecule that actually carries out the matrix-forming activities of TGF-β.

TGF-β is a part of a very large superfamily of proteins that are involved in development, growth, and differentiation *(22)*. Besides TGF-β itself (there are three different forms in man), other well-known members of this family are the bone morphogenic proteins, activin, inhibin, and Mullerian inhibitory substance. TGF-β plays two very prominent roles in inflammation and repair. TGF-β is a very potent inhibitor of immune reactivity, and it suppresses the activation of the immune system *(23)*. Indeed, in knockout mice that lack the TGF-β1 gene, offspring die early in postnatal life from a massive inflammatory reaction. The second major role of TGF-β is in matrix formation and wound healing, in which TGF-β strongly induces—directly or indirectly—the expression of many connective tissue molecules including collagen, elastin, fibronectin, and some proteoglycans, whereas it suppresses the expression of connective tissue degrading enzymes such as collagenase and related MMPs. TGF-β also increases the expression of proteinase inhibitors that act on both the metalloenzyme class of proteinases (tissue inhibitor of metalloproteinases) and the serine proteinase class, such as plasminogen activator inhibitor-1. Thus, it is no surprise that TGF-β expression is often associated with fibrosis and excessive scarring *(24)*. Administration of TGF-β has been shown to accelerate repair in many wound models, and clinical trials of TGF-β2 and TGF-β3 have been conducted as a treatment for chronic wounds.

TGF-β has a complex biology, because it is secreted from cells as a latent factor, and it is sequestered by a class of molecules called latent TGF-β binding proteins *(25)*. Unlike most of the other growth factors, TGF-β and its family members signal, in part, through the assembly of two distinct receptors that signal to the nucleus, in part, through a rather direct pathway that involves molecules known as SMADs *(26)*.

The insulin-like growth factor (IGF)-I and IGF-II are small proteins structurally related to insulin. They each have their own cognate receptor. Insulin itself can interact with the IGF-1 receptor but at about 100-fold higher concentrations. IGF-1 is a growth factor often associated with bone development as an important downstream target of the action of growth hormone. There are significant circulating levels by IGF-1, but it also can be produced locally. IGF-2 binds to a receptor also known as the mannose-6 phosphate receptor. IGF-II expression is more closely associated with development than with tissue repair. IGF-I bioavailability and action is thought to be tightly regulated by a group of molecules known as the IGF binding proteins (IGF-BPs).

Various members of the IGF-BPs can either facilitate the activity of IGF on its receptor or act as sequestering agents to prevent action. Much of the regulation of IGF could thus be at the level of IGF-BP control *(27)*. IGF-1 may be more limited in availability in diabetic wounds *(28)*. Hepatocyte growth factor/scatter factor is another example of a paracrine growth factor that is produced, in large part, by fibroblasts and interacts with the c-Met receptor on epithelial and vascular endothelial cells. This factor has a number of interesting properties, including the stimulation of cell migration and the production of other, angiogenic factors such as VEGF. It has been shown to enhance wound healing in a diabetic mouse model *(29,30)*.

All of these growth factors are proteins, and therefore their production is dictated by the activity of distinct genes. However, regulation occurs at many levels of growth factor action. First, many of these growth factors are synthesized as larger precursor molecules that are biologically inactive until cleared or released. Second, a number of them are expressed in various isoforms whose structure is regulated by alternative splicing during transcription. Third, alternative splicing generates receptor diversity, particularly in the case of FGF. Fourth, unlike endocrine hormones, these proteins are not generally to be found freely circulating in tissue fluid or plasma. Instead they are frequently associated with other molecules, including those of the extracellular matrix, by either electrostatic interactions or more specific protein–protein interactions. Specific examples include the very tight binding of FGF family members to positively charged proteoglycans such as the heparan sulfate proteoglycans *(31,32)*. TGF-β binds to a cell surface proteoglycan, betaglycan, and has also been reported to interact with a small matrix proteoglycan, decorin, and a component of the elastic fibers, fibrillin. Fibrillin is in turn a member of a larger family of molecules known as the latent TGF-β binding proteins *(25)*. The implication of these observations is that the mere evidence that a growth factor gene is expressed at a tissue site or its addition it to a tissue target does not ensure that the biologically active molecule will reach its appropriate receptor and evoke a tissue response.

CELLULAR COMPONENTS OF THE INFLAMMATORY SYSTEM

Platelets

These cells play a critical role in hemostasis and wound healing. Although platelets are fragments of mature megakaryocytes, they act as independent cells at sites of tissue injury. Aggregation of platelets is predominantly induced by exposure of circulating platelets to collagen. Platelets bind to the collagen through a specific integrin receptor and begin several steps in their irreversible progression toward formation of a thrombus. Many small molecules are released, in particular byproducts of arachidonic acid metabolism. These molecules are released after activation of enzymes at the platelet surface that modify the structure of phospholipids in the plasma membrane. These biologically active molecules, which include the prostaglandins and leukotrienes, have important effects on underlying vascular endothelial and smooth muscle cells. The platelets, once adherent to the fibrin clot and underlying collagen, will, over the course of several minutes, begin to undergo the process of clot retraction. Simultaneously with these events, the platelet releases two important classes of biologically active molecules: first, it releases additional proteins that facilitate cell adhesion and cell migration, including thrombospondin and fibromodulin; second, the platelet granule is a potent source of several growth factors, especially PDGF, TGF-β, EGF, and TGF-α. Thus, extracts of platelets and blood serum are extremely rich in agents which promote wound repair. Deficiencies of platelets lead to impaired blood coagulation and reduced wound healing.

PDGF (becaplermin) is the only pharmaceutical available for treatment of diabetic foot ulcers, whereas several formulations of autologous platelet extracts have been used as part of diabetic wound-healing protocols *(33)*.

Neutrophils

Once blood loss is controlled by fibrin clot formation and platelet activation, the inflammatory system comes into play. By activation of specific adhesive molecules on the vascular endothelial surface, neutrophils bind to endothelium and rapidly move from the luminal surface of vessels into tissue space. Activation can occur through a number of signals, including cell–cell adhesion or the presence of small, soluble signal molecules. Neutrophils play a critical role in debridement and control of infection. Neutrophil activation leads to the release of reactive oxygen species through the actions of enzymatic pathways leading to production of superoxide free radicals and peroxide. These oxidants have extremely potent antimicrobial activity. To some extent, host cells are protected from the action of these reactive oxygen species by enzymatic systems such as superoxide dismutase and catalase. The second important activity of the neutrophil is the release of several proteinases of the serine proteinase class (trypsin-like enzymes). These include elastase, cathepsin, and proteinases. Each of these enzymes has broad substrate specificity and can bring about massive degradation of proteins in the local environment. The activity of these enzymes is normally counterbalanced by the presence of circulating serine proteinase inhibitors such as α1-antiproteinase, α2-antichymotrypsin, and α2-macroglobulin as well as local expression of secretory leukocyte protease inhibitor. Deficiencies in proteinase inhibitors can lead to an imbalance and excess tissue destruction. The neutrophil also expresses a specific form of collagenase, MMP-8, and it also expresses growth factors such as TGF-β.

Normally, the neutrophil has a limited life-span in the wound-healing process. Many spent neutrophils are found in the overlying wound exudate or the eschar. Neutrophil abundance declines with the removal of foreign material and infectious organisms.

Monocytes

Shortly after neutrophil invasion, the next wave of inflammatory cells to normally enter the wound site is the mononuclear phagocyte. These cells, which circulate as monocytes, rapidly differentiate into macrophages on entry into the tissue space, and they play a crucial role in the coordination of cell activities by their expression of growth factors and cytokines. These cells also continue the process of debridement by engulfment of foreign particles; however, most of the enzymatic activity of macrophages is secreted intracellularly into lysosomal vacuoles. Variations in the extracellular environment for macrophage activation can lead to expression of different classes of cytokines. For example, infection may simulate the expression of tumor necrosis factor-α and interleukin molecules, which tend to perpetuate the inflammatory process. On the other hand, appropriate signals will stimulate macrophages to express a wide variety of growth factors including FGF, TGF-β, and VEGF. The macrophage does express a number of important proteinases involved in wound remodeling, including collagenase and metalloelastase (MMP-12).

Lymphocytes

The classical components of the immune system, lymphocytes are not prominently active in acute wounds, although T-cell involvement in chronic lesions is often seen. These immune effectors can have important modulatory activity on the wound healing process *(34)*, but they appear to play a small role in early restoration of tissue architecture.

Mast Cells

These resident tissue cells that act as a component of the inflammatory system are often activated by allergic or immunological stimuli, but they can also play a role in tissue repair *(35)*. Mast cells and their products have been implicated in a number of chronic fibrotic states. These cells are capable of releasing a variety of cytokines and they are known to express a unique set of proteinases of the serine proteinase class.

SEQUENTIAL EVENTS IN THE WOUND REPAIR CASCADE

Under normal circumstances, wound repair is a highly orchestrated progression of events that involves the interaction of the elements described in the preceding sections. Because of the different cell populations and signals involved in each of the stages, it is often convenient to divide this orchestral work into different movements. As one might imagine the first elements in the healing process involve hemostasis, particularly in the case of traumatic injury. The damaged tissue quickly releases tissue factor and other stimuli such as exposed collagen that activate the coagulation pathway leading to production of a fibrin clot and the accumulation of circulating platelets that generate a complete thrombus. These hemostatic events, together with vasoconstriction, driven by arachidonic acid metabolites, eventually stop blood flow. The trapping of both serum proteins and the discharged contents of platelet granules provides the clotting reaction a rich bed on which cellular invasion may begin to take place.

This initial wound material has been termed the provisional matrix by Clark *(36)*. In molecular terms, this matrix consists of fibrin and serum proteins. The growth factors are released from platelets together with adhesion factors such as thrombospondin, fibromodulin, and the important adhesive protein fibronectin. As cells begin to migrate out of the normal, surrounding tissue to attempt to restore the damaged architecture, this is the first substrate that cells will see. Obviously, appropriate integrin receptors must be generated on the cell surface of migratory cells to recognize these novel substrates as compared to the normal, intact matrix surrounding the cells.

INFLAMMATION

The formation of the provisional matrix is accompanied by an acute inflammatory response. The first waves of inflammatory cells to reach the injury site are the neutrophils, with their potent antibacterial and tissue debridement repertoire. Neutrophil extravasation begins almost immediately as vascular endothelial cell surfaces surrounding the injury site begin to express adhesive molecules such as VCAM and E-selectin, which in turn interact with circulating leukocyte cell surface molecules. After a gradual slowing down of rolling movement within the smaller channels, these cells will eventually come to adhere to sites where they then diapedese through spaces between endothelial cells or move out into the tissue space through the openings of ruptured capillaries. Under normal circumstances, the flux of neutrophils is rapidly terminated, and as necrotic material is degraded these spent cells move upward out of the wound together with their destroyed contents to become part of the eschar. Excessive infection or foreign material may lead to the accumulation of a cellular exudate or—in the worst case—an abscess. The next cell in succession of inflammatory cells is the macrophage, which acts as the key coordinating factor in many of these wounds. Experiments in which animals have been depleted of macrophages show markedly reduced ability to mount a tissue repair response.

Appropriate inflammation and the appropriate function of inflammatory cells have generally been considered indispensable for successful wound healing. Landmark studies in the early 1970s and 1980s demonstrated that immune cells, particularly macrophages, are critical to wound healing, and the ability of macrophages to modulate angiogenesis and fibroplasia has been firmly established (37–39). However, recent gene knockout studies in the mouse call these findings into question (67). There is little argument that proper leukocyte activity assists in microbial decontamination of wounds. In addition, there are several logical arguments in support of a role for leukocytes in healing, even for sterile wounds. First, phagocytic leukocytes, as well as lymphocytes, produce multiple growth factors that promote the repair process. Second, the cellular death and tissue remodeling that occurs during injury and repair probably requires phagocytic clearance for complete resolution. Finally, studies in a variety of model systems suggest that several specific inflammatory cytokines and molecules, including chemokines and nitric oxide, are critical to wound healing (40–46).

The Sequence of Inflammation Following Tissue Injury

Immediately following injury, innate immune cells at the site of injury initiate an inflammatory response. Cells of the innate immune system, including mast cells, resident macrophages, and some specialized T-lymphocyte populations, stand at the ready, acting as sentinels to respond quickly to tissue damage or microbes. In the skin, keratinocytes are often considered a part of the immune sentinel system as well, as this cell type can quickly respond to stimuli and produces several proinflammatory mediators (47). The response of the innate immune cells to injury is rapid, and an abundance of proinflammatory mediators are produced within the first hour following insult. The mediators produced by resident innate immune cells in response to injury or insult trigger vascular responses, including vasodilation, endothelial cell activation, and increased vascular permeability. Further, early mediators also assist in recruiting the first wave of circulating leukocytes from the bloodstream into the injured tissue. The pattern of leukocytic infiltration into wounds is similar in progression to other acute inflammatory conditions. Neutrophils are the first leukocyte to be recruited in response to chemotactic mediators derived from platelets and resident innate immune cells, and perhaps by activation of complement *(34)*. If the wound is contaminated, microbial products may also serve as leukocyte chemoattractants. Within a day or two of injury, circulating monocytes also enter the wound and differentiate into mature tissue macrophages *(48)*. Macrophages become the most abundant leukocyte in the wound at this stage. Macrophages are thought to play an integral role in the successful outcome of wound healing through the generation of growth factors that promote cell proliferation and protein synthesis *(49)*. Macrophages also respond to neutrophils and their products, and can recognize and ingest apoptotic neutrophils *(50,51)*. The mast cell also increases in density in the wound bed, with most of the infiltration originating from the adjacent tissue *(52)*. As the leukocyte density within the wound increases, the leukocytes that have been recruited into the wound produce large amounts of cytokines and chemoattractants, amplifying the inflammatory response. In the late inflammatory phase of wound repair, T-lymphocytes appear in the wound bed, and may support the resolution and remodeling of the wound *(53,54)*.

Excessive Inflammation in Diabetic Wounds

Poorly healing wounds, including those of individuals with diabetes, often are characterized by a prolonged and dysregulated inflammatory phase *(55–58)*. In mice, the impaired wound healing that is seen in diabetic animals includes a sustained induction of chemokines and a prolonged persistence of neutrophils and macrophages at the site of the injury *(55)*. The excessive neutrophil content of poorly healing wounds, along with the ability of neutrophils to destroy tissue, has suggested that neutrophils might negatively influence repair. Neutrophils do produce a variety of growth factors that could promote revascularization and repair of injured tissue *(59)*. However, they also produce many enzymes that can induce substantial tissue damage. Neutrophil proteases, such as elastase and cathepsin G, can degrade most components of the extracellular matrix as well as proteins as diverse as clotting factors, complement, immunoglobulins, and cytokines *(60,61)*. Because the extracellular matrix serves as a supporting scaffold for infiltrating cells, modification of the extracellular matrix by neutrophils could have important consequences for repair. A reduction in neutrophil content, therefore, seems likely to improve healing outcomes if bacterial burden is not excessive. This concept has been demonstrated in animal models, as wound closure is accelerated in neutropenic diabetic mice *(62)*.

A number of additional recent studies in several systems bolster the concept that leukocytes can be detrimental to the process *(63–67)*. One remarkable example is that of wound repair in the early fetus. In contrast to adult skin, in which injury repair results in a fibrous scar, the skin of an early to midgestation fetus exhibits rapid and scarless regeneration *(68)*. Remarkably, early fetal wounds exhibit very little, if any, inflammatory response, and also demonstrate specific changes in the levels of members of the TGF family that appear to correlate with the lack of scar formation *(69–72)*. Scarless repair and altered growth factor production in fetal wounds does not appear to be a function of the fetal environment, as adult skin transplanted into a fetal environment maintains a scar-forming phenotype in response to injury *(73)*. Factors intrinsic to fetal skin, including the inflammatory response, appear to be the most important factors in creating the ideal repair phenotype that is seen in this tissue. Interestingly, more recent studies suggest that reduced inflammation can lead to improved outcomes in adult animals as well. Wounds that are produced in the PU.1 null mouse, a mouse that lacks both macrophages and functioning neutrophils, exhibit little inflammation, and heal quickly with reduced scarring *(67)*.

Together, then, these contemporary investigations of wound inflammation suggest that the therapeutic modulation of leukocyte function might improve wound-healing outcomes. Given the immune dysregulation observed in wounds of persons with diabetes, this therapeutic approach seems likely to have special utility in patients with diabetes. The challenge of such an approach will be to support optimal repair whereas maintaining adequate protection from infection.

GRANULATION TISSUE AND EPITHELIZATION

Within 3–4 days, inflammation has begun to subside and the provisional matrix begins to be replaced by the characteristic organ of tissue repair, granulation tissue. This is a highly cellular, highly vascularized mixture of fibroblasts, endothelial cells, and macrophages that advances into the provisional matrix and begins to lay down a more permanent extracellular matrix that provides much greater mechanical integrity to the wound site. The key processes that occur during granulation tissue formation are (1) fibroplasia, the accumulation of collagen and other matrix molecules; and (2) angiogenesis, the formation of a rich capillary bed to supply the rapidly growing extracellular matrix with adequate nutrient supply. Under normal circumstances, granulation tissue is a transient facet of wound repair, often progressing within less than a week to mature scar tissue. Granulation tissue formation and regression is a classic example of rapid cell growth and cell death. Granulation tissue has some unusual characteristics as compared to normal surrounding connective tissue. It is not innervated and therefore insensate. Its rich vascular supply and the presence of a large number of inflammatory cells provide high resistance to infection. The name granulation tissue reflect cobbled surface texture of this material in healing excisional wounds as capillary buds begin to form from underlying intact connective tissue.

Concurrent with the formation of granulation tissue in superficial wounds is the reformation of an intact epithelial (epidermal) sheet. The epidermis has remarkable self-renewing properties inherent in its growth pattern. When a defect occurs in the epidermis, there is rapid transformation of basal keratinocytes at the wound margin to switch to a migratory phenotype. These basal keratinocytes express connective tissue degrading enzymes which seem to facilitate the movement of migrating cells out over the newly deposited/exposed extracellular matrix to rapidly cover the granulation, tissue, thus insuring a barrier to infection, and to further fluid loss. The activated epidermis is also a rich source of growth factors. Intact epidermis also contains many stored cytokines and growth factors such as IL-1 and TGF-β. Damage or irritation to the skin surface promotes the release of these highly active molecules to act on adjacent epidermis and underlying connective tissue structures. Likewise, injury to the deeper dermal tissues can activate the expression of molecules that stimulate epidermal growth: the keratinocyte growth factors (FGF-7, -10). The extracellular matrix of intact and damaged tissue will also serve as a source for many bound growth factors as hydrolytic enzymes are released during the course of wound repair and remodeling. The breakdown of these structures is likely to release additional growth factor stores into the wound site. Indeed, extracellular matrix molecules may serve as an excellent delivery system for many different kinds of growth factors.

ANGIOGENESIS

The development of a new capillary bed, or angiogenesis, is a visible component of the proliferative phase of repair (74). Neovascularization provides oxygen and nutrient support to the rapidly proliferating cells within healing wounds, and promotes granulation tissue formation. Angiogenesis in wounds follows an orderly and carefully regulated pattern. During the proliferative phase of wound healing, capillary growth continues until the capillary density reaches nearly three times that of uninjured normal tissue (75). During the resolution phase of repair, most of the new capillaries regress, leaving behind a residual vascularity that is similar or slightly higher than uninjured tissue (76). Such carefully regulated growth and regression of vessels occurs in adult mammals in only a few physiological circumstances, including wound healing, uterine cycling, follicular development in the ovary, and lactation in the female breast (77). This pattern is in direct contrast to the dysregulated capillary growth that is a feature of many pathological diseases, including malignant tumors, retinopathies, and psoriasis (78).

Neovascularization within wounds, as in all tissues, depends on many factors, including levels of growth factors, cell–cell interactions, cell–extracellular matrix interactions, and the activity of proteases (79–81). One critical factor in all angiogenic processes is the balance between soluble proangiogenic and antiangiogenic factors that act directly on endothelial cells (82). In both physiological angiogenesis, such as the healing wound, and pathological angiogenesis, such as malignant tumors, the net angiogenic stimulus at any particular point is believed to rely on the equilibrium between positive and negative mediators. Studies in healing wounds have demonstrated the importance of two key proangiogenic factors in stimulating this process. FGF-2 is abundant in wounds, as it is both released from its sequestered location within the extracellular matrix and actively synthesized in the healing wound (83,84). FGF-2 levels diminish during the first few days after injury, at which time the dominant proangiogenic factor switches to vascular endothelial growth factor, or VEGF. VEGF is a potent, directly acting angiogenic factor that is capable of stimulating endothelial cell migration and activation in vitro, and angiogenesis in vivo (85,86).

Vasculogenesis is a newer concept in wound healing. It is a process in which new blood vessels are formed by recruitment of precursors (endothelial progenitor cells) from the blood and hence the bone marrow. This phenomenon, together with the ability of VEGF to drive the process, offers an alternative method for creating new vasculature at sites of ischemia (20,87). Angiogenesis has been described to be impaired in the healing wounds of diabetic animals, and some studies suggest that the topical application of proangiogenic factors such as VEGF may improve healing outcomes in patients with diabetes *(88,89)*. Interestingly, though, several recent studies seem to indicate that robust angiogenesis is not a critical determinant of repair, and inhibition of angiogenesis alone does not appear to negatively impact healing *(90,91)*. One possible explanation for this puzzle might be that proangiogenic factors have effects well beyond a simple stimulation of endothelial cell growth and differentiation. Indeed, VEGF application to wounds has been shown to mobilize stem cells from the bone marrow *(89)*. In addition, several cell types other than endothelial cells, such as smooth muscle cells and leukocytes, have now been described to also have receptors for proangiogenic factors, and activation of these cells might influence healing *(92–95)*. In short, the application of proangiogenic factors may promote wound healing in many ways beyond enhanced vascularity.

FIBROPLASIA

The final phase of wound repair involves the formation of a scar. This occurs as the loosely woven, highly cellular granulation tissue gradually transforms into predominantly collagen-rich and less vascularized extracellular matrix. There is progressive reduction in capillary diameter and density, and the orientation of collagen fibers within granulation tissue will begin to change from a random organization to one that is more perpendicular to the wound site. Only after many weeks or months will collagen fiber organization eventually approach the concentration, orientation and fiber thickness of surrounding normal tissue. Thus it is quite easy to distinguish scar tissue at a microscopic level even after superficial signs of its presence have disappeared. Scar formation is often characterized by the phenomenon of wound contraction. This is a process that is driven by cellular elements within the connective tissue. Both fibroblasts and the more specialized myofibroblasts have contractile proteins within them that, under appropriate simulation, will act through integrin receptors to pull on the extracellular matrix and draw the margins of the wound toward one another. In pathological states, wound contracture occurs, which is a disfiguring and disabling wound repair phenomenon. A further characteristic of the scar formation phase of wound repair is the extensive remodeling of the extracellular matrix and cellular organization. The wound is hardly a static site. There is intense turnover of various components or building blocks of the system as the area transforms from a weak but efficiently formed fibrin clot into a strong but histologically distinguishable scar tissue. This remodeling is accomplished by the highly controlled expression of various extracellular matrix proteinases.

Traumatic injury can irreversibly destroy many structures in damaged tissue. In the skin, the extent of regeneration depends largely on the depth of the injury. Superficial injuries which only scrape off the upper layers of the epidermis will still leave behind many epidermal appendages such as sweat glands and hair follicles that can, in turn, serve as reservoirs for regeneration of new epidermis. As a consequence, superficial scrapes rapidly resurface not only from the wound margins but from all these internal sources. Deeper traumatic wounds or burns that remove or destroy these epidermal appendages result in the irreversible loss of these structures from the skin. Scar tissue is characterized by a more disorganized weave to the collagen fiber bundles, differences in capillary density, altered pigmentation of the epidermis, and a markedly diminished content and organization of elastic fibers.

PATHOBIOLOGY OF WOUND REPAIR

There are three highly significant pathologies that occur in the area of wound healing: nonhealing wounds, excessive healing, and the specialized response of tissues to burns. Nonhealing wounds or ulcers can arise from a variety of sources. Nevertheless, they share some important common features. First, ulcers all fail to develop an underlying connective tissue structure. Second, the lack of this important groundwork for cell organization results in impaired overgrowth of epithelium. Third, there is often reduced angiogenesis and reduced fibroplasia. Fourth, there is the persistent presence of inflammatory cells: neutrophils or macrophages. Fifth, because of this persistent failure to restore tissue integrity, the chronic wound is often a site of persistent bacterial infection, which in itself can stimulate inappropriate inflammatory cell responses.

There are a wide variety of clinical subtypes of nonhealing wounds which are not precisely enough distinguished at the biochemical level to allow classification. Many of these conditions arise as a result of transient or chronically impaired vascular supply. In the former case, local ischemia caused by pressure, other kinds of physical injury or even chemical injury can lead to the loss of oxygen and tissue perfusion, leading to local cell necrosis and tissue death. Reperfusion may exacerbate the injury. Under many circumstances, ischemia leads to the progressive replacement of damaged tissue by scar tissue with loss of important mechanical and physiological properties.

In the skin, nonhealing wounds classically form on the extremities and over bony processes as the result of either unrelieved pressure or repeated trauma. There is frequently a failure of both granulation tissue formation and epithelial overgrowth. Currently there is insufficient information on levels of active growth factors at sites of chronic nonhealing wounds. It is likely that either growth factor abundance or bioavailability is severely reduced in chronic wounds. Growth factor expression is reduced in diabetic wounds. For this reason a number of growth factors are being used in clinical trials to remedy nonhealing wounds.

The present evidence points to proteolytic degradation in the lesion environment as a major cause of wound-healing failure *(96)*. A variety of proteinases, including elastase and some of the metalloproteinases, are capable of degrading not only adhesive substrates for cell migration but also signaling molecules such as growth factors and cytokines *(97)*. In addition, excess proteolysis may cause a release of high levels of breakdown products of connective tissue that inappropriately activate inflammatory cell processes. Thus, much attention is being given to the development of appropriate proteinase inhibitors for control of certain forms of nonhealing wounds. It should be noted however, that necrotic tissue is an important negative factor in prolonging nonhealing wound. It is well recognized that extensive and aggressive debridement of such wounds is essential to stimulate healing. For this reason a number of manufacturers have developed protease formulations that have varying degrees of ability to discriminate between necrotic and living tissue.

Excessive Healing

Uncontrolled overgrowth at various phases of the repair process is an important aspect of wound repair pathobiology. Examples of wounds locked in the earliest phases of repair are pyogenic granuloma/pyoderma granulosum and other chronic inflammatory conditions of skin and other organs. Little is known about the mechanism which brings about these conditions, but certainly many of the inflammatory states are owing to immunological stimuli.

Uncontrolled growth of scar tissue can take two forms. In hypertrophic scarring there is an excess growth of scar tissue within the wound margins, which may project well above the plane of the skin. These sites usually contain overabundant collagen and may be hypervascularized. Hypertrophic scars are commonly associated with second- and third-degree burns in which their lateral extent may provoke the formation of excessive contractures. Physical forces seem to play an important role in generating these types of scars, because coverage of injured areas with skin substitutes or splinting of the wound with a variety of films can often moderate the effects. Hypertrophic scars are known to contain fibroblasts that have abnormal growth factor responses and growth factor production profiles. It is quite likely that fibroblasts within the hypertrophic scar represent a subpopulation that has excess fibrotic tendencies owing to the overproduction of molecules such as TGF-β and a higher sensitivity to fibrogenic stimulation by this molecule. Presently, the only antagonist being evaluated in clinical trials is interferon-α. It is likely that further studies will attempt to address the problem more directly with TGF-β antagonists or perhaps molecules that block the action of the downstream effector, CTGF.

The other well-known cutaneous scar pathology is the keloid. This is an intriguing condition in which cutaneous injury results in scar formation that takes on the appearance of a benign tumor. Keloids grow beyond the lateral margins of the wound, and they are usually restricted in location to the upper trunk, face, neck, and ears. This regional variation emphasizes the heterogeneity of skin cell populations. There is also a predilection to keloid formation in many darker skinned races. There is also evidence of familial inheritance of the keloid tendency. Current studies are under way to attempt to map the keloid gene. The consequences of excessive healing in organs other than skin can be far more life threatening. Pulmonary, renal, and hepatic fibrosis all have marked effects of appropriate mechanical or secretory function in these tissues. The formation of surgical adhesions and is also an excess response to injury. Scarring occurs subsequent to ischemic injury of various organs and it leads to major health complications in coronary artery insufficiency and in stroke.

EXPERIMENTAL MODELS OF WOUND HEALING

Experimental Diabetes

The simplest method of creating a diabetic model in small animals is by chemical destruction of the pancreatic islets. In the rat and mouse, streptozotocin produces a rapid and profound hypoinsulinemia and hyperglycemia that is intended to mimic type 2 diabetes *(98)*. Animals cannot be maintained more than a few weeks to months in this state without insulin treatment, and wound healing is dramatically inhibited. Genetic models of type 2 diabetes include the db/db and ob/ob mouse mutations, which correspond to the deletion of the leptin receptor and leptin, respectively. Both of these mutants exhibit a high level of obesity that is consistent with the role of leptin in adipogenesis. Interestingly, leptin is expressed in wounds and it appears to have some anti-inflammatory properties *(56,99)*. Although both strains are diabetic, the lack of leptin signaling and the high obesity create a more complex physiological model. Other obesity models in the rat may hold more promise as type 2 diabetic analogs *(100)*. The nonobese diabetic mouse *(101–104)* is considered a reasonable model of type 1 diabetes, because it is late in onset and linked to autoimmunity. However, it is a more expensive and time-consuming model because the disease occurs after several months. Although there are several other rodent strains that exhibit diabetic complications, they have not been routinely used for wound-healing evaluation.

Diabetes can also be induced in larger animals. Alloxan is the appropriate chemotherapeutic agent for pancreatic islet destruction in the rabbit. Interestingly, these animals are much more tolerant of the hyperglycemic state and survive several months without insulin therapy. The diabetic state has also been induced in pigs *(105)*.

Granulation Tissue and Angiogenesis

The filling and revascularization phases of wound repair are readily modeled in a variety of synthetic wounds. Among the most popular are so-called wound chambers, which can be either sponges, implantable cages made up of plastic or metal, or a sponge-like tissue equivalent into which cells will invade. This type of model has many advantages because it can define a wound space of fixed dimensions. In most of these models, trauma and hemorrhage is minimal, so that the wound repair process is initiated by exudation of plasma into the enclosed space followed by formation of a fibrin clot. Release of fibrin degradation products leads to subsequent, transient phases of inflammation granulation tissue formation and initiation of scar formation. Usually, such implants are less useful for studies of later phases of wound remodeling, except the capsule that surrounds such implants is a valuable index of tendency toward fibrosis.

Irritant Injection

The precursor to the wound chamber model was the implantation of materials, which induced a more robust inflammatory response. This includes a wide variety of foreign materials, including cotton pellets, carrageenan, and other irritants, or even simply the formation of an air bubble or blister. Because these are chronic inflammatory models, they are more strongly driven by neutrophil and macrophage-mediated processes than are the pure wound chamber models. They may be more useful therefore for studying pathobiologies associated with those inflammatory cells.

Implanted Biomaterials

A number of new biomatrix molecules have been used for specialized repair assays. These include collagen sponges which actually fit very nicely with the other wound chamber models, and a novel biomatrix known under the trade name of Matrigel™. This material is the product of secretion by embryonic chrondrosarcoma cells, and it contains most of the components of the basement membrane. It has been used by a number of laboratories as a substrate for identifying angiogenic events independent of fibroplasia. The drawback of Matrigel is that it not a highly purified material. Under normal circumstances, many cytokines and growth factor activities have been identified in the matrix of this biomaterial. Protocols that allow partial purification may reduce background problems.

Excisional Wounds

The excisional wound is, for many investigators still the *sine qua non* of wound-repair assays. A relatively large portion of epidermis and/or dermis is removed from one or more sites on the experimental animal, and wound healing is monitored by various parameters, including the rate of closure of the wound, the rate of granulation tissue formation, and the changing biochemical character of granulation and scar tissue forming within the wound space. As discussed earlier, excisional wounds can be either full or partial thickness. Full-thickness wounds have more robust granulation tissue formation and heal only from the margins and the base. However, they also heal by contraction. Partial thickness wounds in animals will rapidly regenerate epidermis from remnant epidermal appendages, but the underlying, remnant dermis will act as a splint to prevent the artifact of wound contraction. Some investigators have taken advantage of wound contraction. In recent studies with recombinant mice, a full-thickness punch wound is made, and rates of contraction can be studied noninvasively over the course of several weeks. Because the mutant mice are usually a precious commodity, this is a useful assay. It is not clear how well differences in wound contraction predict to rates of healing in man.

For the study of epithelialization, one can also use the partial thickness injury as a good model. An alternative that is used often in transgenic and other mutant mice is stripping the tail skin with adhesive tape. This only damages the epidermis and leaves the dermis completely intact. The results may be analyzed by microscopic examination.

Incisional Biomechanics

The linear incision is still the key experimental tool for examining long-term effects of treatment on connective tissue formation. Incisions can be produced in a variety of sites and either left to close by secondary intention or closed with sutures or staples. Wound strength is then measured after excision of the injury site in a biomechanical testing device. Among useful parameters that can be derived are breaking strength, breaking energy, and elastic modulus. In addition, it is possible to gain some inference about the degree of cross-linking of the extracellular matrix by comparing the strength of wounds that have been preserved with or without formaldehyde fixation. The incision, at least that enclosed by primary intention, is not as suitable a model for examining histological effects of treatments, because the volume of granulation tissue is relatively small. Likewise, biochemical determinations are extremely difficult in this type of model.

Chronic Wounds

Generation of chronic wound models in a humane fashion is a challenge to the experimenter. For example, it has been extremely difficult to develop a model for true pressure sores in any laboratory species. Reports of success have been obtained by using greyhound dogs which have a very thin skin or using pigs in which the hindlimb is immobilized but placed in a cast that applies pressure. Constantine and Bolton have described an ischemic lesion that can be produced in guinea pigs by insertion of a rubber plug under the skin that is then ligated externally for several hours to produce a dermal infarct *(106)*. Chemical models may be somewhat easier to generate. Our laboratory, for example has capitalized on information first provided by Rudolph that the chemotherapeutic agent, adriamycin, produces a chronic lesion when injected into the dermis. Using this type of model, wounds in rats and rabbits persist for up to 60 days. A second model generated in this laboratory utilizes the toxicity of the venom of the brown recluse spider. This toxin causes the intense aggregation and eventual activation of neutrophils at sites of injection, leading to a massive, localized hemorrhage and tissue necrosis. Such lesions also are extremely persistent, although the mechanism by which they develop is quite different from other burns. Thermal burns are certainly slow to heal in animal models. With high temperature burns, on has a combination of the effects of complete denaturation of the local site, coagulation of adjacent vascular supply by heat, and collateral, thermal effects that extend beyond the zone of acute damage. The extent of burning is easily controlled by temperature and the pressure of the applied heat source. Freezing burns or cryosurgical burns have a somewhat different nature, because the proteins of the killed tissue remain in a relatively native state. As a result there is quite a difference in terms of the kind of inflammatory reactions that occur in thermal as opposed to cryogenic burns. These burn models are most widely used to examine the effects of debriding agents because the major inhibitory effect is often the larger burden of excess tissue at the injury site.

SUMMARY

The process of wound healing is a complex cascade of cell interactions that leads to restoration of tissue integrity. In the diabetic extremity, healing is markedly slowed by a persistent inflammatory process and by reduced signaling and responsiveness of the target tissue. Healing is particularly compromised by poor macro- and microvascular circulation. Infection exacerbates the chronicity of the diabetic wound. Modern technologies are attempting to reverse this increasingly prevalent complication by surgical or pharmacological stimulation of vascularization, devices and molecules that promote tissue growth, and better understanding of the fundamental physiological features of the diabetic wound.

ACKNOWLEDGMENT

Supported by grants from the NIA (JMD), NIDDK (JMD), NIGMS (LAD), and the Department of Veterans Affairs (JMD).

REFERENCES

1. Majno G. *The Healing Hand: Man and Wound in the Ancient World,* Harvard University Press, Cambridge, 1991.
2. Needham AE. *Regeneration and Wound Healing*, John Wiley & Sons, New York, 1952.
3. Clark RAF, Henson PM. *The Molecular and Cellular Biology of Wound Repair*, 1st ed., Plenum, New York, 1988.
4. Davidson JM, Benn SI. Regulation of angiogenesis and wound repair: interactive role of the matrix and growth factors, in *Cellular and Molecular Pathogenesis* (Sirica AE, ed.), 2nd ed., Lippincott-Raven, New York, 1996, pp. 79–107.
5. Jyung RW, Mustoe TA. Growth factors in wound healing, in *Clinical Applications of Cytokines: Role in Pathogenesis and Therapy* (Gearing A, Rossio J, Oppenheim J, eds.), Oxford University Press, New York, 1992, pp. 307–328.
6. Hay ED (ed.). *Cell Biology of Extracellular Matrix*, 2nd ed., Plenum Press, New York, 1991.
7. Debelle L, Tamburro AM. Elastin: molecular description and function. *Int J Biochem Cell Biol* 1999;31(2):261–272.
8. Goova MT, Li J, Kislinger T, et al. Blockade of receptor for advanced glycation end-products restores effective wound healing in diabetic mice. *Am J Pathol* 2001;159(2):513–525.

9. Santana RB, Xu L, Chase HB, Amar S, Graves DT, Trackman PC. A role for advanced glycation end products in diminished bone healing in type 1 diabetes. *Diabetes* 2003; 52(6):1502–1510.

10. Wear-Maggitti K, Lee J, Conejero A, Schmidt AM, Grant R, Breitbart A. Use of topical sRAGE in diabetic wounds increases neovascularization and granulation tissue formation. *Ann Plast Surg* 2004;52(5):519–521, discussion 22.

11. Ahmed N. Advanced glycation endproducts—role in pathology of diabetic complications. *Diabetes Res Clin Pract* 2005;67(1):3–21.

12. Kim BM, Eichler J, Reiser KM, Rubenchik AM, Da Silva LB. Collagen structure and nonlinear susceptibility: effects of heat, glycation, and enzymatic cleavage on second harmonic signal intensity. *Lasers Surg Med* 2000;27(4):329–335.

13. Ghohestani RF, Li K, Rousselle P, Uitto J. Molecular organization of the cutaneous basement membrane zone. *Clin Dermatol* 2001;19(5):551–562.

14. Nanney LB, King LE, Jr. Epidermal growth factor and transforming growth factor-α, in *The Molecular and Cellular Biology of Wound Repair* (Clark RAF, ed.), 2nd ed., Plenum, New York, 1996, pp. 171–194.

15. Bennett NT, Schultz GS. Growth factors and wound healing: biochemical properties of growth factors and their receptors. *Am J Surg* 1993;165(6):728–737.

16. Abraham JA, Klagsbrun M. Modulation of wound repair by members of the fibroblast growth factor family, in *The Molecular and Cellular Biology of Wound Repair* (Clark RAF, ed.), 2nd ed., Plenum, New York, 1996:195–248.

17. Werner S, Breeden M, Hübner G, Greenhalgh DG, Longaker MT. Induction of keratinocyte growth factor expression is reduced and delayed during wound healing in the genetically diabetic mouse. *J Invest Dermatol* 1994;103(469–473):473.

18. Senger DR, Van de Water L, Brown LF, et al. Vascular permeability factor (VPF, VEGF) in tumor biology. *Cancer Metastasis Rev* 1993;12(3–4):303–324.

19. Carmeliet P, Collen D. Molecular analysis of blood vessel formation and disease. *Am J Physiol* 1997;273(5 Pt 2):H2091–H2104.

20. Isner JM, Walsh K, Symes J, et al. Arterial gene transfer for therapeutic angiogenesis in patients with peripheral artery disease. *Hum Gene Ther* 1996;7(8):959–988.

21. Frazier K, Williams S, Kothapalli D, Klapper H, Grotendorst GR. Stimulation of fibroblast cell growth, matrix production, and granulation tissue formation by connective tissue growth factor. *J Invest Dermatol* 1996;107(3):404–411.

22. Chin D, Boyle GM, Parsons PG, Coman WB. What is transforming growth factor-beta (TGF-beta)? *Br J Plast Surg* 2004;57(3):215–221.

23. Wahl SM, Swisher J, McCartney-Francis N, Chen W. TGF-beta: the perpetrator of immune suppression by regulatory T cells and suicidal T cells. *J Leukoc Biol* 2004;76(1):15–24.

24. Leask A, Abraham DJ. TGF-beta signaling and the fibrotic response. *FASEB J* 2004;18(7): 816–827.

25. Hyytiainen M, Penttinen C, Keski-Oja J. Latent TGF-beta binding proteins: extracellular matrix association and roles in TGF-beta activation. *Crit Rev Clin Lab Sci* 2004;41(3):233–264.

26. Schiller M, Javelaud D, Mauviel A. TGF-beta-induced SMAD signaling and gene regulation: consequences for extracellular matrix remodeling and wound healing. *J Dermatol Sci* 2004;35(2):83–92.

27. Baxter RC. Signalling pathways involved in antiproliferative effects of IGFBP-3: a review. *Mol Pathol* 2001;54(3):145–148.

28. Blakytny R, Jude EB, Martin Gibson J, Boulton AJ, Ferguson MW. Lack of insulin-like growth factor 1 (IGF1) in the basal keratinocyte layer of diabetic skin and diabetic foot ulcers. *J Pathol* 2000;190(5):589–594.

29. Yoshida S, Matsumoto K, Tomioka D, et al. Recombinant hepatocyte growth factor accelerates cutaneous wound healing in a diabetic mouse model. *Growth Factors* 2004;22(2):111–119.

30. Bevan D, Gherardi E, Fan TP, Edwards D, Warn R. Diverse and potent activities of HGF/SF in skin wound repair. *J Pathol* 2004;203(3):831–838.

31. Powers CJ, McLeskey SW, Wellstein A. Fibroblast growth factors, their receptors and signaling. *Endocr Relat Cancer* 2000;7(3):165–197.

32. Nissen NN, Shankar R, Gamelli RL, Singh A, DiPietro LA. Heparin and heparan sulphate protect basic fibroblast growth factor from non-enzymic glycosylation. *Biochem J* 1999;338(Pt 3):637–642.

33. Knighton DR, Ciresi K, Fiegel VD. Classification and treatment of chronic, nonhealing wounds. *Ann Surg* 1986;204(3):322–330.

34. Park JE, Barbul A. Understanding the role of immune regulation in wound healing. *Am J Surg* 2004;187(5A):11S–16S.

35. Maurer M, Theoharides T, Granstein RD, et al. What is the physiological function of mast cells? *Exp Dermatol* 2003;12(6):886–910.

36. Clark RA, Lanigan JM, DellaPelle P, Manseau E, Dvorak HF, Colvin RB. Fibronectin and fibrin provide a provisional matrix for epidermal cell migration during wound reepithelialization. *J Invest Dermatol* 1982;79(5):264–249.

37. Leibovich SJ, Ross R. The role of the macrophage in wound repair. A study with hydrocortisone and antimacrophage serum. *Am J Pathol* 1975;78(1):71–100.

38. Hunt TK, Knighton DR, Thakral KK, Goodson WH, 3rd, Andrews WS. Studies on inflammation and wound healing: angiogenesis and collagen synthesis stimulated in vivo by resident and activated wound macrophages. *Surgery* 1984;96(1):48–54.

39. Kovacs EJ, DiPietro LA. Fibrogenic cytokines and connective tissue production. *FASEB J* 1994;8(11):854–861.

40. DiPietro LA, Polverini PJ, Rahbe SM, Kovacs EJ. Modulation of JE/MCP-1 expression in dermal wound repair. *Am J Pathol* 1995;146(4):868–875.

41. DiPietro LA, Burdick M, Low QE, Kunkel SL, Strieter RM. MIP-1alpha as a critical macrophage chemoattractant in murine wound repair. *J ClinInvest* 1998;101(8):1693–1698.

42. Stallmeyer B, Kampfer H, Kolb N, Pfeilschifter J, Frank S. The function of nitric oxide in wound repair: inhibition of inducible nitric oxide-synthase severely impairs wound reepithelialization. *J Invest Dermatol* 1999;113(6):1090–1098.

43. Yamasaki K, Edington HD, McClosky C, et al. Reversal of impaired wound repair in iNOS-deficient mice by topical adenoviral-mediated iNOS gene transfer. *J Clin Invest* 1998;101(5):967–971.

44. Lee PC, Salyapongse AN, Bragdon GA, et al. Impaired wound healing and angiogenesis in eNOS-deficient mice. *Am J Physiol* 1999;277(4 Pt 2):H1600–H1608.

45. Gallucci RM, Simeonova PP, Matheson JM, et al. Impaired cutaneous wound healing in interleukin-6-deficient and immunosuppressed mice. *FASEB J* 2000;14(15):2525–2531.

46. Devalaraja RM, Nanney LB, Du J, et al. Delayed wound healing in CXCR2 knockout mice. *J Invest Dermatol* 2000;115(2):234–244.

47. Kupper TS, Fuhlbrigge RC. Immune surveillance in the skin: mechanisms and clinical consequences. *Nat Rev Immunol* 2004;4(3):211–222.

48. Ross R, Odland G. Human wound repair. II. Inflammatory cells, epithelial-mesenchymal interrelations, and fibrogenesis. *J Cell Biol* 1968;39(1):152–168.

49. Rappolee DA, Mark D, Banda MJ, Werb Z. Wound macrophages express TGF-alpha and other growth factors in vivo: analysis by mRNA phenotyping. *Science* 1988;241(4866):708–712.

50. Meszaros AJ, Reichner JS, Albina JE. Macrophage phagocytosis of wound neutrophils. *J Leukoc Biol* 1999;65(1):35–42.

51. Daley JM, Reichner JS, Mahoney EJ, et al. Modulation of macrophage phenotype by soluble product(s) released from neutrophils. *J Immunol* 2005;174(4):2265–2272.
52. Artuc M, Hermes B, Steckelings UM, Grutzkau A, Henz BM. Mast cells and their mediators in cutaneous wound healing—active participants or innocent bystanders? *Exp Dermatol* 1999;8(1):1–16.
53. Barbul A, Shawe T, Rotter SM, Efron JE, Wasserkrug HL, Badawy SB. Wound healing in nude mice: a study on the regulatory role of lymphocytes in fibroplasia. Surgery 1989;105(6):764–769.
54. Barbul A, Breslin RJ, Woodyard JP, Wasserkrug HL, Efron G. The effect of in vivo T helper and T suppressor lymphocyte depletion on wound healing. *Ann Surg* 1989;209(4):479–483.
55. Wetzler C, Kampfer H, Stallmeyer B, Pfeilschifter J, Frank S. Large and sustained induction of chemokines during impaired wound healing in the genetically diabetic mouse: prolonged persistence of neutrophils and macrophages during the late phase of repair. *J Invest Dermatol* 2000;115(2):245–253.
56. Goren I, Kampfer H, Podda M, Pfeilschifter J, Frank S. Leptin and wound inflammation in diabetic ob/ob mice: differential regulation of neutrophil and macrophage influx and a potential role for the scab as a sink for inflammatory cells and mediators. *Diabetes* 2003;52(11):2821–2832.
57. Angele MK, Knoferl MW, Ayala A, et al. Trauma-hemorrhage delays wound healing potentially by increasing pro-inflammatory cytokines at the wound site. *Surgery* 1999;126(2):279–285.
58. Pierce GF. Inflammation in nonhealing diabetic wounds: the space-time continuum does matter.[comment]. *Am J Pathol* 2001;159(2):399–403.
59. Taichman NS, Young S, Cruchley AT, Taylor P, Paleolog E. Human neutrophils secrete vascular endothelial growth factor. *J Leukoc Biol* 1997;62(3):397–400.
60. Briggaman RA, Schechter NM, Fraki J, Lazarus GS. Degradation of the epidermal-dermal junction by proteolytic enzymes from human skin and human polymorphonuclear leukocytes. *J Exp Med* 1984;160(4):1027–1042.
61. Dovi JV, Szpaderska AM, DiPietro LA. Neutrophil function in the healing wound: adding insult to injury? *Thromb Haemost* 2004;92(2):275–280.
62. Dovi JV, He LK, DiPietro LA. Accelerated wound closure in neutrophil-depleted mice. *J Leukoc Biol* 2003;73(4):448–455.
63. Ashcroft GS, Yang X, Glick AB, et al. Mice lacking Smad3 show accelerated wound healing and an impaired local inflammatory response.[see comment]. *Nat Cell Biol* 1999;1(5): 260–266.
64. Ashcroft GS, Lei K, Jin W, et al. Secretory leukocyte protease inhibitor mediates non-redundant functions necessary for normal wound healing. *Nat Med* 2000;6(10): 1147–1153.
65. Redd MJ, Cooper L, Wood W, Stramer B, Martin P. Wound healing and inflammation: embryos reveal the way to perfect repair. *Philos Trans R Soc Lond B Biol Sci* 2004;359(1445):777–784.
66. Wilgus TA, Vodovotz Y, Vittadini E, Clubbs EA, Oberyszyn TM. Reduction of scar formation in full-thickness wounds with topical celecoxib treatment. *Wound Repair Regen* 2003;11(1):25–34.
67. Martin P, D'Souza D, Martin J, et al. Wound healing in the PU.1 null mouse-tissue repair is not dependent on inflammatory cells. *Curr Biol* 2003;13(13):1122–1128.
68. Cowin AJ, Brosnan MP, Holmes TM, Ferguson MW. Endogenous inflammatory response to dermal wound healing in the fetal and adult mouse. *Dev Dyn* 1998;212(3):385–393.
69. Whitby DJ, Ferguson MW. Immunohistochemical localization of growth factors in fetal wound healing. *Dev Biol* 1991;147(1):207–215.

70. Lin RY, Sullivan KM, Argenta PA, Meuli M, Lorenz HP, Adzick NS. Exogenous transforming growth factor-beta amplifies its own expression and induces scar formation in a model of human fetal skin repair. *Ann Surg* 1995;222(2):146–154.

71. Cowin AJ, Holmes TM, Brosnan P, Ferguson MW. Expression of TGF-beta and its receptors in murine fetal and adult dermal wounds. *Eur J Dermatol* 2001;11(5):424–431.

72. Shah M, Foreman DM, Ferguson MW. Neutralisation of TGF-beta 1 and TGF-beta 2 or exogenous addition of TGF-beta 3 to cutaneous rat wounds reduces scarring. *J Cell Sci* 1995;108(Pt 3):985–1002.

73. Longaker MT, Whitby DJ, Ferguson MW, Lorenz HP, Harrison MR, Adzick NS. Adult skin wounds in the fetal environment heal with scar formation. *Ann Surg* 1994;219(1):65–72.

74. Battegay EJ. Angiogenesis: mechanistic insights, neovascular diseases, and therapeutic prospects. *J Mol Med* 1995;73(7):333–346.

75. Swift ME, Kleinman HK, DiPietro LA. Impaired wound repair and delayed angiogenesis in aged mice. *Lab Invest* 1999;79(12):1479–1487.

76. Brown NJ, Smyth EA, Reed MW. Angiogenesis induction and regression in human surgical wounds. *Wound Repair Regen* 2002;10(4):245–251.

77. Iruela-Arispe ML, Dvorak HF. Angiogenesis: a dynamic balance of stimulators and inhibitors. *Thromb Haemost* 1997;78(1):672–677.

78. Folkman J. Angiogenesis in cancer, vascular, rheumatoid and other disease. *Nat Med* 1995;1(1):27–31.

79. Clark RA, Tonnesen MG, Gailit J, Cheresh DA. Transient functional expression of alphaVbeta 3 on vascular cells during wound repair. *Am J Pathol* 1996;148(5):1407–1421.

80. Jang YC, Arumugam S, Gibran NS, Isik FF. Role of alpha(v) integrins and angiogenesis during wound repair. *Wound Repair Regen* 1999;7(5):375–380.

81. Chakraborti S, Mandal M, Das S, Mandal A, Chakraborti T. Regulation of matrix metalloproteinases: an overview. *Mol Cell Biochem* 2003;253(1–2):269–285.

82. Folkman J. Angiogenesis and angiogenesis inhibition: an overview. *Exs* 1997;79:1–8.

83. Nissen NN, Polverini PJ, Koch AE, Volin MV, Gamelli RL, DiPietro LA. Vascular endothelial growth factor mediates angiogenic activity during the proliferative phase of wound healing. *Am J Pathol* 1998;152(6):1445–1452.

84. Nissen NN, Polverini PJ, Gamelli RL, DiPietro LA. Basic fibroblast growth factor mediates angiogenic activity in early surgical wounds. *Surgery* 1996;119(4):457–465.

85. Dvorak HF, Brown LF, Detmar M, Dvorak AM. Vascular permeability factor/vascular endothelial growth factor, microvascular hyperpermeability, and angiogenesis. *Am J Pathol* 1995;146(5):1029–1039.

86. Ferrara N. Vascular endothelial growth factor and the regulation of angiogenesis. *Recent Prog Horm Res* 2000;55:15–35.

87. Asahara T, Masuda H, Takahashi T, et al. Bone marrow origin of endothelial progenitor cells responsible for postnatal vasculogenesis in physiological and pathological neovascularization. *Circ Res* 1999;85(3):221–228.

88. Kirchner LM, Meerbaum SO, Gruber BS, et al. Effects of vascular endothelial growth factor on wound closure rates in the genetically diabetic mouse model. *Wound Repair Regen* 2003;11(2):127–131.

89. Galiano RD, Tepper OM, Pelo CR, et al. Topical vascular endothelial growth factor accelerates diabetic wound healing through increased angiogenesis and by mobilizing and recruiting bone marrow-derived cells. *Am J Pathol* 2004;164(6):1935–1947.

90. Nanney LB, Wamil BD, Whitsitt J, et al. CM101 stimulates cutaneous wound healing through an anti-angiogenic mechanism. *Angiogenesis* 2001;4(1):61–70.

91. Jacobi J, Tam BY, Sundram U, et al. Discordant effects of a soluble VEGF receptor on wound healing and angiogenesis. *Gene Ther* 2004;11(3):302–309.

92. Wang H, Keiser JA. Vascular endothelial growth factor upregulates the expression of matrix metalloproteinases in vascular smooth muscle cells: role of flt-1. *Circ Res* 1998;83(8):832–840.
93. Ancelin M, Chollet-Martin S, Herve MA, Legrand C, El Benna J, Perrot-Applanat M. Vascular endothelial growth factor VEGF189 induces human neutrophil chemotaxis in extravascular tissue via an autocrine amplification mechanism. *Lab Invest* 2004;84(4):502–512.
94. Barleon B, Sozzani S, Zhou D, Weich HA, Mantovani A, Marme D. Migration of human monocytes in response to vascular endothelial growth factor (VEGF) is mediated via the VEGF receptor flt-1. *Blood* 1996;87(8):3336–3343.
95. Sawano A, Iwai S, Sakurai Y, et al. Flt-1, vascular endothelial growth factor receptor 1, is a novel cell surface marker for the lineage of monocyte-macrophages in humans. *Blood* 2001;97(3):785–791.
96. Abatangelo G, Donati L, Vanscheidt W (eds.). *Proteolysis in Wound Repair*, Springer-Verlag, Heidelberg, 1996.
97. Trengove NJ, Stacey MC, MacAuley S, et al. Analysis of the acute and chronic wound environments: the role of proteases and their inhibitors. *Wound Repair Regen* 1999;7(6): 442–452.
98. Davidson JM. Animal models for wound repair. *Arch Dermatol Res* 1998;290(Suppl): S1–S11.
99. Murad A, Nath AK, Cha ST, Demir E, Flores-Riveros J, Sierra-Honigmann MR. Leptin is an autocrine/paracrine regulator of wound healing. *FASEB J* 2003;17(13):1895–1897.
100. Bauer BS, Ghahary A, Scott PG, et al. The JCR:LA-cp rat: a novel model for impaired wound healing. *Wound Repair Regen* 2004;12(1):86–92.
101. Keswani SG, Katz AB, Lim FY, et al. Adenoviral mediated gene transfer of PDGF-B enhances wound healing in type I and type II diabetic wounds. *Wound Repair Regen* 2004;12(5):497–504.
102. Rodgers KE, Espinoza T, Felix J, Roda N, Maldonado S, diZerega G. Acceleration of healing, reduction of fibrotic scar, and normalization of tissue architecture by an angiotensin analogue, NorLeu3-A(1–7). *Plast Reconstr Surg* 2003;111(3):1195–1206.
103. Beer HD, Longaker MT, Werner S. Reduced expression of PDGF and PDGF receptors during impaired wound healing. *J Invest Dermatol* 1997;109(2):132–138.
104. Darby IA, Bisucci T, Hewitson TD, MacLellan DG. Apoptosis is increased in a model of diabetes-impaired wound healing in genetically diabetic mice. *Int J Biochem Cell Biol* 1997;29(1):191–200.
105. Zhang L, Zalewski A, Liu Y, et al. Diabetes-induced oxidative stress and low-grade inflammation in porcine coronary arteries. *Circulation* 2003;108(4):472–478.
106. Constantine BE, Bolton LL. A wound model for ischemic ulcers in the guinea pig. *Arch Dermatol Res* 1986;278(5):429–431.

5
Induced Regeneration of Skin and Peripheral Nerves

Eric C. Soller, MSME and Ioannis V. Yannas, PhD

INTRODUCTION

Acute or chronic injury to an organ is followed by a spontaneous healing process. Injury to the mammalian fetus is reversible during early stages of gestation; the spontaneous wound response is capable of restoring the structure and function of the original organ (regeneration). In contrast, the unimpaired response of adults to severe injury is an irreversible process leading to closure of the injured site by contraction and formation of scar, a nonphysiological tissue (repair). The consequences of irreversible healing at the organ scale are far reaching: they often result in an essentially nonfunctional organ.

Numerous approaches have been investigated to restore the loss of organ function in adults following irreversible injury. These strategies include transplantation, autografting, implantation of permanent prostheses, use of stem cells, in vitro synthesis, and regenerative medicine (1). The last of these strategies is also referred to as induced organ regeneration, or the recovery of physiological structure and function of non-regenerative tissues in an organ (de novo synthesis) by use of elementary reactants, such as biologically active scaffolds, either unseeded or seeded with cells.

There is accumulating evidence that the spontaneous healing process of an injured organ in the adult mammal can be modified to yield a partially or completely regenerated organ. Regenerative medicine is an emerging field of study involving the implantation of biomaterials to facilitate formation (regeneration) of tissue in vivo. This field is undergoing rapid growth at this time, as evidenced by observation of regeneration or reported progress in on-going research efforts in a wide range of organs including skin (2), conjunctiva (3), peripheral nerves (4), bone (5), heart valves (6) articular cartilage (7), urological organs (8), and the spinal cord (9).

The basic outline of a hypothetical mechanism for induced organ regeneration has become clear. It relies on regenerative studies in three organs (skin, conjunctiva, and peripheral nerves), which started much earlier and have progressed much further than research in other organs. From these studies a pattern has emerged, based on two observations: (1) regeneration was successfully induced, at least partially, when contraction was blocked, following grafting with a class of scaffolds that were characterized by a very highly specific structure (collectively referred to as "regeneration templates") and (2) when a class of "inactive scaffolds" with slightly different properties than their biologically

From: *The Diabetic Foot, Second Edition*
Edited by: A. Veves, J. M. Giurini, and F. W. LoGerfo © Humana Press Inc., Totowa, NJ

active counterparts was used, regeneration was thwarted and vigorous contraction ensued. The available data support the hypothesis of contraction blocking as a plausible mechanism for induced organ regeneration in the adult mammal. In almost all such processes the critical reactant supplied by the investigators was a scaffold, a highly porous, degradable macromolecular solid that has a specific contraction-blocking activity as well as the ability to mimic the in vivo environment, and particularly the stroma, of the organ.

In this chapter, we present elements of a theory of induced regeneration, which is organ nonspecific. We proceed by discussing, in order, the macroscopic outcome of irreversible healing in adults, the evidence for induced regeneration, the association between contraction blocking and regeneration, and a proposed mechanism for the regenerative activity of certain scaffolds.

Most regeneration data available to date come from acute wound models which prove to be far more amenable to control by the investigator than chronic wound models. When healing is unimpaired, the adult mammalian spontaneous healing response to severe acute injury is contraction and scar synthesis. Nevertheless, the results of a recent clinical study suggest that the discussion in this chapter is relevant to severe chronic wounds, as discussed in ref. *10*. The Integra Dermal Regeneration Template (DRT®) was studied with 111 patients as a method of closure for select refractory pathological wounds. Patients were treated predominantly in an outpatient setting with an average healing time of 7 months. Detailed indications for the use of Integra DRT in the treatment of chronic wounds (classified by both anatomy and pathology/diagnosis) have been presented *(10)*.

The majority of available induced regeneration data comes from skin *(11–18)* and peripheral nerve models *(19–27)*, these are the two organs that have been studied most extensively in this respect to date. A limited amount of data concerning regeneration of the conjuctiva also exists; the reader will be referred to the literature for details *(28)*. Skin wounds can be studied with relative ease and for this reason studies of skin wound healing comprise the bulk of quantitative wound healing data in the literature. In organs other than skin, wound healing has been studied mostly qualitatively. Nevertheless, the observations made so far form a body of evidence that suggests certain strong similarities, as well as identifying differences, between wound healing in skin and in less studied organs, such as peripheral nerves. Taken together, the wealth of regenerative data for these two very different organs has aided the development of a general theory of induced regeneration that is not organ specific *(1)*.

IRREVERSIBLE INJURY IN SKIN AND NERVES

The complex inflammatory response of the adult mammal to injury is increasingly elucidated by on-going research at the cellular and molecular level. Although the formation of an accurate mechanistic perspective of wound healing is essential both in understanding the effect of current clinical treatment and in the development of emergent therapies (indeed, such a mechanistic perspective is presented elsewhere in this volume), an examination of the macroscopic outcome of healing also provides a uniquely valuable viewpoint. An introductory phenomenological discussion of spontaneous wound healing at the tissue level provides a framework that (1) forms a focus for future discussion of detailed cellular/molecular mechanisms and (2) facilitates the derivation of concepts and rules of induced regeneration that may conceivably apply to almost any organ in the body.

Macroscopic Outcomes of Healing: Repair vs Regeneration

When exposed to injury, in the form of either acute trauma or chronic insult, the organism mounts a spontaneous wound-healing process that typically closes the discontinuity in organ mass caused by the injury in a matter of days. Two macroscopic outcomes to injury have been observed experimentally, regeneration and repair. These fundamentally different processes are clearly distinguished by the identity of tissue present in the final state, i.e., the tissue that has been displaced or synthesized to close the injury. In the early mammalian fetus and in many species of amphibians, wound healing is largely reversible and proceeds via spontaneous regeneration, a process that restores the structure and physiological function through synthesis of the missing organ structures *(1)*. Certain adult urodeles exhibit an impressive capacity for spontaneous regeneration: replacement of an amputated appendage occurs by direct outgrowth of the severed cross-section (epimorphic regeneration), a reversible process *(29)*.

In clear contrast, severe injury to normal adult mammalian tissue typically results in an irreversible healing response. Spontaneous healing of severe skin wounds proceeds via repair, in which the wound closes with a combination of tissue deformation and translation (collectively referred to as contraction) and synthesis of a nonphysiological tissue (scar) in place of the normally functioning tissue that has been injured *(1)*. By replacing the lost organ mass with scar, the injured organ is condemned, whereas the organism is spared as a result of the healing process. The immediate consequence of irreversible injury is a loss of normal organ function. On a broader scale skin injury may have additional detrimental effects, such as loss of mobility and lack of social acceptance following formation of disfiguring scars from burns. It appears that nearly all adult mammalian organs can be injured irreversibly, the extent of irreversibility seems to depend both on the identity of the tissue injured and the severity of the injury *(1)*.

Regenerative Similarity of the Tissue Triad

Standard pathology texts describe three generic tissue types that comprise the majority of organs in the body: epithelia, basement membrane, and stroma *(1,30–32)* (Fig. 1). Collectively, we will refer to these three tissue types as the tissue triad. This classification provides a useful framework for comparing the regenerative capacity of specific tissue types from one organ to another. The composition of each member of the triad is markedly different. Epithelial tissue forms a completely cellular covering on every surface, tube, and cavity in the body, performing a wide array of vital functions including protection, secretion, absorption, and filtration. As epithelial tissue is devoid of extracellular matrix (ECM) and blood vessels, it is sustained by the diffusion of nutrients from the underlying vascular connective tissue, or stroma. With the exception of the liver, epithelia is separated from the underlying stroma by the basement membrane (basal lamina), a very thin, noncellular tissue layer, comprising exclusively ECM. The stroma is a connective tissue layer that is vascularized, containing both cells and ECM.

The skin, as one example, consists of the epidermis (epithelia) attached to the basement membrane and the underlying dermis (stroma). Considerable evidence from peripheral nerve studies indicates that Schwann cells function as epithelial cells following synthesis

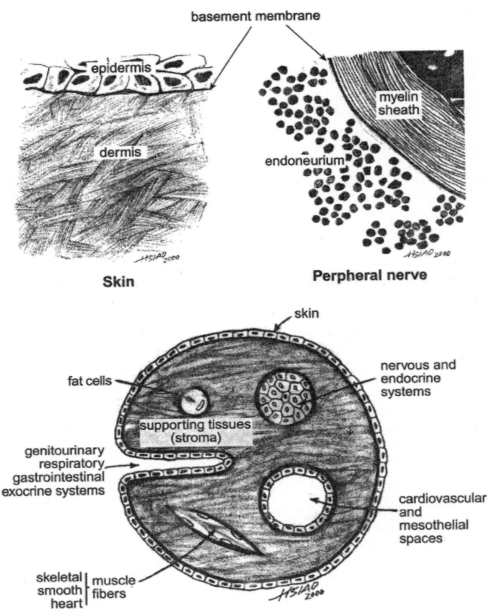

Fig. 1. (Top) The tissue triad structure in skin and peripheral nerves. The basement membrane (basal lamina), a thin noncellular layer consisting of extracellular matrix, separates the cellular, nonvascular epithelia (epidermis, myelin sheath) from the stroma (dermis, endoneurium) which contains cells, ECM, and blood vessels. Epithelia and basement membrane regenerate spontaneously; stroma does not. (Bottom) Illustration of the tissue triad layers in mammalian anatomy. Stromal tissues include bone, cartilage, and their associated cell types as well as elastin and collagen. Epithelial tissues are those that line the genitourinary, respiratory, and gastrointestinal tracts as well as surfaces of the mesothelial cells in body cavities, and include muscle fibers, fat cells, and endothelial cells in the cardiovascular system. [(*1*); bottom sketch adapted from ref. *32*.]

of a completely cellular layer (myelin sheath) around axons. Nerve fibers (Schwann cell-axon units) are attached to a basement membrane which separates them from the outlying endoneurial stroma, a tissue consisting of vascularized ECM. Further evidence for the epithelial nature of the myelin sheath comes from the observed polarity of Schwann cells which is very similar to that of keratinocytes (KC), the epithelial cells that form the epidermis in skin. In each case, one epithelial cell surface is firmly attached to a basement membrane and another is part of the epithelial tissue, endowed in each case with function unique to the respective organ, which characterizes the epidermis (in the case of skin) or the nerve fiber insulation of peripheral nerves *(33)*. Tissues that are "regeneratively similar" appear in different organs yet share a common spontaneous healing response, be it regeneration or repair. The spontaneous healing behavior of each layer of the tissue triad in skin and peripheral nerves is well documented and will be briefly reviewed.

Partial- or full-thickness injury to the epithelial layer of either of the two organs (the epidermis in skin and myelin sheath in peripheral nerves, respectively) results in spontaneous regeneration of the injured tissue by remaining epithelial cells in the defect (provided the stroma is still intact to facilitate epithelial cell spreading) *(1,34–37)*. Following nerve crushing with myelin disruption but with no injury to the endoneurium, the myelin sheath regenerates spontaneously and no contraction is observed. Similarly, epidermal excision is a reversible injury that closes exclusively by spontaneous regeneration rather than contraction. The epidermis in skin and the myelin sheath in peripheral nerves exhibits spontaneous regeneration, a reversible healing response leading to a full recovery of structure and function, and are therefore regeneratively similar *(1)*. Injuries that interrupt the continuity of the basement membrane in both organs also exhibit spontaneous regeneration by epithelial cells; basement membranes are regeneratively similar in the two organs. However, when a wound is severe enough to cause injury to the stroma of either organ (the dermis in skin or the endoneurial stroma in peripheral nerves), the organism achieves wound closure by a combination of contraction and scar synthesis (irreversible healing response) *(38)*. The dermis and nonneuronal peripheral nervous tissue heal by repair; because they are both nonregenerative, they are considered to be regeneratively similar.

In summary, when the spontaneous regenerative capacity of corresponding tissue types in skin and peripheral nerves is directly compared, a useful similarity emerges *(1)*. Epithelia and basement membrane are regeneratively similar tissue layers, exhibiting a reversible healing response even in the case of severe injury. Likewise, the stroma in both organs is distinctly nonregenerative. Hence, the central objective of induced organ regeneration is synthesis of the nonregenerative stroma.

EXPERIMENTAL CONSIDERATIONS

Importance of an Anatomically Well-Defined Defect

The appropriate experimental volume for studies of induced organ regeneration is the anatomically well-defined defect *(1)*. As discussed earlier of the differential regenerative capacity of the various tissue triad layers calls for an experimental injury that is free of nonregenerative tissue. In this manner, the effects of an exogenous regenerative agent on the potential synthesis of nonregenerative tissue can be evaluated without ambiguity.

In addition, the experimental volume should also have well-defined anatomical boundaries to reduce contributions from extraneous healing processes occurring elsewhere in the organ (e.g., caused by collateral damage during the surgical procedure) and to improve the reproducibility of the surgical protocol from one animal to the next as well as between independent laboratories. The treatment of the defect should include prevention of loss of extravascular tissue fluid (exudate), which contains important growth factors and regulators that are crucial both to regeneration and to repair. Inability to prevent exudate loss from the injured site radically affects the outcome of both spontaneous and induced healing processes in both skin and peripheral nerves *(39–41)*. Physical containment is also necessary to prevent detrimental extraneous processes, such as bacterial infection in skin, from interfering with the outcome of the healing response.

For studies of induced regeneration in skin, the most widely used well-defined defect is the dermis-free full thickness wound in the rodent or swine. In the case of peripheral nerves, the tubulated, fully transected peripheral nerve in the rat or mouse has been studied extensively *(1)*. Both the introduction of various grafts or sheet-like covers to skin defects and tubulation to transected nerves using a variety of materials typically impart significant activity that either assists or hinders regeneration; their use must be controlled carefully.

Synthetic Protocol: In Vitro or In Vivo?

A detailed comparison of the synthetic regeneration processes carried out in vitro and in vivo shows that in studies of skin and peripheral nerves, various protocols for in vitro synthesis have so far resulted largely in the formation of epithelia and the associated basement membrane but not the physiological stroma. In contrast, several protocols conducted in vivo have yielded not only the physiological epithelia and basement membrane, but a near-physiological stroma as well. The following section highlights these observed cases of induced regeneration.

OVERVIEW OF INDUCED ORGAN REGENERATION

Three adult organs have been induced to regenerate partially with the aid of certain insoluble substrates (scaffolds) that were optionally seeded with cells. Studies that started in the early 1970s in the Fibers and Polymers Laboratory, Massachusetts Institute of Technology have shown that the adult mammal can be induced to regenerate selected organs that have been accidentally lost or excised. In every case it had been established previously that the excised adult organ in question does not regenerate spontaneously; i.e., in the absence of experimental intervention, the adult excised site generally closed spontaneously by contraction and scar formation rather than by regeneration.

The three anatomical sites that were induced to regenerate partially were:

1. Full-thickness skin wounds, with epidermis and dermis completely excised, in the adult guinea pig, adult swine, and adult human;
2. Full-thickness excision of the conjunctiva, with complete excision of the stroma, in the adult rabbit; and
3. The fully transected rat sciatic nerve, with stumps initially separated by an unprecedented gap (as of 1985) of 15 mm (later 22 mm and recently 30 mm).

Table 1
Constitutive Tissues of Skin, Peripheral Nerves, and Conjunctiva That Were Induced to Regenerate in Adults

Organ	Regeneration observed	Regeneration observed	Regeneration not studied
Skin (guinea pig, swine, human) *(1)*	Keratinized epidermis, basement membrane, dermis, nerve endings, blood vessels	Appendages (e.g., hair follicles, sweat glands)	
Peripheral nerve (mouse, rat, cat, monkey, human)	Myelin sheath, nerve fibers (large and small diameter), blood vessels, endoneurial stroma?		Endoneurial stroma? perineurium
Conjunctiva (rabbit)	Epithelia, conjunctival stroma		Basement membrane

Adapted from ref. *104*

A summary of induced regeneration data for the constitutive tissues of each organ is presented in Table 1. Observations of induced regeneration in adults made over the years have been tested repeatedly by morphological and functional tests, as follows:

1. Confirmation of partial regeneration of skin (including both dermis and epidermis) was made by histological, immunohistochemical, ultrastructural, and functional studies *(11–18,42)*; and
2. Confirmation of regeneration of the conjunctiva (including the conjunctival stroma) was made using histological data *(28)*; and
3. Confirmation of regeneration of peripheral nerves was made using both morphological and functional (electrophysiological and neurological) data *(19–27)*.

The available evidence in the above studies strongly supports the conclusion that these severely injured anatomical sites did not close by contraction and scar formation. Nevertheless, induced regeneration observed to date is described as "partial" because perfectly physiological organs have not yet been regenerated. Regenerated skin was histologically and functionally different from scar and identical to physiological skin in almost all respects (including a physiological epidermis, well-formed basement membrane, well-formed capillary loops at the rete ridges of the dermal–epidermal junction, nerve endings with confirmed tactile and heat–cold feeling, and a physiological dermis); however, the regenerate lacked certain organelles (hair follicles, sweat glands, and so on). Evidence for the induced regeneration of partial skin is presented in Fig. 2. Supportive data for induced regeneration of peripheral nerves are presented in Fig. 3.

The Defect Closure Rule

Careful review of the literature suggests that not more than three distinct processes are used to close an anatomically well-defined defect (dermis-free defect) in skin wounds, contraction originating from the edges of the defect, scar formation by stromal fibroblasts (followed by epithelialization of scar), and regeneration.

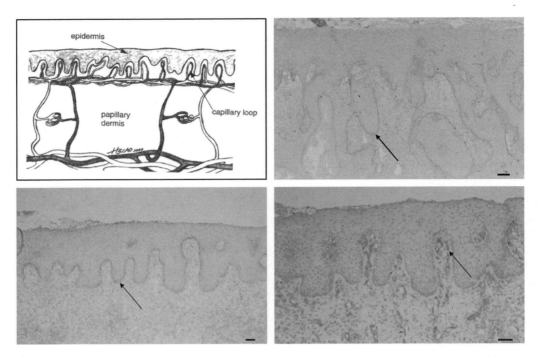

Fig. 2. (Top left) A diagram of physiologically normal skin shows characteristic rete ridges at the dermoepidermal junction and the vascular network (capillary loops) characteristic of the subepidermal region *(4)*. (Top right) As early as 12 days after grafting a full-thickness skin wound with a keratinocyte-seeded dermis regeneration template, anchoring fibrils were observed in the regenerating basement membrane (arrow). The basal surface epithelium and the periphery of the epithelial cords are labeled with type-VII collagen immunostaining, identifying the anchorage structures at the dermoepidermal interface. Bar: 150 μm. (Bottom left) As early as 35 days after grafting a full-thickness skin wound with a keratinocyte-seeded DRT, a confluent hemidesmosomal staining pattern is observed at the dermoepidermal junction (arrow) by immunostaining for the $\alpha_6\beta_4$-integrin. The pattern observed in the regenerating skin is identical to that observed in physiological skin. Bar: 100 μm. (Bottom right) A full-thickness skin wound grafted with a keratinocyte-seeded DRT was observed to regenerate many of the structure observed in normal skin. Immunostaining for Factor VIII 35 days after grafting revealed that capillary loops had formed in the rete ridges of the regenerated dermis (arrow) similar to those observed in physiological skin. Bar: 75 μm. *(17)*.

Continuous kinetic data are rarely available in regeneration experiments and often difficult to compare from one study to another. One approach to studying the regenerative activity of exogenous agents on the healing process is to establish two standardized configuration states and to evaluate the total change that is caused during this fixed period in the healing process. In the absence of kinetic data, the defect closure rule bridges the gap by presenting a quantitative description of the healing process through comparison of snapshots of the initial and final stages of wounding. The initial state of configuration is the anatomical description of the recently generated defect, characterized by the loss of structural continuity in one or more tissues, the beginning of exudate flow, and the loss of physiological homeostatic control of the organ. As defect healing progresses, the original area, A_0, eventually diminishes spontaneously because of one

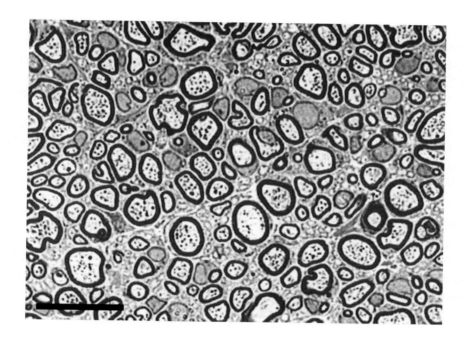

Fig. 3. Evidence of partial nerve regeneration using an optimally degraded collagen-based nerve regeneration template. Optimal degradation rate was described by an implant half-life of 3 weeks. The light micrograph shows regenerated axon morphology observed in cross-sections at the midpoint of the regenerated nerve trunk (middle of the 15-mm gap). The number of axons with diameter larger than 6 µm (A fibers; control conduction velocity) is maximum above, and the myelin sheath is very well defined, indicative of maximum quality of regeneration at this intermediate level of scaffold degradation rate. Bar: 25 µm *(81)*.

or more of the three processes mentioned above. The area of the closed defect (the closed wound) comprises tissues that result either from contraction (fractional amount, %C), scar formation (%S), or regeneration (%R). Therefore, the configuration of the final state can be described by the following simple relation:

$$C + S + R = 100 \qquad (1)$$

Eq. 1 states that the defect closure in any organ can be described by only three outcomes: contraction, scar formation (neuroma or fibrosis), and regeneration (partial or total).

For the idealized case of early fetal wound healing (spontaneous regeneration), contraction and scarring is absent ($C, S = 0$) and

$$R = 100 \qquad \text{(regeneration)}$$

For normal defect closure in adult mammals in response to irreversible injury (repair), regeneration is absent ($R = 0$) and

$$C + S = 100 \qquad \text{(repair)}$$

The literature describes several assays to determine the configuration of the final state (recently closed defect) *(1)*. Functional assays can be used to qualitatively identify the physiological nature of the tissue and assist in providing a quantitative measure of its incidence in the final state in terms of the numerical values of these three quantities (*C*, *S*, or *R*?). The defect closure rule may be interpreted as a conservation principle: provided that the magnitude of two individual terms (*C* and *S* for example) has been determined, the magnitude of the remaining process may be calculated. Defect closure data are expressed using the following convention: [%*C*, %*S*, %*R*].

The defect closure rule is useful in evaluating the activity of unknown reactants as inductive agents of regeneration. This quantitative description of the structure and function of the injured organ at its final state has shed interesting light on the relationship between the characteristic elements of the adult healing response (contraction or scar synthesis, or both) and regeneration.

Prevalence of Contraction During Spontaneous Healing

In the skin, the defect closure rule has been used to approximate data on the configuration of the final state following spontaneous healing of the anatomically well-defined defect (dermis-free defect) in several species. In all cases, it was ensured that the contribution of regeneration to defect closure was negligible (*R* = 0). Skin contraction was measured directly as the reduction in initial wound surface area by inward (centripetal) movement of skin from the margins of the wound. Scar formation was studied qualitatively by histology or quantitatively by use of laser light scattering (to measure the average degree of collagen fiber orientation). Values for the percentage of initial defect area closed by epithelialized scar (*S*) were determined using the simplified defect closure rule for repair (*S* = 100–*C*).

The contribution of the various methods of defect closure in anatomically well-defined defects is species dependent. In rodents, in which the integument is mobile, contraction is by far the main engine of closure of skin wounds, whereas scar formation has been shown to be quantitatively much less important.

The spontaneous healing of a full-thickness skin wound in the guinea pig is characteristic of several rodents and lagomorphs (rabbits), and results in the following final state configuration: [91, 9, 0] *(11,12,42)*. In general, *C* >> *S* and defect closure for adult rodents and rabbits reduces to *C* approx 100. Alternatively, the approximation of the final state is expressed as [100, 0, 0].

In humans, in which the integument is tethered more securely onto subcutaneous tissues, contraction and scar formation contribute approximately equally to wound closure. Experimentally, the spontaneous healing of full-thickness skin defects in the humans (*R* = 0) results in a final state represented by [37, 63, 0] *(43)*.

In the absence of direct quantitative observations, histological analysis was used to describe the closure of the fully transected peripheral nerve in the adult rat. Spontaneous healing results in reduction of the initial area of cross-sections of nerve trunks by 95% with neuroma formation (neural scar) accounting for the remaining 5%. The resulting estimation of the final state configuration is [95, 5, 0] *(25)*.

The contraction of a wide array of organs in response to trauma is well documented in both animals and humans, yet these reports are almost exclusively of a qualitative nature *(44–64)*. With very few exceptions the sole organ in which contraction has been studied systematically to date is the skin. Despite the dearth of widespread quantitative data, the prevalence of contraction must not be overlooked; it appears to be a critical outcome of the spontaneous healing response throughout the adult organism.

The Antagonistic Relation Between Contraction and Regeneration

The characteristic elements of the adult healing response (contraction or scar synthesis, or both) must be controlled in order for induced regeneration to occur. Extensive data, including empirical data on the final state of the defect in response to various reactants, suggest that during healing of a severe injury, contraction antagonizes regeneration *(1)*.

Induced regeneration of skin, a peripheral nerve trunk, and the conjunctival stroma was accompanied in each case by direct observation of a significant reduction in contraction as a mode of defect closure. Conjunctival and peripheral nerve regeneration studies were guided by earlier studies of skin regeneration. Partial skin was first induced to regenerate in the adult guinea pig. The spontaneous healing behavior of the untreated dermis-free defect in this organism resulted in a final configuration of [91, 9, 0]. Grafting an identical well-defined skin defect with a highly porous polymer of type-I collagen and chondroitin 6-sulfate (referred to as a DRT) (Fig. 4A), abolished scar synthesis and led to the regeneration of a small mass of dermis and subsequent synthesis of an overlying epidermis within the defect. In the context of the defect closure rule, the regenerative activity of the DRT on the configuration of the final state was as follows:

$$[92, 8, 0] \rightarrow [89, 0, 11] \qquad \text{(DRT)}.$$

In addition, the DRT led to a significant delay in wound contraction over 25 days *(40,41)*.

When a DRT seeded with KC was grafted into an identical defect, the result was more pronounced:

$$[91, 9, 0] \rightarrow [28, 0, 72] \qquad \text{(DRT + KC)}.$$

KC-seeded DRTs accomplished rapid wound closure through partial regeneration of skin (simultaneous synthesis of a physiological dermis and epidermis, described earlier), and completely arrested contraction at 35–40 days *(11,42)*.

The cell-free DRT that induces partial skin regeneration comprises the regenerative component of the two-layer device (Integra DRT®, Integra Life Sciences, Plainsboro, NJ) approved by the Food and Drug Administration (FDA) for restoration of a physiological epidermis and dermis in patients suffering from severe burns as well as those undergoing plastic and reconstructive surgery of the skin, as described in early studies *(15,65,66)*. Growth factors *(67,68)*, epidermal cell suspensions, and cell sheets *(69)* exhibited negligible regenerative activity when added to full-thickness skin wounds in other rodent models. These reactants did not significantly alter the configuration of the final state or the extent of contraction delay. Similarly, a number of synthetic polymer scaffolds *(70,71)*, failed to induce physiological dermis (or skin) regeneration. These observations focus attention on the mechanism of scaffold regenerative activity, to be discussed later.

Quantitative studies of induced regeneration of peripheral nerves were conducted in the adult rat. The spontaneous healing behavior of the untreated transected peripheral nerve in this organism resulted in a final configuration that was estimated using histological analysis to be [95, 5, 0]. Insertion of the fully transected nerve stumps into a silicone tube filled with a collagen-based tubular regeneration template (referred to as a Nerve Regeneration Template or NRT, Fig. 4B) resulted in reduced contraction (as determined by histological analysis of cross-sectional areas of regenerates) and partial

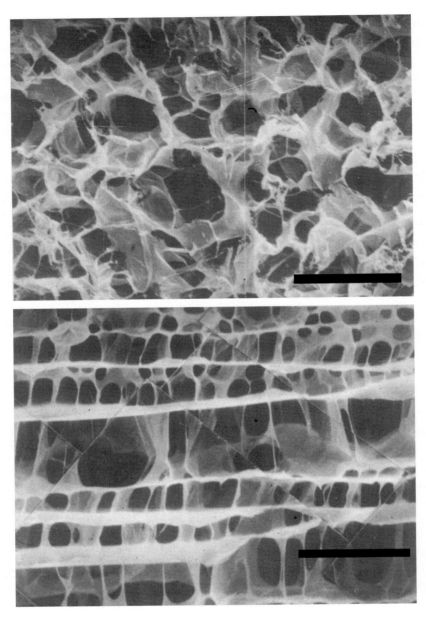

Fig. 4. (A, top) A scaffold that has induced regeneration of the dermis in animals and humans. Composition: graft copolymer of type-I collagen and chondroitin 6-sulfate. Scanning electron micrograph. Pore channel orientation is almost completely random. Average pore diameter, 80 μm *(4)*. **(B,** bottom) Peripheral nerve was induced to regenerate across a 15-mm gap (and eventually longer gaps) in the rat sciatic nerve using this scaffold as a bridge between the two stumps inside a silicone tube. In later studies the chemical composition of this scaffold was changed to GAG-free type-I collagen. Pore channel orientation along major nerve axis. Scanning electron micrograph. Average pore diameter, 20 μm *(104)*.

regeneration over an unprecedented gap length *(25,26)*. Contraction was abolished and the quality of regeneration improved significantly when the NRT was used in conjunction with a degradable collagen tube. In the context of the defect closure rule, the regenerative activity of the NRT in each experimental configuration can be evaluated by inspecting the characteristics of the final state, as follows (the arrow indicates the change observed following use of the scaffold):

$$[95, 5, 0] \rightarrow [53, 0, 47] \qquad \text{(NRT in silicone tube),}$$

$$[95, 5, 0] \rightarrow [0, 0, 100] \qquad \text{(NRT in collagen tube).}$$

The relative importance of each method of defect closure (*C*, *S*, and *R*) changes during animal development. A sharp change occurs during the fetal–adult transition in mammals (roughly during the third trimester of gestation), in which contraction replaces regeneration as the dominant method of closure *(72–74)*. Similarly, as amphibian development progresses, contraction becomes a more prominent method of wound closure, as regeneration recedes and scar formation becomes more evident *(75,76)*.

Although scar has been widely considered the key barrier to regeneration in adults, quantitative study reveals that contraction is the dominant mode of spontaneous closure in skin and peripheral nerve defects. Studies of induced regeneration in skin, peripheral nerves using analogs of the ECM indicate that scar formation is a process that is secondary to contraction: in studies of induced regeneration in these organs, when contraction was even slightly inhibited, scar formation was totally abolished *(1)*.

$$[92, 8, 0] \rightarrow [89, 0, 11] \qquad \text{(DRT),}$$

$$[91, 9, 0] \rightarrow [28, 0, 72] \qquad \text{(skin, DRT + KC),}$$

$$[95, 5, 0] \rightarrow [53, 0, 47] \qquad \text{(peripheral nerve, NRT in silicone tube),}$$

$$[95, 5, 0] \rightarrow [0, 0, 100] \qquad \text{(peripheral nerve, NRT in collagen tube).}$$

Suppression of contraction in certain cases of impaired healing, for example, following use of pharmacological agents, such as steroids, or application of devices, for example, use of mechanical splints or full-thickness skin grafts, was not accompanied by regeneration, indicating that suppression of contraction alone did not suffice to induce regeneration *(1)*.

The available evidence supports the theory that selectively suppressed contraction in adult defects is required, but not sufficient to induce regeneration of skin and peripheral nerves. This can be expressed in the context of the defect closure (Eq. 1) rule as follows:

$$\Delta R > 0 \text{ and } S \rightarrow 0 \quad \text{if } \Delta C < 0 \qquad (2)$$

This condition describes an antagonistic relationship between contraction and regeneration in the closure of a defect. It suggests that successful induced regeneration strategies consist of reactants that block contraction without blocking other aspects of the healing process.

Repair: Mechanism of Contraction

Similarities in the mechanistic hypotheses for inducing regeneration of skin and peripheral nerves originate in their common response to irreversible injury. Both organs spontaneously respond to injury by recruiting contractile cells that, if not properly suppressed, drive closure of the defect by contraction and scar synthesis rather than by regeneration. Contraction of skin defects starts from a cell cluster at the edge of the defect and later extends across the entire defect area. In peripheral nerves, contraction primarily results from the activity of a circumstantial sheath of contractile cells.

The Contractile Fibroblast is the Main Cell Type Associated With Contraction

The well-documented, macroscopic contraction that drives the closure of skin defects finds its origin at the cellular scale, arising from the individual contribution of contractile forces generated by differentiated myofibroblasts (MFB) *(75,77–83)*. The current consensus is that MFB present in the granulation tissue following skin wounding derive directly from fibroblasts and comprise an intermediate, contractile, cellular phenotype between the fibroblast and the smooth muscle cell *(77)*. There is also evidence that undifferentiated fibroblasts may contribute to macroscopic contraction by applying traction to the ECM very soon after coming into contact with it *(47,61,84–88)*.

In response to external tension, fibroblasts exert sustained isometric force on their surrounding environment via a rho/rho-kinase-mediated, actomyosin contractile apparatus *(89–91)*. This three-dimensional, transcellular structure consists of bundles of actin and nonmuscle myosin microfilaments called "stress fibers."

Of the many ultrastructural and biochemical factors that distinguish MFB from their fibroblast precursors, the most useful operational distinction of MFB differentiation is expression of the α-smooth muscle actin (SMA) phenotype *(75–78)*. Stress fibers of immature MFB (called proto-MFB) contain only β- and γ-cytoplasmic actins *(77)*. Additionally, differentiated MFB exhibit stress fibers typically arranged parallel to the long axis of the cell, nuclei which consistently show multiple indentations or deep folds, and two cell-matrix adhesion macromolecules (vinculin and fibronectin) *(92,93)*.

Simplistically, the myofibroblast differentiation process can be described as a positive feedback loop that requires the concurrent action of at least three factors: the cytokine transforming growth factor (TGF)-β_1, the presence of mechanical tension, and the ED-A splice variant of cellular fibronectin (an ECM component) *(77)*. Fibroblasts respond to the development of mechanical tension by upregulating TGF-β_1 production and expressing the α-SMA isoform; in turn, α-SMA expression strengthens the contractile apparatus and increases tension development *(77)*.

Mechanism of Scaffold Regenerative Activity

Not surprisingly, scaffolds that induce regeneration of partial skin (Fig. 4A) possess a highly specific structure that is distinctly different in pore structure and degradation rate from scaffolds that regenerate peripheral nerves (Fig. 4B). The nature and duration of the contractile response as well as the structure of the two organs differ greatly as do the values for several of the structural parameters of the early scaffolds that were used to control contraction and induce regeneration in each organ. The scaffolds have a common ligand identity resulting from an identical chemical composition (type-I collagen/GAG, 98/2 w/w ratio) yet they differ in average pore diameter (higher in the case of the DRT), the pore channel orientation (axial for the nerve guide, random for the DRT), and degradation rate (a higher average molecular weight between cross-links, M_c [kDa] in the nerve guide leads to faster degradation).

In skin wounds, the mechanism of induced regeneration has been elucidated through careful modulation of the DRT's structural properties that impart contraction blocking activity. DRTs that actively block contraction in skin wounds (and induce regeneration) have structural properties that accomplish three main processes: (1) inhibition of TGF-β synthesis, leading to downregulation of myofibroblast recruitment following severe injury; (2) blocking orientation of MFB axes in the plane of the defect in which macroscopic contraction is observed, and (3) ensuring that the DRT's contraction blocking properties persist for the duration of the interim myofibroblast contractile response but not so long as to interfere with key regenerative processes.

1. Downregulation of TGF-β synthesis. The quaternary structure of collagen fibers is a requirement for the aggregation of platelets, an early component of the wound response. Platelet aggregation initiates a cascade of events that include the release of the cytokine TGF-β_1, one of the main inductors of the myofibroblast phenotype. Collagen fibers in the DRT maintain their tertiary (triple helical) structure but are practically free of banding. In this manner the DRT disrupts platelet aggregation within the defect, reducing production of TGF-β_1, and the recruitment of contractile MFB to the wound site *(94)*.

2. Blocking orientation of MFB axes in the plane of the wound. Contraction blocking requires extensive MFB binding onto a sufficiently large scaffold surface by specific integrin–ligand interactions. When other structural properties are held constant, a scaffold's ligand density increases with decreasing average pore size (the specific surface area of the scaffold available for attachment is increased). An appropriate ligand density is necessary to disrupt extensive MFB–ECM binding responsible for the onset of macroscopic contraction in skin wounds. When MFB bind to specific DRT integrins that are distributed evenly in a three-dimensional, interconnecting porous network, the axes of their contractile apparatus become disoriented. At the cellular level, the randomized configuration of the preferential contractile axes, which individual MFB adopt in the presence of DRT approximately cancels the macroscopic mechanical forces that lead to two-dimensional contraction and scar synthesis in ungrafted skin wounds. When the pore diameter of DRT is increased much beyond the level of 120 µm, the effective DRT ligand density drops to a value that does not provide sufficient binding of MFB and the contraction-blocking activity of the scaffold is lost *(1,94,95)*. Similarly, a minimal average pore size exists that is necessary to ensure MFB migration inside the scaffold. If the pore size is too small, MFB will not infiltrate the scaffold, MFB–DRT ligand bonds will not be formed, and MFB contractile activity will not be canceled *(14)*. Experimentally, the highly linear orientation of myofibroblast axes that is characteristic of the macroscopic contractile response in ungrafted skin wounds is negligible in the presence of DRT *(96)*.

3. Duration of DRT in an undegraded state over the entire contraction process. In its optimal configuration, the DRT accomplishes isomorphous tissue replacement, in which the regenerate (dermis) is synthesized at a rate which is of the same order as the rate of degradation of the DRT. The scaffold must persist in an undegraded (insoluble) state over a period that matches the length of the contraction process in skin wounds, thereby ensuring that TGF-β_1 synthesis is downregulated and MFB axes are disoriented and macroscopic contraction is blocked. The optimal half-life of degradation (t_b) for DRT in vivo is 14 days, roughly matching the irreversible contraction response in ungrafted wounds (t_h). When the scaffold degraded at a slower rate ($t_b \gg 14$ days), the persisting DRT interfered with synthesis of the regenerate and scar formed around the scaffold. When the half-life of the DRT was significantly lower than the half-life of the contractile response ($t_b \ll 14$ days) the DRT had little effect on blocking contraction or scar synthesis and regeneration was not observed *(14)*. In summary, DRT dramatically blocks contraction when inducing skin regeneration. Scaffolds that are close in structure to DRT but do not block contraction, do not induce regeneration. There is evidence that DRT prevents recruitment of MFB and formation of oriented structures of MFB, two processes that characterize spontaneous healing in the adult mammal, over the duration of the normal contraction process.

DISCUSSION AND CONCLUSIONS

The experimental protocols that were used by several independent investigators to induce synthesis of elements of skin and peripheral nerves both in vitro and in vivo were analyzed in an effort to identify the minimal reactants required for organ regeneration. Despite the structural differences between the two organs, the simplest reactants required for induced regeneration of either skin or peripheral nerves were found to be similar. The empirical evidence supports the conclusion that partial synthesis of either skin or peripheral nerves requires only the implantation of a scaffold with the requisite structure, appropriately seeded with epithelial cells dissociated from the organ of interest. The scaffold should possess a minimal density of specific ligands for contractile cells and an optimal persistence time in the insoluble state *(1)*. Exogenous reactants utilized widely in many regeneration protocols, notably cytokines and stromal cells (fibroblasts), were redundant. Although the experimental evidence derives only from the two organs that have been studied extensively to date in this context, the conclusions reached earlier may be interpreted as a "transorgan" approach for future regeneration efforts.

The clinical significance of induced regeneration studies is readily apparent. Two regenerative devices have been approved thus far by the FDA, one each for the regeneration of skin and peripheral nerves; increasingly, these devices are establishing themselves as a viable alternative to autografting.

In 1996, the FDA approved the Integra DRT (DRT, described briefly earlier), as an urgent treatment modality for patients suffering from severe burns. Because that time, DRT has been approved by regulatory agencies in several other countries and more than 13,000 burn patients worldwide have been treated. In 2002, the FDA approved DRT for a second application: restorative or reconstructive surgery of skin scars. The efficacy of DRT for the induced regeneration and treatment of chronic and pathological deep skin ulcers (chronic skin wounds) has been established *(10)*. DRT has been studied recently by several clinical investigators *(97–103)*.

In 2001, Neuragen® (Integra), an early version of the collagen-based tubular devices that have been described above was approved for the regeneration of peripheral nerves. Till date this devices have been used to treat more than 1000 individuals suffering from paralysis of the extremities. Further studies have identified an optimized version of the device: a cell-permeable collagen tube with controlled degradation rate, higher cell permeability, and an overall superior quality of regeneration (Fig. 3).

Severe wounds in several organs in adults heal primarily by contraction, the same mechanism by which skin and apparently peripheral nerves heal in adults. Contraction blocking in skin and apparently in peripheral nerves is associated with induced regeneration. The available data suggest, therefore, the possibility that the mechanism of contraction blocking by scaffolds is similar in these two organs. It now becomes possible to seriously consider the prospect that the adult organism can be enabled to regenerate most of its organs.

REFERENCES

1. Yannas IV. *Tissue and Organ Regeneration in Adults*. Springer, New York, 2001.
2. Butler CE, Orgill DP. Simultaneous in vivo regeneration of neodermis, epidermis, and basement membrane. *Adv Biochem Eng Biotechnol* 2005;94:23–41.

3. Hatton MP, Rubin PAD. Conjunctival regeneration. *Adv Biochem Eng Biotechnol* 2005;94:125–140.
4. Zhang M, Yannas IV. Peripheral nerve regeneration. *Adv Biochem Eng Biotechnol* 2005; 94:67–89.
5. Mistry AS, Mikos AG. Tissue engineering for bone regeneration. *Adv Biochem Eng Biotechnol* 2005;94:1–22.
6. Rabkin-Aikawa E, Mayer JE Jr, Schoen FJ. Heart valve regeneration. *Adv Biochem Eng Biotechnol* 2005;94:141–178.
7. Kinner B, Capito RM, Spector M. Regeneration of articular cartilage. *Adv Biochem Eng Biotechnol* 2005;94:91–123.
8. Atala A. Regeneration of urologic tissues and organs. *Adv Biochem Eng Biotechnol* 2005; 94:179–208.
9. Verma P, Fawcett J. Spinal cord regeneration. *Adv Biochem Eng Biotechnol* 2005; 94:43–66.
10. Gottlieb ME, Furman J. Successful management and surgical closure of chronic and pathological wounds using Integra®. *J Burns Surg Wound Care* 2004;3(1):4.
11. Yannas IV, Burke JF, Orgill DP, Skrabut EM. Wound tissue can utilise a polymeric template to synthesise a functional extension of skin. *Science* 1982;215:174–176.
12. Yannas IV, Burke JF, Orgill DP, Skrabut EM. Regeneration of skin following closure of deep wounds with a biodegradable template. *Trans Soc Biomater* 1982;5:24–27.
13. Yannas IV, Orgill DP, Skrabut EM, Burke JF. Skin regeneration with a bioreplaceable polymeric template, in *Polymeric Materials and Artificial Organs*, (Gebelein CG, ed.), American Chemical Society, Washington, DC, 1984, pp. 191–197.
14. Yannas IV, Lee E, Orgill DP, Skrabut EM, Murphy GF. Synthesis and characterization of a model extracellular matrix which induces partial regeneration of adult mammalian skin. *Proc Natl Acad Sci USA* 1989;86:933–937.
15. Burke JF, Yannas IV, Quniby WC Jr, Bondoc CC, Jung WK. Successful use of a physiologically acceptable artificial skin in the treatment of extensive burn injury. *Ann Surg* 1981;194:413–428.
16. Murphy GF, Orgill DP, Yannas IV. Partial dermal regeneration is induced by biodegradable collagen-glycosaminoglycan grafts. *Lab Invest* 1990;62:305–313.
17. Compton CC, Butler CE, Yannas IV, Warland G, Orgill DP. Organized skin structure is regenerated in vivo from collagen-GAG matrices seeded with autologous keratinocytes. *J Invest Dermatol* 1998;110:908–916.
18. Butler CE, Yannas IV, Compton CC, Correia CA, Orgill DP. Comparison of cultured and uncultured keratinocytes seeded into a collagen-GAG matrix for skin replacements. *Br J Plast Surg* 1999;52:127–132.
19. Yannas IV, Orgill DP, Silver J, Norregaard TV, Zervas NT, Schoene WC. Polymeric template facilitates regeneration of sciatic nerve across 15 mm gap. *Trans Soc Biomater* 1985;8:146.
20. Yannas IV, Orgill DP, Silver J, Norregaard TV, Zervas NT, Schoene WC. Regeneration of sciatic nerve across 15 mm gap by use of a polymeric template, in *Advances in Biomedical Polymers* (Gebelein CG, ed.), Plenum Publishing Corporation, New York, 1987, pp. 1–9.
21. Chang A, Yannas IV, Perutz S, et al. Electrophysiological study of recovery of peripheral nerves regenerated by a collagen-glycosaminoglycan copolymer matrix, in *Progress in biomedical polymers* (Gebeelin CG, Dunn RL, eds.), Plenum, New York, 1990, pp. 107–119.
22. Chang AS-P, Yannas IV. Peripheral nerve regeneration, in *Neuroscience Year* (Smith B, Adelman G, eds.), Birkhauser, Boston, 1992.
23. Chamberlain LJ, Yannas IV, Arrizabalaga A, Hsu H-P, Norregarrd TV, Spector M. Early peripheral nerve healing in collagen and silicone tube implants: myofibroblasts and the cellular response. *Biomaterials* 1998;19:1393–1403.

24. Chamberlain LJ, Yannas IV, Hsu H-P, Strichartz G, Spector M. Collagen-GAG substrate enhances the quality of nerve regeneration through collagen tubes up to level of autograft. *Exp Neurol* 1998;154:315–329.
25. Chamberlain LJ, Yannas IV, Hsu H-P, Spector M. Connective tissue response to tubular implants for peripheral nerve regeneration: the role of myofibroblasts. *J Comp Neurol* 2000;417:415–430.
26. Chamberlain LJ, Yannas IV, Hsu H-P, Strichartz GR, Spector M. Near-terminus axonal structure and function following rat sciatic nerve regeneration through a collagen-GAG matrix in a ten-millimeter gap. *J Neurosci Res* 2000;60:666–677.
27. Spilker MH. Peripheral nerve regeneration through tubular devices. PhD Thesis, Massachusetts Institute of Technology, Cambridge, MA, 2000.
28. Hsu WC, Spilker MH, Yannas IV, Rubin PAD. Inhibition of conjunctival scarring and contraction by a porous collagen-GAG implant. *Invest Opthamol Vis Sci* 2000;41:2404–2411.
29. Goss RJ. Regeneration versus repair, in *Wound Healing: Biochemical and Clinical Aspects* (Cohen IK, Diegelmann RF, Lindblad WJ, eds.), Saunders, Philadelphia, PA, 1992, pp. 20–39.
30. Martinez-Hernandez A. Repair, regeneration, and fibrosis, in *Pathology* (Rubin E, Farber JL, eds.). JB Lippincott-Raven, Philadelphia, PA, 1998, pp.66–95.
31. Burkitt HG, Young B, Heath JW, Kilgore J. *Wheater's Functional Histology*, 2nd ed., Churchill Livingstone, Edinburgh, 1993.
32. Vracko R. Basal lamina scaffold-anatomy and significance for maintenance of orderly tissue structure. *Am J Pathol* 1974;77:313–346.
33. Bunge RP, Bunge MB. Interrelationship between Schwann cell function and extracellular matrix production. *Trends Neurosci* 1983;6:499.
34. Fu SY, Gordon T. The cellular and molecular basis of peripheral nerve regeneration. *Mol Neurobiol* 1997;14;67–116.
35. Stenn KS, Malhotra R. Epithelialization, in *Wound Healing: Biochemical and Clinical Aspects* (Cohen IK, Diegelmann RF, Lindblad WJ, eds.), Saunders, Philadelphia, PA, 1992, pp. 115–127.
36. Haber RM, Hanna W, Ramsay CA, Boxall LB. Cicatricial junctional epidermolysis bullosa. *J Am Acad Dermatol* 1985;12; 836–844.
37. Ikeda K, Oda Y, Tomita K, Nomura S, Nakanishi I. Isolated Schwann cells can synthesize the basement membrane in vitro. *J Electron Microsc (Tokyo)* 1989;38;230–234.
38. Uitto J, Mauviel A, McGrath J. The dermal–epidermal basement membrane zone in cutaneous wound healing, in *The Molecular and Cellular Biology of Wound Repair* (Clark RAF, ed.), 2nd ed., Plenum, New York, 1996, pp. 513–560.
39. Winter GD. Epidermal regeneration studied in the domestic pig, in *Epidermal Wound Healing* (Maibach HL, Rovee DT, eds.), Year Book Medical Publishers, Chicago, IL, 1972, pp. 71–112.
40. De Medinacelli L, Wyatt RJ, Freed WJ. Peripheral nerve reconnection: mechanical, thermal, and ionic conditions that promote the return of function. *Exp Neurol* 1983;81:469–487.
41. Terzis JK. *Microreconstruction of Nerve Injuries*. WB Saunders, Philadelphia, PA, 1987.
42. Yannas IV, Burke JF, Warpehoski M, et al. Prompt, long-term functional replacement of skin. *Trans Am Soc Artif Intern Organs* 1981;27:19–22.
43. Ramirez AT, Soroff HS, Schwartz MS, Mooty J, Pearson E, Raben MS. *Surg Gynecol Obstet* 1969;128(2):283–293.
44. Oppenheimer R, Hinman F Jr. Ureteral regeneration: contracture vs. hyperplasia of smooth muscle. *J Urol* 1955;74:476–484.
45. Kiviat MD, Ross R, Ansell JS. Smooth muscle regeneration in the ureter. *Am J Pathol* 1973;72:403–416.
46. Bulut T, Bilsel Y, Yanar H, et al. The effects of beta-aminopropionitrile on colonic anastomosis in rats. *J Invest Surg* 2004;17(4):211–219.

47. Dahners LE, Banes AJ, Burridge KWT. The relationship of actin to ligament contraction. *Clin Orthop* 1986;210:246–251.
48. Wilson CJ, Dahners LE. An examination of the mechanism of ligament contracture. *Clin Orthop* 1988;227:286–291.
49. Unterhauser FN, Bosch U, Zeichen J, Weiler A. Alpha-smooth muscle actin containing contractile fibroblastic cells in human knee arthrofibrosis tissue. *Arch Orthop Trauma Surg* 2004;124(9):585–591.
50. Zeinoun T, Nammour S, Sourov N, Luomanen M. Myofibroblasts in healing laser excision wounds. *Lasers Surg Med* 2001;28(1):74–79.
51. Delaere PR, Hardillo J, Hermans R, Van Den Hof B. Prefabrication of composite tissue for improved tracheal reconstruction. *Ann Otol Rhinol Laryngol* 2001;110(9):849–860.
52. Schmidt MR, Maeng M, Kristiansen SB, Andersen HR, Falk E. The natural history of collagen and alpha-actin expression after coronary angioplasty. *Cardiovasc Pathol* 2004; 13(5):260–267.
53. Levine D, Rockey DC, Milner TA, Breuss JM, Fallon JT, Schnapp LM. Expression of the integrin alpha8beta1 during pulmonary and hepatic fibrosis. *Am J Pathol* 2000;156(6):1927–1935.
54. Rudolph R, Van de Berg J, Ehrlich P. Wound contraction and scar contracture, in *Wound Healing: Biochemical and Clinical Aspects* (Cohen IK, Diegelmann RF, Lindblad WJ, eds.),WB Saunders Company, Philadelphia, PA, 1992, pp. 96–114.
55. Peacock EE Jr. Wound healing and wound care, in *Principles of Surgery* (Schwartz SI, Shires GT, Spencer FC, Storer EH, eds.), McGraw-Hill, New York, 1984.
56. Chou TD, Lee WT, Chen SL, et al. Split calvarial bone graft for chemical burn-associated nasal augmentation. *Burns* 2004;30(4):380–385.
57. Holmes W, Young JZ. Nerve regeneration after immediate and delayed suture. *J Anat (London)* 1942;77:63–96.
58. Weiss P. The technology of nerve regeneration: a review. Sutureless tabulation and related methods of nerve repair. *J Neurosurg* 1944;1:400–450.
59. Weiss P, Taylor AC. Further experimental evidence against "neurotropism" in nerve regeneration. *J Exp Zool* 1944;95:233–257.
60. Sunderland S. The anatomy and pathology of nerve injury. *Muscle Nerve* 1990;13:771–784.
61. Krishnan KG, Winkler PA, Muller A, Grevers G, Steiger HJ. Closure of recurrent frontal skull base defects with vascularized flaps—a technical case report. *Acta Neurochir (Wien)* 2000;142(12):1353–1358.
62. Cornelissen AM, Maltha JC, Von den Hoff JW, Kuijpers-Jagtman AM. Local injection of IFN-gamma reduces the number of myofibroblasts and the collagen content in palatal wounds. *J Dent Res* 2000;79(10):1782–1788.
63. Wong TTL, Daniels JT, Crowston JG, Khaw PT. MMP inhibition prevents human lens epithelial cell migration and contraction of the lens capsule. *Br J Ophthalmol* 2004;88(7):868–872.
64. Ivarsen A, Laurberg T, Moller-Pedersen T. Characterisation of corneal fibrotic wound repair at the LASIK flap margin. *Br J Ophthalmol* 2003;87(10):1272–1278.
65. Heimbach D, Luterman A, Burke J, et al. Artificial dermis for major burns. *Ann Surg* 1988;208:313–320.
66. Stern R, McPherson M, Longaker MT. Histologic study of artificial skin used in the treatment of full-thickness thermal injury. *J Burn Care Rehabil* 1990;11:7–13.
67. Greenhalgh DG, Sprugel KH, Murray MJ, Ross R. PDGF and FGF stimulate wound healing in the genetically diabetic mouse. *Am J Pathol* 1990;136:1235–1246.
68. Puolakkainen PA, Twardzik DR, Ranchalis JE, Pankey SC, Reed MJ, Gombotz WR. The enhancement in wound healing by transforming growth factor-β1 (TGF-β1) depends on the topical delivery system. *J Surg Res* 1995;58:321–329.
69. Billingham RE, Reynolds J. Transplantation studies on sheets of pure epidermal epithelium and epidermal cell suspensions. *Br J Plast Surg* 1952;5:25–36.

70. Hansbrough JF, Morgan JL, Greenleaf GE, Bartel R. Composite grafts of human keratinocytes grown on a polyglactin mesh-cultured fibroblast dermal substitute function as a bilayer skin replacement in full-thickness wounds on athymic mice. *J Burn Care Rehabil* 1993;14:485–494.

71. Cooper ML, Hansbrough JF, Spielvogel RL, Cohen R, Bartel RL, Naughton G. In vivo optimization of a living dermal substitute employing cultured human fibroblasts on a biodegradable polyglycolic acid or polyglactin mesh. *Biomaterials* 1991;12:243–248.

72. Lorenz HP, Adzick NS. Scarless skin wound repair in the fetus. *West J Med* 1993; 159:350–355.

73. Mast BA, Neslon JM, Krummel TM. Tissue repair in the mammalian fetus, in *Wound Healing: Biochemical and Clinical Aspects* (Cohen IK, Diegelmann RF, Lindblad WJ, eds.), WB Saunders Company, Philadelphia, PA, 1992.

74. Martin P. Wound healing: aiming for perfect skin regeneration. *Science* 1996;276:75–81.

75. Stocum DL. *Wound Repair, Regeneration and Artificial Tissues*, RG Landes Co., Austin, TX, 1995.

76. Yannas IV, Colt J, Wai YC. Wound contraction and scar synthesis during development of the amphibian *Rana catesbeiana. Wound Repair Regen* 1996;4:31–41.

77. Desmouliere A, Chaponnier C, Gabbiani G. Tissue repair, contraction, and the myofibroblast. *Wound Repair Regen* 2005;13(1):7–12.

78. Frangos JA (ed.) *Physical Forces and the Mammalian Cell*. Academic Press, New York, 1993.

79. Freyman TM, Yannas IV, Yokoo R, Gibson LJ. Fibroblast contraction of a collagen-GAG matrix. *Biomaterials* 2001;22:2883–2891.

80. Freyman TM, Yannas IV, Pek Y-S, Yokoo R, Gibson LJ. Micromechanics of fibroblast contraction of a collagen-GAG matrix. *Exp Cell Res* 2001;269:140–153.

81. Harley BA, Spilker MH, Wu JW, et al. Optimal degradation rate for collagen chambers used for regeneration of peripheral nerves over long gaps. *Cells Tissues Organs* 2004;176:153–165.

82. Racine-Samson L, Rockey DC, Bissell DM. The role of alpha1beta1 integrin in wound contraction. A quantitative analysis of liver myofibroblasts in vivo and in primary culture. *J Biol Chem* 1997;272:30,911–30,917.

83. Rudolph R, Abraham J, Vecchione T, Guber S, Woodward M. Myofibroblasts and free silicon around breast implants. *Plast Reconstr Surg* 1978;62:185–196.

84. Davison SP, McCaffrey TV, Porter MN, Manders E. Improved nerve regeneration with neutralization of transforming growth factor-beta1. *Laryngoscope* 1999;109:631–635.

85. Delaere PR, Hardillo J, Hermans R, Van Den Hof B. Prefabrication of composite tissue for improved tracheal reconstruction. *Ann Otol Rhinol Laryngol* 2001;110(9):849–860.

86. Ehrlich HP, Keefer KA, Myers RL, Passaniti A. Vanadate and the absence of myofibroblasts in wound contraction. *Arch Surg* 1999;134:494–501.

87. Ehrlich HP, Gabbiani G, Meda P. Cell coupling modulates the contraction of fibroblast-populated collagen lattices. *J Cell Physiol* 2002;184:86–92.

88. Eyden B. Electron microscopy in the study of myofibroblastic lesions. *Semin Diagn Pathol* 2003;20:13–24.

89. Amano M, Chihara K, Kimura K, et al. Formation of actin stress fibers and focal adhesions enhanced by Rho-kinase. *Science* 1997;275(5304):1308–1311.

90. Hall A. Rho GTPases and the actin cytoskeleton. *Science* 1998;279(5350):509–514.

91. Kimura K, Ito M, Amano M, et al. Regulation of myosin phosphatase by Rho and Rho-associated kinase (Rho-kinase). *Science* 1996;273(5272):245–248.

92. Serini G, Bochaton-Piallat M-L, Ropraz P, et al. The fibronectin domain ED-A is crucial for myofibroblastic phenotype induction by transforming growth factor-beta1. *J Cell Biol* 1998;142:873–881.

93. Dugina V, Fontao L, Chaponnier C, Vasiliev J, Gabbiani G. Focal adhesion features during myofibroblast differentiation are controlled by intracellular and extracellular forces. *J Cell Sci* 2001;114:3285–3296.

94. Yannas IV. Models of organ regeneration processes induced by templates. *Ann N Y Acad Sci* 1997;831:280–293.

95. Yannas IV. Studies on the biological activity of the dermal regeneration template. *Wound Repair Regen* 1998;6:518–524.

96. Troxel K. Delay of skin wound contraction by porous collagen-GAG matrices. PhD Thesis, Massachusetts Institute of Technology, Cambridge, MA, 1994.

97. Dantzer E, Queruel P, Salinier L, Palmier B, Quinot JF. Dermal regeneration template for deep hand burns: clinical utility for both early grafting and reconstructive surgery. *Br J Plast Surg* 2003;56(8):764–774.

98. Young RC, Burd A. Pediatric upper limb contracture release following burn injury. *Burns* 2004;30(7):723–728.

99. Blanco NM, Edwards J, Zamboni WA. Dermal substitute (Integra) for open nasal wounds. *Plast Reconstr Surg* 2004;113(7):2224, 2225.

100. Navsaria HA, Ojeh NO, Moiemen N, Griffiths MA, Frame JD. Reepithelialization of a full-thickness burn from stem cells of hair follicles micrografted into a tissue-engineered dermal template (Integra). *Plast Reconstr Surg* 2004;113(3):978–981.

101. Abai B, Thayer D, Glat PM. The use of a dermal regeneration template (Integra) for acute resurfacing and reconstruction of defects created by excision of giant hairy nevi. *Plast Reconstr Surg* 2004;114(1):162–168.

102. Frame JD, Still J, Lakhel-LeCoadou A, et al. Use of dermal regeneration template in contracture release procedures: a multicenter evaluation. *Plast Reconstr Surg* 2004;113(5):1330–1338.

103. Heitland A, Piatkowski A, Noah EM, Pallua N. Update on the use of collagen/glycosaminoglycate skin substitute-six years of experiences with artificial skin in 15 German burn centers. *Burns* 2004;30(5):471–475.

104. Yannas IV. Facts and theories of organ regeneration. *Adv Biochem Eng Biotechnol* 2005;93:1–31.

6

Diabetic Neuropathy

Solomon Tesfaye, MD, FRCP

INTRODUCTION

Polyneuropathy is one of the commonest complications of the diabetes and the commonest form of neuropathy in the developed world. Diabetic polyneuropathy encompasses several neuropathic syndromes, the most common of which is distal symmetrical neuropathy, the main initiating factor for foot ulceration. The epidemiology of diabetic neuropathy has recently been reviewed in reasonable detail (1). Several clinic- (2,3) and population-based studies (4,5) show surprisingly similar prevalence rates for distal symmetrical neuropathy, affecting about 30% of all people with diabetes. The EURODIAB prospective complications study, which involved the examination of 3250 patient with type 1 from 16 European countries, found a prevalence rate of 28% for distal symmetrical neuropathy (2). After excluding those with neuropathy at baseline, the study showed that over a 7-year period, about one-quarter of patients with type 1 diabetes developed distal symmetrical neuropathy; age, duration of diabetes, and poor glycemic control being major determinants (6). The development of neuropathy was also associated with potentially modifiable cardiovascular risk factors such as serum lipids, hypertension, body mass index, and cigaret smoking (6). Furthermore, cardiovascular disease at baseline carried a twofold risk of neuropathy, independent of cardiovascular risk factors (6). Based on recent epidemiological studies, correlates of diabetic neuropathy include increasing age, increasing duration of diabetes, poor glycemic control, retinopathy, albuminuria, and vascular risk factors (1,2,4,6). The differing clinical presentation of the several neuropathic syndromes in diabetes suggests varied etiological factors.

CLASSIFICATION

Clinical classification of the various syndromes of diabetic peripheral neuropathy has proved difficult. The variation and overlap in etiology, clinical features, natural history, and prognosis has meant that most classifications are necessarily oversimplified and none has proved capable of accounting for all these factors. Nevertheless, attempts at classification stimulate thought concerning the etiology of the various syndromes and also assist in the planning of management strategy for the patient.

Clinical manifestations (7) and measurement (8,9) of somatic neuropathy have recently been reviewed. There are a number of classifications for diabetic polyneuropathy. Based on the various distinct clinical presentations to the physician, Ward recommended a classification of diabetic polyneuropathy depicted in Table 1 (10). This practical approach to

From: *The Diabetic Foot, Second Edition*
Edited by: A. Veves, J. M. Giurini, and F. W. LoGerfo © Humana Press Inc., Totowa, NJ

Table 1
The Varied Presentations of the Neuropathic
Syndromes Associated With Diabetes

Chronic insidious sensory neuropathy
Acute painful neuropathy
Proximal motor neuropathy
Diffuse symmetrical motor neuropathy
The neuropathic foot
Pressure neuropathy
Focal vascular neuropathy
Neuropathy present at diagnosis
Treatment induced neuropathy
Hypoglycemic neuropathy

Adapted from ref. *10* with permission.

Table 2
Classification of Diabetic Neuropathy

Symmetrical neuropathies	Asymmetrical neuropathies
Distal sensory and sensory-motor neuropathy	Mononeuropathy
Large-fiber type of diabetic neuropathy	Mononeuropathy multiplex
Small-fiber type of diabetic neuropathy	Radiculopathies
Distal small-fiber neuropathy	Lumbar plexopathy or radiculoplexopathy
"Insulin neuropathy"	Chronic inflammatory demyelinating
Chronic inflammatory demyelinating polyradiculoneuropathy (CIDP)	polyradiculoneuropathy

Adapted from ref. *14* with permission.

the classification of diabetic neuropathies provides the clinician to have workable, crude definitions for the various neuropathic syndromes, and also assists in the management of the patient.

More recently, Watkins and Edmonds *(11)* have suggested a classification for diabetic polyneuropathy based on the natural history of the various syndromes, which clearly separates them into three distinct groups:

1. Progressive neuropathies are associated with increasing duration of diabetes and with other microvascular complications. Sensory disturbance predominates and autonomic involvement is common. The onset is gradual and there is no recovery.
2. Reversible neuropathies have an acute onset, often occurring at the presentation of diabetes itself, and are not related to the duration of diabetes or other microvascular complications. There is spontaneous recovery of these acute neuropathies.
3. Pressure palsies although are not specific to diabetes only, they tend to occur more frequently in patients with diabetes than in the general population. There is no association with duration of diabetes or other microvascular complications of diabetes.

Another method of classifying diabetic polyneuropathy is by considering whether the clinical involvement is symmetrical or asymmetrical. However, the separation to symmetrical and asymmetrical neuropathies, although useful in identifying distinct entities and perhaps providing clues to the varied etiologies, is an oversimplification of the truth as there is a great overlapping of the syndromes. This method was originally suggested by Bruyn and Garland *(12)*, and later modified by Thomas *(13)*. More recently, Low and Suarez *(14)* have further modified this classification (Table 2).

SYMMETRICAL NEUROPATHIES

Distal Symmetrical Neuropathy

This is the commonest neuropathic syndrome and what is meant in clinical practice by the phrase "diabetic neuropathy." There is a "length-related" pattern of sensory loss, with sensory symptoms starting in the toes and then extending to involve the feet and legs in a stocking distribution. In more severe cases, there is often upper limb involvement, with a similar progression proximally starting in the fingers. Although the nerve damage can extend over the entire body including the head and face, this is exceptional. Subclinical neuropathy detectable by autonomic function tests is usually present. However, clinical autonomic neuropathy is less common. Autonomic neuropathy is considered in more detail on pages 118–121. As the disease advances, overt motor manifestations such as wasting of the small muscles of the hands and limb weakness become apparent. However, subclinical motor involvement detected by magnetic resonance imaging appears to be common, and thus motor disturbance is clearly part of the functional impairment caused by distal symmetrical neuropathy *(15)*.

The main clinical presentation of distal symmetrical neuropathy is sensory loss which the patient may not be aware of, or may be described as "numbness" or "dead feeling." However, some may experience a progressive buildup of unpleasant sensory symptoms *(16)* including tingling (paraesthesiae); burning pain; shooting pains down the legs; lancinating pains; contact pain often with daytime clothes and bedclothes (allodynia); pain on walking often described as "walking barefoot on marbles," or "walking barefoot on hot sand"; sensations of heat or cold in the feet; and persistent achy feeling in the feet and cramp-like sensations in the legs. Occasionally pain can extend above the feet and may involve the whole of the legs, and when this is the case there is usually upper limb involvement also. There is a large spectrum of severity of these symptoms. Some may have minor complaints such as tingling in one or two toes; others may be affected with the devastating complications such as "the numb diabetic foot," or severe painful neuropathy that does not respond to drug therapy.

Diabetic neuropathic pain is characteristically more severe at night, and often prevents sleep *(17,18)*. Some patients may be in a constant state of tiredness because of sleep deprivation *(17)*. Others are unable to maintain full employment *(17–19)*. Severe painful neuropathy can occasionally cause marked reduction in exercise threshold so as interfere with daily activities *(17,20)*. This is particularly the case when there is an associated disabling, severe postural hypotension resulting from autonomic involvement *(11)*. Not surprisingly therefore, depressive and symptoms are not uncommon *(17,20)*. Although, subclinical autonomic neuropathy is commonly found in patients with distal symmetrical neuropathy *(21)*, symptomatic autonomic neuropathy is uncommon.

It is important to appreciate that many subjects with distal symmetrical neuropathy may not have any of the above symptoms, and their first presentation may be with a foot ulcer. This underpins the need for carefully examining and screening the feet of all diabetic people, in order to identify those at risk of developing foot ulceration. The insensate foot is at risk of developing mechanical and thermal injuries, and patients must therefore be warned about these and given appropriate advice regarding foot care. A curious feature of the neuropathic foot is that both numbness and pain may occur, the so-called painful, painless leg *(22)*. It is indeed a paradox that the patient with a large foot ulcer may also have severe neuropathic pain. In those with advanced neuropathy, there may be sensory ataxia. The unfortunate sufferer is affected by unsteadiness on walking, and even falls particularly if there is associated visual impairment because of retinopathy.

Neuropathy is usually easily detected by simple clinical examination *(23)*. Shoes and socks should be removed and the feet examined at least annually and more often if neuropathy is present. The most common presenting abnormality is a reduction or absence of vibration sense in the toes. As the disease progresses there is sensory loss in a "stocking" and sometimes in a "glove" distribution involving all modalities. When there is severe sensory loss, proprioception may also be impaired, leading to a positive Romberg's sign. Ankle tendon reflexes are lost and with more advanced neuropathy, knee reflexes are often reduced or absent.

Muscle strength is usually normal early during the course of the disease, although mild weakness may be found in toe extensors. However, with progressive disease there is significant generalized muscular wasting, particularly in the small muscles of the hand and feet. The fine movements of fingers would then be affected, and there is difficulty in handling small objects. Wasting of dorsal interossei is however usually because of the entrapment of the ulnar nerve at the elbow. The clawing of the toes is believed to be owing to unopposed (because of wasting of the small muscles of the foot) pulling of the long extensor and flexor tendons. This scenario results in elevated plantar pressure points at the metatarsal heads that are prone to callus formation and foot ulceration. Deformities such as a bunion can form the focus of ulceration and with more extreme deformities, such as those associated with Charcot arthropathy *(24)*, the risk is further increased. As one of the most common precipitants to foot ulceration is inappropriate footwear, a thorough assessment should also include examination of shoes for poor fit, abnormal wear, and internal pressure areas or foreign bodies.

Autonomic neuropathy affecting the feet can cause a reduction in sweating and consequently dry skin that is likely to crack easily, predisposing the patient to the risk of infection. The "purely" neuropathic foot is also warm because of the arterio/ venous shunting first described by Ward *(23)*. This results in the distension of foot veins that fail to collapse even when the foot is elevated. It is not unusual to observe a gangrenous toe in a foot that has bounding arterial pulses, as there is impairment of the nutritive capillary circulation because of arteriovenous shunting. The oxygen tension of the blood in these veins is typically raised *(25)*. The increasing blood flow brought about by autonomic neuropathy can sometimes result in neuropathic edema, which is resistant to treatment with diuretics but may respond to treatment with ephedrine *(26)*.

Small-Fiber Neuropathy

The existence "small-fiber neuropathy" as a distinct entity has been advocated by some authorities *(27,28)*, usually within the context of young patients with type 1. A prominent feature of this syndrome is neuropathic pain, which may be very severe, with relative sparing of large-fiber functions (vibration and proprioception). The pain is described as burning, deep and aching. The sensation of pins and needles (paraesthesiae) is also often experienced. Contact hypersensitivity may be present. However, rarely, patients with small-fiber neuropathy may not have neuropathic pain, and some may occasionally have foot ulceration. Autonomic involvement is common, and severely affected patients may be disabled by postural hypotension and/or gastrointestinal symptoms. The syndrome tends to develop within a few years of diabetes as a relatively early complication.

On clinical examination there is little evidence of objective signs of nerve damage, apart from a reduction in pinprick and temperature sensation, which are reduced in a "stocking" and "glove" distribution. There is relative sparing of vibration and position sense (because of relative sparing of the large diameter Aβ-fibers). Muscle strength is usually normal and reflexes are also usually normal. However, autonomic function tests are frequently abnormal and affected male patients usually have erectile dysfunction. Electrophysiological tests support small-fiber dysfunction. Sural sensory conduction velocity may be normal, although the amplitude may be reduced. Motor nerves appear to be less affected. Controversy still exists as to whether small-fiber neuropathy is a distinct entity or an earlier manifestation of chronic sensory motor neuropathy (27,28). Said et al. (27) studied a small series of subjects with this syndrome and showed that small-fiber degeneration predominated morphometrically. Veves et al. (29) found a varying degree of early small-fiber involvement in all diabetic polyneuropathies which was confirmed by detailed sensory and autonomic function tests. It is unclear, therefore, whether this syndrome is in fact distinct or merely represents the early stages of distal symmetrical neuropathy that has been detected by the prominence of early symptoms.

Differential Diagnosis of Distal Symmetrical Neuropathy

Diabetic peripheral neuropathy presents in a similar way to neuropathies of other causes, and thus the physician needs to carefully exclude other common causes before attributing the neuropathy to diabetes. Absence of other complications of diabetes, rapid weight loss, excessive alcohol intake, and other atypical features in either the history or clinical examination should alert the physician to search for other causes of neuropathy. Table 3 shows differential diagnoses for distal symmetrical neuropathy.

Natural History of Distal Symmetrical Neuropathy

Although distal symmetrical neuropathy is common in clinical practice, there are few prospective studies that have looked at its natural history, which remains poorly understood. This may partly be owing to our inadequate knowledge regarding the pathogenesis of distal symmetrical neuropathy, although several mechanisms have been suggested (30–32), and the list of potential mechanisms is constantly growing. Unlike in diabetic retinopathy and nephropathy, the scarcity of simple, accurate, and readily reproducible methods of measuring neuropathy further complicates the problem (8,9). One study (33) reported that neuropathic symptoms remain or get worse over a 5-year period in patients with chronic distal symmetrical neuropathy. A major drawback of this study was that it involved highly selected patients from a hospital base. A more recent study reported improvements in painful symptoms over 3.5 years (34). Neuropathic pain was assessed using a visual analog scale, and small-fiber function by thermal limen, heat pain threshold, and weighted pinprick threshold. At follow-up 3.5 years later, one-third of the 50 patients at baseline had died or were lost to follow-up. Clearly this is a major drawback. There was symptomatic improvement in painful neuropathy in the majority of the remaining patients. Despite this

Table 3
Differential Diagnosis of Distal Symmetrical Neuropathy

Metabolic	Neoplastic disorders
Diabetes	Bronchial or gastric carcinoma
Amyloidosis	Lymphoma
Uremia	Infective or inflammatory
Myxedema	Leprosy
Porphyria	Guillain-Barre syndrome
Vitamin deficiency (thiamin, B_{12}, B_6, pyridoxine)	Lyme borreliosis
Drugs and chemicals	Chronic inflammatory
Alcohol	demyelinating polyneuropathy
Cytotoxic drugs, for example, Vincristine	Polyarteritis nodosa
Chlorambucil	Genetic
Nitrofurantoin	Charcot-Marie-Tooth disease
Isoniazid	Hereditary sensory neuropathies

symptomatic improvement, however, small-fiber function as measured by the above tests deteriorated significantly. Thus, there was a dichotomy in the evolution of neuropathic symptoms and neurophysiological measures.

Are Painful and Painless Neuropathies Distinct Entities?

One of the complexities of distal symmetrical neuropathy is the variety of presentation to the clinician *(16)*. A relative minority present with pain as the predominant symptom *(35)*. There is controversy concerning whether the clinical, neurophysiological, peripheral nerve hemodynamic/morphometric findings are distinctly different in subjects with painful and painless diabetic neuropathy *(16)*. Young et al. *(36)* reported that patients with painful neuropathy had a higher ratio of autonomic (small-fiber) abnormality to electrophysiological (large-fiber) abnormality. In contrast, they found that electrophysiological parameters were significantly worse in patients with foot ulceration compared with those with painful neuropathy. They concluded that in distal symmetrical neuropathy, the relationship between large- and small-fiber damage is not uniform, and that there may be different etiological influences on large- and small-fiber neuropathy in subjects with diabetes, with the predominant type of fiber damage determining the form of the presenting clinical syndrome *(36)*. This view is supported by the study of Tsigos et al. *(37)*, who also suggested that painful and painless neuropathies represent two distinct clinical entities with little overlap. However, a contrary view was expressed by Veves et al. *(38)* who found that painful symptoms were frequent in diabetic neuropathy, irrespective of the presence or absence of foot ulceration, and that these symptoms may occur at any stage of the disease. They concluded that there is a spectrum of presentations from varying degrees of painful neuropathy to predominantly painless neuropathy associated with foot ulceration, and that much overlap is present *(38)*. The author's clinical observations support this view, as painful symptoms are often similarly present in patients with and without foot ulceration, suggesting that painless and painful neuropathy represent extreme forms of the same syndrome. Thus, an important clinical point is that the neuropathic foot with painful symptoms is just as vulnerable to foot ulceration as the foot with absence of painful neuropathic symptoms. The crucial determining factor is elevation of vibration perception threshold *(39)* and not the presence or absence of painful symptoms. Indeed, the "painful–painless" foot with ulceration, is frequently observed in the diabetic foot clinic, a phenomenon first described by Ward *(22)*.

Acute Painful Neuropathies

These are transient neuropathic syndromes characterized by an acute onset of pain in the lower limbs. Acute neuropathies present in a symmetrical fashion and are relatively uncommon. Pain is invariably present and is usually distressing to the patient, and can sometimes be incapacitating. There are two distinct syndromes, the first of which occurs within the context of poor glycemic control, and the second with rapid improvements in metabolic control.

Acute Painful Neuropathy of Poor Glycemic Control

This phenomenon occurs usually in patients with type 1 or -2 diabetes who have poor glycemic control. There is no relationship to the presence of other chronic diabetic complications. There is often an associated severe weight loss *(40)*. Ellenberg coined the description of this condition as "neuropathic cachexia" *(41)*. Patients typically develop persistent burning pain associated with allodynia (contact pain). The pain is most marked in the feet but often affects the whole of the lower extremities. As in chronic distal symmetrical neuropathy, the pain is typically worse at night although persistent pain during daytime is also common. The pain is likened to "walking on burning sand" and there may be a subjective feeling of the feet being "swollen." Patients also describe intermittent bouts of stabbing pain that shoot up the legs from the feet ("peak pain"), superimposed on the background of burning pain ("background pain"). Not surprisingly, these disabling symptoms often lead to depression.

On examination, sensory loss is usually surprisingly mild or even absent. There are usually no motor signs, although ankle jerks may be absent. Nerve conduction studies are also usually normal or mildly abnormal. Temperature discrimination threshold (small-fiber function) is however, affected more commonly than vibration perception threshold (large-fiber function) *(42)*. There is complete resolution of symptoms within 12 months, and weight gain is usual with continued improvement in glycemic control with the use of insulin. The lack of objective signs should not raise the doubt that these painful symptoms are not real. Many patients feel that people including health care professionals do not fully appreciate their predicament.

Acute Painful Neuropathy of Rapid Glycemic Control (Insulin Neuritis)

The term "insulin neuritis" was coined by Caravati *(43)* who first described the syndrome of acute painful neuropathy of rapid glycemic control. The term is a misnomer as the condition can follow rapid improvement in glycemic control with oral hypoglycemic agents, and "neuritis" implies a neural inflammatory process for which there is no evidence. The author has therefore recommended that the term "acute painful neuropathy of rapid glycemic control" be used to describe this condition *(44)*.

The natural history of acute painful neuropathies is an almost guaranteed improvement *(40)* in contrast to chronic distal symmetrical neuropathy *(33,34)*. The patient presents with burning pain, paraesthesiae, allodynia, often with a nocturnal exacerbation of symptoms, and depression may be a feature. There is no associated weight loss, unlike acute painful neuropathy of poor glycemic control. Sensory loss is often mild or absent, and there are no motor signs. There is little or no abnormality on nerve conduction studies, but there is impaired exercise-induced conduction velocity increment *(44,45)*. There is usually complete resolution of symptoms within 12 months.

On sural nerve biopsy, typical morphometric changes of chronic distal symmetrical neuropathy but with active regeneration, were observed *(46)*. In contrast, degeneration of both myelinated and unmyelinated fibers was found in acute painful neuropathy of poor glycemic control *(40)*. A recent study looking into the epineurial vessels of sural nerves in patients with acute painful neuropathy of rapid glycemic control demonstrated marked arteriovenous abnormality including the presence of proliferating new vessels, similar to those found in the retina *(44)*. The study suggested that the presence of this fine network of epineurial vessels may lead to a "steal" effect rendering the endoneurium ischemic, and the authors also suggested that this process may be important in the genesis of neuropathic pain *(44)*. These findings were also supported by studies in experimental diabetes which demonstrated that insulin administration led to acute endoneurial hypoxia, by increasing nerve arteriovenous flow, and reducing the nutritive flow of normal nerves *(47)*. Further work needs to address whether these observed sural nerve vessel changes resolve with the resolution of painful symptoms.

ASYMMETRICAL NEUROPATHIES

Asymmetrical or focal neuropathies are well-recognized complications of diabetes. They have a relatively rapid onset and complete recovery is usual. This contrasts with chronic distal symmetrical neuropathy, in which there is usually no improvement in symptoms 5 years after onset *(48)*. Unlike chronic distal symmetrical neuropathy they are often unrelated to the presence of other diabetic complications *(8–11)*. Asymmetrical neuropathies are more common in men and tend to predominantly affect older patients *(48,49)*. A careful history is therefore mandatory in order to identify any associated symptoms that might point to another cause for the neuropathy. A vascular etiology has been suggested by virtue of the rapid onset of symptoms and the focal nature of the neuropathic syndromes *(50)*.

Proximal Motor Neuropathy (Femoral Neuropathy, Amyotrophy, and Plexopathy)

The syndrome of progressive asymmetrical proximal leg weakness and atrophy was first described by Garland *(51)*, who coined the term "diabetic amyotrophy." This condition has also been named as "proximal motor neuropathy," "femoral neuropathy," or "plexopathy." The patient presents with severe pain which is felt deep in the thigh, but can sometimes be of burning quality and extend below the knee. The pain is usually continuous and often causes insomnia and depression *(52)*. Both patients with type 1 and type 2 over the age of 50 years are affected *(51–54)*. There is an associated weight loss, which can sometimes be very severe, and can raise the possibility of an occult malignancy.

On examination there is profound wasting of the quadriceps with marked weakness in these muscle groups, although hip flexors and hip abductors can also be affected *(55)*. Thigh adductors, glutei, and hamstring muscles may also be involved. The knee jerk is usually reduced or absent. The profound weakness can lead to difficulty from getting out of a low chair or climbing stairs. Sensory loss is unusual, and if present indicates a coexistent distal sensory neuropathy.

It is important to carefully exclude other causes of quadriceps wasting such as nerve root and cauda equina lesions, and the possibility of occult malignancy causing proximal myopathy syndromes such as polymyocytis. MR imaging of the lumbo-sacral spine is now mandatory in order to exclude focal nerve root entrapment and other pathologies. An erythrocyte sedimentation rate, an X-ray of the lumbar/sacral spine, a chest X-ray, and ultrasound of the abdomen may also be required. Cerebrospinal fluid protein is often elevated. Electrophysiological studies may demonstrate increased femoral nerve latency and active denervation of affected muscles.

The cause of diabetic proximal motor neuropathy is not known. It tends to occur within the background of diabetic distal symmetrical neuropathy *(56)*. Some have suggested that the combination of focal features superimposed on diffuse peripheral neuropathy may suggest vascular damage to the femoral nerve roots, as a cause of this condition *(57)*.

As in distal symmetrical neuropathy, there is scarcity of prospective studies that have looked at the natural history of proximal motor neuropathy. Coppack and Watkins *(52)* have reported that pain usually starts to settle after about 3 months, and usually settles by 1 year, whereas the knee jerk is restored in 50% of the patients after 2 years. Recurrence on the other side is a rare event. Management is largely symptomatic and supportive. Patients should be encouraged and reassured that this condition is likely to resolve. There is still controversy regarding whether the use of insulin therapy influences the natural history of this syndrome. Some patients benefit from physiotherapy that involves extension exercises aimed at strengthening the quadriceps. The management of pain in proximal motor neuropathy is similar to that of chronic or acute distal symmetrical neuropathies (*see* "Management of Diabetic Neuropathy").

Cranial Mononeuropathies

The commonest cranial mononeuropathy is the third cranial nerve palsy. The patient presents with pain in the orbit, or sometimes with a frontal headache *(50,58)*. There is typically ptosis and ophthalmoplegia, although the pupil is usually spared *(59,60)*. Recovery occurs usually over 3 months. The clinical onset and time-scale for recovery, and the focal nature of the lesions on the third cranial nerve, on postmortem studies suggested an ischemic etiology *(50,61)*. It is important to exclude any other cause of third cranial nerve palsy (aneurysm or tumor) by CT or MR scanning, in which the diagnosis is in doubt. Fourth, sixth, and seventh cranial nerve palsies have also been described in subjects with diabetes, but the association with diabetes is not as strong as that with third cranial nerve palsy.

Truncal Radiculopathy

Truncal radiculopathy is well recognized to occur in diabetes. It is characterized by an acute onset pain in a dermatomal distribution over the thorax or the abdomen *(62)*. The pain is usually asymmetrical, and can cause local bulging of the muscle *(63)*. There may be patchy sensory loss and other causes of nerve root compression should be excluded. Some patients presenting with abdominal pain have undergone unnecessary investigations such as barium enema, colonoscopy, and even laparotomy, when the diagnosis could easily have been made by careful clinical history and examination. Recovery is usually the rule within several months, although symptoms can sometimes persist for a few years.

Pressure Palsies

Carpal Tunnel Syndrome

A number of nerves are vulnerable to pressure damage in diabetes. In the Rochester diabetic neuropathy study, which was a population-based epidemiological study, Dyck et al. *(64)* found electrophysiological evidence of median nerve lesions at the wrist in about 30% of subjects with diabetes, although the typical symptoms of carpel tunnel syndrome occurred in less than 10%. The patient typically has pain and paraesthesia in the hands, which sometimes radiate to the forearm and are particularly marked at night. In severe cases clinical examination may reveal a reduction in sensation in the median territory in the hands, and wasting of the muscle bulk in the thenar eminence. The clinical diagnosis is easily confirmed by median nerve conduction studies and treatment involves surgical decompression at the carpel tunnel in the wrist. There is generally good response to surgery, although painful symptoms appear to relapse more commonly than in the nondiabetic population *(65)*.

Ulnar Nerve and Other Isolated Nerve Entrapments

The ulnar nerve is also vulnerable to pressure damage at the elbow in the ulnar groove. This results in wasting of the dorsal interossei, particularly the first dorsal interossius. This is easily confirmed by ulnar electrophysiological studies, which localize the lesion to the elbow. Rarely, the patients may present with wrist drop resulting from radial nerve palsy after prolonged sitting (with pressure over the radial nerve in the back of the arms), whereas unconscious during hypoglycemia or asleep after an alcohol binge.

In the lower limbs the common peroneal (lateral popliteal) is the most commonly affected nerve. The compression is at the level of the head of the fibula and causes foot drop. Unfortunately complete recovery is not usual. The lateral cutaneous nerve of the thigh is occasionally also affected with entrapment neuropathy in diabetes. Phrenic nerve involvement in association with diabetes has also been described, although the possibility of a pressure lesion could not be excluded *(64)*.

PATHOGENESIS OF DISTAL SYMMETRICAL NEUROPATHY

Despite considerable research, the pathogenesis of diabetic neuropathy remains undetermined *(30–32)*. Morphometric studies have demonstrated that distal symmetrical neuropathy is characterized by pathological changes including:

1. axonal loss distally, with a "dying back" phenomenon *(27)*,
2. a reduction in myelinated fiber density *(67)*, and
3. focal areas of demyelination on teased fiber preparations *(27)*.

Nerve regenerative activity may also be seen with the emergence of "regenerative clusters" *(68)*, containing groups of myelinated axons and nonmyelinated axons sprouts.

Table 4
Proposed Hypotheses of Diabetic Peripheral Nerve Damage

Chronic hyperglycaemia
Nerve microvascular dysfunction
Increased free radical formation
Polyol pathway hyperactivity
PKC hyperactivity
Nonenzymatic glycation
Abnormalities of nerve growth

However, the small and unmyelinated fibers that make up around 80% of all nerve fibers have proved more difficult to assess.

Historically, there have been two distinct views regarding the pathogenesis of distal symmetrical neuropathy. The first view regards metabolic factors *(69)* to be primarily important in the pathogenesis of distal symmetrical neuropathy, the second contends that vascular factors *(32)* be the determining etiological factors for neuropathy (Table 4). However, most authorities now agree that the truth is probably in the middle and that both metabolic and vascular factors are important. Evidence for this comes from recent work that has demonstrated an interaction between some of the proposed metabolic hypotheses of peripheral nerve damage and the vascular endothelium *(32)*. Figure 2 shows current thinking with regard to the pathogenesis of diabetic neuropathy.

Chronic Hyperglycemia

Over the past decade, at least three large prospective studies have conclusively demonstrated that there is now little doubt that chronic hyperglycemia is implicated in the pathogenesis of diabetic neuropathy. The EURODIAB prospective study *(6)*, the Diabetes control and complications trial *(70)*, and more recently the United Kingdom prospective diabetes study *(71)* have demonstrated that poor glycemic control is related to the increased prevalence of neuropathy in patients with diabetes and that improved glycemic control may prevent/reverse distal symmetrical neuropathy. However, there are major gaps in our understanding of how exactly the effects of chronic hyperglycemia result in nerve damage.

Oxidative Stress

Hyperglycemia leads to an increase in free radical generation as a result of several metabolic derangements including nonenzymatic glycation and polyol pathway hyperactivity. Moreover the capacity to neutralize free radicals is also reduced because of several metabolic abnormalities including NADPH depletion as a result of polyol pathway hyperactivity *(72)*. Thus, oxidative stress may impair nerve function by direct toxic effect or by reducing nitric oxide and hence nerve blood flow. Recent studies in rats with experimental diabetes have shown that free radical scavengers may improve nerve conduction velocity abnormalities *(73)* although these findings need to be proven in human diabetic neuropathy. Future studies may also explore an alternative to free radical scavenging i.e., preventing free radical formation in the first place.

Increased Polyol Pathway Flux

In 1966, Gabbay et al. postulated that polyol pathway hyperactivity as a mechanism which could link hyperglycemia to neuropathy *(74)*. It was proposed that hyperglycemia led to sorbitol accumulation in the peripheral nerve because of increased conversion from glucose, via the enzyme aldose reductase. This is supported by the demonstration of elevated sorbitol levels in diabetic nerves *(75,76)*. Elevated sorbitol levels are associated with depletion of myoinositol, which is important in phosphoinositide metabolism, and reduction in $Na^+ K^+$-ATPase which has an important role of intracellular and extracellular sodium; hence, nerve membrane potential *(75,76)*. Indeed aldose reductase inhibitors administered to either animals *(77)* or man *(78)* result in an improvement in nerve conduction velocity. Some improvement in nerve fiber count has also been reported *(79)*, but there is no unequivocal demonstration of amelioration of symptoms and clinical signs in humans. Thus, there is as yet, no convincing evidence for the use of these agents in routine clinical practice particularly when one considers the possibility of side effects long term. A number of studies are currently taking place with newer and possibly more potent aldose reductase inhibitors, in "early" neuropathy, as in advanced neuropathy the nerve is highly disorganized and is unlikely to respond to treatment. The long-term safety of these drugs remains an important issue of concern for many clinicians.

Nonenzymatic Glycation

Glucose is highly reactive and free amino groups on proteins may be nonenzymatically glycated. From this reversible step there follows a series of reactions that are progressively irreversible; Amadori products and then advanced glycation end products (AGEs). Nonenzymatic glycosylation of proteins has been demonstrated in brain tubulin and peripheral nerve *(80,81)*. This process may be an important initiating factor for nerve demyelination *(68)* by interfering with axonal transport. AGE can also absorb ("quench") nitric oxide, a potent vasodilator, and hence lead to impaired nerve blood flow *(82)*. Aminoguanidine, which inhibits AGE formation, has been demonstrated to improve nerve conduction deficits and blood flow in experimental diabetes *(83)*, although its role in human diabetic neuropathy is still undetermined.

Neurotrophic Factors

Various neurotrophic factors support the growth and differentiation neurones. Among these neurotrophic agents are insulin-like growth factors-I and -II and the neurotrophin family. The neurotrophin family includes nerve growth factor (NGF), the levels of which are found to be reduced in experimental diabetes *(84)*. NGF treatment corrects some aspects of sensory neuropathy related to small-fiber dysfunction in diabetic rats. A recent clinical trial looking into the effect of parental NGF in human diabetic neuropathy was stopped because of lack of effect, and therefore the precise role of neurotrophic factors in human diabetic neuropathy and the potential use of trophic intervention in diabetic neuropathy remain undetermined.

Protein Kinase C Activation

Diabetes results in hyperactivity of vascular protein kinase C (PKC), in particular for the β-isoform *(85)*. Increased synthesis of diacylglycerol from glucose activates PKC. PKC activation is associated with abnormalities in vascular function seen in preclinical models of diabetes. In rats with streptozotocin diabetes, retinal blood flow is decreased in parallel with an increase in retinal PKC activity. PKC inhibitor treatment corrected deficits in retinal perfusion and prevented the early glomerular hyperfiltration and increased urinary albumin excretion in diabetic rats *(85)*. Moreover, a PKC inhibitor has recently been shown to correct nerve conduction velocity and perfusion deficits and to protect endothelial dependent relaxation, in diabetic rats *(86)*. There is currently a clinical trial of a PKC inhibitor in subjects with early distal symmetrical neuropathy taking place and the results are awaited.

Vascular Factors

The view that microvessel disease may be central to the pathogenesis of diabetic neuropathy is not new *(87)*. Severe neural microvascular disease has been demonstrated in subjects with clinical diabetic neuropathy *(88)*. Several workers have reported basal membrane thickening of endoneurial capillaries, degeneration of pericytes and hypoplasia, and swelling of endothelial cells and sometimes vessel closure (Fig. 3). The degree of microvascular disease has been correlated with the severity of neuropathy by Malik and colleagues *(89)*.

In vivo studies looking at the exposed sural nerve in human subjects have demonstrated epineurial arteriovenous shunting, which appears to result in a "steal" phenomenon diverting blood from the nutritive endoneurial circulation *(44,90)*. The consequent impairment of nerve blood flow causes a fall in endoneural oxygen tension *(91)*. In addition, several other studies provide indirect evidence supporting a vascular etiology for diabetic neuropathy. Strenuous exercise increases nerve blood flow, and thereby increases nerve conduction velocity by an average of 4 m/second in nonneuropathic subjects with diabetes *(45)*. However, this significant increase in nerve conduction velocity, with exercise, is absent *(45)* in neuropathic subjects as the nerve microvasculature is severely diseased *(90)*. Moreover, there is a strong correlation between nerve conduction velocity and lower limb transcutaneous oxygenation measurements in diabetes; macrovascular disease appears to exacerbate neuropathy and surgical restoration of perfusion improves nerve conduction velocity *(92)*. A recent epidemiological study has also found a strong correlation between diabetic neuropathy and cardiovascular risk factors including; body weight, hypertension, smoking, and reduced HDL cholesterol *(6)*.

In addition to human studies impairment of blood flow has been found to be an early feature in rats with streptozotocin diabetes. Several vasodilators have also been found to enhance nerve blood flow and nerve function in diabetic animals *(72)*. In human diabetic neuropathy ACE inhibitors have been found to improve nerve function *(93,94)*. The presence of severe microvascular changes in subjects with acute painful neuropathy of rapid glycemic control (insulin neuritis), hitherto thought to be purely metabolic in origin, provides an even more compelling evidence for the importance of microvascular factors in the pathogenesis of distal symmetric neuropathy *(44)*.

A number of metabolic derangements brought about by the diabetic state mentioned earlier (Table 4) have an impact on nerve perfusion, the vascular endothelium being a major target *(32)*. Oxidative stress, activation of the PKC system, and nonenzymatic glycation lead to reduced nerve nitric oxide. Occlusion of endoneural capillaries and the presence of hemorrheological abnormalities associated with diabetes further exacerbate the impairment of nerve blood flow leading to nerve hypoxia and hence nerve structural and functional abnormalities (Fig. 1).

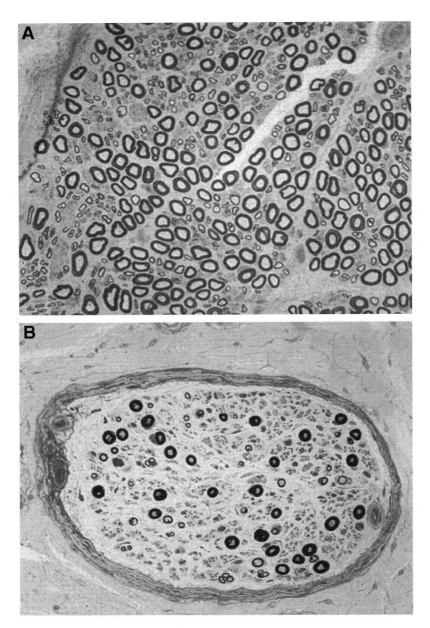

Fig. 1. Sural nerve biopsies from a healthy control (**A**) and a neuropathic patient (**B**). A considerable loss of myelinated nerve fibers can be seen in the neuropathic patient.

AUTONOMIC NEUROPATHY

Abnormalities of autonomic function are very common in subjects with longstanding diabetes, however, clinically significant autonomic dysfunction is uncommon. Several systems are affected (Table 5). Autonomic neuropathy has a gradual onset and is slowly progressive. The prevalence of diabetic autonomic neuropathy depends on the type of

Table 5
Autonomic Neuropathy

Autonomic neuropathy	Gastrointestinal
Cardiovascular	Gastroparesis
Resting tachycardia	Diarrhea
Heart rate abnormalities	Constipation
Edema	Dermatological
Postural hypotension	Gustatory sweating
Arrhythmias	Dry skin
Sudden death	Sudomotor dysfunction
Genitourinary	Arteriovenous shunting
Erectile dysfunction	Neurological
Retrograde ejaculation	Pupillary dysfunction
Atonic bladder	Respiratory
Bladder infection	Bronchoconstrictor dysfunction
Abnormal renal sodium handling	
Nephropathy	

population studied, and a number of tests of autonomic function employed. In the EURODIAB study the prevalence of autonomic neuropathy defined as the presence of two abnormal cardiovascular autonomic function tests, was 23%, and the prevalence increased with age, duration of diabetes, glycemic control, and presence of cardiovascular risk factors, in particular hypertension *(95)*.

Cardiovascular Autonomic Neuropathy

Cardiovascular autonomic neuropathy causes postural hypotension, change in peripheral blood flow, and may be a cause of sudden death.

Postural Hypotension

It is now generally accepted that a fall in systolic blood pressure of >20 mmHg is considered abnormal *(95)*. Coincidental treatment with tricyclic antidepressants for neuropathic pain, and diuretics may exacerbate postural hypotension, the chief symptom of which is dizziness on standing. The symptoms of postural hypotension can be disabling for some patients who may not be able to walk for more than a few minutes. In clinical practice the severity of dizziness does not correlate with the postural drop in blood pressure. There is increased mortality in subjects with postural hypotension, although the reasons for this are not fully clear. The management of subjects with postural hypotension poses major problems, and for some patients there may not be any satisfactory treatment. Current treatment includes improving glycemic control, advising patients to get up from the sitting or lying position slowly, treatment with fludrocortisone whereas carefully monitoring urea and electrolytes, and the use of support stockings. In severe cases "antigravity or space suits" which may compress the lower limbs, the α-1 adrenal receptor agonist, midodrine or occasionally octreotide may be effective.

Table 6
Reference Values for Cardiovascular Function Tests

	Normal	Borderline	Abnormal
Heart rate tests			
Heart rate response to standing up (30:15 ratio)	≥1.04	1.01–1.03	≤1
Heart rate response to deep breathing (maximum minus minimum heart rate)	≥15 beats/minute	11–14 beats/minute	≤10 beats/minute
Heart rate response to Valsalva maneuver (Valsalva ratio)	≥1.21	–	≤1.20
Blood pressure (BP) tests			
BP response to standing up (fall in systolic BP)	≤10 mmHg	11–29 mmHg	≥30 mmHg
BP response to sustained hand-grip (increase in diastolic BP)	≥16 mmHg	11–15 mmHg	≤10 mmHg

Changes in Peripheral Blood Flow

Autonomic neuropathy can cause arteriovenus shunting, with prominent veins in the neuropathic leg *(23)*. Leg-vein oxygen tension *(25)* and capillary pressure *(96)* are increased in the neuropathic leg resulting from sympathetic denervation. Thus, in the absence of peripheral vascular disease the neuropathic foot is warm, and this may be one of the factors that cause osteopenia associated with the development of Charcot neuroarthropathy *(24)*.

Cardiovascular Autonomic Function Tests

Five cardiovascular autonomic function tests are now widely used for the assessment of autonomic function. These tests are noninvasive, and do not require sophisticated equipment (all that is required is an electrocardiogram machine, an aneroid pressure gauge attached to a mouthpiece, a hand-grip dynamometer, and sphygmomanometer). Table 6 shows reference list for cardiovascular autonomic function test *(97)*.

Gastrointestinal Autonomic Neuropathy

Gastroparesis

Autonomic neuropathy can affect the upper gastrointestinal system by reducing esophageal motility (dysphagia and heartburn), and gastroparesis (reduced gastric emptying, vomiting, swings in blood sugar) *(98)*.

Management of diabetic gastroparesis includes optimization of glycemic control, the use of antiemetics (metoclopramide and domperidone), the use of the cholinergic agent which stimulates oesophageal motility (erythromycin which may enhance the activity of the gut peptide, motilin). Gastric electrical stimulation has recently been introduced as a treatment option in patients with drug refractory gastroparesis to increase the quality of life by alleviating nausea and vomiting frequencies *(99)*. Improvement in diabetic control has also been reported by one study *(100)*.

The diagnosis of gastroparesis is often made on clinical grounds by the evaluation of symptoms and sometimes the presence of succussion splash, whereas barium swallow and follow-through, and gastroscopy may reveal a large food residue in the stomach. Gastric motility and emptying studies can sometimes be performed in specialized units, and may help with diagnosis.

Severe gastroparesis causing recurrent vomiting, is associated with dehydration, swings in blood sugar and weight loss, and is therefore an indication for hospital admission. The patient should be adequately hydrated with intravenous fluids and blood sugar should be stabilized by intravenous insulin, antiemetics could be given intravenously and if the course of the gastroparesis is prolonged, total parenteral nutrition or feeding through a gastrostomy tube may be required.

Autonomic Diarrhea

The patient may present with diarrhea which tends to be worse at night, or alternatively some may present with constipation. Both the diarrhea and constipation respond to conventional treatment. Diarrhea associated with bacterial overgrowth may respond to treatment with a broad spectrum antibiotic such as erythromycin, tetracycline, or ampicillin.

Abnormal Sweating

Increased sweating usually affecting the face, and often brought about by eating (gustatory sweating) can be very embarrassing to patients. There may also be reduced sweating in the feet of affected patients, which can cause dry feet that are at risk of fissuring and hence infection. Unfortunately, there is no totally satisfactory treatment for gustatory sweating, although the anticholinergic drug poldine may be useful in a minority of patients.

Abnormalities of Bladder Function

Bladder dysfunction is a rare complication of autonomic neuropathy involving the sacral nerves. The patient presents with hesitancy of micturition, increased frequency of micturition, and in serious cases with urinary retention associated with overflow incontinence. Such a patient is prone to urinary tract infections. Ultrasound scan of the urinary tract, intravenous urography, and urodynamic studies may be required. Treatment maneuvers include mechanical methods of bladder emptying by applying suprapubic pressure, or the use of intermittent self-catheterization. Anticholinesterase drugs such as neostigmine or peridostigmine may be useful. Long-term indwelling catheterization may be required in some, but this unfortunately predisposes the patient to urinary tract infections and long-term antibiotic prophylaxis may be required.

MANAGEMENT OF DIABETIC NEUROPATHY

The two chief presentations of diabetic neuropathy are pain *(16)* and the numb foot which predisposes the patient to foot ulceration. The problems associated with the numb foot are discussed in detail elsewhere in this book. The treatment scenario for painful neuropathy is less than satisfactory as currently available treatment approaches are highly symptomatic and often ineffective *(16)*. As the pathological processes leading to diabetic nerve damage become to clear, potential therapeutic agents that have the capacity to prevent or reverse the neuropathic process, will emerge.

A careful history and examination of the patient is essential in order to exclude other possible causes of leg pain such as peripheral vascular disease, prolapsed intervertebral disks, spinal canal stenosis, and corda aquina lesions *(16)*. Unilateral leg pain should arouse a suspicion that the pain may be because of lumbar-sacral nerve root compression. These patients may well need to be investigated with a lumbar-sacral magnetic resonance imaging. Other causes of peripheral neuropathy such as excessive alcohol intake and B_{12} deficiency *(16)*. Where pain is the predominant symptom the quality and severity should be assessed. Neuropathic pain can be disabling in some patients and an empathic approach is essential. In general patients should be allowed to express their symptoms freely without too many interruptions. The psychological support of the patient's painful neuropathy is an important aspect of the overall management of the pain.

Glycemic Control

There is now little doubt that good blood sugar control prevents/delays the onset of diabetic neuropathy *(6,70,71)*. In addition, painful neuropathic symptoms are also improved by improving metabolic control, if necessary with the use of insulin in type 2 diabetes *(101)*. The first step in the management of painful neuropathy is a concerted effort aimed at improving glycemic control *(102)*.

Tricyclic Compounds

Tricyclic compounds are now regarded as the first line treatment for painful diabetic neuropathy *(18,102)*. A number of double blind clinical trials have confirmed their effectiveness beyond any doubt. As these drugs do have unwanted side effects such as drowsiness, anticholinergic side effects such as dry mouth and dizziness resulting from postural hypotension in those that have autonomic neuropathy, patients should be started on imipramine or amitriptyline at a low dose (25–50 mg taken before bed), the dose gradually titrated if necessary up to 150 mg/day. The mechanism of action of tricyclic compounds in improving neuropathic pain is not known, but their effect does not appear through their antidepressant property, as they appear to be effective even in those with a depressed mood *(103)*.

Anticonvulsants

Anticonvulsants, including carbamazepine, phenytoin, gabapentin *(104)*, more recently pregabalin *(105)* have also been found effective in the relief of more severe neuropathic pain. Unfortunately treatment with anticonvulsants is often complicated with troublesome side effects such as sedation, dizziness and ataxia, and therefore treatment should be started at a relatively low dose and gradually increased to maintenance dose of these drugs, when carefully looking for side effects. However, pregabalin and gabapentin appear to have less unwanted side effects and are hence better tolerated *(104,105)*.

Topical Capsaicin

Topical capsaicin (0.075%) applied sparingly three to four times per day to the affected area has also been found to relieve neuropathic pain. Topical capsaicin works by depleting substance "P" from nerve terminals, and there may be worsening of neuropathic symptoms for the first 2–4 weeks of application *(106)*.

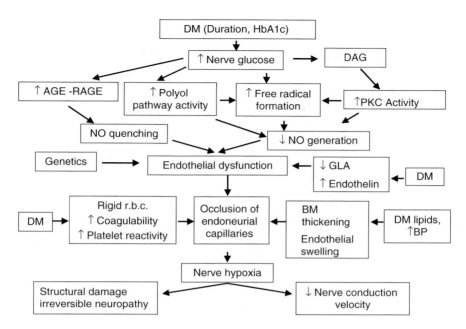

Fig. 2. Metabolic and vascular factors in the pathogenesis of diabetic distal symmetrical neuropathy.

Intravenous Lignocaine and Oral Mexiletine

Intravenous lignocaine at a dose of 5 mg/kg body wt with another 30 minutes with a cardiac monitor *in situ*, has also been found to be effective in relieving neuropathic pain for up to 2 weeks *(107)*. This form of treatment is useful in subjects that are having severe pain which is not responding to the above agents, although it does necessitate bringing the patient into hospital for a few hours. Oral mexiletine, which has similar structure to lignocaine, may have a beneficial effect at reducing neuropathic pain, although in the author's experience treatment is disappointing.

α-Lipoic Acid

Infusion of the antioxidant α-lipoic acid at a dose of 600 mg intravenously per day over a 3-week period (5–5–4 days), has also been found to be useful in reducing neuropathic pain *(108)*.

Opiates

The opiate derivative tramadol has been found effective in relieving neuropathic pain *(109)*. Recently, the combination of morphine and gabapentin was found to be more effective than either in the management of neuropathic pain *(110)*.

Management of Disabling Painful Neuropathy Not Responding to Pharmacological Treatment

Neuropathic pain can sometimes be extremely severe, interfering significantly with patients' sleep and daily activities. Unfortunately some patients are not helped by conventional pharmacological treatment. Such patients pose a major challenge for they are

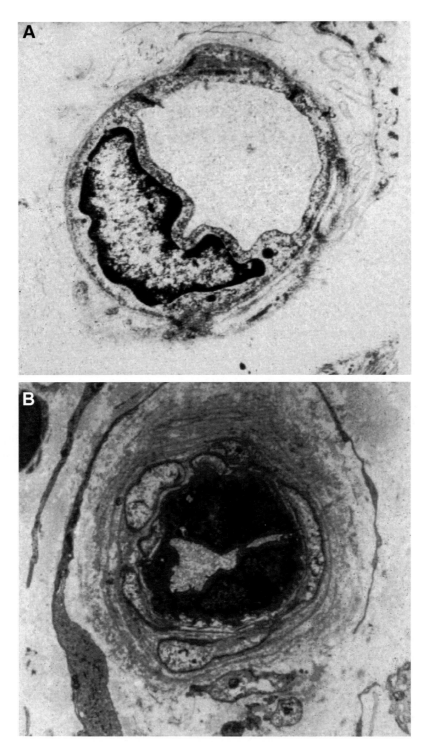

Fig. 3. Photomicrographs of endoneurial capillaries from sural nerve biopsies showing a normal (**A**) capillary from a subject with diabetes without neuropathy and a closed capillary from a subject with chronic diabetic neuropathy (**B**) showing endothelial cell proliferation and basement membrane thickening (Pictures from Dr. RA Malik).

severely distressed and sometimes wheelchair bound. A recent study has demonstrated that such patients may respond to electrical spinal cord stimulation which relieves both background and peak neuropathic pain *(19)*. This form of treatment is particularly advantageous, as the patient does not have to take any other pain relieving medications, with all their side effects. A recent follow-up of patients fitted with electrical spinal cord stimulators found that stimulators continued to be effective 5 years after implantation. Transcutaneous electrical nerve stimulation may also be beneficial for the relief of localized neuropathic pain in one limb.

REFERENCES

1. Shaw JE, Zimmet PZ. The epidemiology of diabetic neuropathy. *Diabetes Rev* 1999; 7:245–252.
2. Tesfaye S, Stephens L, Stephenson J, et al. The prevalence of diabetic neuropathy and its relation to glycemic control and potential risk factors: the EURODIAB IDDM Complications Study. *Diabetologia* 1996;39:1377–1384.
3. Young MJ, Boulton AJM, Macleod AF, Williams DRR, Sonksen PH. A multicentre study of the prevalence of diabetic peripheral neuropathy in the United Kingdom hospital clinic population. *Diabetologia* 1993;36:150–154.
4. Maser RE, Steenkiste AR, Dorman JS, et al. Epidemiological correlates of diabetic neuropathy. Report from Pittsburgh Epidemiology of Diabetes Complications Study. *Diabetes* 1989;38:1456–1461.
5. Ziegler D. Diagnosis, staging and epidemiology of diabetic peripheral neuropathy. *Diabetes Nutr Metab* 1994;7:342–348.
6. Tesfaye S, Chaturvedi N, Eaton SEM, Witte D, Ward JD, Fuller J. Vascular risk factors and diabetic neuropathy. *New Engl J Med* 2005;352:341–350.
7. Tesfaye S. Diabetic neuropathy: achieving best practice. *Br J Vasc Dis* 2003;3:112–117.
8. Eaton SEM, Tesfaye S. Clinical manifestations and measurement of somatic neuropathy. *Diabetes Rev* 1999;7:312–325.
9. Scott LA, Tesfaye S. Measurement of somatic neuropathy for clinical practice and clinical trials. *Curr Diab Rep* 2001;1:208–215.
10. Ward JD. Clinical features of diabetic neuropathy, in *Diabetic Neuropathy* (Ward JD, Goto Y, eds.). Wiley, Chichester, UK, 1990, pp. 281–296.
11. Watkins PJ, Edmonds ME. Clinical features of diabetic neuropathy, in *Textbook of Diabetes*, Volume 2 (Pickup J, Williams G eds.). 1997, pp. 50.1–50.20.
12. Bruyn GW, Garland H. Neuropathies of endocrine origin, in *Handbook of Clinical Neurology* (Vinken PJ, Bruyn GW eds.). Volume 8, North-Holland Publishing Co., Amsterdam, 1970, p. 29.
13. Thomas PK. Metabolic neuropathy. *J Roy Coll Phys (Lond)* 1973;7:154–174.
14. Low PA, Suarez GA. Diabetic neuropathies. *Baillieres Clin Neurol* 1995;4(3):401–425.
15. Andersen H, Jakobsen J. Motor function in diabetes. *Diabetes Rev* 1999;7:326–341.
16. Witte DR, Tesfaye S, Chaturvedi N, et al. Risk factors for cardiac autonomic neuropathy in type 1 diabetes mellitus. *Diabetologia* 2005;48:164–171.
17. Watkins PJ. Pain and diabetic neuropathy. *Br Med J* 1984;288:168, 169.
18. Tesfaye S, Price D. Therapeutic approaches in diabetic neuropathy and neuropathic pain, in *Diabetic Neuropathy* (Boulton AJM ed.). 1997, pp. 159–181.
19. Tesfaye S, Watt J, Benbow SJ, Pang KA, Miles J, MacFarlane IA. Electrical spinal cord stimulation for painful diabetic peripheral neuropathy. *Lancet* 1996;348:1696–1701.
20. Quattrini C, Tesfaye S. Understanding the impact of painful diabetic neuropathy. *Diabetes Metab Res Rev* 2003;Suppl. 1:S1–S8.
21. Ewing DJ, Borsey DQ, Bellavere F, Clarke BF. Cardiac autonomic neuropathy in diabetes: comparison of measures of R-R interval variation. *Diabetologia* 1981;21:18–24.

22. Ward JD. The diabetic leg. *Diabetologia* 1982;22:141–147.
23. Ward JD, Simms JM, Knight G, Boulton AJM, Sandler DA. Venous distension in the diabetic neuropathic foot (physical sign of arterio-venous shunting). *J R Soc Med* 1983;76:1011–1014.
24. Rajbhandari SM, Jenkins R, Davies C, Tesfaye S. Charcot neuroarthropathy in diabetes mellitus. *Diabetologia* 2002;45:1085–1096.
25. Boulton AJM, Scarpello JHB, Ward JD. Venous oxygenation in the diabetic neuropathic foot: evidence of arterial venous shunting? *Diabetologia* 1982;22:6–8.
26. Edmonds ME, Archer AG, Watkins PJ. Ephedrine: a new treatment for diabetic neuropathic oedema. *Lancet* 1983;i:548–551.
27. Said G, Slama G, Selva J. Progressive centripital degeneration of axons in small-fibre type diabetic polyneuropathy. A clinical and pathological study. *Brain* 1983;106:791.
28. Vinik AI, Park TS, Stansberry KB, Pittenger GL. Diabetic neuropathies. *Diabetologia* 2000;43:957–973.
29. Veves A, Young MJ, Manes C, et al. Differences in peripheral and autonomic nerve function measurements in painful and painless neuropathy: a clinical study. *Diabetes Care* 1994;17: 1200–1202.
30. Ward JD, Tesfaye S. Pathogenesis of diabetic neuropathy, in *Textbook of Diabetes* (Pickup J, Williams G eds.). Vol. 2, 1997, pp. 49.1–49.19.
31. Tesfaye S, Malik R, Ward JD. Vascular factors in diabetic neuropathy. *Diabetologia* 1994;37:847–854.
32. Cameron NE, Eaton SE, Cotter MA, Tesfaye S. Vascular factors and metabolic interactions in the pathogenesis of diabetic neuropathy. *Diabetologia* 2001;44:1973–1988.
33. Boulton AJM, Armstrong WD, Scarpello JHB, Ward JD. The natural history of painful diabetic neuropathy—a 4 year study. *Postgrad Med J* 1983;59:556–559.
34. Benbow SJ, Chan AW, Bowsher D, McFarlane IA, Williams G. A prospective study of painful symptoms, small fibre function and peripheral vascular disease in chronic painful diabetic neuropathy. *Diabet Med* 1994;11:17–21.
35. Chan AW, MacFarlane IA, Bowsher DR, Wells JC, Bessex C, Griffiths K. Chronic pain in patients with diabetes mellitus: comparison with non-diabetic population. *Pain Clin* 1990;3:147–159.
36. Young RJ, Zhou YQ, Rodriguez E, Prescott RJ, Ewing DJ, Clarke BF. Variable relationship between peripheral somatic and autonomic neuropathy in patients with different syndromes of diabetic polyneuropathy. *Diabetes* 1986;35:192–197.
37. Tsigos C, White A, Young RJ. Discrimination between painful and painless diabetic neuropathy based on testing of large somatic nerve and sympathetic nerve function. *Diabet Med* 1992;9:359–365.
38. Veves A, Manes C, Murray HJ, Young MJ, Boulton AJM. Painful neuropathy and foot ulceration in diabetic patients. *Diabetes Care* 1993;16:1187–1189.
39. Young MJ, Breddy JL, Veves A, Boulton AJ. The prediction of diabetic neuropathic foot ulceration using vibration perception thresholds. A prospective study. *Diabetes Care* 1994; 17(6):557–560.
40. Archer AG, Watkins PJ, Thomas PJ, Sharma AK, Payan J. The natural history of acute painful neuropathy in diabetes mellitus. *J Neurol Neurosurg Psychiatry* 1983;46:491–496.
41. Ellenberg M. Diabetic neuropathic cachexia. *Diabetes* 1974;23:418–423.
42. Guy RJC, Clark CA, Malcolm PN, Watkins PJ. Evaluation of thermal and vibration sensation in diabetic neuropathy. *Diabetologia* 1985;28:131.
43. Caravati CM. Insulin neuritis: a case report. *Va Med Mon* 1933;59:745–746.
44. Tesfaye S, Malik R, Harris N, et al. Arteriovenous shunting and proliferating new vessels in acute painful neuropathy of rapid glycemic control (insulin neuritis). *Diabetologia* 1996;39:329–335.
45. Tesfaye S, Harris N, Wilson RM, Ward JD. Exercise induced conduction velocity increment: a marker of impaired nerve blood flow in diabetic neuropathy. *Diabetologia* 1992;35:155–159.

46. Llewelyn JG, Thomas PK, Fonseca V, King RHM, Dandona P. Acute painful diabetic neuropathy precipitated by strict glycemic control. *Acta Neuropathol (Berl)* 1986;72:157– 163.

47. Kihara M, Zollman PJ, Smithson IL, et al. Hypoxic effect of endogenous insulin on normal and diabetic peripheral nerve. *Am J Physiol* 1994;266:E980–E985.

48. Clements RS, Bell DSH. Diagnostic, pathogenic and therapeutic aspects of diabetic neuropathy. *Spec Top Endocrinol Metab* 1982;3:1–43.

49. Matikainen E, Juntunen J. Diabetic neuropathy: epidemiological, pathogenetic, and clinical aspects with special emphasis on type 2 diabetes mellitus. *Acta Endocrinol Suppl (Copenh)* 1984;262:89–94.

50. Asbury AK, Aldredge H, Hershberg R, Fisher CM. Oculomotor palsy in diabetes mellitus: a clinicopathological study. *Brain* 1970;93:555–557.

51. Garland H. Diabetic amyotrophy. *Br Med J* 1955;2:1287–1290.

52. Coppack SW, Watkins PJ. The natural history of femoral neuropathy. *QJ Med* 1991;79:307–313.

53. Casey EB, Harrison MJG. Diabetic amyotrophy: a follow-up study. *Br Med J* 1972;1:656.

54. Garland H, Taverner D. Diabetic myelopathy. *Br Med J* 1953;1:1405.

55. Subramony SH, Willbourn AJ. Diabetic proximal neuropathy. Clinical and electromyographic studies. *J Neurol Sci* 1982;53:293–304.

56. Bastron JA, Thomas JE. Diabetic polyradiculoneuropathy: clinical and electromyographic findings in 105 patients. *Mayo Clin Proc* 1981;56:725–732.

57. Said G, Goulon-Goeau C, Lacroix C, Moulonguet A. Nerve biopsy findings in different patterns of proximal diabetic neuropathy. *Ann Neurol* 1994;33:559–569.

58. Zorilla E, Kozak GP. Ophthalmoplegia in diabetes mellitus. *Ann Intern Med* 1967;67: 968–976.

59. Goldstein JE, Cogan DG. Diabetic ophthalmoplegia with special reference to the pupil. *Arch Ophthalmol* 1960;64:592–600.

60. Leslie RDG, Ellis C. Clinical course following diabetic ocular palsy. *Postgrad Med J* 1978; 54:791, 792.

61. Dreyfuss PM, Hakim S, Adams RD. Diabetic ophthalmoplegia. *Arch Neurol Psychiatry* 1957;77:337–349.

62. Ellenberg M. Diabetic truncal mononeuropathy—a new clinical syndrome. *Diabetes Care* 1978;1:10–13.

63. Boulton AJM, Angus E, Ayyar DR, Weiss R. Diabetic thoracic polyradiculopathy presenting as abdominal swelling. *BMJ* 1984;289:798, 799.

64. Dyck PJ, Kratz KM, Karnes JL, et al. The prevalence by staged severity of various types of diabetic neuropathy, retinopathy, and nephropathy in a population-based cohort: the Rochester Diabetic Neuropathy Study. *Neurology* 1993;43:817–824.

65. Clayburgh RH, Beckenbaugh RD, Dobyns JH, Carpal tunnel release in patients with diffuse peripheral neuropathy. *Hand Surg* 1987;12A:380–383.

66. White JES, Bullock RF, Hudgson P, Home PD, Gibson GJ. Phrenic neuropathy in association with diabetes. *Diabet Med* 1992;9:954–956.

67. Malik RA. The pathology of diabetic neuropathy. *Diabetes* 1997;46 (Suppl. 2):S50–S53.

68. Bradley JL, Thomas PK, King RH, et al. Myelinated nerve fibre regeneration in diabetic sensory polyneuropathy: correlation with type of diabetes. *Acta Neuropathol (Berl)* 1995;90:403–410.

69. Stevens MJ, Feldman EL, Thomas T, Greene DA. Pathogenesis of diabetic neuropathy, in *Contemporary Endocrinology: Clinical Management of Diabetic Neuropathy* (Veves A, ed.). Humana Press, Totowa NJ, 1998, pp. 13–48.

70. Diabetes Control and Complications Trial Research Group. The effect of intensive diabetes therapy on the development and progression of neuropathy. *Ann Intern Med* 1995;122: 561–568.

71. United Kingdom Prospective Diabetes Study Group. Intensive blood glucose control with sulphonylureas or insulin compared with conventional treatment and risk of complications in patients with type 2 diabetes. *Lancet* 1998;352:837–853.

72. Cameron NE, Cotter MA. The relationship of vascular changes to metabolic factors in diabetes mellitus and their role in the development of peripheral nerve complications. *Diabetes Metab Rev* 1994;10:189–224.

73. Cameron NE, Cotter MA, Archbald V, Dines KC, Maxfield EK. Anti-oxidant and pro-oxidant effects on nerve conduction velocity, endoneurial blood flow and oxygen tension in non-diabetic and streptozotocin-diabetic rats. *Diabetologia* 1994;37:449–459.

74. Gabbay KH, Merola LO, Field RA. Sorbitol pathway: presence in nerve and cord with substrate accumulation in diabetes. *Science* 1966;151:209–210.

75. Dyck PJ, Zimmerman BR, Vilan TH, et al. Nerve glucose, fructose, sorbitol, myo-inositol, and fiber degeneration in diabetic neuropathy. *N Engl J Med* 1988;319:542–548.

76. Ward JD, Baker RWR, Davis B. Effect of blood sugar control on the accumulation of sorbitol and fructose in nervous tissue. *Diabetes* 1972;21:1173–1178.

77. Tomlinson DR, Moriarty RJ, Mayer H. Prevention and reversal of defective axonal transport and motor nerve conduction velocity in rats with experimental diabetes by treatment with addose reductase inhibitor Sorbinil. *Diabetes* 1984;33:470–476.

78. Judzewitsch RG, Jaspan JB, Polonsky KS, et al. Aldose reductase inhibition improves nerve conduction velocity in diabetic patients. *N Engl J Med* 1983;308:119–125.

79. Sima AAF, Bril V, Nathaniel V, McEwen TAG, Greene DA. Regeneration and repair of myelinated fibres in sural nerve biopsy specimens from patients with diabetic neuropathy treated with sorbinil. *N Engl J Med* 1988;319:548–555.

80. Williams SK, Howarth NL, Devenny JJ, Bitensky MW. Structural and functional consequences of increased tubulin glycosylation in diabetes mellitus. *Proc Natl Acad Sci USA* 1982;79:6546–6550.

81. Vlassara H, Brownlee M, Cerami A. Accumulation of diabetic rat peripheral nerve myelin by macrophages increases with the presence of advanced glycosylation end products. *J Exp Med* 1984;160:197.

82. Bucala R, Cerami A, Vlassara H. Advanced glycosylation end products in diabetic complications. Biochemical basis and prospects for therapeutic intervention. *Diabetes Rev* 1995;3:258–268.

83. Kihara J, Schmelzer JD, Poduslo JF, Curran GL, Nickander KK, Low PA. Aminoguanidine effects on nerve blood flow, vascular permeability, electrophysiology and oxygen free radicals. *Proc Natl Acad Sci USA* 1991;88:6107–6111.

84. Hellweg R, Hartung HD. Endogenous levels of nerve growth factor (NGF) are altered in experimental diabetes mellitus: a possible role for NGF in the pathogenesis of diabetic neuropathy. *J Neurosci Res* 1990;26:258–267.

85. Koya D, King GL. Protein kinase C activation and the development of diabetic complications. *Diabetes* 1998;47:859–866.

86. Cameron NE, Cotter MA, Lai K, Hohman TC. Effects of protein kinase C inhibition on nerve function, blood flow and Na+, K+ ATPase defects in diabetic rats. *Diabetes* 1997;46 (Suppl. 1):31A.

87. Fagerberg SE. Diabetic neuropathy: a clinical and histological study on the significance of vascular affections. *Acta Med Scand* 1959;164 (Suppl. 345):5–81.

88. Giannini C, Dyck PJ. Ultrastructural morphometric abnormalities of sural nerve endoneurial microvessels in diabetes mellitus. *Ann Neurol* 1994;36:408–415.

89. Malik RA, Newrick PG, Sharma AK, et al. Microangiopathy in human diabetic neuropathy: relationship between capillary abnormalities and the severity of neuropathy. *Diabetologia* 1998;32:92–102.

90. Tesfaye S, Harris N, Jakubowski J, et al. Impaired blood flow and arterio-venous shunting in human diabetic neuropathy: a novel technique of nerve photography and fluorescein angiography. *Diabetologia* 36:1266–1274.

91. Newrick PG, Wilson AJ, Jakubowski J, Boulton AJM, Ward JD. Sural nerve oxygen tension in diabetes. *Br Med J* 1986;193:1053, 1054.

92. Young MJ, Veves A, Smith JV, Walker MG, Boulton AJM. Restoring lower limb blood flow improves conduction velocity in diabetic patients. *Diabetologia* 1995;38:1051–1054.

93. Reja A, Tesfaye S, Harris ND, Ward JD. Is ACE inhibition with lisinopril helpful in diabetic neuropathy? *Diabetic Med* 1995;12:307–309.

94. Malik RA, Williamson S, Abbott CA, et al. Effect of the angiotensin converting enzyme inhibitor trandalopril on human diabetic neuropathy: a randomised controlled trial. *Lancet* 1998;352:1978–1981.

95. Kempler P, Tesfaye S, Chaturvedi N, et al. The prevalence of autonomic neuropathy and potential risk factors: the EURODIAB IDDM Complications Study. *Diabetic Med* 2002;19:900–909.

96. Rayman G. Diabetic neuropathy and micro circulation. *Diabetes Rev* 1999;7:261–274.

97. Ewing DJ, Martyn CN, Young RJ, Clarke BF. The value of cardiovascular autonomic function tests: ten years experience in diabetes. *Diabetes Care* 1985;8:491–498.

98. Horowitz M, Fraser R. Disordered gastric motor function in diabetes mellitus. *Diabetologia* 1994;37:543–551.

99. Lin Z, Forster J, Sarosiek I, McCallum RW. Treatment of diabetic gastroparesis by high-frequency gastric electrical stimulation. *Diabetes Care* 2004;27(5):1071–1076.

100. van der Voort IR, Becker JC, Dietl KH, Konturek JW, Domschke W, Pohle T. Gastric electrical stimulation results in improved metabolic control in diabetic patients suffering from gastroparesis. *Exp Clin Endocrinol Diabetes* 2005;113(1):38–42.

101. Boulton AJM, Drury J, Clarke B, Ward JD. Continuous subcutaneous insulin infusion in the management of painful diabetic neuropathy. *Diabetes Care* 1982;5:386–390.

102. Boulton AJM, Malik RA, Arezzo JC, Sosenko JM. Diabetic somatic neuropathies. *Diabetes Care* 2004;27:1458–1486.

103. Max MB, Culnane M, Schafer SC, et al. Amitriptyline relieves diabetic neuropathy pain in patients with normal or depressed mood. *Neurology* 1987;37:596–598.

104. Backonja M, Beydoun A, Edwards KR, et al. Gabapentin for the symptomatic treatment of painful neuropathy in patients with diabetes mellitus: a randomised controlled trial. *JAMA* 1998;280:1831–1836.

105. Lesser H, Sharma U, LaMoreaux L, Poole RM. Pregabalin relieves symptoms of painful diabetic neuropathy: a randomized controlled trial. *Neurology* 2004;63(11):2104–2110.

106. Capsaicin Study Group. The effect of treatment with capsaicin on daily activities of patients with painful diabetic neuropathy. *Diabetes Care* 1992;15:159–165.

107. Kastrup J, Angelo H, Petersen P, Dejgard A, Hilstead J. Treatment of chronic painful neuropathy with intravenous lidocaine infusion. *Br Med J* 1986;292:173.

108. Zeigler D, Hanefeld M, Ruhnau KJ, et al. Treatment of symptomatic diabetic peripheral neuropathy with anti-oxidant alpha-lipoic acid: a 3-week multicentre randomised controlled trial (ALADIN Study). *Diabetologia* 1995;38:1425–1433.

109. Harati Y, Gooch C, Swenson M, et al. Double-blind randomized trial of tramadol for the treatment of the pain of diabetic neuropathy. *Neurology* 1998;50(6):1842–1846.

110. Gilron I, Bailey JM, Tu D, Holden RR, Weaver DF, Houlden RL. Morphine, gabapentin, or their combination for neuropathic pain. *N Engl J Med* 2005;352(13):1324–1334.

7

Microvascular Changes in the Diabetic Foot

Thanh Dinh, DPM and Aristidis Veves, MD, DSc

INTRODUCTION

It has been nearly half a century since the concept of "small vessel disease" was introduced as a unique entity in the microvasculature of the patient with diabetes. This misconception was arrived at through a retrospective histological study demonstrating the presence of periodic acid Schiff-positive material occluding the arterioles in amputated limb specimens of patients with diabetes *(1)*. From these observations, Goldenberg and his colleagues deduced that the deposits in the small and medium-sized arterioles were the hallmark of vascular disease in the patient with diabetes. Perpetuation of this erroneous idea led to the belief that preferential occlusion of the small vessels in the patient with diabetes produced a poorer prognosis with limited revascularization options.

Since then, numerous studies have successfully refuted the notion of "small vessel disease." In a blinded, prospective analysis of amputated limbs, periodic acid Schiff staining showed a similar meager pattern of occlusive disease in both diabetic and nondiabetic limbs at the arteriole level *(2)*. Using a sophisticated casting technique, Conrad also demonstrated a lack of significant occlusive disease at the arteriole level in both the patients with and without diabetes *(3)*. Furthermore, vascular reactivity in the vessels of patients with diabetes has been shown to be comparable to those of patients without diabetes based on physiological studies involving the administration of a papaverine (a vasodilator) into femoro-popliteal bypass grafts *(4)*. These data, coupled with a vast clinical experience of nearly three decades of successful arterial reconstruction in patients with diabetes, have thoroughly dispelled the notion of diabetic "small vessel disease" *(5)*.

However, recent work suggests that although an occlusive disease of the microcirculation does not exist, the microcirculation (predominantly capillaries and arterioles) is impaired in the patient with diabetes. In simplest terms, microvascular dysfunction in diabetes may be described by an increased vascular permeability and impaired autoregulation of blood flow and vascular tone. It is postulated that metabolic derangements as a result of hyperglycemia and insulin resistance work synergistically to cause microvascular dysfunction. Consequently, these metabolic alterations produce functional and structural changes at multiple levels within the arteriolar and capillary level.

From: *The Diabetic Foot, Second Edition*
Edited by: A. Veves, J. M. Giurini, and F. W. LoGerfo © Humana Press Inc., Totowa, NJ

STRUCTURAL CHANGES IN THE MICROCIRCULATION

Basement Membrane Thickening

Structurally, the most notable changes in the microcirculation involve thickening of the basement membrane and an observed reduction in the capillary size *(6,7)*. However, the density of the skin capillaries does not differ from healthy subjects *(8)*. These structural changes are more pronounced in the legs, likely the result of increased hydrostatic pressures in that part of the body *(9)*. The extent of basement membrane thickening has also been observed to be related to the level of glycemic control, with increased basement thickening in poorly controlled patients with diabetes *(10)*.

In the diabetic foot, basement membrane thickening has been demonstrated in the muscle capillaries *(11)*. The sequence of events leading to basement membrane thickening begins with the increased hydrostatic pressure and shear force in the microcirculation. This is thought to evoke an injury response on the part of the microvascular endothelium with subsequent release of extravascular matrix proteins. Subsequently, thickening of the basement membrane with arteriolar hyalinosis occurs *(12)*.

Because changes in the basement membrane can affect numerous cellular functions, such as vascular permeability, cellular adhesion, proliferation, differentiation, and gene expression, alterations in its components may cause vascular dysfunctions. Thickening of the basement membrane impairs the normal exchange of nutrients and activated leukocyte migration between the capillary and interstitium. Furthermore, the elastic properties of the capillary vessel walls are diminished, limiting their ability to vasodilate *(13)*. As a result, the normal hyperemic response to injury is impaired, limiting the compensatory arteriolar dilatation in response to local injury, resulting in a reduced hyperemic response *(14)*. It is important to note that basement membrane thickening does not appear to lead to narrowing of the capillary lumen, instead arteriolar blood flow is observed at normal levels or even increased despite these changes *(15)*.

FUNCTIONAL CHANGES IN THE MICROCIRCULATION

The observed failure of the microcirculation to vasodilate in response to injury has been described as a functional ischemia and has been demonstrated to be a result of a number of factors at play in the microcirculation of the patient with diabetes. Alteration in the microcirculation of the foot has been postulated to be an important factor in the poor wound healing associated with chronic diabetic foot ulcerations. Recent work from our unit has addressed these changes, with specific emphasis placed on the changes in the diabetic foot microcirculation, nerve function, and muscle metabolism.

DIABETIC FOOT MICROCIRCULATION

The resting total skin microcirculation in the diabetic foot is comparable with that of the nondiabetic foot, when peripheral neuropathy is absent. However, when neuropathy is present, the capillary blood flow has been shown to be reduced *(16,17)*. This may indicate a maldistribution of blood flow to the skin, with a resultant functional ischemia. As previously mentioned, the hyperemic response is impaired in the diabetic microcirculation, thereby failing to achieve maximal blood flow following injury. Development of new techniques to evaluate the microcirculation has expanded our understanding of these functional changes. Therefore, review of these techniques may be of particular importance.

Methods of Evaluating the Microcirculation of the Feet

Recent technological advances over the past decade have enabled us to evaluate the functional microcirculation of the feet. Methods such as laser Doppler flowmetry, flow-video microscopy, cannulation measurements of capillary pressure, and transcutaneous oxygen tension measurements have all been used. The most commonly used technique, and the one used in our lab, for evaluating blood flow in the skin remains laser Doppler flowmetry.

Laser Doppler Flowmetry

This method is considered the most widely accepted technique for evaluating capillary blood flow in the skin microcirculation based on its ease of use and reproducibility. Presently employed in our unit, this method uses a red laser light that is transmitted to the skin though a fiberoptic cable. The frequency shift of light back-scattered from the moving red blood cells beneath the probe tip is used to give a measure of the superficial microvascular perfusion *(17)*.

There are two types of laser probes available for use with this method, a single-point laser probe or a real-time laser scanner. The single-point laser probe measures the microvascular blood flow at a single point in the skin, and has been used for evaluating the hyperemic response to a heat stimulus, or for evaluating the nerve–axon-related hyperemic response. Measurement of the hyperemic response to a heat stimulus is performed by first taking baseline blood flow measurements. Next, the skin is heated to 44°C for 20 minutes using a small brass heater, or in our experience, maintaining the ambient room temperature at this level. Following this, the maximum blood flow is determined by the magnitude of blood flow change in response to heat.

In conjunction with the technique of iontophoresis and the addition of a second probe, the single-point laser probe method can be used to assess the integrity of the nerve–axon reflex. The technique of iontophoresis involves the delivery of a vasoactive substance (acetylcholine chloride or sodium nitroprusside [SNP]) transdermally with a low-voltage current (200 µA) in order to effect vasodilation. In the two single-point laser probe technique, the first probe is exposed to acetylcholine, in order to measure the blood flow to a specified area of skin. The second probe is situated in close proximity (5 mm) to the first probe, and consequently measures the indirect effect of the iontophoresed acetylcholine. The indirect effect of the acetylcholine results from stimulation of the C-nociceptive nerve fibers and therefore, the nerve–axon reflex hyperemic response.

The method of laser scanning also uses the technique of iontophoresis to evaluate the endothelium-dependent microvascular reactivity. More specifically, a device consisting of two chambers that accommodate two single-point laser probes are applied to the skin. A small quantity (<1 mL) of the vasoactive substance is placed in the chamber whereas a second nonactive electrode is placed 10–15 cm away from the chamber. A constant current of 200 µA is applied, creating movement of the solution toward the skin, causing vasodilation. Iontophoresis of acetylcholine chloride measures the endothelium-dependent vasodilation, whereas SNP measures the endothelium-independent vasodilation.

Following iontophoresis of the vasoactive substance, the adhesive device is removed and the area of skin is scanned with a laser Doppler scanner. The laser Doppler perfusion imager uses 1-mW helium–neon laser beam of 633-nm wavelength to sequentially scan the area of skin. Increased blood flow at the skin level is recorded by the scanner and expressed in volts. This technique has been validated against direct measurements of the capillary flow velocity with consistent measurements achieved.

Flow-Video Microscopy

Flow-video microscopy enables measurements of capillary blood flow along with such parameters as average flow velocity, peak postocclusive hyperemic flow velocity, and the response to other physiological maneuvers. With the use of an image-shearing monitor, the capillary red cell column width is calculated. This is performed by lighting mercury vapor onto skin that has previously been brushed with a thin film of oil or varnish in order to limit the scattering of light. The image of the moving blood elements can then be recorded with a low-light sensitive video system *(18)*. More recently, a digitized system has been developed that is capable of recording continuous capillary blood flow. Measurements are then calculated through an integrated software program. However, this method may underestimate the true capillary lumen resulting from the unvisualized marginal plasma layer.

Capillary Pressure Measurements

The measurement of capillary pressure involves direct cannulation of a single vessel. Following cannulation of the vessel, the transmitted pressure can be measured manometrically or through use of an electronic device. This invasive technique is capable of detecting small changes in the capillary pressure as low as 1–2 mmHg. Additionally, it has the added benefit of being able to measure the capillary pressure continuously. However, the procedure can be complex and may require significant expertise.

Transcutaneous Oxygen Tension Measurements

The measurement of oxygen transcutaneously can be performed based on the fact that oxygen is capable of diffusing throughout the body tissue and skin. Although the rate of diffusion is very low at normal surface body temperature, application of heat to a localized area can sufficiently enhance the flow of oxygen through the dermis to allow for noninvasive measurement of the capillary oxygen level. However, these measurements can be inaccurate as they appear to fluctuate with the skin temperature and room temperature.

MICROVASCULAR REACTIVITY IN THE DIABETIC FOOT

Functional changes in the microcirculation appear to impact the ability of the microcirculation to vasodilate in periods of stress or injury. Clinical examination of the neuropathic diabetic foot with an ulcer may demonstrate a warm foot with palpable pulses and distended veins. Although there appears to be no reduction in blood flow to the foot, the blood flow to the skin microcirculation may be reduced *(19,20)* through shunting of blood from the nutritional capillaries to the subpapillary arteriovenous shunts of a much lower resistance *(21)*.

As these shunts are innervated by sympathetic nerves, the existence of diabetic autonomic neuropathy with sympathetic denervation may lead to opening of these shunts with a resultant augmentation of the maldistribution of blood between the nutritional capillaries and subpapillary vessels *(8,22)*. Ultimately, arteriovenous shunting further aggravates the functionally ischemic foot, as evidenced by studies using venous occlusion plethysmography, Doppler sonography, and venous oxygen tension measurements *(23)*.

Much work has been done in the past decade to investigate why the microvasculature in diabetes fails to respond appropriately to stress and injury. The recent development of noninvasive techniques that can reliably quantify blood flow in the skin microcirculation and evaluate endothelial function has made it possible to study changes in microvascular function in patients with diabetes. Those findings will be discussed in detail.

Endothelial Dysfunction

The vascular endothelium plays an important role in controlling the microvascular tone by synthesizing and releasing substances such as prostacyclin, endothelin, prostaglandins, and nitric oxide that modulate the vasomotor tone and prevent thrombosis. Nitric oxide is the most important vasodilator substance responsible for endothelium-dependent vasodilation. After its secretion from the endothelium it diffuses to the adjacent smooth muscle cells and stimulates the guanylate cyclase enzyme which leads to smooth muscle relaxation and vasodilation *(24)*.

There is substantial evidence that endothelial function is abnormal in patients with both type 1 (insulin-dependent) and type 2 (noninsulin-dependent) diabetes mellitus *(25,26)*. As a result, the causes of endothelial function have been postulated to include both hyperglycemia and hyperinsulinemia as possible mediators of abnormal endothelium-dependent responses. The significance of endothelial dysfunction on the micro- and macrocirculation and the variety of proposed mechanisms affecting normal function will be discussed in further detail.

Endothelium-Dependent Vasodilation

The majority of studies agree that the endothelium-dependent vasodilation in the large vessels is impaired in diabetes, irrespective of the presence or absence of long-term complications *(25–29)*. Initial studies of endothelium-dependent vasodilation used venous occlusion plethysmography whereas subsequent studies employed flow-mediated vasodilation, a noninvasive technique. Through these techniques, endothelium-dependent vasodilation has been shown to be impaired in adolescents with type 1 diabetes, a population that is generally spared from the micro and macrovascular complications of diabetes *(30)*. This finding suggests that endothelial dysfunction is present before the development of these vascular complications and may play an important role in their development. Finally, endothelial function in type 1 diabetes has been shown to be associated with total cholesterol, red cell folate, blood glucose levels, and duration of diabetes *(31–33)*.

In the past decade, extensive research effort has focused on the relationship of type 2 diabetes and vascular disease. Thus, it is currently well established that the endothelium-dependent vasodilation are impaired in both the micro- and macrocirculation in type 2 diabetes. Furthermore, there is almost universal agreement that changes in the endothelial function precedes the development of diabetes and is present in the prediabetic stage. It is also of interest that endothelial dysfunction is associated with insulin resistance in subjects without diabetes, suggesting a cause–effect relationship of these two conditions.

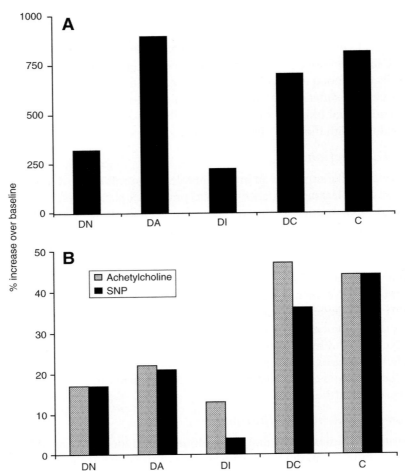

Fig. 1. (A) The maximal hyperemic response to heating of foot skin at 44°C for at least 20 min (expressed as the percentage of increase over baseline flow measured by a single-point laser probe) is reduced in the diabetic patient with neuropathy (DN) and in diabetic patients with neuropathy and peripheral vascular disease (DI) when compared with diabetic patients with Charcot arthropathy (DA), patients with diabetes without complications (DC), and normal control subjects (C) ($p < 0.001$). **(B)** The response to iontophoresis of acetylcholine and sodium nitroprusside (expressed as the percentage of increase over baseline flow measured by laser scanner imager). The response to acetylcholine is equally reduced in the DN, DI, and DA groups when compared with the DC and C groups ($p < 0.001$). The response to SNP was more pronounced in the DI group and also reduced in the DN and DA groups compared with the DC and C groups ($p < 0.001$) *(26)*.

Findings from our unit further corroborate impairment of endothelium-dependent vasodilation in patients with diabetes. We have evaluated the effect of neuropathy and hypoxia on foot circulation on five groups of patients, patients with diabetes and neuropathy, patients with neuropathy and clinical signs of vascular disease, patients with diabetes and Charcot neuroarthropathy, nonneuropathic patients with diabetes, and healthy controls. *(27)* (Fig. 1). The endothelial-dependent vasodilation was studied by using laser Doppler imaging to measure the vasodilatory response to iontophoresis of acetylcholine. Administration of acetylcholine directly stimulates the production of nitric oxide, resulting in vasodilation. We found that the vasodilatory response to acetylcholine was reduced in patients with neuropathy, neuropathy and vascular disease, and Charcot neuroarthropathy, whereas no difference was found between nonneuropathic subjects and the healthy controls. Additionally, the vasodilatory response was not diminished in subjects with neuropathy and vascular disease in comparison with subjects with neuropathy alone.

Interestingly enough, impairment in the microcirculation was found to be present in the absence of large vessel disease. These findings implied that the main reason for reduced microvascular reactivity was the presence of neuropathy, as indicated by the fact that no abnormalities were found in the nonneuropathic patients with diabetes. Further support for this claim is provided by the findings that the coexistence of neuropathy and vascular disease did not result in a greater decrease in endothelium-dependent vasodilation than that resulting from neuropathy alone.

Endothelium-Independent Vasodilation

Regarding the endothelium-independent vasodilation, which evaluates the function of the vascular smooth muscle cell, the majority of published studies have been conflicting. However, it should be emphasized that most of the early studies that demonstrated no impairment of endothelium-independent vasodilation in type 1 diabetes composed of a small number of subjects whereas the power analysis was mainly based on the results from the endothelial function. Thus, the possibility of not detecting a difference because of methodological problems cannot be excluded. Despite contrary initial reports, there is mounting evidence that endothelium-independent vasodilation is impaired in type 1 diabetes, even in diabetes without secondary complications *(34,35)*.

In the presence of secondary complications such as microalbuminuria in type 1 diabetes, there exists conflicting data on the function of endothelium-independent vasodilation. An early study found that endothelium-independent vasodilation is normal in the presence of microalbuminuria *(36)*, whereas subsequent work has revealed that endothelium-independent vasodilation dysfunction was present in the absence of microalbuminuria, potentially predicting the development of microalbuminuria in type 1 diabetes and other cardiovascular complications *(37–40)*.

Endothelium-independent vasodilation in type 2 diabetes has also met with contradictory early results. However, most studies agree that endothelium-independent vasodilation in type 2 diabetes is unchanged in the macrocirculation, and diminished, along with impairment of the vascular smooth muscle function, in the microcirculation *(41,42)*. Of note, these changes were also found in patients with type 2 diabetes without secondary complications of the disease *(42)*.

In our unit, endothelium-independent vasodilation was also found to be decreased in patients with diabetes *(17)*. (Fig. 1) The endothelium-independent vasodilation was studied using laser Doppler imaging to measure the vasodilatory response to iontophoresis of SNP. This response was most severely reduced in diabetic patients with vascular disease, suggesting that the endothelium-independent response may be spared. Because acetylcholine stimulates the production of nitric oxide, it was surmised that an impaired nitric oxide production was responsible for the impaired vasodilatory response observed.

Mechanisms of Endothelial Dysfunction

In 1980, Furchgott and Zawadzki *(43)* discovered that arterial vasodilation was dependent on an intact endothelium and its release of a substance they called endothelium-derived relaxing factor, which causes arterial smooth muscle relaxation in response to acetylcholine and other vasodilators. Later identified as endothelial-derived nitric oxide (EDNO), its roles include activation of vascular smooth muscle guanylatecyclase, elevation of cGMP levels, and may increase Na^+, K^+-ATPase activity *(44)*. In addition to acetylcholine, there appear to be a number of substances that produce EDNO-mediated vasodilation. These other substances appear to cause vasodilary effects through the nitric oxide pathway, with insulin mediating the vasodilation through modulating the synthesis and release of EDNO *(45,46)*.

A variety of mechanisms have been proposed for endothelial dysfunction, principally abnormalities in the EDNO pathway. The main mechanisms that are involved include the activation of protein kinase C (PKC), the increased vasoconstrictor protanoids, reduction in Na^+, K^+-ATPase activity, poly (adenosine diphosphate [ADP]-ribose) polymerase (PARP) activation, alterations in oxidative stress, and advanced glycosylated end products (AGEs).

Increased vascular permeability is another characteristic abnormality observed as a result of endothelial dysfunction in diabetes. This can occur as early as 4–6 weeks after the onset of diabetes and is probably caused by a loss of integrity in the tight junctions between the endothelial cells *(47)*. Increased activation of PKC, a key player in intercellular signal transduction for hormone and cytokines, may be the result of hyperglycemia. PKC inhibitors have also been used to restore impaired vascular reactivity, lending support to the role of increased PKC activation in endothelial dysfunction *(41)*. Finally, PKC activation can also regulate vascular permeability and neovascularization via the expression of growth factors, such as vascular endothelial growth factor (VEGF)/vascular permeability factor.

Experimental studies in diabetic animals have also indicated that abnormal endothelial production of vasoconstrictor prostanoids may be a cause of endothelial cell dysfunction. Increased levels of thromboxane (TXA_2) and prostaglandin (PGH_2) have been isolated from segments of diabetic vascular tissue. In human studies, however, the role of vasoconstrictor prostanoids is less clear. Flow-dependent vasodilation in healthy subjects, which may be used as an index of endothelial function is unaffected by aspirin, thus demonstrating that it is entirely mediated by EDNO and independent of vasoactive prostanoids *(48)*.

Na^+, K^+-ATPase is an integral component of the sodium pump and is involved in the maintenance of cellular integrity and functions of contractility, growth, and differentiation. Therefore, impairment of this mechanism can lead to vascular dysfunction. It is well established that activity of the Na^+, K^+-ATPase is generally decreased in the vascular tissues of patients with diabetes.

Recent work has also shed light on the role of PARP in endothelial function *(49)*. PARP is a nuclear enzyme that responds to oxidative DNA damage by activating an inefficient cellular metabolic cycle, often leading to cell necrosis. Interestingly, PARP activation has been observed in patients with diabetes as well as those healthy patients at risk for developing diabetes. This finding suggests that changes in the microcirculation resulting from PARP activation may begin in the prediabetic state.

In a study performed in our unit *(45)*, nondiabetic controls were compared with three groups: those with type 2 diabetes, those with glucose intolerance only, and those with a family history of type 2 diabetes but no intolerance themselves. PARP activation was higher in all three diabetes-associated groups than in the healthy controls. The activation of PARP was associated with changes in the vascular reactivity of the skin microcirculation in from biopsies taken from these subjects, supporting the hypothesis that PARP activation contributes to changes in microvascular reactivity. Further study is required to prove this association and possible benefits from inhibiting this activation.

It has recently been proposed that oxidative stress contributes to the development of diabetic vascular complications, through an increased production of oxygen-derived free radicals. This increased production in diabetes directly inactivates endothelium-derived nitric oxide, thereby reducing the bioavailability of EDNO *(50)*. In animal models, endothelium-derived free radicals impaired EDNO-mediated vasodilation. In human studies, administration of vitamin E (400 IU/day), a potent free radical scavenger, had no apparent effect on cardiovascular outcomes in patients with diabetes with complications *(51)*. However, early studies showed that high-dose vitamin E (1800 IU/day) normalized hemodynamic abnormalities, suggesting that administration of an antioxidant may reduce the risks of diabetic vascular complications *(52)*. Later studies involving long-term high-dose vitamin E found no beneficial effects on endothelial function or left ventricular function in patients with type 1 and patients with type 2 diabetes *(53)*. Furthermore, high-dosage vitamin E was also associated with worsening in some vascular reactivity measurements when compared with control subjects.

AGEs result from a nonenzymatic reaction when proteins are exposed to hyperglycemic environments. The resultant Shiff bases can be rearranged to form Amadori products, AGEs, and reactive oxygen species. Increased AGE levels have been found in patients with diabetes and may contribute to the increased vascular permeability of diabetes, because blockade of a specific receptor for AGE reverses diabetes-mediated vascular hyperpermeability *(54)*. Furthermore, the generated reactive oxygen species have been shown to cause severe disturbances in the regulation of coronary flow and cellular hemostasis, leading to the severe macrovascular lesions typically observed in diabetic patients after more than 10 years of disease *(55)*. Interestingly, inhibition of reactive oxygen species also prevents the generation of AGE products, suggesting that the autoxidative process plays an important role in the complex reaction cascade leading to AGE.

Biochemical Markers of Endothelial Dysfunction

When the endothelium has been injured, a number of vasoactive substances are produced in response. As a result, these biochemical markers, such as von Willebrand factor (vWF) and cellular adhesion molecules, have been employed to evaluate endothelial dysfunction. vWf, a multimeric glycoprotein mainly synthesized by endothelial cells, is involved in platelet adhesion and aggregation and acts as the carrier of coagulation factor VIII in plasma. Increased levels of vWf, reflecting activation of or damage to endothelial cells, have been described in association with atherosclerosis and diabetes. Initial studies in patients with diabetes have demonstrated increased plasma levels of vWF *(56)*. Furthermore, these elevations preceded the development of albuminuria and peripheral nerve dysfunction. Therefore, it has been suggested that vWF could be used as a predictive indicator of vascular complications.

Cellular adhesion molecules are expressed on endothelial cells in response to inflammation and facilitate the adhesion of circulating leukocytes to their surface. Increased

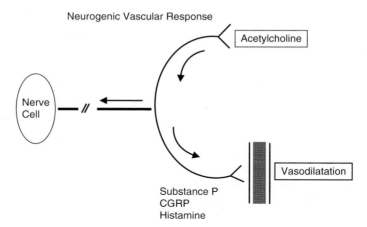

Fig. 2. Stimulation of the C-nociceptive nerve fibers leads to antidromic stimulation of the adjacent C fibers, which secrete substance P, calcitonin gene-related peptide and histamine that cause vasodilation and increased blood flow.

levels of soluble intercellular adhesion molecule (sICAM) in healthy individuals have been linked with a higher risk of future cardiovascular complications *(57)*. Furthermore, both sICAM and soluble vascular cell adhesion molecule levels have been reported to be higher in patients with diabetes and in some instances, individuals with impaired glucose tolerance *(58,59)*.

In vitro studies of sICAM and soluble vascular cell adhesion molecule demonstrated that these biochemical markers were expressed by endothelial cells following a short period of incubation in high glucose conditions *(60)*, lending support that hyperglycemia plays a role in activation of these molecules. Furthermore, a direct correlation has been detected between vascular cell adhesion molecule (VCAM)-1 and VEGF, suggesting that cellular adhesion and neovascularization may be linked processes *(61)*.

Nerve–Axon Reflex

Nerve dysfunction contributes to the diminished vasodilatory response observed in diabetes. Under normal conditions, the ability to increase blood flow to the skin depends on the existence of an intact neurogenic vascular response. This response is referred to as Lewis' triple flare response and begins with stimulation of C-nociceptive nerve fibers, leading to antidromic stimulation of the adjacent C fibers (Fig. 2). These fibers then secrete substance P, calcitonin gene-related peptide, and histamine, causing vasodilation and increased blood flow to the injured tissues. Typically, this response is equal to one-third of the maximal vasodilatory capacity.

Measurements in the diabetic neuropathic foot have shown that this neurovascular response is impaired, leading to a significant reduction in blood flow under conditions of stress. Thus, the diabetic neuropathic foot fails to respond to injury or infection in the usual manner, providing a plausible explanation for the clinically observed lack of hyperemia in the infected or injured diabetic foot. It has been postulated that the observed reduction in the nerve–axon reflex-related vasodilation in diabetic neuropathy is related to both impaired C-nociceptive fiber function and impaired ability of the microvasculature to respond to vasomodulators secreted by these fibers *(62)*.

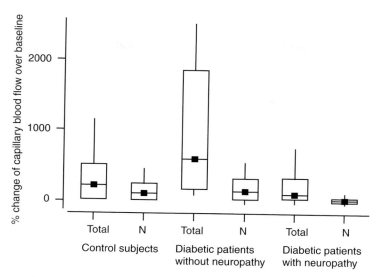

Fig. 3. Total and neurovascular (N) change in skin blood flow in response to acetylcholine at the foot level. The median, first quartile, and third quartile and the range are shown. The total response is significantly lower in neuropathic diabetic patients than it is in control subjects and diabetic patients without neuropathy ($p < 0.01$). The percentage contribution of neurovascular response to the total response is also significantly lower in neuropathic diabetic patients than in control subjects and diabetic patients without neuropathy ($p < 0.01$) *(64)*.

Evidence for this vasodilatory impairment related to the presence of diabetic neuropathy is provided by studies in our lab that used the previously described single-point laser probe technique to evaluate the nerve–axon-related vasodilatory response. The indirect response to the iontophoresis of acetylcholine was significantly reduced in diabetic patients with neuropathy, diabetic patients with neuropathy and peripheral vascular disease, and diabetic patients with Charcot arthropathy, compared with patients with diabetes without complications or healthy subjects *(45)*. The abnormality in axon-related vascular reactivity is believed to further aggravate the abnormalities in the microcirculation, and a vicious cycle ensues *(17)*. Subsequently, involvement of the C-nociceptive fibers in diabetes not only leads to impaired pain perception, but also to impaired vasodilation under conditions of stress.

The contribution of the nerve–axon reflex-related vasodilation response to the total endothelium-dependent and endothelium-independent vasodilation was also studied in a group of patients with diabetes and a group of healthy control subjects *(63)*. The nerve–axon-related response in healthy subjects was found to be 35% of the total response at the forearm level and 29% at the foot level. By contrast, response to SNP, a substance that does not specifically excite the C-nociceptive fibers was 13% at the level of the forearm and 12% at the level of the foot. This indicates that the presence of a non-specific galvanic response may also be responsible.

In the presence of diabetic neuropathy, the total response was reduced to 8%, a significant reduction in comparison with the healthy controls (Fig. 3). These findings indicate that although the neurovascular response is an important factor in the skin microcirculation, it is not the sole nor dominant pathway through which vasodilation is achieved *(64)*. However, the presence of neuropathy appears to render the diabetic foot functionally ischemic, as blood flow fails to increase under periods of stress.

CONCLUSION

In conclusion, although an occlusive disease of the microcirculation does not exist, functional impairment of the microcirculation in diabetes may contribute to secondary complications such as foot infections and ulcerations. Microcirculation to the diabetic foot suffers both structural and functional derangements. Nerve–axon-related microvascular reactivity is clearly impaired in the diabetic population and there is a growing belief that both the failure of the vessels to dilate and the impairment of the nerve-axon reflex are major causes for impaired wound healing in patients with diabetes. Further studies are necessary to clarify the precise etiology of observed endothelial dysfunction in diabetic and neuropathic patients and to identify the possible potential therapeutic interventions to prevent or to retard its progression.

REFERENCES

1. Goldenberg S, Joshi R. Nonatheromatous peripheral vascular disease of the lower extremity in diabetes mellitus. *Diabetes* 1959;8:261–273.
2. Strandness D, Gibbons G. Combined clinical and pathological study of diabetic and nondiabetic peripheral arterial disease. *Diabetes* 1964;13:366–372.
3. Conrad M. Large and small artery occlusion in diabetics and nondiabetics with severe vascular disease. *Circulation* 1967;36:83–91.
4. Barner H, Kaiser G, Willman V. Blood flow in the diabetic leg. *Circulation* 1971;43:391–394.
5. LoGerfo F, Coffman J. Current concepts. Vascular and microvascular disease of the foot in diabetes. Implications for foot care. *N Engl J Med* 1984;311:1615–1619.
6. Jaap AJ, Shore AC, Stockman AJ, Tooke JE. Skin capillary density in subjects with impaired glucose tolerance and patients with type 2 diabetes. *Diabetes Med* 1996;13:160–167.
7. Rayman G, Malik RA, Sharma AK, Day JL. Microvascular response to tissue injury and capillary ultrastructure in the foot skin of type I diabetic patients. *Clin Sci* 1995;89:467–474.
8. Malik RA, Newrick PG, Sharma AK, et al. Microangiopathy in human diabetic neuropathy: relationship between capillary abnormalities and the severity of neuropathy. *Diabetologia* 1989;32:92–102.
9. Williamson JR, Kilo C. Basement membrane physiology and pathophysiology, in *International Textbook of Diabetes Mellitus* (Alberti KGMM, DeFronzo RA, Keen H, Zimmet P, eds.), Volume 2, John Wiley, Chichester, 1992, pp. 1245–1265.
10. Raskin P, Pietri A, Unger R, Shannon WA Jr. The effect of diabetic control on skeletal muscle capillary basement membrane width in patients with type 1 diabetes mellitus. *N Engl J Med* 1983;309:1546–1550.
11. Rayman G, Williams SA, Spencer PD, et al. Impaired microvascular hyperaemic response to minor skin trauma in type I diabetes. *BMJ* 1986;292:1295–1298.
12. Tilton RG, Faller Am, Burkhardt JK, et al. Pericyte degeneration and acellular capillaries are increased in the feet of human diabetes. *Diabetologia* 1985;28:895–900.
13. Tooke JE. Microvascular function in human diabetes: a physiological perspective. *Diabetes* 1995;44:721–726.
14. Parving H, Viberti G, Keen H, et al. Hemodynamic factors in the genesis of diabetic microangiopathy. *Metabolism* 1983;32:943–949.
15. Flynn MD, Tooke JE. Aetiology of diabetic foot ulceration: a role for the microcirculation? *Diabet Med* 1992;8:320–329.

16. Jorneskog G, Brismar K, Fagrell B. Skin capillary circulation severely impaired in toes of patients with IDDM, with and without late diabetic complications. *Diabetologia* 1995;38:474–480.
17. Veves A, Akbari CM, Primavera J, et al. Endothelial dysfunction and the expression of endothelial nitric oxide synthetase in diabetic neuropathy, vascular disease and foot ulceration. *Diabetes* 1998;47:457–463.
18. Rendell M, Bergman T, O'Donnell G, et al. Microvascular blood flow, volume, and velocity measured by laser Doppler techniques in IDDM. *Diabetes* 1989;38:819–824.
19. Flynn MD, Williams SA, Tooke AE. Clinical television microscopy. *J Med Eng Technol* 1989;13:278–284.
20. Boulton AJM, Scarpello JHB, Ward JD. Venous oxygenation in the diabetic neuropathic foot: evidence of arteriovenous shunting? *Diabetologia* 1981;22:6–8.
21. Murray HJ, Boulton A. The pathophysiology of diabetic foot ulceration. *Clin Pediatr Med Surg* 1995;12:1–7.
22. Conrad MC. *Functional Anatomy of the Circulation to the Lower Extremities*, Year Book Medical Publishers, Chicago, 1971, pp. 60–75.
23. Flynn MD, Tooke JE. Diabetic neuropathy and the microcirculation. *Diabetes Med* 1995;12:298–301.
24. Edmonds ME, Roberts VC, Watkins PJ. Blood flow in the diabetic neuropathic foot. *Diabetologia* 1982;22:141–147.
25. Palmer RMJ, Ashton DS, Moncada S. Vascular endothelial cells synthesize nitric oxide from L-arginine. *Nature* 1998;333:664–666.
26. Williams SB, Cusco JA, Roddy M, Johnstone MY, Creager MA. Impaired nitric oxide-mediated vasodilation in patients with non-insulin-dependent diabetes mellitus. *J Am Coll Cardio* 1996;27:567–574.
27. Johnstone MT, Creager SJ, Scales KM, et al. Impaired endothelium-dependent vasodilation in patients with insulin-dependent diabetes mellitus. *Circulation* 1993;88:2510–2516.
28. Caballero AE, Arora S, Saouaf R, et al. Micro- and macro-vascular reactivity is impaired in subjects at risk for type 2 diabetes. *Diabetes* 1999;48:1863–1867.
29. Morris SJ, Shore AC, Tooke JE. Responses of the skin microcirculation to acetylcholine and sodium nitroprusside in patients with NIDDM. *Diabetologia* 1995;38:1337–1344.
30. Elhadd TA, Kennedy G, Hill A, et al. Abnormal markers of endothelial cell activation and oxidative stress in children, adolescents and young adults with type 1 diabetes with no clinical vascular disease. *Diabetes Metab Res Rev* 1999;15:405–411.
31. Sarman B, Farkas K, Toth M, Somogyi A, Tulassay Z. Circulating plasma endothelin-1, plasma lipids and complications in type 1 diabetes mellitus. *Diabetes Nutr Metab* 2000;13:142–148.
32. Woo KS, Chook P, Lolin YI, Sanderson JE, Metreweli C, Celermajer DS. Folic acid improves arterial endothelial function in adults with hyperhomocystinemia. *J Am Coll Cardiol* 1999;34:2002–2006.
33. Karamanos B, Porta M, Songini M, et al. Different risk factors of microangiopathy in patients with type I diabetes mellitus of short versus long duration. The EURODIAB IDDM Complications Study. *Diabetologia* 2000;43:348–355.
34. Singh TP, Groehn H, Kazmers A. Vascular function and carotid intimal-medial thickness in children with insulin-dependent diabetes mellitus. *J Am Coll Cardiol* 2003;41:661–665.
35. Koitka A, Abraham P, Bouhanick B, Sigaudo-Roussel D, Demiot C, Saumet JL. Impaired pressure-induced vasodilation at the foot in young adults with type 1 diabetes. *Diabetes* 2004;53:721–725.
36. Lambert J, Aarsen M, Donker AJ, Stehouwer CD. Endothelium-dependent and -independent vasodilation of large arteries in normoalbuminuric insulin-dependent diabetes mellitus. *Arterioscler Thromb Vasc Biol* 1996;16:705–711.

37. Stehouwer CD, Fischer HR, van Kuijk AW, Polak BC, Donker AJ. Endothelial dysfunction precedes development of microalbuminuria in IDDM. *Diabetes* 1995;44:561–564.

38. Dogra G, Rich L, Stanton K, Watts GF. Endothelium-dependent and independent vasodilation studies at normoglycaemia in type I diabetes mellitus with and without microalbuminuria. *Diabetologia* 2001;44:593–601.

39. Meeking DR, Cummings MH, Thorne S, et al. Endothelial dysfunction in type 2 diabetic subjects with and without microalbuminuria. *Diabet Med* 1999;16:841–847.

40. McVeigh GE, Brennan GM, Johnston GD, et al. Impaired endothelium-dependent and independent vasodilation in patients with type 2 (non-insulin-dependent) diabetes mellitus. *Diabetologia* 1992;35:771–776.

41. Watts GF, O'Brien SF, Silvester W, Millar JA. Impaired endothelium-dependent and independent dilatation of forearm resistance arteries in men with diet-treated non-insulin-dependent diabetes: role of dyslipidaemia. *Clin Sci* 1996;91:567–573.

42. Furchgott RF, Zawadzki JV. The obligatory role of endothelial cells in the relaxation of arterial smooth muscle by acetylcholine. *Nature* 1980;288:373–376.

43. Palmer RM, Ferrige AG, Moncada S. Nitric oxide release accounts for the biologic activity of endothelium-derived relaxing factor. *Nature* 1987;327:524–526.

44. Scherrer U, Randin D, Vollenweider P, Vollenweider L, Nicod P. Nitric oxide release accounts for insulin's vascular effects in humans. *J Clin Invest* 1994;94:2511–2515.

45. Taddei S, Virdis A, Mattei P, et al. Effect of insulin on acetylcholine-induced vasodilation in normotensive subjects and patients with essential hypertension. *Circulation* 1995;92:2911–2918.

46. Arora S, Smakowski P, Frykberg RG, et al. Differences in foot and forearm skin microcirculation in diabetic patients with and without neuropathy. *Diabetes Care* 1998;21:1339–1344.

47. Williamson JR, Chang K, Tilton RG, et al. Increased vascular permeability in spontaneously diabetic BB/W rats and in rats with mild versus severe streptozotocin-induced diabetes. *Diabetes* 1987;36:813–821.

48. Joannides R, Haefeli WE, Linder L, et al. Nitric oxide is responsible for flow-dependent dilatation of human peripheral conduit arteries in vivo. *Circulation* 1995;91:1314–1319.

49. Szabo C, Zanchi A, Komjati K et al. Poly (ADP-Ribose) polymerase is activated in subjects at risk of developing type 2 diabetes and is associated with impaired vascular reactivity. *Circulation* 2002;106:2680–2686.

50. Wolff SP, Dean RT. Glucose autoxidation and protein modification: the role of oxidative glycosylation in diabetes. *Biochem J* 1987;245:234–250.

51. The Heart Outcomes Prevention Evaluation Study Investigators. Vitamin E supplementation and cardiovascular events in high-risk patients. *N Engl J Med* 2000;342:154–160.

52. Bursell SE, Clermont AC, Aiello LP, et al. High-dose vitamin E supplementation normalizes retinal blood flow and creatinine clearance in patients with type 1 diabetes. *Diabetes Care* 1999;22:1245–1251.

53. Panayiotis A, Khaodhiar L, Caselli A, et al. The effect of vitamin E on endothelial function of micro- and macrocirculation and left ventricular function in type 1 and type 2 diabetic patients. *Diabetes* 2005;54:204–211.

54. Makita Z, Radoff S, Rayfield EJ. Advanced glycosylation end products in patients with diabetic nephropathy. *N Engl J Med* 1991;325:836–842.

55. Schernthaner G. Cardiovascular mortality and morbidity in type-2 diabetes mellitus. *Diabetes Res Clin Pract* 1996;33:S3–S14.

56. Verrotti A, Greco R, Basciani F, Morgese G, Chiarelli F. von Willebrand factor and its propeptide in children with diabetes. Relation between endothelial dysfunction and microalbuminuria. *Pediatr Res* 2003;53:382–386.

57. Ridker PM, Hennekens CH, Roitman-Johnson B, Stamofer MJ, Allen J. Plasma concentration of soluble intercellular adhesion molecule 1 and risks of future myocardial infarction in apparently healthy men. *Lancet* 1998;351:88–92.

58. Ferri C, Desideri G, Baldoncini R, et al. Early activation of vascular endothelium in nonobese, nondiabetic essential hypertensive patients with multiple metabolic abnormalities. *Diabetes* 1998;47:660–667.
59. Otosuki M, Hashimoto K, Morimoto Y, Kishimoto T, Kasayama S. Circulating vascular cell adhesion molecule-1 (V CAM-1) in atherosclerotic NIDDM patients. *Diabetes* 1997;46: 2096–2101.
60. Altannavch TS, Roubalova K, Kucera P, Andel M. Effect of high glucose concentrations on expression of ELAM-1, VCAM-1 and ICAM-1 in HUVEC with and without cytokine activation. *Physiol Res* 2004;53:77–82.
61. Vinik AI, Erbas T, Park TS, Stansberry KB, Scanelli JA, Pittenger GL. Dermal neurovascular dysfunction in type 2 diabetes. *Diabetes Care* 2001;24:1468–1475.
62. Hernandez C, Burgos R, Canton A, Garcia-Arumi J, Segura RM, Simo R. Vitreous levels of vascular cell adhesion molecule and vascular endothelial growth factor in patients with proliferative diabetic retinopathy: a case-control study. *Diabetes Care* 2001;24:516–521.
63. Hamdy O, Abou-Elenin K, LoGerfo FW, Horton ES, Veves A. Contribution of nerve-axon reflex-related vasodilation to the total skin vasodilation in diabetic patients with and without neuropathy. *Diabetes Care* 2001;24:344–349.
64. Parkhouse N, LeQueen PM. Impaired neurogenic vascular response in patients with diabetes and neuropathic foot lesions. *N Engl J Med* 1988;318:1306–1309.

8

Clinical Features and Diagnosis
of Macrovascular Disease

Chantel Hile, MD, Nikhil Kansal, MD, Allen Hamdan, MD, and Frank W. LoGerfo, MD

INTRODUCTION

Atherosclerotic peripheral vascular disease in patients with diabetes is a major factor in the progression of diabetic foot pathology. The rate of lower extremity amputation in the diabetic population is 15 times that seen in the nondiabetic population (1). A number of factors conspire in the patient with diabetes, each of which synergistically contributes to this extremely high amputation rate. Peripheral neuropathy, infection, microvascular changes, and macrovascular changes all have complex interplay. Peripheral neuropathy leads to structural and sensory changes within the foot, making the limb injury-prone. In addition, once it occurs, that injury is often not easily detectable and heals slowly if at all. Microvascular changes are nonocclusive changes in the microcirculation that lead to impairment of normal cellular exchange, again preventing easy healing. Infection in patients with diabetes can often be aggressive and polymicrobial. Macrovascular disease, atherosclerosis of the peripheral arteries, contributes to poor perfusion of the extremities. Although the underlying pathogenesis of atherosclerotic disease in patients with diabetes is similar to that noted in patients without diabetes, there are some significant differences. It is important to realize that the diabetic foot is more susceptible to moderate changes in perfusion than the nondiabetic foot, resulting in a greater sensitivity to atherosclerotic occlusive disease. Compounding this scenario is the fact that patients with diabetes are noted to have a fourfold increase in the prevalence of atherosclerosis as well as a propensity for accelerated atherosclerosis. This chapter will review the pathobiology and anatomic distribution of occlusive disease in the patient with diabetes, the usual clinical presentation of peripheral vascular disease, and the various diagnostic modalities useful in planning treatment. It will conclude with a diagnostic and treatment protocol that can be used in patients presenting with this multifactorial disease process.

PATHOLOGY OF ATHEROSCLEROSIS IN DIABETES

Understanding of the basic pathology of atherosclerosis in patients with diabetes has evolved considerably over the last 15 years. One fundamental concept that has been disproved is the commonly held belief that patients with diabetes are prone to "small vessel disease." This popular misconception, in which the arterioles of the ankle and foot are

From: *The Diabetic Foot, Second Edition*
Edited by: A. Veves, J. M. Giurini, and F. W. LoGerfo © Humana Press Inc., Totowa, NJ

thought to be preferentially affected by atherosclerotic occlusive disease, originated from a paper by Goldenberg *(2)*. In his retrospective review of amputation specimens from patients with and without diabetes, Goldenberg used periodic acid-Schiff staining to histologically examine the peripheral vasculature. Deposits that stained positive in the arterioles of the foot and ankle were noted to be unique to the diabetic specimens. These deposits were interpreted as being atherosclerotic lesions and were felt to be the principle cause of the poor outcome seen in patients with diabetes. The prevailing belief became that patients with diabetes were not candidates for distal revascularization because the "small vessels" (arterioles) were somehow preferentially involved in the occlusive process.

Further work in an attempt to categorize and quantify whether there was a diffuse and unique type of atherosclerosis between patients with and without diabetes was evaluated by a number of research studies. In a prospective analysis of amputation specimens, this time with blinded histological review, Strandness and coworkers *(3)* used periodic acid-Schiff staining and showed that there was no difference in the atherosclerotic pattern between patients with and without diabetes. Both groups were noted to have a paucity of occlusive disease at the arteriolar level. In another prospective study, using a sophisticated casting technique for evaluating the peripheral vasculature, Conrad *(4)* confirmed the similar characteristics of arteriolar atherosclerosis in both groups of patients. To dispel the theory that the peripheral vascular bed in patients with diabetes was less "reactive," Barner *(5)* measured the flow rate in femoropopliteal bypass grafts in the two groups. By infusing papavarine into the outflow vascular bed, he was able to assess any difference in vessel reactivity; again, no difference was noted between patients with and without diabetes. It is clear from these studies that a unique "small vessel" occlusive pattern does not exist in patients with diabetes. The label of "unreconstructable disease" has led to many unnecessary amputations in the diabetic population.

There are, however, some aspects of atherosclerotic peripheral vascular disease, which are different from that noted in the nondiabetic population. As has already been mentioned, patients with diabetes have a fourfold higher prevalence of atherosclerosis and this occlusive disease is known to progress at a more rapid rate. It is also noteworthy that diabetic patients with the sequelae of atherosclerotic disease often present at an earlier age than their counterparts without diabetes. In addition, patients with diabetes often have a unique distribution of atherosclerosis at the arterial level. Unlike in their counterparts without diabetes, occlusive disease in patients with diabetes has a distinct propensity to occur in the infrageniculate vessels in the calf. The affected arteries, namely the anterior tibial artery, posterior tibial artery, and peroneal artery, are more severely affected and are more likely to present with occlusion in patients with diabetes (Figs. 1 and 2). Although these arteries are preferentially affected, the proximal arteries to the level of the popliteal artery are often spared in patients with diabetes. Equally important is the observation that the arteries of the foot, namely the dorsalis pedis artery, are commonly spared from the occlusive disease (Fig. 3). These patterns are generalizations, and it is important to mention that some patients with diabetes present with atherosclerotic lesions very similar to those seen in patients without diabetes.

These observations have had a crucial impact in the way that peripheral vascular disease in patients with diabetes is approached. Based in part on the expected presence of the so-called small vessel disease, in the past, patients with diabetes were not treated

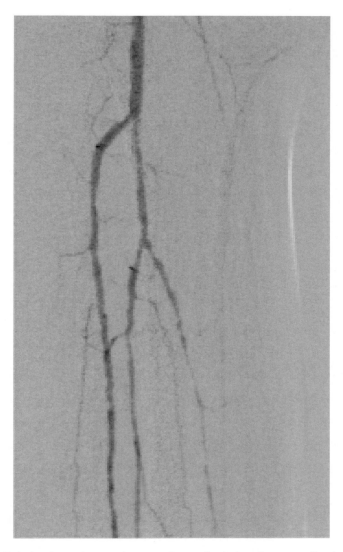

Fig. 1. This digital subtraction angiogram shows the below-knee popliteal artery and tibial arteries in a patient with diabetes. The diffuse pattern of atherosclerotic disease is typical of the type seen in this population.

as aggressively as they are currently. Because patients with diabetes were thought to have occlusive disease at the arteriolar level, bypass to patent vessels proximal to the foot was thought to be futile. Now, as our understanding of the disease process has evolved, so has our treatment protocol. Understanding that, in patients with diabetes, calf vessels are more severely affected by atherosclerosis whereas the pedal vessels are spared, we have been able to modify our approach to the evaluation and treatment of patients with diabetes. A more aggressive approach to identifying pedal arteries suitable for bypass along with aggressive measures to control local infection has radically changed the prognosis of peripheral vascular disease in the diabetic foot.

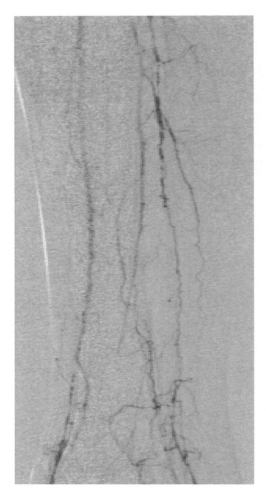

Fig. 2. This is a more distal film of the same patient in Fig. 1. It is evident that there are no patent tibial arteries. The blood flow to the foot in this patient is entirely dependent on the small collateral vessels that are seen. In the past, with this angiogram, this patient would not have been considered a candidate for bypass. Now, however, it is known that the pedal arteries in diabetic patients with this type of disease must be visualized. Many of these patients are found to have pedal arteries amenable to bypass procedures (*see* Figs. 3, 6, and 7).

CLINICAL PRESENTATION

In order to appreciate the differences in the presentation of peripheral vascular disease in patients with diabetes, it is important to understand its presentation in patients without diabetes. Atherosclerotic disease is manifest by a continuum of signs and symptoms that can be divided into categories. These categories in order of increasing severity are: claudication, rest pain, and tissue loss. These categories represent the normal evolution of symptoms in the nondiabetic population with peripheral vascular disease. Because of the effects of diabetic neuropathy, this progression of symptoms may be absent in patients with diabetes. This topic is further detailed in another chapter.

Claudication is defined as ischemic muscle pain resulting from inadequate blood flow. This lack of tissue perfusion is owing to proximal arterial occlusive disease resulting in

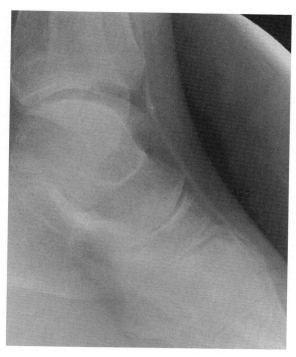

Fig. 3. This is a lateral view of the foot (nonsubtraction) of a diabetic patient with severe tibial artery occlusive disease. This patient had no patent tibial vessels to which bypass could be performed. Note the location and patency of the artery on the dorsum of the foot. This is the dorsalis pedis artery and is an excellent target artery for bypass.

diminished blood flow to large muscle groups. For example, claudication of the thigh and buttocks is a result of occlusive disease of the aortoiliac system, whereas claudication of the calf results from superficial femoral artery occlusion. Calf claudication is a common initial presenting symptom. The pain is characteristic, involving the calf muscles, and is usually described as "cramping" in nature. It is often aggravated by exercise, and relieved by several minutes of rest. Often helpful in tracking the progression of claudication is the patient's ability to quantify the amount of distance they are able to walk before becoming symptomatic. This distance is noted as the "initial claudication distance." This assessment is extremely valuable in clinical practice for the follow-up of patients with peripheral vascular disease. As a result of the rich collateral network of blood supply to the lower extremity, occlusive disease at two levels is usually required to cause claudication. This does not hold true for patients with diabetes, however, because they are more susceptible than nondiabetics to small changes in tissue perfusion. Therefore, it is not uncommon for patients with diabetes to present with symptoms resulting from vascular occlusive disease localized to one level, whereas nondiabetics will often have multilevel disease by the time they become symptomatic. Claudication is an important early sign of peripheral vascular disease, which should always be elicited in a patient's history. Careful follow-up and monitoring of claudication can identify patients with worsening occlusive disease before the progression to more severe pathology. Most patients, about 75%, will remain stable regarding their claudication, i.e., the distance they can walk does not lessen over time. Of patients with diabetes with claudication, operative treatment or amputations are required in only 1% of patients per year.

Rest pain is another symptom of peripheral vascular disease and is an indication of severe occlusive disease. It is characterized as a "burning pain" involving either the forefoot or the region of the metatarsal heads. Unlike claudication, rest pain is constant, occurs even at rest (most commonly at night with leg elevation), and is relieved only by dependent hanging of the extremity. Patients will often dangle the affected leg off the side of the bed at night in order to gain relief. Rest pain is often an ominous sign of severely progressive occlusive disease. Unfortunately, secondary to peripheral neuropathy, diabetics may not develop rest pain, or it may be confused with the pain of neuropathy. The absence of this hallmark clinical sign may lead to a delay in the diagnosis of severe ischemia of the foot.

Tissue loss is the most severe presentation of vascular disease, and can be broken-down into two separate types: foot ulceration and gangrene. Ulceration is the most common presentation of peripheral vascular disease in patients with diabetes. The increased incidence of foot ulceration in diabetics is resulting from the synergistic effects of the various other contributing factors as discussed early in this chapter. It is important to realize that ulceration in patients with diabetes is rarely owing to ischemia alone; a fact that should be kept in mind when devising treatment strategy. All patients with diabetes presenting with foot ulceration should be evaluated for peripheral vascular disease. Gangrene seen in patients with and without diabetes is quite similar. The gangrenous extremity is a hallmark of severe vascular occlusive disease. The diagnosis is established at clinical exam. The affected extremity appears black and shriveled, is insensate, and has no motor function. Gangrene as defined does not include the presence of infection, and as such, is of little systemic consequence in the affected patient. This is not the case when the gangrenous tissue is secondarily infected, or the so-called wet gangrene. This separate clinical entity is characterized by the classical findings of gangrene, with the addition of signs of invasive infection: fever, chills, leukocytosis, erythema, cellulitis, pus, abscess, or osteomyelitis. In contrast to uninfected or "dry gangrene," wet gangrene poses a surgical emergency.

Any discussion regarding the presentation of peripheral vascular disease would not be complete without the mention of infection as a presenting symptom. Although less common in the nondiabetic population, infection can be the first sign of peripheral ischemia in patients with diabetes. In addition, infection associated with ulceration and gangrene is also more common in patients with diabetes. These infections are often aggressive, polymicrobial, cause significant tissue destruction, and are the most common cause of amputation in the diabetic foot. In terms of presentation, it is crucial to realize that the signs of infection may be subtle. Because the normal immune response to infection is altered in patients with diabetes, patients with massive invasive infection may not manifest with classic signs such as fever, chills, leukocytosis, or even cellulitis. In fact, many diabetic patients with foot infection may present merely with hyperglycemia, or simply an increase in their insulin requirement. It is because of these factors that the index of suspicion for foot infection in patients with diabetes should always be high.

DIAGNOSIS AND EVALUATION

The cornerstone in the evaluation of patients with diabetes and peripheral vascular disease remains the physical exam. Our experience has shown that the absence of pedal pulses, either dorsalis pedis or posterior tibial, is an indication of advanced occlusive

Table 1
Diagnostic Criteria for Peripheral Arterial Disease
Based on Ankle–Brachial Index Measurements

0.91–1.30	Normal
0.70–0.90	Mild obstruction
0.40–0.69	Moderate obstruction
<0.40	Severe obstruction

disease. Palpation of the peripheral pulses should include the femoral, popliteal, and pedal vessels. Although this is a skill that takes time to develop, when an examination is performed by an experienced person, absence of both pedal pulses is a clear marker of vascular disease. Beyond physical exam there is a myriad of noninvasive and invasive diagnostic modalities available to the clinician. Noninvasive modalities are preferred for screening and initial workup and include ankle–brachial indices, pulse volume recordings (PVR), segmental pressures, toe pressures, and transcutaneous oxygen measurements. There are many conflicting arguments regarding the efficacy and reproducibility of these methods. The continued controversy, along with the inapplicability of many of these tests in patients with diabetes, has hampered their usefulness. Magnetic resonance angiography (MRA) and computed tomographic angiography (CTA) are two relatively noninvasive tests, yet are being considered as alternatives to the more invasive digital subtraction angiography. They have significant limitations, and have yet to be accepted as replacements of conventional angiography. The only invasive diagnostic test in the evaluation of vascular disease is digital subtraction angiography. This is currently considered the "gold standard" in the assessment of occlusive disease.

Noninvasive measurements in patients with peripheral vascular disease can often yield a large amount of information regarding the location and severity of occlusive lesions. Unfortunately, many of these modalities are either altered by the diabetic process, or simply cannot be performed consistently on the diabetic foot. Ankle–brachial index is an easily measurable way to compare the systolic pressure of the upper extremity to that of the affected lower extremity. Using a Doppler probe and a blood pressure cuff, the systolic pressure in the pedal arteries (dorsalis pedis or posterior tibial) is taken. The higher of these two measurements is compared with a similarly taken brachial artery systolic pressure (again, the highest brachial pressure is used). A ratio (ankle–brachial) of less than 1 is considered a sign of impaired flow to the extremity (Table 1). Because of the arterial wall medial calcification that occurs in patients with diabetes, the arteries are often less compressible than similar arteries at the same pressure. As a result, this measurement is often falsely elevated and unreliable. In some patients with diabetes, this process is so severe that the cuff pressure cannot occlude the arteries; these vessels are referred to as "noncompressible." It is for this reason that this measurement can have limited clinical applicability in patients with diabetes. Nevertheless, the ADA Consensus Statement recommends a screening ABI be done on all patients with diabetes over 50 years of age and, if normal, repeated every 5 years. Those diabetic patients with risk factors for peripheral arterial disease should be screened with an ABI no matter the age *(6)*.

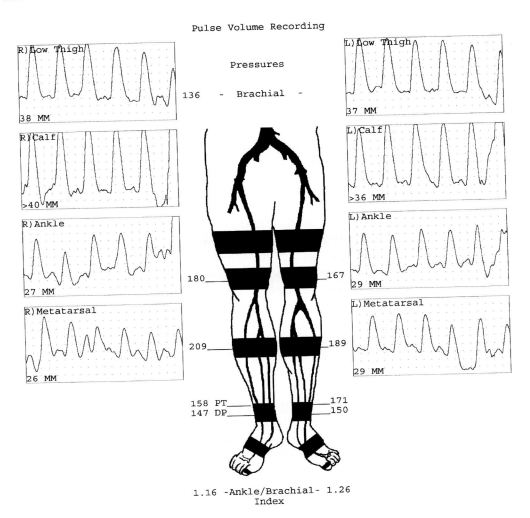

Pulse Volume Recording

Pressures

136 - Brachial -

180 _____ / _____ 167

209 _____ / _____ 189

158 PT _____ / _____ 171
147 DP _____ / _____ 150

R) Low Thigh
38 MM

R) Calf
>40 MM

R) Ankle
27 MM

R) Metatarsal
26 MM

L) Low Thigh
37 MM

L) Calf
>36 MM

L) Ankle
29 MM

L) Metatarsal
29 MM

1.16 -Ankle/Brachial- 1.26
Index

Fig. 4. This is an example of a pulse-volume recording (PVR) data sheet. Included are the segmental pressures (along-side the diagram) and the ankle–brachial indices (ABIs; bottom of diagram). This patient is diabetic and was noted to have elevated segmental pressures (the absolute pressure increases distally) and elevated ABIs (both ABIs are greater than 1). Because medial wall calcification often causes elevation of these two measurements, PVRs are utilized to assess the presence or absence of true occlusive disease. Note that the amplitude of the waveforms is maintained from the thigh to the metatarsal level. This indicates that this patient does not have significant vascular occlusive disease.

The technique of measuring segmental pressures from the high thigh down to the foot is a popular method for assessing the location of occlusive lesions. This test is performed by placing a series of pressure cuffs at various levels along the affected extremity. The systolic pressure measurements at each level are an indication of the amount of tissue perfusion at that level. A drop in the pressure from one level to the next is predictive of an occlusive lesion within the arterial system between those two levels (Figs. 4 and 5). Unfortunately, this measurement is also affected by the arterial wall calcification in patients with diabetes, and as a result is often not reliable in this population.

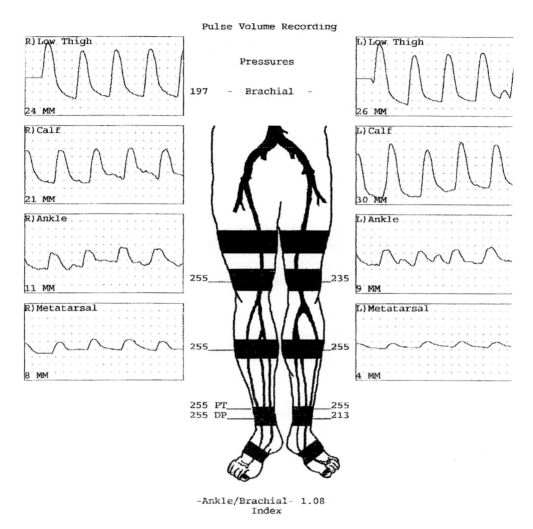

Fig. 5. This PVR recording is also taken from a patient with diabetes. As in Fig. 6, this patient is noted to have elevated segmental pressures and ABIs. The difference is that this patient clearly has "dampening" of the waveforms on both extremities beginning at the level of the ankle. This decrease in amplitude of the tracing suggests that an occlusive vascular lesion exists between the level of the calf and ankle. As you can see, the results of this test are merely qualitative, and do not provide an objective quantification of the extent of vascular disease present.

As it became increasingly evident that the vasculature of the foot was spared the changes noted in the more proximal vessels of the calf, measurement of digital toe pressures was initiated. Subsequent study has confirmed that toe pressures are not hampered by the coexistence of diabetes. In fact, Vincent and Towne *(7)* showed that toe pressure was an "accurate hemodynamic indicator of total peripheral arterial obstructive disease" in patients with diabetes. Generally, a toe pressure less than 40 mmHg predicts healing difficulties. Although this methodology can be a useful adjunct in the evaluation of vascular disease in the diabetic foot, its use is often obviated by the presence of ulceration, gangrene, or amputation of the toe, and unfamiliarity with its use at some hospitals.

PVR are an assessment of the flow characteristics within the arterial system. A series of air plethysmography cuffs are placed at the toe, ankle, calf, low thigh, and high thigh. These cuffs detect the small change in diameter of the leg during systole and diastole. This change with each heartbeat is recorded as a waveform (Figs. 4 and 5). A progression from "triphasic" to "monophasic" or "dampened waveform" would be indicative of occlusive disease and a waveform less than 4 at the toe level indicate an extent of ischemia such that tissue healing is unlikely. The advantage of this method is the fact that it is not hampered by arterial wall calcification (Fig. 5). For patients with a normal ABI but clear claudication symptoms, a reasonable option is the treadmill functional test. Patients whose symptoms truly are because of claudication will have a higher than 20 mmHg drop in ankle pressure after a period of exercise. Although PVR testing does confer some information, it is mostly a qualitative rather than quantitative examination, and is difficult to use as an absolute or objective reference regarding the severity of the disease.

Transcutaneous oxygen measurements are used to evaluate the amount of tissue perfusion in patients with vascular disease. This method had been used to predict the healing potential of a diseased extremity, i.e., to determine if the patient would be able to heal a wound that either exists, or would be created by performing a surgical procedure. The test is performed by placing a probe over the metatarsal region of the affected foot. After equilibrating to a specific temperature, the oxygen level is determined. Enthusiasm for this measurement has been hampered by the large degree of variability noted in the measurements. Many different factors, including the site of measurement and the temperature, affect the oxygen reading; but in a review of multiple factors, no one factor could account for the variability (8). Another review noted that the transcutaneous oxygen tension (TcPO2) was lower in diabetics than nondiabetics when comparing groups with similar disease severity (9).

Although there is some literature supporting the use of TcPO2 in the evaluation of the diabetic foot (10), results are difficult to interpret. This has led to a "gray-zone" of values without a significantly predictive scale. Rule of thumb is that a value of less than 30 mmHg is associated with poor healing. The continued evaluation of this modality may lead to a better understanding of its importance.

The "gold standard" in the evaluation of diabetic patients with peripheral vascular disease is digital subtraction angiography. The results of conventional angiography have been greatly enhanced with the advent of digital subtraction technology (Figs. 3 and 6). This technology, by subtracting away the bone and soft tissue to better visualize the contrast column, allows the radiographer to follow the contrast bolus over a greater period of time and allows for selection of the optimal images. This has resulted in greater visualization of the distal and pedal vessels. The most important aspect for a radiographer to understand, especially in patients with diabetes, is that even in the presence of tibial vessel occlusion, priority must be given to visualizing the pedal anatomy. Angiograms are often terminated prematurely in these situations with the misconception that tibial occlusion represents "unreconstructable disease." Two views (anteroposterior and lateral) of the foot should be obtained and care should be taken to avoid excessive plantar flexion of the foot during the exam as this may impede flow to the dorsalis pedis artery (Fig. 7). The prevailing concern with the use of angiography is the risk of renal failure in diabetic patients with preexisting renal insufficiency. The most important factor in the

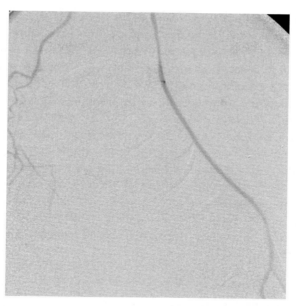

Fig. 6. This is the same patient seen in Fig. 3 viewed using digital subtraction technology. This technology allows improved visualization of difficult to see arteries, especially in situations in which blood flow is diminished.

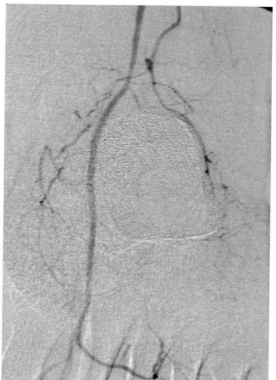

Fig. 7. This is an AP view of the foot of the patient seen in Figs. 3 and 6. The widely patent dorsalis pedis artery is well visualized and can be seen feeding the pedal arch. It is mandatory to obtain a lateral and AP view angiogram of the foot when evaluating the pedal vasculature.

prevention of renal failure in these patients has been the use of hydration prior to obtaining the angiogram *(11)*. When renal failure does occur, it is almost always reversible *(12)*, but may delay the arterial reconstructive surgery for several days while the creatinine returns to baseline. Recent data suggest that sodium bicarbonate infusion prior to contrast exposure may be even more effective than normal saline hydration *(13)* and *N*-acetylcysteine treatment preceding and following contrast exposure has also been shown to help prevent contrast nephropathy *(14)*.

MRA and spiral CTA have been investigated as alternatives to conventional angiography. The ability of MRA to provide information without the risks related to catheterization, nephrotoxicity and radiation exposure makes it an attractive option. MRA using "2D time of flight" was used to assess the distal lower extremity vasculature in diabetics in comparison to digital subtraction angiography *(15)*. Although MRA was shown to have acceptable sensitivity and specificity in the evaluation of the tibial vessels, it was not ideal for identifying patent pedal vessels. The three areas that are prone to error by MRA are as follow:

1. The bifurcation of the peroneal artery;
2. The plantar arch; and
3. Retrograde flow into the lateral plantar artery.

These shortcomings are especially significant in the diabetic population in whom the pedal vessels are often a target of revascularization. Weighing the pluses and minuses of this study, the American Diabetes Association endorsed its use with the caveat that X-ray angiography remains the gold standard for vascular imaging *(6)*.

The role of CTA in the evaluation of peripheral vascular disease has also been investigated. Some reviews *(16)* have reported an accuracy of 95%. Confounding items such as overlapping leg veins and vessel wall calcification can contribute to inaccurate CTA readings. This modality is also limited by the amount of contrast required to image the entire length from the distal aorta to the foot. For this reason, studies evaluating CTA have not included the pedal vessels in their evaluation, and to do so would likely require prohibitively high contrast levels. The combination of inaccuracy with calcification and the inability to visualize the pedal vessels makes CTA an ineffective means of evaluating vascular disease in the diabetic.

Overall, noninvasive diagnostic tests are quite useful in the evaluation of nondiabetic patients with peripheral vascular disease. Unfortunately, these tests are easy to misinterpret in patients with diabetes. The combination of peripheral neuropathy and medial arterial wall calcification limits the ability to accurately diagnose and predict the location or severity of occlusive disease by noninvasive methods. Because the traditional approach to the work-up of peripheral vascular disease is not adequate in the patient with diabetes, a separate algorithm in the management of these patients is required.

TREATMENT PROTOCOL

The approach to the diabetic patient with signs and symptoms of vascular occlusive disease is separate from that utilized in the nondiabetic population. Patients being evaluated with diabetic foot complications should be considered at high risk both for the development and progression of atherosclerotic occlusive disease. In lieu of the previously discussed shortcomings of noninvasive testing, we place emphasis on the presence

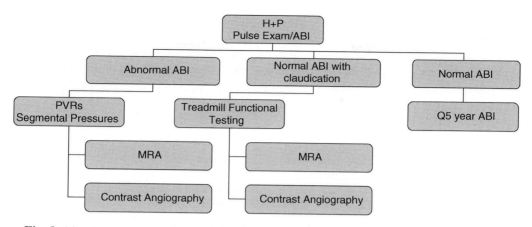

Fig. 8. Algorithm for assessing peripheral vascular disease in the patient with diabetes (based on recommendations laid out in the 2003 ADA Consensus Statement [6]).

or absence of pedal pulses (Fig. 8). As a general rule, if a patient has a diabetic foot ulcer and nonpalpable pulses, he or she is regarded as having a significant component of ischemia. If the ulcer does not heal with conservative measures or if bone, joint, or tendon is involved, digital subtraction arteriography should be performed.

The management of a patient that presents with an ischemic diabetic foot should be approached in a premeditated and stepwise fashion. The initial priority is the prompt and thorough drainage and/or debridement of any infected or necrotic tissue. This may be accomplished by simple incision and debridement of an abscess, or may require more extensive procedures. The goal of these procedures, whether extensive soft tissue debridement or partial amputation is the final result, is the complete eradication of an ongoing source of sepsis. Multiple trips to the operating suite may be needed to insure adequate results. Again, one must keep in mind that the signs of continued infection in diabetics can be blunted and their diagnosis requires a high level of suspicion. Once the infection is controlled, the next step is determining the level of ischemia. This step should not be delayed, and can be pursued even in the presence of active infection. As was previously mentioned, the absence of pedal pulses is a good predictor of the need for angiography, especially in the setting of tissue loss, poor healing, or gangrene. Once angiography is complete, planning for revascularization is undertaken. Even in the face of tibial and peroneal occlusion, the pedal vessels should be evaluated for patency. The fundamental goal of any revascularization in the diabetic foot should be restoration of pulsatile blood flow to the foot. The priority of bypass vessels should be to those arteries with direct runoff into the foot (anterior and posterior tibial arteries), however; results of bypass to the peroneal artery are also excellent. Once revascularization has been accomplished, attention can then again be turned to the repair of the initial foot lesion. Secondary revision or closure may be required, and may be carried out as a separate procedure.

The care and management of the patient with diabetes presenting with the sequelae of peripheral vascular disease is a complex undertaking. A thorough knowledge of the pathobiology associated with this disease is essential. All aspects of the care of these patients, from presentation to diagnosis to treatment, must be tailored to patients with diabetes. As the evolution of our understanding of this disease process has evolved, so has our ability to effect improvement in outcome. Patients presenting with diabetic foot complications exacerbated by atherosclerotic occlusive disease are now treated very aggressively. The use of distal bypass grafting in appropriate patients has led to improved results and an optimistic prognosis for the diabetic population.

REFERENCES

1. Armstrong DG, Lavery LA. Diabetic foot ulcers: prevention, diagnosis and classification. *Am Fam Phys* 1998;57(6):1325–1332.
2. Goldenberg SG, Alex M, Joshi RA, et al. Nonatheromatous peripheral vascular disease of the lower extremity in diabetes mellitus. *Diabetes* 1959;8:261–273.
3. Strandness DE, Priest RE, Gibbons GE. Combined clinical and pathologic study of diabetic and nondiabetic peripheral arterial disease. *Diabetes* 1964;13:366–372.
4. Conrad MC. Large and small artery occlusion in diabetics and nondiabetics with severe vascular disease. *Circulation* 1967;36:83–91.
5. Barner HB, Kaiser GC, Willman VL. Blood flow in the diabetic leg. *Circulation* 1971;43: 391–394.
6. Peripheral Arterial Disease in People with Diabetes, American Diabetes Association Consensus Statement. *Diabetes Care*, 2003;26(12):3333–3341.
7. Vincent DG, Salles-Cunha SX, Bernhard VM, Taine JB. Noninvasive assessment of toe systolic pressures with special reference to diabetes mellitus. *J Cardiovasc Surg* 1983;24(1):22–28.
8. Boyko EJ, Afroni JF. Predictors of transcutaneous oxygen tension in the lower limbs of diabetic subjects. *Diabet Med* 1996;13:549–554.
9. Rooke TW, Osmundson PJ. The influence of age, sex, smoking, and diabetes on lower limb transcutaneois oxygen tension in patients with arterial occlusive disease. *Arch Intern Med* 1990;150:129–132.
10. Eke CC, Bunt TJ, Killeen JD. A prospective evaluation of transcutaaneois oxygen measurements in the management of diabetic foot problems. *J Vasc Surg* 1995;22(4):485–490.
11. Solomon R, Werner C, et al. Effects of saline, mannitol, and furosemide on acute decreases in renal function by radiocontrast agents. *N Engl J Med* 1994;331:1416–1420.
12. Parfrey PS, Griffiths SM, Barret BJ, et al. Contrast material-induced renal failure in patients with diabets mellitus, renal insufficiency, or both: a prospective controlled study. *N Engl J Med* 1989;320:143.
13. Merten GJ, Burgess WP, Gray LV, et al. Prevention of contrast-induced nephropathy with sodium bicarbonate. *JAMA* 2004;291(19):2328–2334.14. Birck R, Krzossk S, et al. Acetylcysteine for prevention of contrast nephropathy: meta-analysis, *Lancet* 2003;362:598–603.
15. McDermott VG, Meakem TJ, Carpenter JP, et al. Magnetic resonance angiography of the distal lower extremity. *Clin Radiol* 1995;50(11):747–746.
16. Lawrence JA, Kim D, Kent KC, et al. Lower extremity spiral CT angiography versus catheter angiograhy. *Radiology* 1995;194(3):903–908.

SUGGESTED READING

1. Kannel WB, McGee DL. Diabetes and glucose tolerance as risk factors for cardiovascular disease: the Framingham study. *Diabetes Care* 1979;2:120–126.
2. Boulton A, Buckenham T, et al. Report of the Diabetic Foot and Amputation Group. *Diabetes Med* 1995;13(9 Suppl 4):S27–S42.

3. Logerfo FW, Moracaccio EF. Etiology and assessment of ischemia in the diabetic. *Ann Chirurgae et Gynaecologiae* 1992;81(2):122–124.
4. LoGerfo FW, Gibbons GW, Pomposelli FB, et al. Trends in the care of the diabetic foot. *Arch Surg* 1992;127(5):617–620.
5. Gils CC, Wheeler LA, Mellstrom M, et al. Amputation prevention by vascular surgery and podiatry collaboration in high-risk diabetic and nondiabetic patients. *Diabetes Care* 1999;22(5):678–683.
6. LoGerfo FW, Gibbons GW. Vascular disease of the lower extremities in diabetes mellitus. *Endocrinol Metab Clin N Am* 1996;25(2):439–445.
7. Chang BB, Shah DM, Darling RC 3rd, Leather RP. Treatment of the diabetic foot from a vascular surgeon's viewpoint. *Clin Orthop Rel Res* 1993;296:27–30.
8. Estes JM, Pomposelli FB. Lower extremity arterial reconstruction in patients with diabetes mellitus. *Diabetes Med* 1996;S43–S46.
9. Akbari CM, LoGerfo FW. Diabetes and peripheral vascular disease. *J Vasc Surg* 1999;30(2):373–384.
10. Bunt TJ, Holloway GA. TcPO2 as an accurate predictor of therapy in limb salvage. *Ann Vasc Surg* 1996;10:224–227.
11. Stevens MJ, Goss DE, Foster AV, et al. Abnormal digital pressure measurements in diabetic neuropathic foot ulceration. *Diabetes Med* 1993;10(10):909–915.
12. Ramsey DE, Manke DA, SumnerDS. Toe blood pressure. A valuable adjunct to ankle pressure measurement for assessing peripheral arterial disease. *J Cardiovasc Surg* 1983;24(1):43–48.
13. Carter SA, Tate RB. Value of toe pulse waves in addition to systolic pressures in the assessment of the severity of peripheral arterial disease and critical limb ischemia. *J Vasc Surg* 1996;24(2):258–265.
14. Ekelund L, Sjoqvist L, Thomas KA, Asberg B. MR angiography of abdominal and peripheral arteries. Techniques and clinical applications. *Acta Radiol* 1996;37(1):3–13.
15. Kramer SC, Gorich J, Aschoff AF, et al. Diagnostic value of spiral-CT angiography in comparison with digital subtraction angiography before and after peripheral vascular intervention. *Angiology* 1998;49(8):599–606.
16. Rieker O, Duber C. Prospective comparison of CT angiography of the legs with intraarterial digital subtraction angiography. *AJR* 1996;166:269–276.

9

Foot Pressure Abnormalities in the Diabetic Foot

Thomas E. Lyons, DPM, Barry I. Rosenblum, DPM, and Aristidis Veves, MD, DSc

INTRODUCTION

For more than 50 years, foot pressure measurements have been used to evaluate many medical conditions. Early techniques to assess plantar foot pressure were simple, innovative methods that provided investigators with semiquantitative data. The introduction of the optical pedobarograph significantly improved the accuracy of foot pressure measurements. Furthermore, computer technologies have allowed accurate and reproducible measurements that can be used not only for research purposes, but also for treating patients with diabetes mellitus.

Foot pressure measurements and plantar ulceration have been extensively researched in the insensate foot *(1–19)*. In western societies, the principal cause of the insensate foot is diabetes mellitus; in other regions of the world, leprosy remains an important contributing factor *(19)*. In fact, the study of patients with Hansen's disease has allowed an understanding of the pathophysiology of the insensate foot and its principles of treatment *(19)*. Moreover, the foot pressure measurements can be clinically valuable in other clinical entities such as rheumatoid arthritis, hallux valgus, and sports medicine.

METHODS OF MEASURING FOOT PRESSURES

Out-of-Shoe Methods

One of the earliest studies to examine foot pressures was that of Beely in 1882 *(20)*. Subjects ambulated over a cloth-filled sack filled with plaster of Paris to produce a footprint. Beely postulated that the plaster would capture the plantar aspect of the foot with the highest load, representing the deepest impression. However, this primitive technique was limited because it represented a crude measurement the total force of the foot creating the impression rather than the dynamic pressures underneath the foot during gait. Moreover, this method was strictly qualitative and therefore susceptible to both inter- and intraobserver unreliability.

In 1930, Morton *(21)* described a ridged, deformable rubber pad, termed the *kinetograph.* This pad made contact with an inked paper placed underneath the foot as the subject ambulated over the pad. The kinetograph examined the relationship between the static and rigid foot deformity and was the first documented attempt to measure foot

From: *The Diabetic Foot, Second Edition*
Edited by: A. Veves, J. M. Giurini, and F. W. LoGerfo © Humana Press Inc., Totowa, NJ

pressures rather than forces. Elftman *(22)* further developed a system that allowed for the observation of dynamic changes in pressure distribution as the subject ambulated. This device was called the *barograph* and consisted of a rubber mat that was smooth on top yet studded with pyramidal projections on the bottom. The mat was placed on a glass plated, and as subjects ambulated over the mat, the area of contact of the projections increased according to changes in the pressures under the foot. A video camera recorded the deformation pattern of the mat from below as the subject walked on the mat.

Harris–Beath Mat

Similarly, in 1947, Harris and Beath *(23)* used a similar method to study foot problems and related foot pressure changes in a large group of Canadian soldiers. Their device used a multilayered inked rubber mat that allowed contact with a piece of paper below. When pressure was applied to the mat with ambulation, the ink escaped from it, thereby staining the paper. Thus, the density of the inked impression was dependent on the applied pressure. By using this technique, Barrett and Mooney *(24)* found high loading under the feet of subjects with diabetes. The major problem with this device, however, was that it could not be calibrated to various degrees of foot pressures and therefore the Harris–Beath Mat would saturate at levels within the normal limits of foot pressures. Furthermore, the amount of ink placed onto the mat could not be standardized. Silvino and associates *(25)*, however, calibrated the Harris–Beath mat by using a contact area of known size and weight, thereby producing both qualitative and semiquantitative data.

Podotrack

A similar device to the Harris–Beath mat is the Podotrack system (Medical Gait Technology, The Netherlands). The system is based on the principles of the Harris–Beath mat. However, the footprint impression is produced by a chemical reaction with carbon paper instead of ink. The Podotrack system has a few advantages over the Harris–Beath mat. For example, there is a standard ink layer that is carbon paper. Furthermore, the system can be calibrated with a scale representing shades of colors corresponding to foot pressures. In 1994, a study reported that the Podotrack system provided reproducible results in 61% of the foot pressure values when compared with those obtained from the pedobarograph *(26)*. Furthermore, the Podotrack and pedobarograph systems were comparatively examined. By placing the Podotrack system on top of the pedobarograph, one could obtain real-time data as subjects ambulated over both systems.

In 1974, Arcan and Brull *(27)* described a system that had the capability of providing more detailed, though semiquantitative, information regarding foot pressure distribution. The apparatus consisted of a rigid transparent platform with optical filters. An optically sensitive elastic material and reflective layer were combined together. Foot pressure measurements were performed either statically or dynamically, and the changes in motion of the foot were recorded using a video camera.

An earlier quantitative technique to measure foot pressures was described by Hutton and Drabble in 1972 *(28)*. Their device consisted of a force plate in which 12 beams were suspended from two load cells. These load cells were attached to several sets of wire strain gauges that permitted the measurement of longitudinal tension. The apparatus was placed onto the walkway because subjects could step on and off the plate during their gait cycle. By using this technique, Scott and colleagues *(29)* scrutinized the load distribution in subjects with and without pes planus (flatfeet) and hallux valgus deformities. The distribution of peak loads was expressed as a percentage of body weight and the results demonstrated that the load of the control subjects was low in the midfoot and high in the forefoot. However, there was considerable variation in loads across the ball of the foot. Conversely, in subjects with pes planus, an increased load was appreciated. In addition, their study reported that subjects who had greater body weight tended to have higher peak loads on the lateral aspect of the foot.

In a later study by Stokes and associates *(18)*, foot pressures, body weight, and foot ulceration in patients with diabetes were examined. Their study was remarkable in that it demonstrated that foot ulcers occurred at sites of maximal load. Furthermore, increased loads in patients with foot ulceration were related to their body weight when they were compared with healthy controls and patients with diabetes without ulcerations.

Subsequently, Ctercteko and colleagues *(17)* developed a computer system that measured vertical foot pressures of the sole on the foot in diabetic patients with and without ulceration and in subjects during ambulation. The system consisted of a load sensitive device divided into 128 strain gauge load cells with a 15 × 15 mm surface area that was built into an 8-m walkway. The foot was divided into eight areas, and the output from each load cell was processed and transmitted into a microcomputer. An evaluation of the data provided quantitative values for the sites of peak force and pressure under the foot and duration of contact time. It demonstrated that in both groups of diabetic subjects, with and without ulceration, a similar pattern of reduced toe loading was noted when compared with control subjects. This resulted in a higher loading at the metatarsophalangeal (MTP) head region, where the majority of ulcerations were present. These results confirmed that foot ulceration occurred at sites of maximal load under the foot.

Optical Pedobarograph

The optical pedobarograph is a device that measures dynamic plantar pressures. The device is based on an earlier system described by Chodera in 1957. The optical pedobarograph consists of an elevated walkway with a glass plate that is illuminated along the edge and covered with a thin sheet of soft plastic *(30)*. The light is then reflected internally within the plate when no pressure is applied. However, when a subject stands or ambulates across the surface, light escapes from the glass at these pressure points and is scattered by the plastic sheet, producing an image of the foot that can be seen below. A monochromatic camera detects the image, and the pressure at any given point can be determined automatically by measuring the intensity of that image at that specific point. This system has high spatial resolution and thereby allows an accurate measurement of high-foot pressures under small areas of the foot with satisfactory precision. The optical barograph is used widely in the examination of high-foot pressures such as in the diabetic foot. Additionally, this system has been used for interventional trials that study the effectiveness of offloading high-pressure areas. However, this system is limited to measurements of barefoot pressures and therefore does not allow the evaluation of in-shoe pressures. Moreover, this system requires substantial space and is not easily portable.

In-Shoe Methods

Over the past two decades, developments in computer technology have enabled microprocessor-like recording devices to measure in-shoe foot pressures. In 1963, Bauman and Brand *(31)* recognized the limitations of barefoot pressure measurements in the insensate and deformed foot. The apparatus they devised was composed of thin pressure-sensitive transducers that were attached to suspected areas of high pressure underneath the foot. Although this method was expensive and elaborate in design, it proved that in-shoe foot pressures were both feasible and indeed useful. In essence, Bauman and Brand laid the foundation for the design of less expensive devices to become available for general use.

ELECTRODYNAGRAM

The aforementioned principles were used in the mid-1970s to develop the electro-dynagram system (EDG System, Langer Biomechanics Group, Deer Park, New York). It is currently used in both clinical and research settings *(32,33)*. This apparatus is a computer-assisted system that uses seven small, separate sensors that adhere to the plantar aspect of the foot. They are attached by cable and relay information into a computer pack carried by the subject, In-shoe and out-of-shoe walking pressures can be evaluated. However, the system is limited because only peak pressures can be measured where the sensors are placed. Hence, this system cannot provide pressure information pertaining to the entire plantar aspect of the foot.

EMED SYSTEM

The EMED system is another computer-assisted and image-generating device that can record both in-shoe and out-of-shoe dynamic foot pressures. Its design is continually updated regularly and permits the examination of the entire plantar aspect of the foot. The system consists of a mat based on the principle that a change in the pressure on a wire causes a similar change on its electrical capacitance, thereby allowing foot pressures to be measured by recording electrical flow through the mat. The device incorporates a sensor area 445×225 mm^2 that has a resolution of 5 mm^2 and can provide measurements with satisfactory reliability. The system has a wide clinical appeal and has been used to scrutinize the asymmetry of plantar pressure distribution in young adults with adults with ankle fractures and diabetic patients with foot ulcerations or Charcot neuroarthropathy *(34)*.

FSCAN SYSTEM

At the author's unit, much study has been conducted using the FSCAN System. This system is a high-resolution, computerized pressure, force, and gait analysis program that was designed according to the principles described previously *(35,36)*. The hardware system collects both static and dynamic plantar pressures data by using either mats (F-Mat™ or HR Mat™) or F-scan in-shoe sensor. The mats measure foot pressures as the subject freely ambulates or stands over the mat without sensor cables that may potentially influence an individual's gait pattern or standing position (Fig.1A,B).

The F-Scan system uses an in-shoe sensor that is ultrathin (0.007 inch/0.15 mm) and flexible. It consists of 960 sensing locations referred to as elements that are distributed

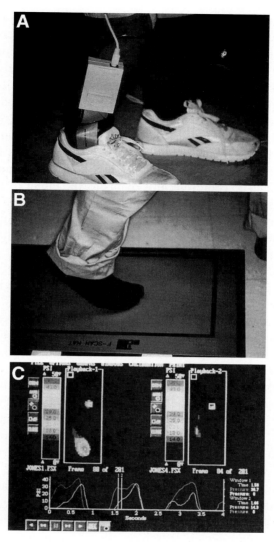

Fig. 1. (A) A subject walking with the FSCAN sensor inserted in his shoes. Changes in the electrical capacitance, which are related to the applied pressures on the sensors during walking, are transmitted via the cable to an IBM compatible computer, in which they are analyzed using the FSCAN software. *(12)*. **(B)** The FSCAN mat, which is based on the same principles used to design the FSCAN sensors, can be used to measure pressures of bare feet. The mat is compatible and is connected to the same apparatus used for in-shoe measurements *(12)*. **(C)** Computer-assisted analysis of a foot step. The highest foot pressures in this subject are seen underneath the heel and the first metatarsal area *(12)*.

uniformly across the entire plantar aspect of the foot *(36,37)*. These sensing elements provide the spatial resolution required for detecting differential pressures exerted over relatively small areas. The unique F-Scan sensor can be trimmed to sizes and inserted into the subject's footwear. The sensor does not interfere with the subject's foot function or reduce the true pressures by accommodating to existing deformities (Fig.1C).

The sensor plugs into a 6-ounce analog-to-digital converter cuff unit about the ankle. This is attached to one or both of the subject's legs. A cable connects the cuff unit to the receiver card placed in the computer for the F-Scan standard system, or to the data logger (receiver) around the waist of the subject. The latter is called F-scan Mobile, the nontethered system. For clinical use, the calibration method entails applying a known load, which is commonly the subject's weight, over the sensing cells. By using the prescribed calibration method, an accuracy method of ±10% may be obtained.

For research use, the scanner system uses an additional calibration technique (via the use of a calibration bladder) called *equilibration*. Equilibration assigns unique calibration curve factors to each sensing cell. It is used to increase the uniformity of sensing cells within a given sensor. Therefore, this dampens the effect of cell-to-cell variation without reducing the spatial resolution. If these additional calibration techniques are followed, the accuracy of the pressure measurement system is within 3–5%. The F-Scan in-shoe system has the capability and option to be upgraded to include a sensor mat that can measure out-of-shoe foot pressures.

This system is advantageous because of its simplicity, easy storage, and reproducibility of data. Satisfactory reproducibility has been reported in the great majority of studies that have used this system. No significant differences in peak pressure were found in eight neuropathic patients with diabetes who had foot pressures measured three times over a short duration, whereas in another study, the coefficient of variation in healthy subjects was 7.8% among separate studies and 2.6% among different steps during the same study *(37,38)*.

The F-Scan sensors, however, have potential limitations. For example, the F-Mat sensor has decreased resolution compared with the in-shoe sensor. Furthermore, because the in-shoe sensor is very thin, it may fail from wrinkling and breakage and thereby yield incorrect data *(35)*. Rose and colleagues *(35)* found that two insole sensors gave different results when used on the same subject. Additionally, there was a decline in sensitivity if the sensor was used 12 times. Altering the shoe insole can also affect foot pressure measurement. However, this is not a limitation but an advantage. Material type, shape, and density affect contact area, load absorption, and force vector orientation, which in return alter force patterns, pressure profiles, and peak values. The high resolution of the F-Scan in-shoe sensor, therefore, allows one to measure the effect of shoe insole alterations useful in everyday clinical practice.

NATURAL HISTORY OF FOOT PRESSURE: ABNORMALITIES IN DIABETES MELLITUS

Foot pressure measurements in patients with diabetes have been attempted for over 30 years. Stokes et al. *(18)* used a segmental force platform to study 37 feet in 22 patients with diabetes. High loads were found at the sites of ulcers. Patients with high loads under the feet were also heavier in weight than those with lower loads. Toe loads in patients with ulcers were found to be reduced. A shift of maximum loads to the lateral foot in neuropathic patients was also reported. In a subsequent study, Ctercteko and colleagues *(17)* confirmed all these findings, except for the lateral shift of maximum loads. Conversely, a medial shift was discovered in their study. In another study, neither a medial nor a lateral shift was found. However, peak pressures under the heel occurred with a lower frequency in all patients with diabetes compared with patients without diabetes *(9)*.

This finding may suggest an early change when foot pressures start rising under the forefoot but still remain within normal limits, as in patients without neuropathy. In previous studies, we have shown that in diabetic neuropathic patients, there is a transfer of high pressures from the heel and the toes to the metatarsal head *(9)*. The main reasons for this transfer are neuropathy and limited joint mobility *(8,9)*. Neuropathy leads to atrophy of the intrinsic musculature of the foot and clawing of the toes, which may result in prominent metatarsal heads under which high pressures occur. Though we realize that forefoot pressures are increased in the feet of patients with diabetic neuropathy, it has also been demonstrated that rearfoot pressures also increase as well especially in moderate-to-severe neuropathy *(39)*. Moreover, a transfer of peak pressures from the rearfoot to the metatarsal heads was noted in patients with diabetic neuropathy *(13)*. Accordingly, it has been demonstrated that the ratio of forefoot to rearfoot pressures is indeed increased in severe diabetic neuropathy *(39)*. This further indicates the inability of the neuropathic foot to distribute foot pressure and avoid the development of high-foot pressures. Additionally, limited joint mobility impairs the ability of the foot to absorb and redistribute the forces related to impact on the ground while walking. Its effects on the foot appear to be global in nature and include reduced motion at the ankle, subtalar, and first metatarsophalangeal joints (MTPJ) *(40)*. Vital musculoskeletal structures such as the Achilles tendon and plantar fascia may also be involved with changes such as shortening and thickening of both structures *(41)*. The foot becomes stiff, rigid, and less able to dampen pressure. Consequently, this contributes to the development of high foot pressures and subsequent ulceration *(9,14)*. Additionally, patients with diabetes mellitus may also have reduced plantar soft tissue thickness *(42,43)*, which further reduces the ability of the foot to mitigate foot pressures. An inverse relationship exists between reduced plantar tissue thickness and elevated foot pressures in some patients with diabetes mellitus *(44)*.

FOOT PRESSURES AND FOOT ULCERATION

Foot ulceration is a significant cause of morbidity in patients with diabetes mellitus and can lead to prolonged lengths of hospital stay. Numerous risk factors for foot ulceration in diabetes have been confirmed. These include limited joint mobility, peripheral neuropathy, vascular disease, and high plantar pressures have been implicated as significant predisposing factors leading to ulceration in population-based and clinical studies seeking to quantify such relationships.

Boulton and associates *(5)* were the first group to employ the optical pedobarograph for research purposes to examine the relationship between high-foot pressures and ulceration. In their study, diabetic patients with and without neuropathy and individuals without diabetes were examined to evaluate the relationships among foot pressures, neuropathy, and foot ulceration. Their results demonstrated that a significantly larger number of patients with diabetic neuropathy had abnormally high-foot pressures compared with controls. Furthermore, patients with a previous history of foot ulceration had high pressures at ulceration sites. Because ulceration occurred at sites of high plantar foot pressures, foot pressure reduction, therefore should lead to a reduced incidence of foot ulceration in neuropathic patients with diabetes.

In a subsequent study performed by the same group, sorbothane shoe inserts were employed in an attempt to evaluate pressure reduction in patients with diabetes *(45)*.

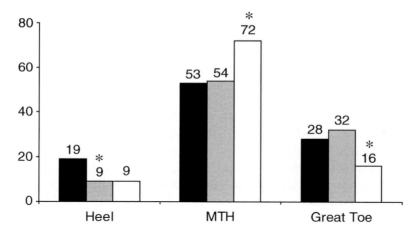

Fig. 2. Histogram demonstrating the distribution of peak pressures under the foot of healthy subjects (black columns), diabetic nonneuropathic patients (gray columns) and neuropathic patients with diabetes (white columns). Peak pressures were more often under the metatarsal heads of the neuropathic patients, whereas they were less often under the heel and great toe. It is also of interest that peak pressures under the heel were less frequent in the nonneuropathic patients ($*p < 0.05$) *(15)*.

Abnormally high-foot pressures were measured in 33% of feet without insoles and in 6% of feet when using the insoles, thereby indicating that special accommodative insoles may help reduce plantar foot pressures in diabetic neuropathic patients.

In a prospective study that lasted 3 year and comprised diabetic patients with long-standing diabetes and neuropathy, Kelly and Coventry *(46)* also examined the long-term changes in plantar foot pressure. Their results demonstrated that important alterations of foot pressure distribution had occurred in a significant number of these subjects, some of whom had developed recurrent ulcerations at these sites of high pressure. Moreover, it was again confirmed that patients with neuropathy and the characteristic intrinsic-minus foot had abnormally high-foot pressures measured at the metatarsal heads *(15)*.

Definite proof that abnormally high pressures in patients with diabetes were related to the development of plantar foot ulceration can be derived from a pivotal prospective study that followed a large number of patients for a mean period of 30 months *(15)*. During this study, plantar ulcers developed in 17% of all feet and in 45% of feet with diabetic neuropathy. All of these ulcerations occurred in patients with high foot pressures at baseline, thereby suggesting that high-foot pressures, especially in neuropathic patients, are predictive for the development of foot ulceration and may be useful for identifying at-risk patients (Fig. 2).

Given the correlation between foot pressures and foot ulceration, a study to evaluate the role between joint mobility and racial affinity in the development of high-foot pressures was performed. This study demonstrated that black subjects without diabetes and patients with diabetes have increased joint mobility compared to Caucasian healthy subjects and patients with diabetes *(16)*. An increase in joint mobility results in lower peak plantar pressures and therefore a lower risk of foot ulceration.

Similarly, the role of neuropathy and high-foot pressures in diabetic foot ulceration was evaluated *(47)*. In a cross-sectional multicenter study, the magnitude of association of several different risk factors for foot ulceration in patients with diabetes mellitus was determined. A cross-sectional group of 251 subjects consisting of Caucasian, Black, and Hispanic races were studied. There was equal distribution of men and women across the entire study population. All patients underwent a complete medical history and lower extremity evaluation for neuropathy and foot pressures. Neuropathic factors were dichotomized (0/1) into 2 high-risk variables: a high vibration perception threshold (hiVPT) >25 V and unable to feel a 5.07 or smaller Semmes–Weinstein monofilament (Hi SWF). The mean dynamic foot pressures of three footsteps were measured using the FSCAN mat system with patients walking in stockings but without shoewear. Maximum plantar pressures were dichotomized into a high pressure variable (Pmax6) indicating those subjects with pressures ≥ 6 kg/cm^2 ($n = 96$). The total of 99 patients had a current or prior history of ulceration at baseline.

The sensor was used in a floor mat system designed to measure barefoot or stocking-foot dynamic pressures. Maximum peak pressures for the entire foot were obtained without regard for specific location by averaging those obtained for three midgait foot steps and were then dichotomized into a high pressure variable indicating those subjects with pressures ≥ 6 kg/cm^2.

With a specific focus on plantar foot pressures, joint mobility and neuropathic parameters consistent with ulceration, this study demonstrated that patients with foot pressures ≥ 6 kg/cm^2 were twice as likely to have ulcerations than those without high pressures, even after adjustment for age, gender, diabetes duration, and racial affinity. In the black and Hispanic groups, significantly lower plantar pressures were demonstrated compared with the Caucasian group. High plantar pressures were relatively infrequent and were not found to be significant predictors of ulceration. Foot pressures ≥ 6 kg/cm^2 were independently associated with ulceration, but to a lesser extent than the neuropathy variables (Tables 1 and 2).

This study demonstrated that the association of high-foot pressures, high vibration perception threshold, and insensitivity to a 5.07 monofilament contributed to the development of foot ulceration. Furthermore, their group demonstrated significant racial difference in joint mobility, associated foot pressures, and the prevalence of ulceration among Caucasian, black, and Hispanic patients. These findings have guided efforts at detecting patients with diabetes at risk of ulceration by incorporating such parameters into screening programs. Foot pressures should be evaluated to detect those neuropathic individuals at risk of ulceration from excessive callus formation or repetitive stress *(9,10)*. Although the two measures of neuropathy have the greater magnitude of effect, foot pressures can still be evaluated to detect those neuropathic individuals at risk of ulceration from excessive plantar callus formation or repetitive stress.

THE ROLE OF FOOT PRESSURES: AS A SCREENING METHOD TO IDENTIFY AT-RISK PATIENTS

Because diabetic foot ulceration is a preventable long-term complication of diabetes mellitus, screening techniques to identify the at-risk patient are probably the most important step in reducing the rate of foot ulceration and lower limb amputation. To this

Table 1
Logistic Regression Results for Risk of Ulceration

	Odds ratio (O.R.)	95% Confidence interval	*p* value
Univariate results			
Age[a]	1.02	1.00–1.03	0.019
Sex[b]	0.26	0.18–0.38	0.000
BMI	0.97	0.94–0.99	0.048
Diabetes duration[a]	1.04	1.02–1.06	0.000
Pulses	0.31	0.18–0.52	0.000
Pmax6	3.9	2.6–5.7	0.000
HiVPT	11.7	7.4–18.4	0.000
HiSWF	9.6	5.02–18.5	0.000
HiRisk	7.4	4.8–11.6	0.000
Multivariate results	(Controlling for age, sex, duration, race)		
Pmax6	2.1	1.32–3.39	0.002
HiVPT	4.4	2.58–7.54	0.000
HiSWF	4.1	1.89–8.87	0.000
HiRisk[c]	4.1	2.48–6.63	0.000

[a] Indicates O.R. per year of increase.
[b] Indicates reduced risk of ulceration in females relative to males.
[c] Indicates multivariate O.R. for interaction term without other neuropathic or pressure variables in model.

Table 2
Multivariate Logistic Regression for Ulceration by Race, Controlling for Age, Sex, and Diabetes Duration

	Odds ratio (O.R.)	95% Confidence interval	*p* value
Caucasian			
Pmax6	7.7	2.07–28.4	0.002
HiVPT	7.4	2.4–22.9	0.001
HiSWF	3.7	1.3–10.3	0.013
Black			
Pmax6	0.53	0.05–5.8	0.608
HiVPT	7.2	1.2–43.7	0.032
HiSWF	19.8	1.1–344.2	0.041
Hispanic			
Pmax6	2.1	0.38–11.5	0.395
HiVPT	6.6	2.3–18.5	0.000
HiSWF[a]	–	–	–

[a] Dropped due to perfect prediction of outcome.

end, various screening techniques have been proposed and are currently in use. These include the evaluation of vibration perception threshold (VPT), foot pressure measurements, joint mobility, and SWF 5.07 testing. Furthermore, a history of previous foot ulceration, Tc PO_2 level of <30 mmHg and the existence of foot deformities have been shown to be risk factors for the development of diabetic foot ulceration. In our unit, a study evaluated plantar pressures and screening techniques to identify people at high risk for diabetic foot ulceration *(48)*. The objective of this study was to compare the specificity, sensitivity, and prospective predictive value of the most commonly used screening techniques for the identification of high risk for foot ulceration in a prospective multicenter fashion. Furthermore, this study aimed to identify as many risk factors as possible and to develop a screening strategy that, by combining the detection of two or more risk factors, would provide the best tool for identifying the at-risk patient.

Two hundred and forty-eight patients from three large diabetic foot centers including our own unit were evaluated in a prospective study. Neuropathy symptom score, neuropathy disability score (NDS), VPT, SWF, joint mobility, peak plantar pressures, and vascular status were evaluated in each of the subjects. Patients were followed up every 6 months for a mean period of 30 months, and all new foot ulcers were recorded. The sensitivity, specificity, and positive predictive value of each risk factor were evaluated.

Foot ulcers developed in 73 patients during the study. Patients who developed foot ulcers were frequently men, had diabetes for a longer duration, and had an inability to detect a 5.07 monofilament. NDS alone had the best sensitivity, whereas the combination of the NDS and the inability to detect a 5.07 monofilament reached a sensitivity of 99%. However, foot pressures had the best specificity, and the best combination was that of NDS and foot pressures.

This study prospectively evaluated the association of several risk factors for foot ulceration. The results demonstrated that a high NDS obtained during a simple stratified clinical examination provided the best sensitivity in identifying patients at risk for foot ulceration, whereas high VPT, the inability to feel a SWF 5.07 and high-foot pressures were independent factors. Furthermore, the combination of NDS and a SWF 5.07 (10 g) could identify all but 1 of 95 ulcerated feet. The use of these two simple methods in clinical practice can assist in identifying the at-risk patient, which is the first step in the prevention of foot ulceration. Foot pressures are often elevated in patients with diabetic neuropathy. However, as an initial tool by itself, the measurement of foot pressures is not very helpful in predicting the development of foot ulceration. This was demonstrated in this study and confirmed in a subsequent study *(49)*. In terms of predicting ulceration, foot pressure measurements are only useful when combined with other modalities making them not very practical as an initial tool. They may be used as a valuable postscreening test in conjunction with assessing the effectiveness of offloading by appropriate footwear.

Although several studies exist evaluating whole foot pressures, there is a paucity of research examining forefoot and rearfoot plantar pressures. In our unit, we measured forefoot and rearfoot pressures separately and examined their validity in predicting foot ulceration *(13)*. Ninety patients with diabetes mellitus were examined, and peak pressures under the rearfoot and forefoot were evaluated using the FSCAN mat system with subjects ambulating without foot wear *(13)*. Significant correlations were found between forefoot peak pressures and age, height, neuropathy disability score, VPT, and force applied on the ground while walking. In contrast, reverse correlations were found between rearfoot peak pressures and measurements of neuropathic severity.

Binary regression analysis demonstrated a higher risk of foot ulceration in patients with high foot pressures. However, no association was found for rearfoot pressure. Thus, peak foot pressure measurements of the forefoot, but not the rearfoot correlate with neuropathy measurements can also predict foot ulceration over 36 months. Moreover, forefoot pressure correlated with the severity of diabetic neuropathy and limited joint mobility. It is also of interest that a negative correlation was found between rearfoot and forefoot pressures. This finding confirms that there is a transfer of peak pressures from the rearfoot to the metatarsal heads in diabetic neuropathy. Additionally, it indicates an inability of the neuropathic foot to distribute pressure and avoid the development of high pressures that eventually leads to the production of foot ulceration under these areas. Therefore, measurement of forefoot peak pressures rather than the whole foot may be more useful for identifying at-risk patients when designing a screening protocol *(13)*.

OFFLOADING THE DIABETIC FOOT: THE ROLE OF FOOTWEAR

Given the high rate of foot ulceration in at-risk patients with diabetes, the need for better preventative methods to offload the foot cannot be more apparent. The effectiveness of footwear in reducing high plantar pressures has been scrutinized using the optical pedobarograph *(5,50–52)*. Several foot pressure studies have examined hosiery and insole materials in the diabetic at-risk population and in patients with rheumatoid arthritis and neuropathy *(12,15,16,50–52)*. Currently available footwear products are constantly evolving. Thus, the lack of uniform data makes the interpretation of pressure reduction studies challenging in both clinical and research settings.

Hosiery

The use of padded hosiery to reduce foot pressures has been evaluated in the literature *(45,51–53)*. In an initial study, the pressure-relieving capacity of specially designed hosiery with padding at the heel and forefoot was tested *(51)*. A significant reduction in peak plantar pressure, up to 30%, was obtained from patients with diabetes who were at risk for ulceration. In a subsequent study, commercially available hosiery, experimental hosiery, and padded socks were evaluated for foot pressure reduction *(52)*. Ten patients who wore experimental padded hosiery for 6 months were tested with an optical pedobarograph. The experimental hosiery continued to provide a significant reduction in forefoot pressures at 3 and 6 months, although the level of reduction was less than that seen at baseline.

Furthermore, commercial hosiery designed as sportswear was examined and compared with experimental hosiery. Although these socks (medium or high-density padding) provided a substantial pressure reduction vs barefoot (10.4% and 17.4%, respectively), this was not as great as that seen with experimental hosiery (27%) *(52)*. Thus, the use of socks designed to reduce pressures on diabetic neuropathic feet may be an effective adjunctive measure for the reduction of foot pressures. Although development of fiber technology and padding distribution continues, the currently available high-density socks are perhaps the best choice of hosiery for protection of the insensate foot.

In another study, in-shoe foot pressures of patients with at-risk feet were compared with healthy subject foot pressures without shoes using the FSCAN system *(14)*. Foot pressures were measured under three conditions in each subject. First, subjects were placed directly in the shoes (S) to measure the pressure between the footwear and the sock. Second, the sensor was taped directly to the barefoot (B), and the subject ambulated wearing both

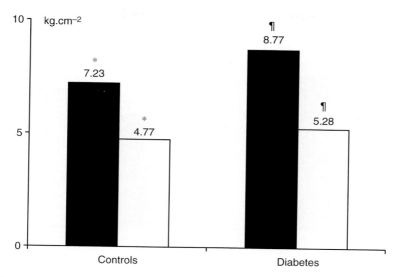

Fig. 3. Foot pressure measurement in healthy control subjects and patients with diabetes while wearing either their socks alone (black column) or both shoes and socks (white columns). Foot pressures with socks alone were significantly lower to the ones measured when ambulating with both shoes and socks in both subjects with diabetes and healthy subjects (*, ¶: $p < 0.02$) *(14)*.

footwear and socks. Finally, the footwear was removed, and each subject ambulated wearing only socks (H). The total force and peak pressure under each foot was measured for each condition.

The results demonstrated that the diabetic group had greater peak pressures compared with the controls and that in both groups a significant pressure reduction was found when subjects ambulated with footwear *(14)*. The study concluded that footwear can offer a cushioning effect and that this property may be further incorporated to design shoewear that can protect against the development of high-foot pressures and foot ulceration (Fig. 3).

Following this study, the authors prospectively examined the effect of using specially padded hosiery in combination with specially fit footwear on providing in-shoe pressure relief *(53)*. Fifty patients at risk for foot ulceration were recruited for the study. All of the patients were provided with three pairs of specially padded hosiery and with two pairs of extra-depth footwear or extra-width running shoes. Dynamic foot pressures were measured at baseline with the patients wearing their regular socks alone, regular footwear and socks, the padded socks, and the new footwear and padded socks. Foot pressures were measured at baseline and subsequent visits over a period of 30 months (Fig. 4).

As initial pressure relief was provided by the new footwear at baseline compared with the patients' own footwear, yet very few differences in peak forces were found among the baseline, interim, and final visits. Moreover, no significant changes in foot pressures were found over a period of 6 months of continuous usage using specifically designed footwear in a group of patients with diabetes at risk for foot ulceration. This also illustrates the importance of making simple recommendations of appropriate footwear

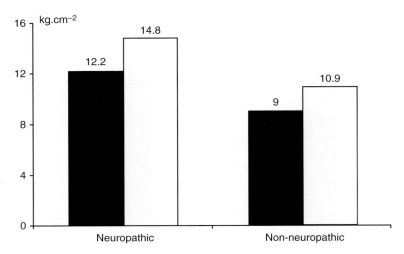

Fig. 4. Changes in the peak foot pressures in neuropathic and nonneuropathic patients over a period of 30 months. The pressures at the end of the study (white columns) were higher compared to the baseline measurements (black columns) in both the neuropathic and nonneuropathic patients *(15).*

in patients at risk for foot ulceration in an effort to provide the most suitable environment for such a foot.

Shoewear

Given the potential of shoes and associated modalities to reduce foot pressures in neuropathic feet and healthy subjects, a discussion of the associated offloading capabilities is warranted. It is anticipated that the use of modern technology may be useful in designing shoes and insoles that will redistribute and reduce foot pressures from areas prone to ulceration.

Shoes are an important consideration for patients at risk for ulceration. They provide protection as a covering for the feet and function as a barrier against toxic substances and thermal extremes. Shoes can also function to decrease plantar foot pressures. For example, noncustom footwear worn by healthy subjects without diabetes decreased foot pressures by 30–35% *(18).* Moreover, greater foot pressure reductions may be observed in patients with elevated foot pressures wearing shoes compared to walking barefoot.

Healing sandals have been employed to decrease plantar pressures in the diabetic foot *(54).* These sandals consist of a postoperative shoe with a thick, soft insole that can be further modified by making the sole rigid with a rocker bottom. The rocker sole is important for the reduction of plantar pressures underneath the forefoot *(2,55).* The soft sole allows for greater pressure distribution beneath the metatarsal heads, whereas the rocker sole alters the mechanics of the forefoot just prior to toe-off, both of which lead to reduced forefoot pressures *(55).*

The postoperative shoe is another modality used in the treatment of plantar foot ulcerations. This shoe is used quite frequently because of its availability; it provides the patient with a gait modifying device. Although it does decrease foot pressures, the postoperative shoe is only minimally effective in the treatment of foot ulcerations compared with other modalities *(54)* and is slightly more effective than a canvas shoe *(56)*. Modifications to the sole and insole may further enhance the effectiveness of the post-operative shoe.

Additionally, half-shoes have been used with success for plantar pressure reduction *(54–56)*. These shoes consist of a postoperative shoe with a large wedge heel that extends just behind the forefoot. The forefoot in the postoperative shoe with a heel of this configuration is kept off the ground. Pressure reduction can be as high as 66% compared with pressures in a baseline canvas shoe *(56)*. Because of the configuration of the heel which is high and wedged in dorsiflexion, instability when ambulating can be a problem. This instability is even more significant with neuropathic patients. Therefore, an ambulatory aid such as a cane or crutches may assist in walking.

Not all shoes relieve foot pressures equally; however, employing materials that significantly reduce foot pressures may prevent the recurrence of ulceration in patients with a prior history of ulceration *(56)*. Shoes that provide a cushion effect reduce plantar pressures *(54,56)*. Leather oxford shoes may decrease plantar pressures in some areas and yet increase pressures in other regions, particularly underneath the lateral metatarsal heads and great toe *(56)*. Therefore, when purchasing a dress shoe, patients should select a softer sole as opposed to a harder sole, which may not afford as much pressure relief. A dress shoe with a rigid sole can be replaced with a softer sole without dramatically altering the appearance of the shoe. Also, selection of a shoe with a removable insole allows for frequent replacement of worn insoles with a new insole and results in a greater cushioning effect.

Running shoes are an option for patients with elevated foot pressures and at-risk feet *(56–58)* (Fig. 5). Also, running shoes are less expensive than extra-depth and custom footwear. They provide a readily available option for obtaining protective shoewear for patients with a reasonably straight foot. Moreover, running shoes may provide a more cosmetically acceptable alternative to extra-depth or custom shoes. Significant pressure reduction can be expected with running shoes. Thirty-nine subjects were studied to evaluate the pressure-reducing effects of running shoewear *(58)*. Three groups of 13 subjects were categorized as having diabetes with neuropathy, diabetes without neuropathy, and those with neither diabetes nor neuropathy. Foot pressures were evaluated while subjects were wearing thin socks and compared with those of subjects wearing leather oxfords and running shoes. A mean decrease in foot pressures of 31% was noted for all three groups while wearing running shoes compared with wearing the socks alone *(58)*.

In another study, 13 patients with diabetes and neuropathy were evaluated in various types of footwear, including the patients' own leather oxfords and extra-depth and running shoes *(59)*. Running shoes were found to decrease mean plantar foot pressures in comparison with the patients' own leather oxfords by 47% at the second and third MTPJ, 29% at the first MTPJ, and 32% at the great toe *(59)*. Running shoes are therefore a viable option for patients at risk for ulceration. For patients with significant foot deformities and prominences other options such as custom footwear must be considered.

Different types of shoes provide various levels of plantar pressure relief. A recent study using a running shoe product found a decrease of between 27% and 38% in plantar pressures compared with a leather oxford product *(60)*. Similarly, another study employing a running shoe demonstrated a reduction of between 29% and 47% in foot pressures compared with leather oxford footwear *(61)*.

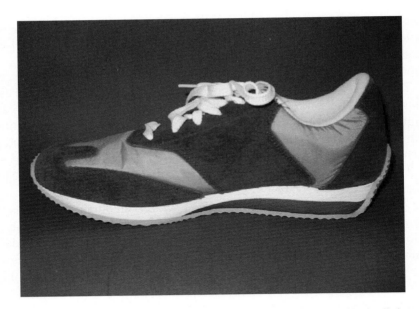

Fig. 5. Running shoes can reduce foot pressures. They are readily available, lightweight, and affordable. The material of the shoe upper is soft and padded on the inside where it interfaces with the foot. A soft sole will reduce foot pressures along with a soft insole that should be removable to allow for frequent replacement.

Note that athletic shoes may not provide the same pressure relief compared with running shoes. For example, cross-trainer-style footwear may not decrease foot pressures compared with running shoes *(38)*. Foot pressures in 32 diabetic patients with neuropathy and histories of recently healed ulcerations were examined. Foot pressures were measured in a canvas oxford and compared with those using an extra-depth shoe, an SAS comfort shoe, and athletic cross-trainer shoes. Measurements were obtained with the manufacturers' insole and with a visco-elastic insole for each shoe type. For patients with a history of ulcerations underneath the metatarsal heads, pressure reduction in all three shoe types were relatively similar as compared to foot pressures in canvas shoe *(38)*.

However, for those patients with a history of great toe ulcers, the extra-depth and comfort SAS shoes decreased foot pressures under the great toe, whereas the cross-trainer shoewear actually increased foot pressures in this area as compared to the canvas oxfords. One may surmise that foot pressure reduction between running shoes and cross-training shoes may be different particularly underneath the great toe. Therefore, patient counseling on the selection and purchase of specific footwear is vital; especially in the marketplace where the vast choices of footwear available may easily overwhelm a patient not familiar with athletic shoes *(38)*.

Extra-depth footwear is another option for the patient with at-risk feet. The extra space in the toe box is particularly useful for patients with forefoot deformities. Extra-depth footwear also decreases foot pressures significantly *(56–58)*. The pressure reduction ability of extra-depth shoewear can be further augmented with the use of specially padded socks as discussed previously *(59,60)* and insoles *(58)*. It is the authors' experience that many extra-depth shoes contain a flat insole with minimal cushioning quality.

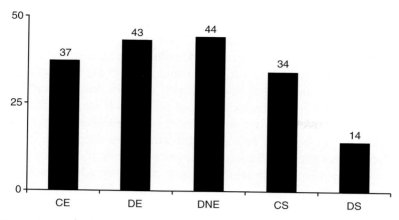

Fig. 6. Percentage of foot pressure relief achieved by the athletic shoes in healthy controls who exercised regularly (CE group), type 1 nonneuropathic diabetic patients who exercised regularly (DE), type 1 diabetic neuropathic patients who exercised regularly (DNE), healthy controls who did not exercise regularly (CS) and patients with diabetes who did not exercise regularly (DS). The highest pressure relief was achieved in the three first groups who consisted of regularly exercising subjects. These data indicate that proper selection of footwear can result to considerable pressure relief *(55)*.

A study evaluating extra-depth shoes demonstrated pressure reduction with the factory insole 16%, 27%, 19%, and 34% at the great toe, first MTPJ, second MTPJ, third MTPJ and heel, respectively *(54)*. With a custom accommodative insole, the pressure reduction was increased to 33, 50, 48, and 49%, respectively *(55)*. In a subsequent study, 32 patients with diabetes and a history of ulceration noted a significant reduction in foot pressures using extra-depth shoes when compared with a baseline of the patient's own canvas oxford. When the factory-constructed insole was replaced with a commercially available insole, a further pressure reduction of 4–15% was observed. Therefore, pressure reduction using extra-depth shoes can easily be augmented with the use of a readily available insole. The pressure reducing ability of extra-depth footwear can be further augmented with specially padded socks *(47)*.

In another study, patients with diabetes who exercised and those who did not were evaluated to determine what effect aerobic exercise might have on foot pressures with and without shoes *(60)*. When participants ambulated without their shoes, the peak pressures were highest in group DNE (diabetic nonexercisers). Foot pressures were also higher in groups CE (healthy exercisers), CS (healthy nonexercisers), and DE (exercisers with diabetes); probably a result of the increased stress of the foot skin and the subsequent callus formation.

However, when foot pressures were measured wearing shoes a different picture emerged. The foot pressures were highest in groups CS and DS, intermediate in group DNE, and lowest in groups CE and DE (Fig. 6). Those who consistently exercised achieved the highest pressure relief. These differences may reflect the ability of regularly exercising individuals to choose comfortable and good quality shoewear. In summary, these results indicate that proper selection of footwear can result in considerable pressure relief.

Insoles and Orthotics

Insoles and orthotics are recommended for the prevention of ulcerations in at-risk feet. *(38,61–64)*. The addition of a material to cushion the plantar aspect of the foot can decrease foot pressures significantly *(5)*. By using a 5-mm thick visco-elastic polymer insole, foot pressure reduction has been reported *(45)*. In another study, 4-mm thick visco-elastic insoles were noted to decrease foot pressures from 5–20% above what was observed with stock insoles of extra-depth, comfort, and athletic shoes *(30)*.

Custom orthotics of both the soft and rigid variety are used to decrease foot pressures *(38,61–64)*. Heat-pressed Plastizote™ insoles decrease foot pressures for diabetic patients by 40–50% *(62)*. Modifications to these insoles by adding arch or metatarsal pads do not increase the pressure reduction significantly *(62)*. However, rigid materials such as polyurethane foot orthoses may reduce plantar pressures by approx 50% *(63)*. Rigid orthotics composed of graphite materials decrease pressures underneath the first metatarsal head and medial heel by approx 30–40% *(63,64)*.

The FSCAN system was employed to measure dynamic pressures at the shoe–foot interface during normal walking with different orthotics *(65)*. This study evaluated the efficacy of pressure redistribution with a Plastizote, Spenco, cork, and plastic foot orthosis as compared with a control (no orthotic). Measurements varied upwards to 18% between sensors and changes in stance time of up to 5% occurred between the orthotics and the control conditions. These results demonstrated the inherent measurement variances of the FSCAN system using numerous orthoses.

Although these variances hindered reliability among the orthoses, statistically significant differences in peak pressure between the orthotics were noted. Plastizote, cork, and plastic foot orthoses were beneficial for decreasing pressure in the forefoot, heel, and second through fifth metatarsal regions. However, these orthotics had the potential to increase the plantar pressures in the midfoot region. In conclusion, the results demonstrated that using an orthotic to relieve pressures in one region of the shoe–foot interface may increase pressures over another region of the plantar surface *(65)*.

Viswanathan et al. also evaluated the effectiveness of different insoles in therapeutic footwear. They evaluated neuropathic patients with diabetes stratified into four groups. Three of the four groups consisted of patients with therapeutic shoes with insoles, each group differing in the composition of the insole. They were compared with a fourth group of similar neuropathic diabetic patients with nontherapeutic footwear. Foot pressures were measured initially and 9 months later and were noted to be significantly reduced along with the rate of development of new ulcerations as compared to the group wearing the nontherapeutic footwear *(66)*.

Interestingly, not all studies support the use of therapeutic footwear in the prevention of foot ulcerations in those patients at risk. A recent study by Reiber et al. *(67)* has demonstrated that therapeutic footwear did not prevent ulceration in their study of diabetic individuals without severe foot deformity. In this study, patients with custom foot insoles fared no better than patients with prefabricated foot insoles and control patients with their usual footwear. All three groups had a similar rate of ulceration. It is important to understand that this does not indicate that therapeutic footwear has less importance than previously thought. It may play just as an important role as ever in patients with severe deformities. It may also mean that the custom insoles in the study were not offloading the sites of increased pressure any better than prefabricated devices or usual footwear but this is difficult to ascertain as pressure measurements between groups was not carried out. Perhaps future studies may investigate the ability of widely dispensed therapeutic footwear to decrease foot pressures by actually measuring foot pressure reduction and correlating this to the ability to decrease risk of ulceration.

SUMMARY

Several methods of measuring and reducing foot pressures including their advantages and limitations have been discussed. Extra-depth footwear, jogging shoes, hosiery, insoles, and orthoses have been shown to decrease plantar foot pressures. Furthermore, these devices can prevent the occurrence and recurrence of foot ulceration. However, when using orthoses or other inserts care must be taken not to increase pressures over another region of the foot.

In the last two decades, the development of intricate computerized systems has revolutionized diabetic foot pressure measurements and made their application possible for daily clinical practice. Foot pressure measurements obtained from out-of-shoe and in-shoe methods may have far-reaching consequences for both research and clinical applications. Moreover, these systems can potentially identify at-risk patients and provide a basis for the implementation of either footwear modifications or surgical intervention. Foot pressure measurement systems are still being developed. Currently, research is in the initial phase of developing methods of measuring in-shoe shear forces. Piezoelectric transducers are currently being evaluated which may be able to measure both vertical and shear forces *(68)*. In the future, computer systems will hopefully become more widely available and may be employed routinely for diabetic foot management and a variety of foot conditions.

SUGGESTED READING

1. Welton EA. The Harris and Beath footprint: interpretation and clinical value. *Foot Ankle* 1992;13:462–468.
2. van Schie CH, Abbott CA, Vileikyte L, et al. A comparative study of Podotrack, a simple semiquantitative plantar pressure measuring device and the optical pedobarograph on the assessment of pressure under the diabetic foot. *Diabet Med* 1999;16:154–159.
3. van Ijzer M. The Podotrack, a new generation Harris mat. *Podopost,* 1993;39–41.

REFERENCES

1. Wagner FW. The diabetic foot. *Orthopedics* 1987;10:163–172.
2. Pollard JP, LeQuesne IP, Tappin JW. Forces under the foot. *J Biomed Eng* 1983;5:37–41.
3. Lang-Stevenson AI, Sharrard WJ, Betts RP, et al. Neuropathic ulcers of the foot. *J Bone Joint Surg Br* 1985;67:438–442.
4. Boulton AJ, Betts RP, Franks CI, et al. The natural history of foot pressure abnormalities in neuropathic diabetic subjects. *Diabetes Care* 1987;5:73–77.
5. Boulton AJ, Hardisty CA, Betts RP, et al. Dynamic foot pressure and other studies as diagnostic and management aids in diabetic neuropathy. *Diabetes Care* 1983;6:26–33.
6. Betts RP, Duckworth TJ. Plantar pressure measurements and prevention of ulceration in the diabetic foot. *J Bone Joint Surg* 1985;67:79–85.

7. Boulton AJ, Veves A, Young MJ. Etiopathogenesis and management of abnormal foot pressures, in *The Diabetic Foot* (Levin ME, O'Neal LW, Bowker JH, eds.), 5th ed. St. Louis, Mosby, 1993, pp 233–246.

8. Fernando DJ, Masson EA, Veves A, et al. Limited joint mobility: relationship to abnormal foot pressures and diabetic foot ulceration. *Diabetes Care* 1991;14:8–11.

9. Veves A, Fernando DJ, Walewski P, et al. A study of plantar pressures in a diabetic clinic population. *Foot* 1991;2:89–92.

10. Young MJ, Cavanagh P, Thomas G, et al. The effect of callus removal on dynamic plantar foot pressures in diabetic patients. *Diabet Med* 1992;5:55–57.

11. Cavanagh PR, Sims DS, Sander LJ. Body mass is a poor predictor of peak plantar pressure in diabetic men. *Diabetes Care* 1991;14:750–755.

12. VM, Veves A. Foot pressure measurement. *Orthop Phys Ther Clin N Am* 1997;6:1–16.

13. Rich J, Veves A. Forefoot and rearfoot plantar pressures in diabetic patients: correlation to foot ulceration. *Wounds* 2000;12(4):82–87.

14. Sarnow MR, Veves A, Giurini JM, et al. In-shoe foot pressure measurements in diabetic patients with at-risk feet and in healthy subjects. *Diabetes Care* 1994;17:1002–1006.

15. Veves A, Murray HJ, Young MJ, et al. The risk of foot ulceration in diabetic patients with high foot pressure: a prospective study. *Diabetologia* 1992;35:660–663.

16. Veves A, Sarnow MR, Giurini JM, et al. Differences in joint mobility and foot pressures between black and white diabetic patients. *Diabet Med* 1995;12:585–589.

17. Ctercteko G, Dhanendran M, Hutton WC, et al. Vertical forces acting on the feet of diabetic patients with neuropathic ulceration. *Br J Surg* 1981;68:608–614.

18. Stokes IA, Furis IB, Hutton WC. The neuropathic ulcer and loads on the foot in diabetic patients. *Acta Orthop Scand* 1975;46:839–847.

19. Brand PW. *Insensitive Feet, a Practical Handbook of Foot Problems in Leprosy*. London, The Leprosy Mission, 1984.

20. Beely F. Zur mechanik des Stehens uber die Bedentung des Fussgewolbes beim Stehen Langenbecks. *Archiv fur klinische Chirurgie* 1882;27:47.

21. Morton DJ. Structural factors in static disorders of the foot. *Am J Surg* 1930;19:315.

22. Elftman H. A cinematic study of the distribution of pressure in the human foot. *Anat Rec* 1934;59:481.

23. Harris RI, Beath T. Army foot survey. Report of national research council of Canada, Ohawa. 1947.

24. Barrett JP, Mooney V. Neuropathy and diabetic pressure lesions. *Orthop Clin North Am* 1973;4:43.

25. Silvino N, Evanski PM, Waugh TR. The Harris and Beath footprinting mat: diagnostic validity and clinical use. *Clin Orthop Relat Res* 1980;(151):265–269.

26. Barnes D: A comparative study of two barefoot pressure measuring systems. BMSc thesis, University of Dundee, 1994.

27. Arcan M, Brull MA. Fundamental characteristics of the human body and foot: the foot-ground pressure pattern. *J Biomech* 1976;9:453–457.

28. Hutton WC, Drabble GE. An apparatus to give the distribution of vertical load under the foot. *Rheumatol Phys Med* 1972;11:313–317.

29. Stott JR, Hutton WC, Stokes IA. Forces under the foot. *J Bone Joint Surg Br* 1973;55B:335–344.

30. Holmes GB, Willits NH. Practical considerations for the use of the pedobarograph. *Foot Ankle* 1991;12(2):105–108.

31. Bauman JH, Brand PW. Measurement of pressure between the foot and shoe. *Lancet* 1963;1:629–632.

32. Duckworth T, Betts RP, Franks CI, et al. The measurement of pressures under the foot. *Foot Ankle* 1992;3(3):130–141.

33. Feehery RV. Clinical applications of the electrodynogram. *Clin Pediatr Med Surg* 1986;3:609–612.
34. Wolf L, Stess R, Graf P. Dynamic foot pressure analysis of the diabetic Charcot foot. *J Am Pediatr Med Assoc* 1991;81:281.
35. Rose N, Feiwell LA, Cracchiolo AC. A method for measuring foot pressure using a high resolution, computerized insole sensor: the effect of heel wedges on plantar pressure distribution and center of force. *Foot Ankle* 1992;13(5):263–270.
36. Pitei D, Edmonds M, Lord M, et al. FSCAN: a new method of in-shoe dynamic measurement of foot pressure. *Diabetic Med* 1993;7(Suppl. 2):S39(abstract).
37. Young CR. The FSCAN system of foot pressure analysis. *Clin Pediatr Med Surg* 1993;10:455–461.
38. Lavery LA, Vela S, Fleischli JG, et al. Reducing plantar pressures in the neuropathic foot. *Diabetes Care* 1997;20:1706–1710.
39. Caselli A, Pham H, Giurini JM, et al. The forefoot-to-rearfoot plantar pressure ration is increased in severe diabetic neuropathy and can predict foot ulceration. *Diabetes Care* 2002;25:1066–1071.
40. Delbridge L, Perry P, Marr S, et al. Limited joint mobility in the diabetic foot: relationship to neuropathic ulceration. *Diabet Med* 1988;5:3333–3337.
41. D'Ambrogi E, Giurato L, D'Agostino M, et al. Contribution of plantar fascia to the increased forefoot pressures in diabetic patients. *Diabetes Care* 2003;26:1525–1529.
42. Goooing AW, Stess RM, Graf PM, et al. Sonography of the sole of the foot: evidence for loss of foot pad thickness in diabetes and its relationship to ulceration of the foot. *Invest Radiol* 1986;2145–2148.
43. Brink T. Induration of the diabetic foot pad: another risk factor for recurrent neuropathic plantar ulcers. *Biomed Technik* 1995;40:205–209.
44. Abouaesha F, van Schie C, Griffiths G, et al. Plantar tissue thickness is related to peak plantar pressure in the high-risk diabetic foot. *Diabetes Care* 2001;24:1270–1274.
45. Boulton AJ, Franks CI, Betts RP, et al. Reduction of abnormal foot pressures in diabetes neuropathy using a new polymer insole material. *Diabetes Care* 1984;7:42–46.
46. Kelly PJ, Coventry MB. Neurotrophic ulcers of the feet: review of 47 cases. *JAMA* 1958;168:388–.
47. Frykberg RG, Lavery LA, Pham H, et al. Role of neuropathy and high foot pressures in diabetic foot ulceration. *Diabetes Care* 1998;21(10):1714–1719.
48. Pham H, Armstrong DG, Harvey C, et al. Screening techniques to identify people at high risk for diabetic foot ulceration: a prospective multicenter trial. *Diabetes Care* 2000;23(5):606–611.
49. Lavery L, Armstrong D, Wunderlich R, et al. Predictive value of foot pressure assessment as part of a population based diabetes disease management program. *Diabetes Care* 2003;26:1069–1073.
50. Veves A, Boulton AJM. The optical pedobarograph. *Clin Pediatr Med Surg* 1993;10: 463–470.
51. Veves A, Masson EA, Fernando DJ, et al. The use of experimental padded hosiery to reduce abnormal foot pressures in diabetic neuropathy. *Diabetes Care* 1989;12:653–655.
52. Veves A, Masson EA, Fernando DJ, et al. Studies of experimental hosiery in diabetic neuropathic patients with high foot pressures. *Diabet Med* 1990;7:324–326.
53. Donaghue VM, Sarnow MR, Giurini JM, et al. Longitudinal in-shoe foot pressure relief achieved by specially designed footwear in high risk diabetic patients. *Diabetes Res Clin Pract* 1996;31:109–114.
54. Giacalone VF, Armstrong DG, Ashry HR, et al. A quantitative assessment of healing sandals and postoperative shoes in offloading the neuropathic diabetic foot. *J Foot Ankle Surg* 1997;36:28–30.

55. Nawoczenski DA, Birke JA, Coleman WC. Effect of rocker sole design on plantar forefoot pressures. *J Am Pediatr Med Assoc.* 1988;78:450–455.
56. Fleischli JG, Lavery LA, Vela SA, et al. Comparison of strategies for reducing pressure at the site of neuropathic ulcers. *J Am Pediatr Med Assoc* 1997;87:466–472.
57. Chanteleau E, Kushner T, Spraul M. How effective is cushioned therapeutic footwear in protecting diabetic feet. *Diabet Med* 1990;7:355–359.
58. Perry JE, Ulbrecht JS, Derr JA, et al. The use of running shoes to reduce plantar pressures in patients who have diabetes. *J Bone J Surg Br* 1995;77A:1819–1827.
59. Kastenbauer T, Sokol G, Auiuger M, et al. Running shoes for relief of plantar pressure in diabetic patients. *Diabet Med* 1998;15:518–522.
60. Veves A, Saouaf R, Donaghue VM, et al. Aerobic exercise capacity remains normal despite impaired endothelial function in the micro- and macrocirculation of physically active IDDM patients. *Diabetes* 1997;46:1846–1852.
61. Lavery LA, Vela SA, Lavery DC, et al. Reducing dynamic foot pressures in high risk diabetic subjects with foot ulcerations. *Diabetes Care* 1996;19:818–821.
62. Ashry HR, Lavery LA, Murdoch DP, et al. Effectiveness of diabetic insoles to reduce foot pressures. *J Foot Ankle Surg* 1997;36:268–271.
63. Albert S, Rinoie C. Effect of custom orthotics on plantar pressure distribution in the pronated diabetic foot. *J Foot Ankle Surg* 1994;33:598-604.
64. Kato H, Takada T, Kawamura T, et al. The reduction and redistribution of plantar pressures using foot orthoses in diabetic patients. *Diabet Res Clin Pract* 1996;31:115–118.
65. Brown M, Rudicel S, Esquenazi A. Measurement of dynamic pressures at the shoe-foot interface during normal walking with various foot orthoses using the FSCAN system. *Foot Ankle Int* 1996;17(3):152–156.
66. Viswanathan V, Madhavan S, Gnanasundaram S, et al. Effectiveness of different types of footwear insoles for the diabetic neuropathic foot. *Diabetes Care* 2004;27:474–477.
67. Reiber GE, Smith DG, Wallace C, et al. Effect of therapeutic footwear on foot reulceration in patients with diabetes: a randomized controlled trial. *JAMA* 2002;287:2552–2558.
68. Personal communication, Dr. Matthew Pepper, University of Kent, Canterbury, Kent, England.

10

Biomechanics of the Diabetic Foot

The Road to Foot Ulceration

C. H. M. van Schie, MSc, PhD and A. J. M. Boulton, MD, FRCP

FOOT FUNCTION

One of the principal functions of the foot is its shock-absorbing capability during heel strike and its adaptation to the uneven surface of the ground during gait. In this function the subtalar joint plays a basic role. The subtalar joint allows motion three planes and is described as pronation (a combination of eversion, abduction, and dorsiflexion) and supination (a combination of inversion, adduction, and plantar flexion) *(1,2)*. The ankle joint is the major point for controlling sagittal plane movements of the leg relative to the foot, which is essential for bipedal ambulation over flat or uneven terrain *(3)*. The midtarsal joint, represents the functional articulation between the hindfoot and midfoot. The inter-relationship of the subtalar and midtarsal joint provides full pronation and supination motions throughout the foot. The first metatarsophalangeal joint (MTPJ) incorporates the first metatarsal head (MTH), the base of the proximal phalanx, and the superior surfaces of the medial and lateral sesamoid bones within a single joint capsule. The main motion of the first MTPJ and the lesser MTPJs is in the sagittal plane (dorsiflexion and plantar flexion). During propulsion the body weight is moving forward over the hallux creating relative dorsiflexion of the first MTPJ. This occurs with the hallux planted firmly on the ground and with the heel lifting for propulsion. The force acting across the first MTPJ approximates body weight, whereas the force across other MTPJs is considerably less *(4)*. Maximum loading of the first MTH and hallux is practically at the same time during stance in normal gait, highlighting the importance of the load-bearing function of both the hallux and first MTH.

During gait, the foot is required to be unstable at first for shock absorption and to adapt to the terrain, whereas during the propulsive phase the foot has to be stable to function as a lever. Foot flexibility and rigidity are mainly controlled with pronation and supination of the subtalar and midtarsal joints. As subtalar joint pronation after heel strike is a major shock-absorbing mechanism, limited joint mobility (LJM) or structural abnormality could compromise flexibility and shock absorption, thereby placing increased stress on the plantar skin surface *(5,6)*. In addition, limited ankle dorsiflexion could result in increased pressure on the forefoot, particularly during the late stance phase of gait, caused by an early heel rise or compensatory pronation *(5,7,8)*.

From: *The Diabetic Foot, Second Edition*
Edited by: A. Veves, J. M. Giurini, and F. W. LoGerfo © Humana Press Inc., Totowa, NJ

GAIT CYCLE

The gait cycle consists of two parts: the stance and the swing phase. The stance or weight-bearing phase can be divided into three parts; the first one is the contact phase initiated by initial contact to toe-off of the opposite limb. Normally, the first area of the foot in contact with the ground is the heel; however, in some cases initial foot contact is with a flat foot. In cases of a midfoot deformity, such as a Charcot joint, the midfoot could be the site of initial contact. The midstance phase begins with opposite-side toe-off and full forefoot loading and terminates with heel-lift. The third phase, the propulsion phase can be further subdivided into two phases: active propulsion and passive lift-off. Active propulsion begins with heel-lift of the support-side and ends with opposite-side heel strike. During this stage the greatest horizontal and vertical forces are directed against the foot and weight bearing is over a relatively small area (forefoot). It is therefore not surprising to find that the highest pressures are usually observed during this part of the stance phase. The passive lift-off begins with opposite heel contact and terminates with support-side toe-off.

Each part of the stance phase is characterized by a rocker action of the foot and ankle. During the contact phase, the heel ("heel rocker") serves as an axis to allow smooth plantar flexion and to make full contact with the ground. During midstance, the ankle ("ankle rocker") allows the tibia to advance forward over the foot, causing relative dorsiflexion of the ankle. This advances the center of pressure from the heel and midfoot to the forefoot. During active propulsion and passive lift-off, the first MTPJ ("the forefoot rocker") allows progression of the limb over the forefoot and accelerates heel-lift.

CHANGES IN THE FOOT CAUSED BY DIABETES

Diabetic foot ulceration occurs as a consequence of the interaction of several contributory factors. Peripheral neuropathy is believed to cause changes in foot function and structure (prominent MTHs), as well as dryness of the skin, which can lead to excessive callus formation (9–11). Another important predictive risk factor for the development of diabetic foot ulceration is high plantar foot pressure (12,13). High foot pressures usually occur at sites with bony prominence, and have been strongly associated with reduced plantar tissue thickness (14,15). In addition, foot deformities are strongly associated with and predictive of increased plantar pressures and foot ulceration (11,16,17). Prominent MTHs have traditionally been attributed to weakness of the intrinsic muscles of the foot leading to toe deformities. Fat cushions under MTHs which are imbedded in the flexor tendons are believed to migrate distally with clawing and hammering of the toes, leaving the MTHs relatively unprotected (18,19). Evidence for atrophy of these muscles has been demonstrated as fatty infiltration in plantar muscles of diabetic patients with a history of foot ulceration (20). However, more recent evidence has shown foot muscle atrophy in patients with diabetic neuropathy although there was no relationship between toe deformities and muscle atrophy, suggesting that intrinsic muscle atrophy is either not the primary causative factor or that loss of foot muscles precedes the development of toe deformities (21,22). In a subsequent study by Bus, it was shown that diabetic neuropathic patients with a toe deformity have a greater reduced sub-MTH padding compared with patients without this deformity, indicating increased probability of high pressure and risk for foot ulcer development at these sites (23).

Charcot arthropathy usually causes gross deformation of the foot, thereby severely affecting functional use of the foot and causing abnormal pressure loading during walking. Peak plantar pressure in patients with Charcot arthropathy were shown to be higher compared with patients with a neuropathic ulcer *(24)*. Patients with partially amputated feet were also shown to exhibit abnormal pressure loading *(25)* and amputation of the hallux greatly increases pressure under the MTHs *(26,27)*. Callus has also been reported to be highly predictive for foot ulceration *(28)*. Callus acts as a foreign body, and its removal leads to reduced plantar pressure in most cases *(29,30)*. Furthermore, neuropathic ulcers are commonly found beneath plantar calluses; therefore, frequent removal of callus is strongly recommended in patients with diabetes. Thus, foot deformity appears to be a strong indicator of abnormal foot loading during walking thereby causing high plantar foot pressures. Alleviation of these high-pressure areas is best achieved with accommodative footwear, including insoles and shoes. It is important to ensure that the altered foot shape is properly fitted and accommodated in the footwear. For many patients normal high street footwear will not meet these criteria.

Limited Joint Mobility

Joint mobility is defined as the range of motion of a joint and is related to age, sex, and ethnic background *(31–33)*. LJM of the foot and ankle has been suggested to increase plantar pressure in patients with diabetes *(34–35)* and to be related to foot ulceration *(36,37)*. The etiology of LJM is unknown, although most evidence favors a relationship with the collagen abnormalities and nonenzymatic glycation of soft tissue that occurs in diabetes, resulting in thickening of skin, tendons, ligaments, and joint capsules, thereby reducing tissue flexibility *(38,39)*. The prevalence of LJM (diagnosed with a positive "prayer sign") has been reported to vary between 49% and 58% for type 1 diabetic patients and between 45% and 52% for patients with type 2 *(40–42)*.

Joint mobility of the subtalar joint was shown to be significantly reduced in the ulcerated foot compared with the contralateral nonulcerated foot in diabetic neuropathic patients *(36)*. The same authors also reported an association between mobility of joints of the hand and foot, indicating that stiffening of joints appears to be a general feature in patients with diabetes. Similarly, ankle dorsiflexion and subtalar range of motion were reduced in diabetic patients with a history of plantar ulceration compared with patients without ulceration and nondiabetic controls *(37)*. In addition, ulceration of the great toe has been associated to a reduced range of motion at the first MTPJ *(8)*. Figure 1 illustrates the relationship between reduced first ray range of motion (first MTH dorsiflexion) and increased pressure at the first MTH in patients with a history of first MTH ulceration as opposed to no apparent relationship for patients with a history of plantar forefoot ulceration not at the first MTH *(8)*.

The suggested explanation for the link between LJM and foot ulceration comes from studies showing a relation between joint mobility at the subtalar and ankle joint and foot pressures *(43)*. Similarly, Andersen and Mogensen *(44)* reported that maximum movements at the ankle were delayed and slowed using an isokinetic dynamometer in long-term patients with type 1 diabetes. In contrast to the above studies, a recent study could not report a clear relationship between joint mobility of the foot (i.e., subtalar, ankle, and first metarsophalangeal joint) and plantar pressures. The only joint mobility measurement related to plantar pressure was the measurement in the hand (extension of the fifth

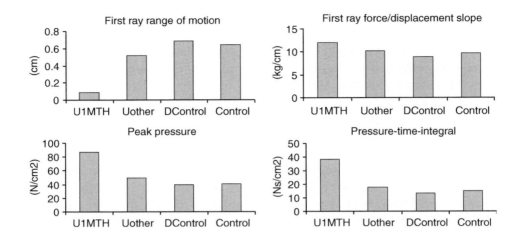

Fig. 1. Range of motion and plantar pressure of first MTH. First ray dorsiflexion was measured as vertical displacement of the first MTH, whereas the second through the fifth MTH were stabilized. The force (up to 8 kg) applied to and the vertical displacement of the first MTH was measured simultaneously. Pressure under the first MTH was measured during barefoot walking at standardized walking velocity. U1MTH, patients with history of ulceration at first MTH; Uother, patients with history of plantar forefoot ulceration not at the first MTH; DControl, diabetic patients without history of foot ulceration; Control, nondiabetic controls. The U1MTH group had a significant stiffer first MTH and higher pressure under the first MTH as compared with the other three groups ($p < 0.05$). (From ref. *8* with permission.)

metacarpophalangeal joint) *(45)*, suggesting that this may be a surrogate marker for diabetic complications in general which could therefore explain the association with increased foot pressures.

Thus, although joint mobility appears to be reduced in patients with diabetes, it is important to note that the relationship with foot ulceration has only been studied retrospectively. The interpretation of this could be that foot ulceration causes stiffening of the joints as opposed to LJM causing foot ulceration. Foot ulcers are frequently healed using casts for off-loading and in addition patients are advised to minimize their level of physical activity while healing the ulcer, these two factors are quite likely to compromise joint mobility.

DEVELOPMENT OF DIABETIC FOOT ULCERATION

Foot ulcers in diabetes result from multiple pathophysiological mechanisms, including roles for neuropathy, peripheral vascular disease, foot deformity, higher foot pressures, and diabetes severity *(46)*. Diabetic neuropathy and peripheral vascular disease are the main etiological factors which predispose to foot ulceration and may act alone, together, or in combination with other factors, such as microvascular disease, biomechanical abnormalities, and an increased susceptibility to infection *(46–49)*. Trauma is needed in addition to neuropathy and vascular disease to cause tissue breakdown. Trauma could be intrinsic, such as repetitive stress from high pressure and/or callus, or extrinsic such as from ill-fitting footwear rubbing on the skin or an object inside the shoe (e.g., drawing

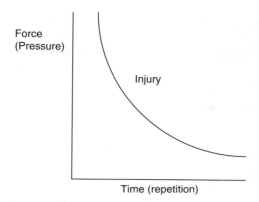

Fig. 2. Inverse relationship between force (pressure) and time (or repetition). As force (pressure) increases, the duration (time) or number (repetition) of force(s) required to cause tissue injury decreases. (From ref. *51* with permission.)

pin and pebble). As trauma, and therefore foot ulceration can be minimized, it is important to identify insensitive feet at risk of ulceration in order to implement preventative care such as the provision of appropriate foot care, education, and referral for podiatry treatment.

Biomechanical Aspects of Foot Ulceration

Ulcer sites are predominantly under the plantar surface of the toes, forefoot, and midfoot, followed by the dorsal surface of the toes and heel *(11)*. As high plantar foot pressures are an important factor in the pathogenesis of diabetic foot ulceration, the proposed mechanism of pressure induced ulcers is discussed next.

Skin is the mechanical link through which intrinsic forces are transmitted to the outside world and environmental forces to the skin and subcutaneous tissue. Ulceration seems to be caused by repetitive and/or excessive pressure on the surface of the insensitive skin leading to tissue damage. If the same pressures occurred in a person with adequate sensation, the person would experience pain and avoid the offending pressures. However, in a person with loss of protective sensation there is no warning of excessive pressures or tissue damage and persistent localized pressures could lead to skin breakdown or ulceration. Foot deformities are usually responsible for these excessive pressures. In addition, healing of plantar ulcers is prevented as long as patients keep walking on their foot wounds, thus highlighting the key issue of mechanical off-loading.

Thus, excessive and/or repetitive pressures appear to be the main causative factor for development of skin breakdown. There are three mechanisms that account for the occurrence of these pressures:

1. Increased duration of pressures,
2. Increased magnitude of pressures, or
3. Increased number of pressures *(50)*.

The first mechanism includes relatively low pressures applied for a long period of time causing ischemia. Prolonged ischemia leads to cell death and wound formation, as has been demonstrated in a classic experiment *(51)*. An inverse relationship was shown between time and pressure and is shown in Fig. 2. High pressures took a relatively short time to cause ulceration whereas low pressures took a relatively long time. Thus, ulceration can develop at very low pressures, but may take a few days to occur. This type of offending pressure and resulting ulcers can occur with ill-fitting footwear, improperly fitted orthotics, or prolonged resting of a heel on a bed or footrest.

The second mechanism of tissue injury includes high pressures acting for a short-time period. This injury only happens if a large force is applied to a relatively small area of skin. This happens, for example, if a person steps on a nail or piece of glass, which is not unusual for diabetic neuropathic patients. Alternatively, a "foot slap" may also conform to this mechanism. A "foot slap" indicates a reduced deceleration of the forefoot after heel strike caused by weak dorsiflexion muscles. It has previously been demonstrated that high rates of tissue deformation lead to cellular death, whereas comparable gradually applied loads do not *(52)*. It is therefore suggested that control of the velocity of the forefoot descending after heel strike by using ankle-foot orthosis could possibly help in prevention of diabetic foot ulcers. The third mechanism of injury comes from repetitions of pressure, which in engineering terms would lead to an equivalent syndrome of mechanical fatigue. Mechanical fatigue is defined as failure of a structure or biological tissue at a submaximal level to maintain integrity resulting from repeated bouts of loading. This type of injury seems to occur in the insensitive skin and subcutaneous tissue of the neuropathic foot.

The body will respond to repeated high pressures or microtrauma with callus formation in order to protect the skin from further damage. However, if callus formation becomes excessive it will contribute to higher pressure, and should therefore be removed at a regular interval *(29,30)*. Although a high level of activity has traditionally been regarded as "repetitive stress" and therefore considered as a risk factor for diabetic foot ulceration, interesting new evidence has shown that patients who were less active were more likely to develop foot ulceration *(53,54)*. In addition, the risk may not be related to the level of activity but the increased variability in physical activity, which was recently shown to be associated with the development of foot ulceration *(55)*.

Thus, not only the magnitude of the plantar pressure is important in causing foot ulceration but also several other factors such as the rate of increase of pressure, duration of high pressure, and the frequency of applied pressure to the skin should be taken into account. In addition, although foot pressures may be high during a barefoot pressure assessment, it is important to keep in mind that it is the combination of footwear, life style factors, tissue characteristics, foot pressures, and level of physical activity, which contribute to the development of foot ulceration. In addition, the effect of physical activity on development of foot ulceration is an area which deserves further exploration.

Plantar Tissue Thickness in Relation to Foot Ulceration

The assessment of plantar tissue thickness in the forefoot has been suggested as an alternative method to pressure measurements. Plantar tissue thickness is strongly associated with plantar pressure, indicating a close relation between the amount of cushioning (soft tissue) available and the pressure distribution over the forefoot *(14,15)*. Similarly, a strong relationship has been demonstrated between tissue thickness and history of ulceration in patients with diabetes *(56,57)*. Qualitative changes of the plantar fat pad have also been observed in the form of a nonspecific fibrotic process beneath the MTH in patients with diabetic neuropathy. This fibrotic tissue affects the intrinsic biomechanical properties of the plantar fat pad to act as a shock absorber and dissipate increased plantar pressures associated with neuropathy *(58)*. Thus, quantity and quality of the plantar cushioning appear to be affected in diabetic neuropathic patients, increasing the risk for developing high pressures, thereby increasing the risk for foot ulceration.

Foot Type and Foot Ulceration

Feet with "abnormal" alignment of the forefoot or rearfoot exhibit a different loading pattern than normally aligned feet. Both nondiabetic and the diabetic planus feet (everted rearfoot, inverted forefoot, and low arch) have shown to experience greater peak pressures than nondiabetic rectus feet (a neutral rearfoot and forefoot with normal arch morphology) *(59)*. This is in agreement with previous reports of an association between type of foot deformity and callus and ulcer location in a group of diabetic patients with active ulceration *(60)*. In this particular study 88% (15/17) of patients with an uncompensated forefoot varus or forefoot valgus (in- or everted forefoot) had ulcers located at the first or fifth MTH. Similarly, an inverted heel position has been associated with lateral ulcers whereas an everted heel position was associated with medial ulcers *(61)*.

Thus, high pressures may not just be caused by the effects of diabetes; therefore, it seems reasonable to hypothesize that diabetic patients with foot-type characteristics that differ from the norm are more likely to develop high foot pressures and ulceration than diabetic patients with normal foot morphology.

INTERVENTIONS TO REDUCE FOOT PRESSURES AND FOOT ULCERATION

Preventive care to reduce the incidence of foot ulceration includes callus debridement as well as provision of pressure reducing insoles and therapeutic footwear. Appropriate management of callus is crucial in patients with diabetes. Callus needs to be removed frequently as it can buildup quickly, with some patients needing debridement as often as every 3–4 weeks or sometimes even more frequently *(30)*. Traditionally, callus is removed when excessively formed under the diabetic foot; however, only a few preliminary studies have addressed how callus buildup can be minimized.

A small randomized placebo-controlled trial showed a reduction in callus grade in patients wearing rigid orthotic in-shoe devices compared with conventional podiatric care *(62)*. The injection of collagen under callus in diabetic patients with previous neuropathic ulceration resulted in a reduced surface area of callus compared with a nontreated control group at 8 months postinjection *(63)*.

The therapeutic use of liquid silicone injections in the foot has been suggested to improve cushioning at callus sites, corns, and localized painful areas *(64)*. In a randomized placebo-controlled trial with diabetic neuropathic patients it was shown that injected liquid silicone decreased peak plantar pressure and callus formation and increased plantar tissue thickness under silicone treated areas *(65)*. This cushioning effect was still significant at 1 year following the injections, although at 2-year follow-up the cushioning properties appeared to be reduced, suggesting that booster injections may be required in certain patients *(66)*. The magnitude of change was greater at injection sites with a lower

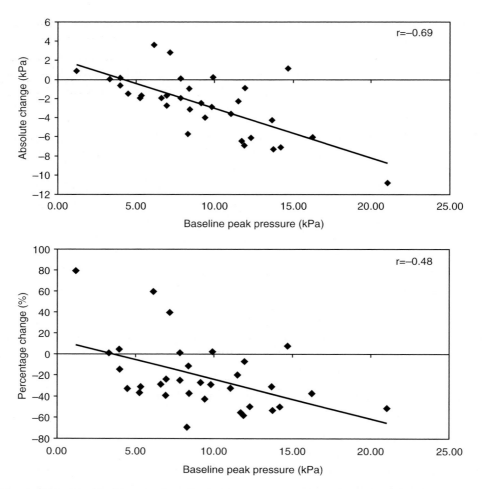

Fig. 3. Relationship between baseline plantar peak pressure and change in peak pressure after silicone injection treatment. Baseline plantar peak pressure was associated with absolute change of pressure (*r* = −0.69), and percentage change of pressure (*r* = −0.48).

baseline thickness and a higher baseline peak pressure (Fig. 3) *(67)*. No side effects were reported in this study and in addition there is a large body of anecdotal evidence to support the safety of this procedure *(64)*. Thus, treatments to reduce foot pressures and the risk of foot ulceration have been developed. However, whether silicone injections can actually prevent foot ulceration needs to be confirmed in larger trials.

Surgical Interventions and Foot Ulceration

Different surgical methods have been suggested and used for reduction of foot pressure and prevention of ulceration. For both reconstructive and prophylactic procedures however, it is imperative to ensure that vascular supply is sufficient to ensure healing.

MTH resection is a surgical technique, which can be used to accelerate wound healing under a MTH area, usually greatly exposed to high pressure. Although pressure reduction was evident in a series of 16 cases at 6–8 weeks following surgery, it is not known whether this procedure may result in a transfer of peak pressure to other areas in the foot in the long-term *(68)*. However, in two different series no recurrent ulcers or transfer lesions were seen during a 6–20-month and a 14 ± 11-month follow-up period *(68,69)*.

Dorsiflexion metatarsal osteotomy has been suggested as an alternative to MTH resection, as this procedure does not violate the MTPJ *(70)*. It elevates prominent MTHs, thereby balancing the MTHs and redistributing weight-bearing forces more evenly across the forefoot, although no pressure data are available to confirm this theory. First MTPJ arthroplasty increases the range of motion at the articulation of the hallux to the first metatarsal and is a technique commonly used to improve healing of ulcers at the hallux. From a 6-month retrospective analysis, this procedure was reported to result in a faster healing rate of ulcers and in fewer recurrent ulcers compared with conservative (nonsurgical) treatment *(71)*.

An Achilles tendon-lengthening (ATL) procedure has been shown to increase ankle dorsiflexion range of motion, decrease forefoot plantar pressure, and reduce the rate of ulcer recurrence in patients with diabetic forefoot ulcers *(72–74)*. The increase in ankle dorsiflexion range of motion was originally thought to lead to subsequent reduction in forefoot pressure. In a recent report plantar pressures were shown to be initially reduced, however to be back at preprocedure levels at 8-month follow-up whereas ankle dorsiflexion range of motion had remained increased *(75)*. From the results of a comprehensive gait-analysis the authors concluded that the initial decrease in forefoot pressure appeared to be caused by a reduced plantar flexion power during gait rather than increased range of ankle motion *(75)*. This procedure did not result in a measurable change in functional limitations, although patients who received ATL and total contact casting reported lower physical functioning 8 months following the procedure compared with patients who received a total contact cast (TCC) only, suggesting that additional physiotherapy may be required in patients receiving ATL *(76)*. Results from a different series described that the most important complication of ATL is the development of a transfer lesion to the heel *(77)*. Although there are risks with every surgical procedure, it is generally accepted that the benefits of the ATL procedure outweigh the risk for patients with recurrent ulcers and limited dorsiflexion at the ankle joint *(76)*.

OFF-LOADING THE DIABETIC FOOT ULCER

Off-loading of the diabetic wound is a key factor in successful wound healing. Several devices have been described in the literature, most of them effective in off-loading and healing wounds. The TCC is generally viewed as the reference standard for off-loading the diabetic wound; however, several useful alternatives exist *(78)*. Although the TCC is probably the most effective in off-loading the wound, the problem with this method is that regular checking the wound is difficult, as this means making a new cast after every check. However new data have demonstrated the successful use of a nonremovable fiberglass casts with a treatment window at the ulcer site, allowing daily inspection of the wound *(79,80)*. The use of a TCC is contraindicated in acutely infected or ischemic foot. Nonetheless, ulcers with moderate ischemia or infection were shown to be effectively treated using a TCC *(81)*. However, when peripheral arterial disease and infection are both present or in case of heel ulcers alternative off-loading methods are required as the outcome was poor in these cases *(81)*. Other devices, such as the removable walkers,

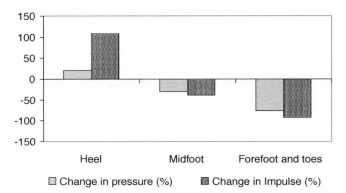

Fig. 4. Change in mean peak plantar pressure and impulse (pressure-time-integral) in the TCC as compared with the shoe condition (cast shoe with a flat 0.5 in. PPT compliant insole). (From ref. *85* with permission.)

Scotchcast boot, half shoes, healing shoes, accommodative dressing, and so on, are equally or not as effective in off-loading; however their main advantage is that regular inspection of the wound is possible. Obviously, this may at the same time also be the main disadvantage, as the possibility to remove the device makes it very easy for patients not to confirm with the off-loading treatment.

The Scotchcast boot is a well-padded plaster boot cut away by the ankle and made removable by cutting away the cast over the dorsum over the foot. Windows are cut under the ulcer and the boot is worn with a cast sandal to increase patients' mobility whereas the cast protects the ulcer from any pressure *(82,83)*. In a retrospective analysis it was observed that healing rates were comparable with using the half shoe *(84)*.

The TCC is a well molded minimally padded cast, which maintains contact with the entire plantar aspect of the foot and lower leg. A large proportion of the pressured reduction achieved in the forefoot of the TCC has shown to be transmitted along the cast wall or to the rearfoot *(85)* (Fig. 4). The advantage of the contact cast over other off-loading methods is that it is highly effective in reducing pressure, immobilization of tissues, and reducing edema and it is not removable by the patient. However, the cast can create secondary lesions, and limits the use of special dressings or topical agents. In addition it requires much expertise and time for application compared with other modalities. It is therefore not always a practical option in some clinics and for certain patients. The use of fiberglass materials with variable rigidity to make a TCC was shown to reduce some of the classic side effects as seen with the traditional TCC, as reduced skin lesions and improved patient acceptability was reported *(79)*.

Although DH Pressure Relief Walkers and Aircast pneumatic walkers (both removable walking casts) were shown to be as effective in reducing plantar foot pressures as the TCC *(86,87)*, a randomized clinical trial showed that TCC healed a higher proportion of wounds in a shorter time compared with a removable cast walker *(88)*.

In contrast, in another trial there was no difference in healing rate between using alternative off-loading methods such as accommodative dressing, a healing shoe and a walking splint compared with using a TCC when controlling for ulcer grade and width *(89)*. In this trial, off-loading method was selected on basis of ulcer location, patient age, and duration of ulceration and treatment was not randomized. The results showed that TCC was more frequently used for ulcers at the metatarsal area and in younger patients with ulcers of longer duration *(89)*.

Recent fascinating results presented the explanation for the importance of off-loading in wound healing. It was demonstrated that pressure relief with a TCC was associated with changes in the histology of neuropathic foot ulcers indicating reduced inflammatory and accelerated repair processes *(90)*. It has also been suggested that the effectiveness of an off-loading device to heal foot ulcers depends completely on whether the device is worn during all weight-bearing activities or not. In a small study it was noted that patients only wore their removable cast walker for 28% of their total daily activity, indicating that this may explain poor healing rates in certain trials *(91)*. These results have led to the development of the instant TCC, which is a removable cast walker wrapped with cohesive bandage or plaster of Paris, making it "irremovable." Recent evidence from preliminary studies on the effectiveness of an irremovable TCC (iTCC) showed that iTTC and TCC resulted in equal healing times, although a second study reported faster healing in a iTCC compared with a removable cast walker *(92,93)*. Even though this promising technique is suggested to address many of the disadvantages of the TCC, it does not change the fact that this type of device is not suitable for all patients and that in addition to off-loading, wound healing needs debridement, treatment of infection, and revascularization if indicated.

The ankle-foot orthosis has been suggested to be a useful alternative to casting techniques in order to off-load the diabetic foot during wound healing and to prevent ulceration *(94)*. It is proposed that an ankle-foot orthosis prevents high-velocity impact between the ground and the plantar surface of the foot, thereby controlling the rate of mechanical loading of the tissues. In fact, most casting techniques indirectly reduce rate of loading of the forefoot by immobilizing the ankle joint. There is only limited evidence of the efficacy of ankle-foot orthosis in ulcer healing and prevention; however, preliminary evidence indicates pressure reductions at ulcer sites ranging from 70% to 92% and significantly reduced loading rates *(94)*.

Thus, several off-loading modalities have been described to prevent (re) ulceration and to improve wound healing. Although the TCC appears to be the reference off-loading method other devices have also shown to be effective in wound healing. The choice of off-loading depends on the patient and clinical situation and therefore more future clinical trials comparing different off-loading methods (i.e., randomized controlled trials) will help to improve clinical decision making in the prevention and treatment of diabetic foot ulcers.

REFERENCES

1. Nester CJ. Review of literature on the axis of rotation at the subtalar joint. *Foot* 1998;8:111–118.
2. Sarrafian SK. Biomechanics of the subtalar joint complex. *Clin Orthop Res* 1993;290:17–26
3. Wernick J, Volpe RG. Lower extremity function and normal mechanics, In *Clinical biomechanics of the lower extremities* (Valmassy RL, ed.), Mosby Year Book, St Louis, 1996, pp. 2–57.
4. Hutton WC, Dhanendran M. The mechanics of normal and hallux valgus feet—a quantitative study. *Clin Orthop Res* 1981;157:7–13.

5. Root ML, Orien WP, Weed JH. Clinical biomechanics: Normal and abnormal function of the foot. Clinical Biomechanics Corp., Los Angeles, 1977,2.

6. Nack JD, Phillips RD. Shock absorption. *Clin Podiatr Med Surg* 1990; 7:391–397.

7. Gibbs RC, Boxer MC. Abnormal biomechanics of feet and their cause of hyperkeratoses. J *Am Acad Dermatol* 1982; 6:1061–1069.

8. Birke JA, Franks BD, Foto JG. First ray joint limitation, pressure, and ulceration of the first metatarsal head in diabetes mellitus. *Foot Ankle* 1995;16:277–284.

9. Boulton AJM (1997) Late sequelae of diabetic neuropathy, In *Diabetic Neuropathy* (Boulton AJM ed.), Marius Press, Lancaster, 1997, pp. 63–76.

10. Mayfield JA, Reiber GE, Sanders LJ, Janisse D, Pogach LM. Preventive foot care in people with diabetes. *Diabetes Care* 1998;21:2161–2177.

11. Reiber GE, Vileikyte L, Boyko EJ, Del Aguila M, Smith DG, Lavery LA, Boulton AJM. Causal pathways for incident lower-extremity ulcers in patients with diabetes from two settings. *Diabetes Care* 1999;22:157–162.

12. Veves A, Murray HJ, Young MJ, Boulton AJM. The risk of foot ulceration in diabetic patients with high foot pressures; a prospective study. *Diabetologia* 1992;35:660–663.

13. Pham H, Armstrong DG, Harvey C, Harkless LB, Giurini JM, Veves A. Screening techniques to identify people at high risk for diabetic foot ulceration. A prospective multicenter trial. *Diabetes Care* 2000;23:606–611.

14. Young MJ, Coffey J, Taylor PM, Boulton AJM. Weight bearing ultrasound in diabetic and rheumatoid arthritis patients. *Foot* 1995;5:76–79.

15. Abouaesha F, van Schie CHM, Griffiths GD, Young RJ, Boulton AJM. Plantar tissue thickness is related to peak plantar pressure in the high-risk diabetic foot. *Diabetes Care* 2001;24:1270–1274.

16. Ahroni JH, Boyko EJ, Forsberg. Clinical correlates of plantar pressure among diabetic veterans. *Diabetes Care* 1999; 22:965–972.

17. Boyko EJ, Ahroni JH, Stensel V, Forsberg RC, Davignon DR, Smith DG. A prospective study of risk factors for diabetic foot ulcer. *Diabetes Care* 1999;22:1036–1042.

18. Boulton AJM, Betts RP, Franks CI, Newrick PG, Ward JD, Duckworth T. Abnormalities of foot pressure in early diabetic neuropathy. *Diabetic Med* 1987;4:225–228.

19. Myerson MS, Shereff MJ. The pathological anatomy of claw and hammer toes. *J Bone Joint Surg* 1989;71-A:45–49.

20. Suzuki E, Kashiwagi A, Hidaka H, et al. 1H- and 31P-magnetic resonance spectroscopy and imaging as a new diagnostic tool to evaluate neuropathic foot ulcers in Type II diabetic patients. *Diabetologia* 2000;43:165–172.

21. Bus SA, Yang QX, Wang JH, Smith MB, Wunderlich R, Cavanagh PR. Intrinsic muscle atrophy and toe deformity in the diabetic neuropathic foot. A magnetic resonance imaging study. *Diabetes Care* 2002;25:1444–1450.

22. Andersen H, Gjerstad MD, Jakobsen J. Atrophy of foot muscles. A measure of diabetic neuropathy. *Diabetes Care* 2004;27:2382–2385.

23. Bus SA, Maas M, Cavanagh PR, Michels RPJ, Levi M. Plantar fat-pad displacement in neuropathic diabetic patients with toe deformity. A magnetic resonance imaging study. *Diabetes Care* 2004;27:2376–2381.

24. Armstrong DG, Lavery LA. Elevated peak plantar pressures in patients who have Charcot arthropathy. *J Bone Joint Surg Am* 1998;80:365–369.

25. Garbalosa JC, Cavanagh PR, Wu G, et al. Foot function in diabetic patients after partial amputation. *Foot and Ankle* 1996;17:43–48.

26. Lavery LA, Lavery DC, Quebedaux-Farnham TL. Increased foot pressures after great toe amputation in diabetes. *Diabetes Care* 1995;18:1460–1462.

27. Quebedeaux Tl, Lavery LA, Lavery DC. The development of foot deformities and ulcers after great toe amputation in diabetes. *Diabetes Care* 1996;19:165–167.

28. Murray HJ, Young MJ, Hollis S, Boulton AJM. The association between callus formation, high pressures and neuropathy in diabetic foot ulceration. *Diabetic Med* 1996;13:979–982.
29. Young MJ, Cavanagh PR, Thomas G, Johnson MM, Murray H, Boulton AJM. The effect of callus removal on dynamic plantar foot pressures in diabetic patients. *Diabetic Med* 1992;9: 55–57.
30. Pitei DL, Foster A, Edmonds M. The effect of regular callus removal on foot pressures. *J Foot and Ankle Surg* 1999;38:251–255.
31. Wordsworth P, Ogilvie D, Smith R, Sykes B. Joint mobility with particular reference to racial variation and inherited connective tissue disorders. *Br J Rheum* 1987;26:9–12.
32. Pountain G. Musculoskeletal pain in Omanis, and the relationship to joint mobility and body mass index. *Br J Rheum* 1992;31:81–85.
33. Vandervoort AA, Chesworth BM, Cunningham DA, Paterson DH, Rechnitzer PA, Koval JJ. Age and sex effects on mobility on the human ankle. *J Gerontol.* 1992;47:M17–M21.
34. Veves A, Sarnow MR, Giurini JM, et al. Differences in joint mobility and foot pressure between black and white diabetic patients. *Diabetic Med* 1995;12:585–589.
35. Frykberg RG, Lavery LA, Pham H, Harvey C, Harkless L, Veves A. Role of neuropathy and high foot pressures in diabetic foot ulceration. *Diabetes Care* 1998;21:1714–1719.
36. Delbridge L, Perry P, Marr S, et al. Limited joint mobility in the diabetic foot: relationship to neuropathic ulceration. *Diabetic Med* 1988;5:333–337.
37. Mueller MJ, Diamond JE, Delitto A, Sinacore DR. Insensitivity, limited joint mobility, and plantar ulcers in patients with diabetes mellitus. *Phys Ther* 1989; 69: 453–462.
38. Crisp AJ, Heathcote JG. Connective tissue abnormalities in diabetes mellitus. *J Roy Coll Phys* 1984;18:132–141.
39. Vlassara H, Brownlee M, Cerami A. Nonenzymatic glycosylation: role in the pathogenesis of diabetic complications. *Clin Chem* 1986;32:B37–B41.
40. Fitzcharles MA, Duby S, Waddell RW, Banks E, Karsh J. Limitation of joint mobility (cheiroarthropathy) in adult noninsulin-dependent diabetic patients. *Ann Rheum Dis* 1984;43:251–257.
41. Pal B, Anderson J, Dick WC, Griffiths ID. Limitation of joint mobility and shoulder capsulitis in insulin- and non-insulin-dependent diabetes mellitus. *Br J Rheum* 1986;25: 147–151.
42. Arkkila PET, Kantola IM, Viikari JSA, Rönnemaa T, Vähätalo MA. Limited joint mobility is associated with the presence but does not predict the development of microvascular complications in Type 1 diabetes. *Diabetic Med* 1996;13:828–833.
43. Mueller MJ, Minor SD, Sahrmann SA, Schaaf JA, Strube MJ. Differences in the gait characteristics of patients with diabetes and peripheral neuropathy compared to age-matched controls. *Phys Ther* 1994;74:299–313.
44. Andersen H., Mogensen PH. Disordered mobility of large joints in association with neuropathy in patients with long-standing insulin-dependent diabetes mellitus. *Diabetic Med* 1996; 14:221–227.
45. Van Schie CHM, Boulton AJM (2000). Joint mobility and foot pressure measurements in Asian and Europid diabetic patients: clues for difference in foot ulcer prevalence (abstract). *Diabetes* 49(Suppl 1):A197.
46. Shaw JE, Boulton AJM (1997) The pathogenesis of diabetic foot problems. An overview. *Diabetes* 46 (Suppl 2):S58–S61.
47. Boulton AJM, Kubrusly DB, Bowker JH, Gadia MT, Quintero L, Becker DM, Skyler JS, Sosenko JM. Impaired vibratory perception and diabetic foot ulceration. *Diabetic Med* 1986;3:335–337.
48. Bild DE, Selby JV, Sinnock P, Browner WS, Braveman P, Showstack JA. Lower-extremity amputation in people with diabetes. Epidemiology and prevention. *Diabetes Care* 1989;12: 24–31.

49. McNeely MJ, Boyko EJ, Ahroni JH, et al. The independent contributions of diabetic neuropathy and vasculopathy in foot ulceration. How great are the risks? *Diabetes Care* 1995;18:216–219.

50. Mueller MJ. Etiology, evaluation, and treatment of the neuropathic foot. *Crit Rev Phys Rehabil Med* 1992;3: 289–309.

51. Kosiak M. Etiology and pathology of ischemic ulcers. *Arch Phys Med Rehabil* 1959;40: 62–69.

52. Landsman AS, Meaney DF, Cargill II RS, Macarak EJ, Thibault LE. High strain tissue deformation. A theory on the mechanical etiology of diabetic foot ulcerations. *J Am Podiatr Assoc* 1995;85:519–527.

53. Maluf KS Mueller MJ. Comparison of physical activity and cumulative plantar tissue stress among subjects with and without diabetes mellitus and a history of recurrent plantar ulcers. *Clinical Biomechanics* 2003;18:567–575

54. Lemaster JW, Reiber GE, Smith DG, Heagerty PJ, Wallace C. Daily weight-bearing activity does not increase the risk of diabetic foot ulcers. *Med Sci Sports Exerc* 2003;35(7): 1093–1099.

55. Armstrong DG, Lavery LA, Holtz-Neiderer K, et al. Variability in activity may precede diabetic foot ulceration. *Diabetes Care* 2004;27:1980–1984.

56. Brink T. Induration of the diabetic foot pad: another risk factor for recurrent neuropathic plantar ulcers. *Biomed Tech* 1995;40:205–209.

57. Gooding GA, Stess RM, Graf PM, Moss KM, Louie KS, Grunfeld C. Sonography of the sole of the foot: evidence for loss of foot pad thickness in diabetes and its relationship to ulceration of the foot. *Invest Radiol* 1986;21:45–48.

58. Brash PD, J Foster, Vennart W, Anthony P, Tooke JE. Magnetic resonance imaging techniques demonstrate soft tissue damage in the diabetic foot. *Diabetic Med* 1999;16: 55–61.

59. Song J, Hillstrom HJ. Effects of foot type biomechanics and diabetic neuropathy on foot function. *Proceedings of the XVIIth International Society of Biomechanics Congress*, 1999, p. 113.

60. Mueller MJ, Minor SD, Diamond JE, Blair VP. Relationship of foot deformity to ulcer location in patients with diabetes mellitus. *Phys Ther* 1990;70:356–362.

61. Bevans JS. Biomechanics and plantar ulcers in diabetes. *Foot* 1992;2:166–172.

62. Colagiuri S, Marsden LL, Naidu V, Taylor L. The use of orthotic devices to correct plantar callus in people with diabetes. *Diabetes Res Clin Prac* 1995;28:29–34.

63. Foster A, Eaton C, Dastoor N, Jones K, Crofton B, Edmonds M. Prevention of neuropathic foot ulceration: a new approach using subdermal injection of collagen (Abstract). *Diabetic Med* 1988;5 (Suppl 5):7.

64. Balkin SW, Kaplan L. Injectable silicone and the diabetic foot: a 25-year report. *Foot* 1991; 2:83–88.

65. Van Schie CHM, Whalley A, Vileikyte L, Wignall T, Hollis S, Boulton AJM. Efficacy of injected liquid silicone in the diabetic foot to reduce risk factors for ulceration. A randomized double-blind placebo-controlled trial. *Diabetes Care* 2000;23:634–638.

66. van Schie CHM, Whalley A, Armstrong DG, Vileikyte L, Boulton AJM. The effect of silicone injections in the diabetic foot on peak plantar pressure and plantar tissue thickness: a 2-year follow-up. *Arch Phys Med Rehabil* 2002;83:919–923.

67. van Schie C, Whalley A, Vileikyte L, Boulton AJM. Efficacy of injected liquid silicone is related to peak plantar foot pressures in the neuropathic diabetic foot. *Wounds* 2002;14(1): 26–30.

68. Patel VG Wieman TJ. Effect of metatarsal head resection for diabetic foot ulcers on the dynamic plantar pressure distribution. *Am J Surg* 1994;167:297–301.

69. Griffiths GD Wieman TJ. Metatarsal head resection for diabetic foot ulcers. *Arch Surg* 1990;125:832–835.

70. Fleischli JE, Anderson RB, Davis WH. Dorsiflexion metatarsal osteotomy for treatment of recalcitrant diabetic neuropathic ulcers. *Foot Ankle Int* 1999;20:80–85.

71. Armstrong DG, Lavery LA, Vazquez JR, et al. Clinical efficacy of the first metatarsophalangeal joint arthroplasty as a curative procedure for hallux interphalangeal joint wounds in patients with diabetes. *Diabetes Care* 2003;26:3284–3287.

72. Armstrong DG, Stacpoole-shea S, Nguyen H, Harkless L. Lengthening of the Achilles tendon in diabetic patients who are at high risk for ulceration of the foot. *J Bone Joint Surg* 1999; 81A:535–538.

73. Lin SS, Lee TH, Wapner KL. Plantar forefoot ulceration with equinus deformity of the ankle in diabetic patients: the effect of tendo-Achilles lengthening and total contact casting. *Orthopedics* 1996;19(5):465–475.

74. Mueller MJ, Sinacore DR, Hastings MK, Strube MJ, Johnson JE. Effect of Achilles tendon lengthening on neuropathic plantar ulcers. A randomized clinical trial. *J Bone Joint Surg Am* 2003;85-A(8):1436–1445.

75. Maluf KS, Mueller MJ, Strube MJ, Engsberg JR, Johnson JE. Tendon Achilles lengthening for the treatment of neuropathic ulcers causes a temporary reduction in forefoot pressure associated with changes in plantar flexor power rather than ankle motion during gait. *J Biomech* 2004;37:897–906.

76. Mueller MJ, Sinacore DR, Hastings MK, Lott DJ, Strube MJ, Johnson JE. Impact of Achilles tendon lengthening on functional imitations and perceived disability in people with a neuropathic plantar ulcer. *Diabetes Care* 2004;27:1559–1564.

77. Holstein P, Lohmann M, Bitsch M, Jørgensen B. Achilles tendon lengthening, the panacea for plantar forefoot ulceration? *Diabetes Metab Res Rev* 2004;20 (Suppl 1):S37–S40.

78. American Diabetes Association: Consensus Development on Diabetic Foot Wound Care. *Diabetes Care* 1999;22:1354–1360.

79. Caravaggi C, Faglia E, De Giglio R, et al. Effectiveness and safety of a nonremovable fibreglass off-bearing cast versus a therapeutic shoe in the treatment of neuropathic foot ulcers. A randomized study. *Diabetes Care* 2003;23:1746–1751.

80. Ha Van G, Siney H, Hartmann-Heurtier A, Jacqueminet S, Greau F, Grimaldi A. Nonremovable, windowed, fibreglass cast boot in the treatment of diabetic plantar ulcers. Efficacy, safety, and compliance. *Diabetes Care* 2003;26:2848–2852.

81. Nabuurs-Franssen MH, Sleegers R, Huijberts MSP, et al. Total contact casting of the diabetic foot in daily practice. A prospective follow-up study. *Diabetes Care* 2005;28:243–247.

82. Jones GR. Walking casts: effective treatment for foot ulcers. *Practical Diabetes* 1991;8: 131, 132.

83. Knowles EA, Boulton AJM. Use of the Scotchcast boot to heal diabetic foot ulcers, in *Proceedings of 5th European Conference of Advanced Wound Care*. McMillan Publishers, London, 1996, pp. 199–201.

84. Chantelau E, Breuer U, Leisch AC, Tanudjaja T, Reuter M. Outpatient treatment of unilateral diabetic foot ulcers with "half shoes". *Diabetic Medicine* 1993;10:267–270.

85. Shaw JE, His WL, Ulbrecht JS, Norkitis A, Becker MB, Cavanagh PR. The mechanism of plantar unloading in total contact casts: implications for design and clinical use. *Foot Ankle Int* 1997;18:809–817.

86. Baumhauer JF, Wervey R, McWilliams J, Harris GF, Shereff MJ. A comparison study of plantar foot pressure in a standardized shoe, total contact cast, and prefabricated pneumatic walking brace. *Foot Ankle Int* 1997;18:26–33.

87. Lavery LA, Vela SA, Lavery DC, Quebedeaux TL. Reducing dynamic foot pressures in high-risk diabetic subjects with foot ulcerations. A comparison of treatments. *Diabetes Care* 1996;19:818–821.

88. Armstrong DG, Nguyen HC, Lavery LA, van Schie CHM, Boulton AJM, Harkless LB. Off-loading the diabetic foot wound. A randomised clinical trial. *Diabetes Care* 2001;24:1019–1022.

89. Birke JA, Pavich MA, Patout CA, Horswell R. Comparison of forefoot ulcer healing using alternative off-loading methods in patients with diabetes mellitus. *Adv Skin Wound Care* 2002;15:210,212–215.
90. Piagessi A, Viacava P, Rizzo L, et al. Semiquantitative analysis of the histopathological features of the neuropathic foot ulcer. Effects of pressure relief. *Diabetes Care* 2003;26(11):3123–3128.
91. Armstrong DG, Lavery LA, Kimbriel HR, Nixon BP, Boulton AJM. Activity patterns of patients with diabetic foot ulceration. Patients with active ulceration may not adhere to a standard pressure off-loading regimen. *Diabetes Care* 2003;26:2595–2597.
92. Katz IA, Harlan A, Miranda-Palma B, et al. A randomized trial of two irremovable off-loading devices in the management of plantar neuropathic diabetic foot ulcers. *Diabetes Care* 2005;28(3):555–559
93. Armstrong DG, Lavery LA, Wu S, Boulton AJM. Evaluation of removable and irremovable cast walkers in the healing of diabetic foot wounds. A randomized controlled trial. *Diabetes Care* 2005;28(3):551–554.
94. Landsman AS and Sage R. Off-loading neuropathic wounds associated with diabetes using an ankle-foot orthosis. *J Am Podiatr Med Assoc* 1997;87:349–357.

11
Clinical Examination of the Diabetic Foot and the Identification of the At-Risk Patient

Stephanie Wu, DPM, MSc, David G. Armstrong, DPM, PhD
Lawrence A. Lavery, DPM, MPH, and Lawrence B. Harkless, DPM

INTRODUCTION

Foot ulceration is one of the most common precursors to lower extremity amputations among persons with diabetes *(1,2)*. Ulcerations are pivotal events in limb loss for two important reasons. They allow an avenue for infection *(3)*, and they can cause progressive tissue necrosis and poor wound healing in the presence of critical ischemia. Infections involving the foot rarely develop in the absence of a wound in adults with diabetes, and ulcers are the most common type of wound in this population *(3)*. Foot ulcers therefore play a central role in the causal pathway to lower extremity amputation *(4)*.

The etiology of ulcerations in persons with diabetes is commonly associated with the presence of peripheral neuropathy and repetitive trauma resulting from normal walking activities to areas of the foot exposed to moderate or high pressure and shear forces *(5)*. Foot deformities, limited joint mobility, partial foot amputations, and other structural deformities often predispose diabetic patients with peripheral neuropathy to abnormal weight bearing, areas of concentrated pressure, and abnormal shear forces that significantly increase their risk of ulceration *(6–8)*. Brand *(9)* theorized that when these types of forces were applied to a discrete area over an extended period they would cause a local inflammatory response, focal tissue ischemia, tissue destruction, and ulceration. Clearly, identification of persons at risk for ulceration is of central importance in any plan for amputation prevention and diabetes care.

By the first quarter of the next millennium, there will be more than 300 million persons with diabetes worldwide *(10)*, the lifetime incidence of these people developing a foot ulcer may be as high as 25% *(11)*. Because most ulcers are entirely avoidable, the concept of prevention takes on an entirely new urgency. In this chapter, we will discuss the key, evidence-based risk factors for ulceration that may be broken down into three practical screening questions to identify patients at highest risk for skin breakdown. We will subsequently discuss seven essential questions to answer when both describing and classifying diabetic foot ulceration. The various classifications for diabetic foot ulcers will also be discussed.

From: *The Diabetic Foot, Second Edition*
Edited by: A. Veves, J. M. Giurini, and F. W. LoGerfo © Humana Press Inc., Totowa, NJ

IDENTIFICATION OF ULCER RISK

Preventing foot complications begins with identifying those at risk. Diabetes is a multifactoral disease and the multidisciplinary approach has been advocated for the comprehensive treatment of diabetes *(12,13)*. Patients with diabetes who present for care should be under the concomitant management of a primary-care physician with appropriate referrals to an endocrinologist, ophthalmologist, renal specialist, vascular surgeon, podiatrist, physical therapist, nutritionist, and a diabetes educator to help ensure adequate care *(11)*. When screening to identify patients at risk for diabetic foot ulcers, there are three key questions that can help identify ulcer risk *(14)*.

1. Does the patient have a previous history of foot amputation, ulceration, or Charcot arthropathy?
2. Is there loss of protective sensation?
3. Is there deformity or limited joint mobility?

Does the Patient Have a Previous History of Foot Amputation, Ulceration, or Charcot Arthropathy?

Primary-care clinicians should inquire about factors known to be associated with foot ulcers such as previous foot ulceration, prior lower extremity amputation, or the presence of neuropathic fractures *(14–16)*. This segment of the population has been shown to have the highest risk of developing subsequent foot ulceration *(14,17)*. It is the easiest risk group to identify, and the group most in need of frequent foot assessment, intensive education, therapeutic shoes, padded stockings, and rigorous blood glucose control. A current ulcer *(16)*, past history of previous ulceration *(16)*, or amputation *(15)* heightens the risk for further ulceration, infection, and subsequent amputation *(4,14,18)*. In general, this may be secondary to three key factors. First, following ulceration, the skin plantar to that site may be less resilient and less well fortified to accept repetitive stress and therefore more prone to subsequent breakdown. Second, persons with a partial foot amputation often develop local foot deformities secondary to biomechanical imbalances that may cause further foci of pressure *(19–21)* (Fig. 1). Certainly, those with a high level amputation such as below or above the knee tend to be much more reliant on their remaining limb for transfer or ambulation and therefore may increase risk for tissue breakdown. Finally, and perhaps most importantly, people with a history of ulceration or amputation have, in general all the risk factors to reulcerate. This is evidenced by the fact that up to 6 in 10 persons with a history of ulceration will develop another one within 1 year of wound healing *(22,23)*.

Is There Loss of Protective Sensation?

Neuropathy is the major component of nearly all diabetic ulcerations *(24)*. Without loss of protective sensation, patients generally will not ulcerate. This is defined as a level of sensory loss that allows patients to jury themselves without recognizing the injury. The consequent vulnerability to physical and thermal trauma increases the risk of foot ulceration sevenfold *(11)*. Patients with neuropathy often wear a hole in their foot much as a sensate patient might wear a hole in our stocking or shoe. Prevention of diabetic foot ulcers begins with screening for loss of protective sensation and substantial evidence supports screening all patients with diabetes to identify those at risk for foot ulceration *(11,25)*. The absence of protective sensation may be determined using

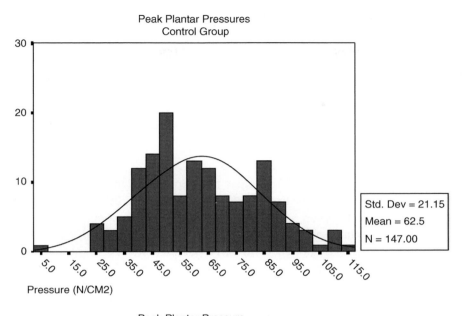

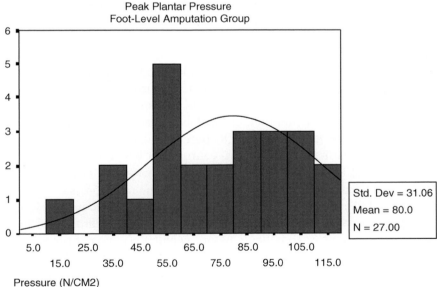

Fig. 1. Plantar pressures are higher following foot-level amputation *(5)*. Partial foot amputation changes the architecture of the foot and therefore may affect its intrinsic stability. These histograms depict a generalized increase in peak plantar pressures in patients with diabetes who have undergone a foot-level amputation.

a tuning fork, a 5.07/10-g Semmes–Weinstein monofilament (SWM) nylon wire, a calibrated vibration perception threshold (VPT) meter, or by a comprehensive physical examination *(16)*. Screening for sensory neuropathy is best determined by clinical examination and the use of several screening tools. Instruments such as the tuning fork, SWM, and VPT are noninvasive and very quick to use in the clinical setting.

Tuning Fork

The conventional tuning fork is an easy and inexpensive tool to assess vibratory sensation. The test is considered positive when the patient loses vibratory sensation whereas the examiner still perceives it *(11)*. Graduated tuning (Rydel–Seiffer) fork have yielded comparable results to the biothesiometer ($r = –0.90$; $p < 0.001$) *(26,27)*. Using the graduated tuning fork, patients indicate first loss of vibration at the plantar hallux as the intersection of two virtual triangles moves on a scale exponentially from 0 to 8 in a mean (AD) of 39.8 (1) seconds *(28)*.

Semmes–Weinstein Monofilament

The 5.07/10-g SWM is one of the most frequently utilized screening tools for identifying loss of protective sensation in the United States *(11,29)*. Although vibratory testing has demonstrated greater sensitivity *(30)*, the inability to perceive the 10 g of force a 5.07-monofilament applied is associated with clinically significant large-fiber neuropathy, and is sensitive enough to identify patient with the highest risk of foot complications *(30,31)*. In three prospective studies, the SWM identified persons at increased risk of foot ulceration with a sensitivity of 66–91%, a specificity of 34–86%, a positive predictive value of 18–39%, and a negative predictive value of 94–95% *(15,32,33)*. The 10-g SWM consists of a plastic handle supporting a nylon filament. It is portable, inexpensive, well tolerated by patients, easy to use, and provides good predictive ability for the risk of ulceration and amputation *(34)*.

There are a number of important concerns regarding the SWM. There is wide variability in the accuracy and durability of SWM sold in the United States. Certain brands of monofilaments are more accurate than others *(35)*. Instruments made in the United Kingdom seem to have better initial accuracy and calibration *(34)*. SWMs experience material failure of the nylon monfilament and become less accurate with repeated measurements. Therefore it is important to purchase calibrated instruments and to replace them on a regular basis. In a clinical setting, it is best for the evaluator to have more than one monofilament available, as after numerous uses without a chance to "recover," the monofilament may buckle at a reduced amount of pressure, thus making it oversensitive and therefore less accurate *(35)*. Longevity and recovery testing results from an independent study suggest that each monofilament, regardless of the brand, will survive usage on approx 10 patients before needing a recovery time of 24 hours before further use *(29,35)*. Furthermore, differences in materials used in manufacture and potentially environmental factors may also change the characteristics of the monofilament *(35,36)*.

In addition, to avoid incorrect diagnosis with the SWM, it is critical that the health-care provider use the device in a consistent manner. Testing via the SWM is administrated with the patient sitting supine in the examination chair with both feet level. It is often advisable to apply the SWM to the patient's hand with his or her eyes open to allow the patient to perceive the sensation of the monofilament application. The patient should then have his or her eyes closed for the actual conduct of the examination and to say "yes" each time that he or she perceives the application of the monofilament. The monofilament device is applied perpendicular to the skin until it bends or buckles from the pressure. It should be left in place for about 1 second then released *(11)*. Authorities recommend that measurements be taken at each of the 10 sites on the foot *(37)*.

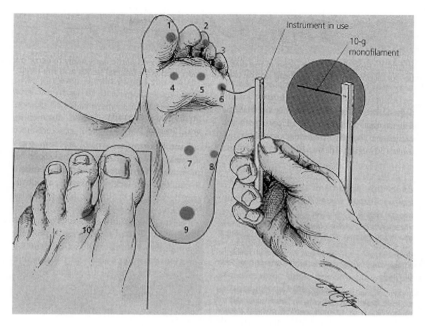

Fig. 2. Use of the 10-g monofilament. Permission must be secured from American Family Physician (printed in March 1998). Sites of testing for 10-g monofilament. Four or more imperceptible sites using a yes–no method of administration may be an optimal combination of sensitivity and specificity for identifying clinically significant loss of protective sensation.

These include the first, third, and fifth digits plantarly; the first, third, and fifth metatarsal heads plantarly; the plantar midfoot medially and laterally; and the plantar heel and the distal first interspace dorsally (Fig. 2). However, testing just four plantar sites on the forefoot, namely the great toe, and base of the first, third, and fifth metatarsals, identifies 90% of patients with loss of protective sensation *(38)*.

Use of a VPT Meter

A VPT meter is another useful adjunct to assist in clinical evaluation of nerve function. It is semiquantitative and is potentially less prone to interoperator variation than the 10-g monofilament device. The VPT meter (also known as Biothesiometer or Neurothesiometer) is a hand-held device with a rubber tactor that vibrates at 100 Hz. The hand-held unit is connected by an electrical cord to a base unit. This unit contains a linear scale that displays the applied voltage, ranging from 0 to 100 V (converted from microns) *(33,39)* (Fig. 3). The device is generally held with the tactor balanced vertically on the pulp of the toe. The voltage amplitude is then increased on the base unit until the patient can perceive a vibration. A mean of three readings (measured in Volts) is generally used to determine the VPT for each foot. In a prospective 4-year study, a VPT of more than 25 V had a sensitivity of 83%, a specificity of 63%, a positive likelihood ratio of 2.2, and a negative likelihood ratio of 0.27 for predicting foot ulceration *(40,41)*.

NEUROPATHY DISABILITY SCORE

The Neuropathy Disability Score is a clinical assessment tool that uses standard clinical tools. These include deep tendon reflexes of achilles tendons, vibration sensation

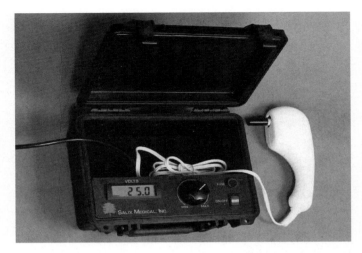

Fig. 3. The vibration perception threshold meter. The vibrating tactor is placed at the distal pulp of the great toe. The amplitude (measured in Volts) is increased on the base unit until the patient feels a vibration. This is termed vibration perception threshold (VPT). A VPT greater than 25 V may be an optimal combination of sensitivity and specificity for identifying clinically significant loss of protective sensation using this device.

with 128 Hz tuning fork, pin prick, hot and cold rods. Use of these instruments, combined into a disability score has proven to be predictive of future diabetic foot complications *(16)*. Furthermore, a gross evaluation of a patient's feet may also provide valuable clues regarding the patient's overall sensorimotor condition. Atrophy of the intrinsic muscles of the hands and feet is an often late-stage condition that is very frequently associated with polyneuropathy (Fig. 4). This condition often leads to prominent digits and metatarsal heads, thus (in the face of sensory loss) leading to a heightened risk for neuropathic ulceration. Similarly, bleeding into callus is not a uncommon condition which is associated with neuropathy.

Is There Deformity or Limited Joint Mobility?

The second causative factor in foot ulceration is excessive plantar pressure from foot deformities. Neuropathy and foot deformity, when combined with repetitive or constant stress, will ultimately lead to failure of the protective integument and ulceration. Characteristically, the highest plantar pressure is associated with the site of ulceration *(5,6,42–44)*. In one study of patients with peripheral neuropathy, 28% with high plantar pressure developed a foot ulcer during a 2.5-year follow-up compared with none with normal pressure *(45)*.

Foot deformity may be defined as any contracture or prominence that cannot be manually reduced. This is a simple, practical definition, which can be used by all clinicians (regardless of specialty) to identify risk. Structural deformity is frequently accompanied by limited joint mobility. Nonenzymatic glycosylation of periarticular soft tissues may limit joint motion in the person with diabetes and neuropathy can lead to atrophy of the intrinsic musculature that can cause hammering of digits *(46–48)* (Fig. 4). Limitation of motion reduces the foot's ability to accommodate for ambulatory ground reactive force

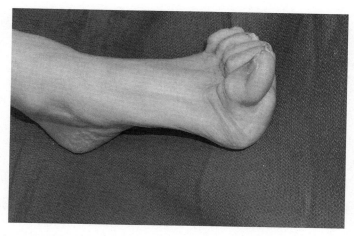

Fig. 4. Intrinsic muscular atrophy and foot deformity. Diabetic peripheral neuropathy also affects motor nerves, often causing atrophy of intrinsic musculature of the hand and foot. When this occurs, the extrinsic musculature work unopposed, thus causing hammering of the toes and retrograde buckling of the metatarsal heads. Thus, both the toes (dorsally) and the metatarsal heads (plantarly) are more prominent and therefore more prone to neuropathic ulceration.

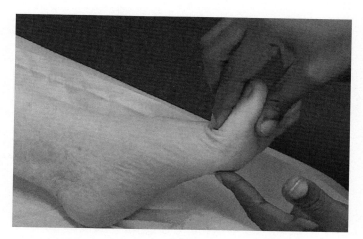

Fig. 5. Evaluation of first metatarsophalangeal joint dorsiflexion (limited joint mobility). Limited joint mobility is frequently encountered in patients with long-standing diabetes. This is most significant in the ankle joint (equinus) and in the forefoot. Less than 50° of dorsiflexion at the first metatarsal phalangeal joint indicates clinically significant limited joint mobility.

and, therefore, increases plantar pressures *(8,49–52)*. We define limited joint mobility as simply less than 50° of nonweight bearing passive dorsiflexion of the hallux *(14,53)* (Fig. 5). Additionally, glycosylation may deleteriously affect the resiliency of the Achilles tendon, thereby pulling the foot into equinus and potentially further increasing the risk for both ulceration and Charcot arthropathy (Fig. 6).

Clinicians should therefore also examine the feet for structural abnormalities including hammer or claw toes, flat feet, bunions and calluses, and reduced joint mobility to help identify pressure points that are susceptible to future ulceration.

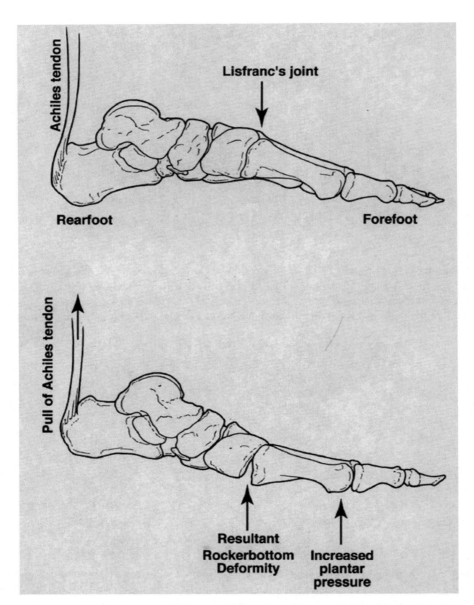

Fig. 6. Equinus and its relationship to elevated forefoot plantar pressure and Charcot arthropathy. Shortening or loss of natural extensibility of the Achilles tendon may lead to pulling of the foot into plantarflexion. This leads to increased forefoot pressure (increasing risk for plantar ulceration) and, in some patients, may be a component of midfoot collapse and Charcot arthropathy.

CUMULATIVE RISK

When these three questions have been answered, one may then begin to assess degree of risk for ulceration. Lavery et al. *(14)* reported that a patient with neuropathy but no deformity or history of ulcer or amputation has a 1.7 times greater risk for ulceration compared with a patient without neuropathy. Neuropathy with concomitant deformity

Table 1
International Consensus on the Diabetic Foot: Risk Categorization

Category	Risk factors	Treatment recommendations	Risk for foot ulcer odds ratio (95% CI)
0	No sensory neuropathy	Evaluation once a year	n/a
1	Sensory neuropathy	Evaluation every 6 months	1.7 (0.7–4.3)
2	Sensory neuropathy or peripheral vascular disease	Evaluation every 2–3 months Therapeutic shoes and insoles	12.1 (5.2–28.3)
	And/or foot deformity	Education of patient and family	
3	Previous ulcer or amputations	Evaluation every 1–2 months Therapeutic shoes and insoles Education of patient and family	36.4 (16.1–82.3)

Foot-risk criteria established by the International Consensus on the Diabetic Foot with cumulative risk for ulceration by foot risk category. CI indicates confidence interval. Low-risk patients are defined as patients with no neuropathy and no previous history of foot ulceration or a partial foot amputation. The International Consensus on the Diabetic Foot and other authors have suggested several similar risk categorization schemes to stratify patients with diabetes in order to apply treatment algorithms according to their risk. As the risk category increases, there is an increased risk of ulceration and amputation *(14,54,57)*.

or limited joint mobility yields a 12.1 times greater risk. Finally, a patient with a history of previous ulceration or amputation has a 36.4 times greater risk for presenting with another ulcer. These three questions compare to the first four categories in the classification system promoted by the international working group on the diabetic foot *(54)* (Table 1) and similar classification systems described by Rith-Najarian and coworkers *(55)* and Armstrong and colleagues *(56)*. Additional studies by Peters and Lavery *(17)* and Mayfield and coworkers *(57)* seem to corroborate this general line of assessment.

CONTRIBUTORY FACTORS

Clinicians should also examine the patient for other contributing risk factors. Cutaneous manifestations associated with diabetes such as dry or fissured skin, calluses, tinea, or onychomycosis should all be noted. Persons with diabetes have a higher rate of onychomycosis and digital interspace tinea infections that can lead to skin disruption *(58,59)*. Footwear should also be inspected to ensure proper fit. Among 699 persons with a foot ulcer, 21% were attributed to rubbing from footwear, 11% were linked to injuries (mostly falls), 4% to cellulites complicating tinea pedis, and 4% to self-inflicted trauma (i.e., when cutting toenails) *(60)*. When present, the callused tissue (as with all callused tissue) should generally be debrided and inspected for the possible presence of underlying neuropathic ulceration or abscess. Failure to do this could lead to exacerbation of the condition by both covering up a potential fluid collection and further increasing plantar pressure *(24,61–66)* (Fig. 7A,B, photo of bleeding into callus and subsequent ulceration).

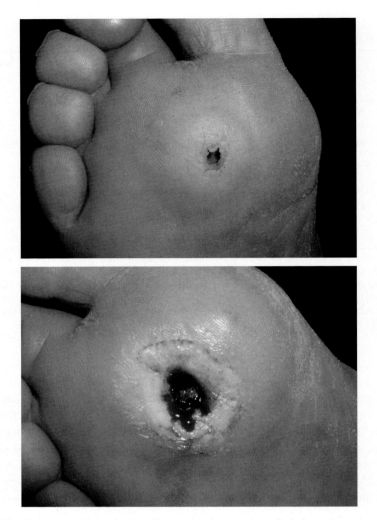

Fig. 7. Hemmorhage into callus and subsequent underlying ulceration.

Although vascular disease is a very important factor that should be assessed thoroughly, it is generally, not frequently a strong risk factor for development of diabetic foot ulceration. It is, however, a powerful risk factor for nonhealing of an ulcer once it is present, and therefore, a risk factor for amputation. This may be true for a number of other comorbid conditions once associated with ulcer development such as renal disease and smoking.

ASSESSMENT FOR AMPUTATION RISK

Three key risk factors for lower extremity amputation include the presence of ulceration, infection, and ischemia and there appears to be a significant overall contribution of wound depth and comorbidities such as infection and/or ischemia to the prevalence of lower limb amputation *(54,67,68)*. However, of these three key factors, ischemia is the only one that can, in and of itself, precipitate a primary amputation. The other two factors listed rely on a host of concomitant or preceding factors to develop. For instance, most ulcers are preceded by neuropathy, deformity, and repetitive stress. In turn, most diabetic foot infections are preceded by an ulcer. Therefore, we will pragmatically discuss assessment for amputation risk in parts: assessment of vascular disease and assessment/classification of diabetic foot ulcers.

VASCULAR EVALUATION

Certainly, macrovascular disease is more common in the diabetic population. It has been reported that patients with peripheral arterial disease (PAD) and diabetes experience worse lower extremity function than those with PAD alone (69). Commensurately, PAD is twice as common in persons with diabetes as in persons without diabetes (70) and is also a major risk factor for lower extremity amputation especially in patients with diabetes (69). However, PAD is not the most common cause of foot ulceration, and is a component factor in only about one-fourth of all cases (71,72). In a recent report, PAD was a component cause in 30% of foot ulcers seen in a two-center study (24). The vessels most often affected in the patient with diabetes are mainly femoropopliteal and smaller vessels in the calf including the posterior tibial, peroneal, and anterior tibial arteries (73). The pedal vessels (digital arteries) are frequently spared and are probably not more commonly involved than in the nondiabetic population (73).

Intermittant claudication is the earliest and the most common symptoms of PAD (69) and may be defined as pain, cramping, or aching in the calves, thighs, or buttocks that appears reproducibly with walking exercise and is relieved by rest (69). Often it may be difficult to make a distinction between diabetic neuropathy as PAD is often more subtle in its presentation in patients with diabetes than those without diabetes. The American Diabetes Association (ADA) consensus statement, the most comprehensive document on this issue, recommends that the initial assessment of PAD in patients with diabetes begins with a thorough medical history and physical examination (69). A thorough walking history is especially important as it will help elicit classic claudication symptoms and variations thereof; furthermore, patients should be asked specifically about these types of symptoms as they are often not reported (69).

Vascular assessment must include palpation of all lower extremity pulses, including femoral, popliteal, posterior tibial, and dorsalis pedis pulses. The palpation of pulses is a learned skill with a high degree of interobserver variability and high false positive and false negative rates (69). The dorsalis pedis pulse has been reported to be absent in 8.1% of healthy individuals and the posterior tibial pulse is absent in 2% (69). The absence of both pedal pulses when assessed by a person experienced in this technique, strongly suggest the presence of vascular disease; however, the presence of palpable pulses does not absolutely exclude peripheral vascular disease. In addition, clinical evidence of dependent rubor, pallor on elevation, absence of hair growth, dystrophic toenails, and cool, dry, fissured skin should also be noted as they may be concomitant signs of vascular insufficiency (69).

Ankle–brachial pressure index (ABPI), in contrast to the variabililty of pulse assessment and the often nonspecific nature of information obtained via history, is an easily reproducible and reasonably accurate method of diagnosing vascular insufficiency in the lower limbs (69). The ABPI is obtained by dividing the ankle systolic pressure by the brachial systolic pressure and is normally between 0.91 and 1.30 (69,74). The blood pressure at the ankle (dorsalis pedis or posterior tibial arteries) is measured using a Doppler ultrasound machine (Huntleigh Nesbit Evans Healthcare, UK). However, a normal ABPI may be deceiving, as medial arterial calcification of the foot vessels results in hardening of the arteries making them and a falsely elevated ABPI.

Because of the high estimated prevalence of PAD in patients with diabetes, the ADA consensus statement issued the following recommendations *(69)*. A screening ABPI be performed in all patients with diabetes >50 years of age; if the results are normal, the test should be repeated every 5 years. A screening ABPI should be considered in patients with diabetes <50 years of age who have other PAD risk factors. These risk factors include smoking, hypertension, hyperlipidemia, or duration of diabetes >10 years.

A diagnostic ABPI should be performed in any patient with symptoms of PAD.

For diabetic patients with either atypical symptoms, or a normal ABPI with typical symptoms of claudication, the ADA consensus statement recommends functional testing with a graded treadmill as patients with claudication will typically exhibit a >20 mmHg drop in ankle pressure after exercise *(69)*.

In the patient with a confirmed diagnosis of PAD, the next step would be a vascular laboratory evaluation of segmental pressures and pulse volume recordings. The ADA consensus statement recommends that these tests be considered for patients with poorly compressible vessels or those with a normal ABI despite a high suspicion of PAD *(69)*. Segmental pressures and pulse volume recordings are determined at the toe, ankle, calf, low thigh, and high thigh. The toe systolic pressure using either a strain-gauge sensor or a photoplethysmograph, with a normal value considered one in excess of 4 kPa *(75,76)*. Segmental pressures help determine lesion location, whereas pulse volume recordings provide qualitative segmental waveform analysis of blood flow *(69)*.

One can also assess peripheral circulation by transcutaneous oxygen tension (normal >40 mmHg) measurement, a noninvasive measurement of limb perfusion *(77)*. Patients with occlusive disease have significantly reduced transcutaneous oxygen tension and this has been used to determine the possibility of ulcer healing and optimal amputation healing. Laboratory assessment of the peripheral circulation includes ultrasonic duplex scanning, color-Doppler flow studies, and magnetic resonance angiogram. Peripheral X-ray angiography is the gold standard for anatomical evaluation of vascular disease in the patient with diabetes and may be used in those intended for vascular reconstruction. All of these modalities, however, have significant limitations, not the least of which may be differences in technique and operator error. Therefore, a combination of modalities and detailed physical examination is always optimal to reliance on laboratory studies in isolation.

RISK FACTORS FOR AMPUTATION: ASSESSING AND CLASSIFYING THE WOUND

Foot ulcers in persons with diabetes are one of the most common precursors to lower extremity amputation. Appropriate care of the diabetic foot ulceration requires a clear, descriptive classification system that may be used to direct appropriate therapy, communicate risk, and possibly predict outcome. Speaking a "common language" when communicating risk in the diabetic foot is therefore essential. This tenet is most important when treating acute diabetic sequelae, such as the diabetic wound. A classification

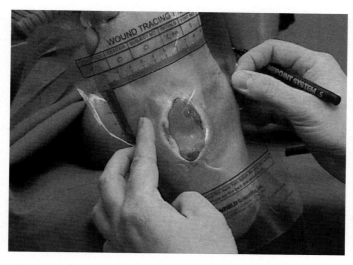

Fig. 8. Tracing the wound using sterile acetate sheet. Wound tracing may yield far more reproducible results in measuring wound size than simply length by width measurement.

system, if it is to be clinically useful, should be easy to use, reproducible, and effective to accurately communicate the status of wounds in persons with diabetes mellitus. There are a variety of variables that could be included in such a system, such as faulty wound healing, compliance issues, quality of wound granulation tissue, host immunity, nutritional status, and comorbidities. However, most of these variables are difficult to measure or categorize and can truly complicate a system. In contrast, three well documented, relatively quantifiable factors associated with poor wound healing and amputation include depth of the wound *(78,79)*, presence of infection, and the presence of concomitant ischemia *(57,68)*.

SEVEN ESSENTIAL QUESTIONS TO ASK WHEN ASSESSING A DIABETIC FOOT WOUND

Although clearly important, a classification system has little value if the clinician employing it does not approach each wound in a step-wise consistent, logical fashion. When employing this approach, the first four questions are useful in terms of their descriptive value. The last three questions are most useful for their predictive qualities.

1. Where is the ulcer located? Location of a wound and its etiology go hand in hand. Generally, wounds on the medial aspect of the foot are caused by constant low-pressure (e.g., tight shoes) whereas wounds on the plantar aspect of the foot are caused by repetitive moderate pressure (e.g., repetitive stress on prominent metatarsal heads during ambulation).
2. How large is the ulcer? Size of the wound plays a key role in determining duration to wound healing. To simplify wound diameter measurements, one may trace the wound on sterile acetate sheeting and tape this tracing into the chart (Fig. 8). The tracing can also be performed on the outer wrapping of an instrument sterilization pack (which would otherwise be discarded). Recently, many centers have begun employing digital photography and computer-driven planimetric wound area calculations. This provides for potentially more consistent, accurate measurements and, ultimately, for comparison of wound healing rates with other centers regionally and beyond. In an evaluation of the reproducibility of wound measurement

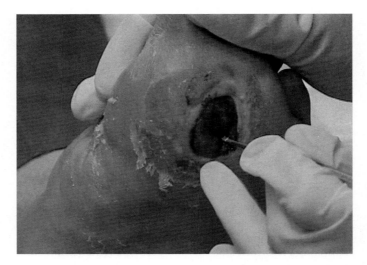

Fig. 9. Use of sterile blunt instrument to probe wound. Probing the wound for both the subdermal dimensions and for involvement of underlying structures is an important part of wound assessment. Palpation of bone in a wound is strongly suggestive of osteomyelitis and should prompt further inspection.

   techniques, Wunderlich and coworkers reported that wound tracing and digital planimetric assessment were by far more reliable than manual measurement of length and width *(80)*.
3. What does the base look like? When describing the base of a wound, one may use terms like granular, fibrotic, or necrotic. One may record the presence or absences of any drainage, which may be described as serous or purulent, with a further description of any odor or color, as necessary.
4. What do the margins look like? The margins tell us about the wound. If adequately debrided and off-loaded, they should be well-adhered to the surface of the underlying subcuticular structures with a gentle slope toward normal epithelium. However, in the inadequately debrided, inadequately off-loaded wound, undermining of the leading edge normally predominates. This is because of the "edge effect" which dictates that an interruption in any matrix (in this case, skin), magnifies both vertical and shear stress on the edges of that interruption. This subsequently causes shearing from the underlying epithelium (making the wound larger by undermining) and increased vertical pressure (making the wound progressively deeper). If appropriately debrided and offloaded, this effect will be mitigated. Nonetheless, the margins of the wound should be classified as undermining, adherent, macerated, and/or nonviable.
       Subsequent to the first questions, which we term "descriptive" come the last three questions which we term "classifiers." These classifiers can then be used to fit a patient into the University of Texas wound classification system. This system has evolved as a significant modification of the Wagner system to include concomitant depth, infection, and ischemia (Figs. 9 and 10). Although both systems have been shown to be predictive of poor outcomes, the UT system has been shown to be significantly more predictive and complete *(67,81)*. Both, however, may be considered useful in a clinical scenario, depending on the preference of the clinician.
5. How deep is the Ulceration?/Are there underlying structures involved? These two questions are so closely related that they are combined into one. There is a possible contribution of depth to ulcer healing times *(82)*. Depth of the wound is the most commonly utilized descriptor in wound classification. Wounds are graded by depth. Grade 0 represents a pre- or

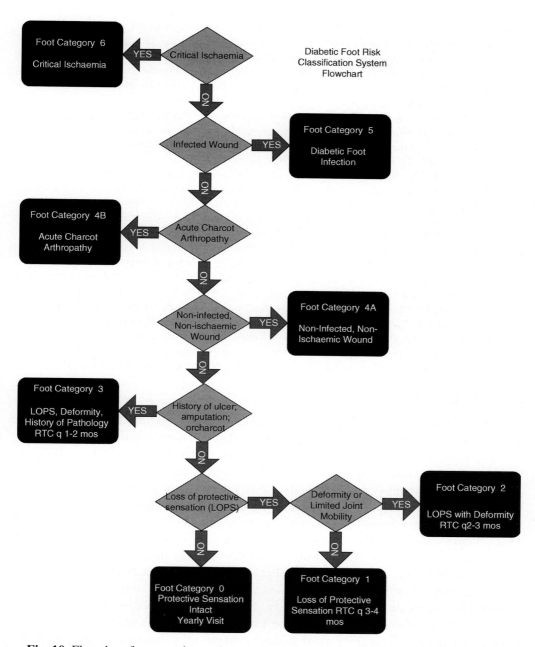

Fig. 10. Flowchart for screening and treatment of the diabetic foot. This flowchart is adapted from the University of Texas Diabetic Foot Risk Classification and International Working Group on the Diabetic Foot Risk Classification Systems. It is designed to comprehensively assess for risk of diabetic foot ulceration and amputation. The clinician begins by asking questions assessing for risk for amputation (ischemia, infection, and ulceration). Subsequently, the clinician may ask questions related to ulcer risk (neuropathy, deformity, history of previous ulcer or amputation).

postulcerative site. Grade 1 ulcers are superficial wounds through the epidermis or epidermis and dermis, but do not penetrate to tendon, capsule, or bone. Grade 2 wounds penetrate to tendon or capsule. Grade 3 wounds penetrate to bone or into a joint. We have known for some time that wounds that penetrate to bone are frequently osteomyelitic *(78)*. Additionally, we have observed that morbid outcomes are intimately associated with progressive wound depth.

Depth of the wound and involvement of underlying structures may best be appreciated through the use of a sterile blunt metallic probe. The instrument is gently inserted into the wound and the dimensions of the wound may be explored. Additionally, bony involvement is typically readily appreciable through this method.

6. Is it infected? The definition of infection is not an easy one. Cultures, laboratory values, and subjective symptoms are all helpful. However, the diagnosis of an infection's genesis and resolution has been and continues to be a clinical one. Although criteria for infection may be something less than clear-cut, there is little question that presence of infection is a prime cause of lower extremity morbidity and frequently eventuates into wet gangrene and subsequent amputation. Therefore, in an effort to facilitate communication and effect consistent results, the foot care team should agree on criteria for this very important risk factor.

7. Is there ischemia? As discussed earlier, identification of ischemia is of utmost importance when evaluating a wound. Ischemic wounds were found to have a longer duration of healing compared with neuropathic wounds without deformities *(82)*. If pulses are not palpable, or if a wound is sluggish to heal even in the face of appropriate off-loading and local wound care, noninvasive vascular studies are warranted followed by a prompt vascular surgery consultation and possible intervention to improve perfusion and thereby effect healing. A flowchart for screening and treatment of the diabetic foot is depicted in Fig. 10.

ULCER CLASSIFICATIONS

Over the past quarter century numerous classification systems have been reported in the medical literature. Most focused primarily on the depth of the ulceration with descriptive wound grades, but local comorbidity such as vascular disease or infection was usually not included. This section aims to chronologically review some of the most commonly described classification systems currently used by a variety of practitioners to stage diabetic foot wounds, and to discuss the outcomes data related to their potential use.

The first standard wound classification system was proposed by Shea *(83)* in 1975. This scheme was designed to assess pressure ulcerations and not diabetic foot ulcerations. The classification was primarily based on wound depth and did not evaluate for infection or ischemia. Because of this, Shea's system is not practical for our purpose. However, Shea's model became the framework for subsequent systems, including the International Association for Enterostomal Therapy system, National Pressure Ulcer Advisory Panel's offering *(84,85)*, and the Yarkony-Kirk classification *(85)*.

One of the most frequently cited diabetic wound classification systems was first described by Meggitt *(86)* in 1976 and popularized by Wagner *(87)* in 1981. The system is based mainly on wound depth and consists of six wound grades. These include grade 0 (intact skin), grade 1 ("superficial ulcer"), grade 2 (deep ulcer to tendon, bone, or joint), grade 3 (deep ulcer with abscess or osteomyelitis), grade 4 ("forefoot gangrene"), and grade 5 ("whole-foot gangrene"). The Meggitt-Wagner Wound Classification System is depicted in Fig. 11.

The classification system contains all three of the key descriptors including depth, infection, and ischemia. However, it does not provide for the description of concomitant

Grade 0:	No ulcer, but high-risk foot (bony Prominences, callus, claw toes, etc.)
Grade 1:	Superficial full-thickness ulcer
Grade 2:	Deep ulcer, may involve tendons, no bone involvement
Grade 3:	Deep ulcer with bone involvements, osteomyelitis
Grade 4:	Localized gangrene, e.g. toes
Grade 5:	Gangrene of whole foot

Fig. 11. Meggitt-Wagner wound classification system.

conditions. Infection is included in only one of the six Meggitt-Wagner ulcer grades, and vascular disease is only included in the last two classification grades. The first three grades are concerned only with depth. It is perhaps for this reason that they are the most commonly used, whereas the last three are largely ignored because of their limited clinical use. Certainly, forefoot and hindfoot gangrene are descriptors of ischemia, but they are end-stage descriptions, and therefore cannot help to guide proactive interventional therapy except frank ablation of the affected site.

Despite its widespread use, evidence of its validity and reliability are lacking *(88,89)*. Calhoun et al. *(89)* evaluated wounds that were infected and retrospectively assigned Wagner grades to them. They found that when wounds were treated according to what they considered a healthy standard of care, then success, which they defined as eradication of infection and prevention of readmission for 1 year, was frequently achieved despite wound grade *(89)*. Van Acker et al. *(90)* found the Wagner classification to have significant association with the duration of healing of the ulcer. Armstrong et al. *(67)* suggested that patients with Wagner stages four and five may be grouped together as the two groups did not have separate prognostic value. In addition these patients are often referred directly to a surgeon for amputation and are rarely seen by the diabetic foot team. The system was adapted to combine medical and surgical elements of therapy to monitor the treatment of diabetic foot infection. Unfortunately, in requiring that wounds be infected as an inclusion criterion, it made assessment of this classification problematic, as Meggitt-Wagner wound grades 0–2 classically have no infection descriptor attached to them. In fact, the only mention of infection in this system occurs in grade 3. It is this fact that causes many to customize this system, such that it often takes on distinctly different regional characteristics. This unfortunately limits its usefulness as a standard diabetic foot classification.

In the 1980s and 1990s many authors including Forrest and Gamborg-Nelson *(91)*, Pecoraro and Reiber *(92)*, Arlt and Protze *(93)*, and Knighton *(94)* proposed their own wound classifications, however, these systems have not gained universal acceptance.

A more recent classification system developed at the University of Texas Health Science Center in San Antonio (UT) has been proposed and implemented. This classification includes three of the most critical predictive elements, namely depth, infection, and vascular status *(54,95–98)*. The classification, integrates a system of wound grade and stage to categorize wounds by severity. It is based around two fundamental questions the clinician asks when assessing a wound: (1) How deep is the wound and (2) Whether the wound infected, ischemic, or both? This formulates into a matrix grade with depth (Question 1) as the longitudinal axis and the presence of infection and/or ischemia (Question 2) as the vertical axis.

Similar to other wound classification systems, the UT system grades wounds by depth. Grade 0 represents a pre- or postulcerative site. Grade 1 ulcers are superficial wounds through either the epidermis or the epidermis and dermis but do not penetrate to tendon, capsule, or bone. Grade 2 wounds penetrate to tendon or capsule but the bone and joints are not involved. Grade 3 wounds penetrate to bone or into a joint. Within each wound grade there are four stages: clean wounds (A), nonischemic infected wounds (B), ischemic wounds (C), and infected ischemic wounds (D).

The Grade 0 Wound

Grade 0 wounds are preulcerative areas or previous ulcer sites that are now completely epithelialized after debridement of hyperkeratosis and nonviable tissue. The diagnosis of a grade 0 wound can be made only after removal of any regional hyperkeratosis, as quite often frank ulcerations may be hidden by overlying calluses. The grade 0-A wound is then a preulcerative area or a completely epithelialized postulcerative are. The grade 0-B wound is a 0-A lesion with associated cellulitis. The grade 0-C wound is a 0-A lesion with concomitant regional signs of ischemia. The grade 0-D wound is a 0-B lesion coupled with a working diagnosis of lower extremity ischemia as defined above.

Although lesions that fall into the grade 0 category do not have a break in the epidermis and may not be classically classified as "wounds," the category is important in the identification of sites that are "at risk" for future ulceration and to monitor and prevent reulceration of newly healed wounds. Twenty-eight to fifty percent of patients with diabetes reulcerate within a year of healing their initial wound *(22)*. An ulcer classification should allow physicians to follow the progression of wounds over time.

The Grade I Wound

Grade I wounds are superficial in nature. They may be either partial or of full thickness, skin wounds without the involvement of tendon, capsule, or bone. The Grade I-A wound is therefore superficial partial or full thickness wound. The Grade I-B wound is an infected superficial wound. As with any neuropathic lesion, Grade I-B wounds should be examined very carefully. By definition, the Grade I-B wound implies superficial infection without involvement of underlying structures. If the wound shows signs of significant purulence or fluctuance, further exploration to expose a higher grade infection is in order. The Grade I-C wound is I-A plus vascular compromise and the Grade I-D wound is the infected I-B wound with concomitant ischemia.

The Grade II Wound

Grade II wounds probe deeper than the Grade I wounds. Grade II wounds may involve tendon or joint capsule but not bone. The reason for the distinct delineation between wounds that probe to bone and those without bone or joint involvement is because of the high correlation between probing to bone and osteomyelitis *(78,99)*.

The II-A wound may therefore probe to tendon or joint capsule, but not bone. The II-B wound is II-A plus infection, again the bone and joint are not involved. The Grade II-C wound is II-A plus ischemia, and the Grade II-D wound correspond to II-B plus ischemia.

The Grade III Wound

A wound that probes to bone is categorized as a grade III wound. The modifiers are then added pending the presence of comorbid factor. The III-A wound probes to bone without local or systemic signs of acute infection. The III-B wound probes to bone with signs of acute infection. The III-C wound is identical to III-A with concomitant ischemia. The III-D wound is characterized by active infection, exposed bone, and vascular insufficiency. The criteria for each of the stages are based on clinical and laboratory data. The working diagnosis of lower extremity ischemia may be based on clinical signs and symptoms such as absence of pedal hair, absent pulses, claudication, rest-pain, atrophic integument, dependent rubor, or pallor on elevation plus one or more of the noninvasive criteria (transcutaneous oxygen measurements of <40 mmHg, ankle-brachial index of <0.80, or absolute toe systolic pressure <45 mm Hg) *(76,97,98,100,101)*.

Clean ulcers may be defined as wounds without local or systemic signs of infection. The clinical diagnosis of infection in persons with diabetes is often difficult and defined by narrow, subtle parameters. Wounds with frank purulence and/or two or more of the following local signs may be classified as "infected": warmth, erythema, lymphangitis, lymphadenopathy, edema, pain, and loss of function. Systemic signs of infection may include fever, chills, nausea, vomiting, or generalized malaise *(102)*. This clinical diagnosis of infection is often obscured by neuropathy and possibly immunopathy. In the insensitive foot, pain and/or loss of function are poor indicators of inflammation and infection *(103)*. Likewise, subjects with diabetes have been shown to posses deficiencies in leukocyte adherence, chemotaxis, phagocytosis, and diapedesis *(104–106)* and often do not have leukocytosis in the presence of acute soft tissue or bone infection *(103,107,108)*. Warmth and edema are less than ideal indicators of infection, as ulcerated sites tend to be warmer and more edematous than the corresponding site contralaterally regardless of the presence of infectious disease *(109)*. However, despite these impediments, diagnosis of a diabetic foot infection remains primarily a clinical one *(107,108)*. The diagnosis and subsequent treatment of infection may also be assisted by laboratory studies or positive deep tissue cultures or wound based curettage *(110)*. When osteomyelitis is suspected, bone biopsy with appropriate pathology and culture studies is still the gold standard for diagnosis.

Armstrong et al. validated the predictive value of the UT classification system in 1998 *(67)* and noted a significant overall trend toward an increased prevalence of amputations as wounds increased in both grade (depth) and stage (comorbidity). For example, patients whose wounds were both infected and ischemic were noted to be almost 90 times more likely to receive a high level amputation compared with patients in a less advanced wound stage, and patients whose wound probed to the underlying bone were more than 11 times as likely to receive a high level amputation *(82)*. Unfortunately the study was retrospective and was not a multicenter trial. In addition, some degree of bias may have been present since the study was carried out by the center that first described the system and the clinicians using it intimately familiar with the system.

Oyibo et al. *(111)* compared the Meggitt-Wagner classification system with the UT system in a multicenter prospective longitudinal case–control study of 194 patients. The study suggested that both the UT and the Wagner classification system correlated similarly with clinical outcome. Both systems associated higher grades with a greater likelihood of an ulcer not healing and a greater chance of limb amputation *(82)*. The trend for grade of the UT classification system was slightly more robust than the trend for grade of the Wagner classification. The inclusion of comorbid factors such as infection

Table 2
The University of Texas Health Science Center San Antonio Diabetic Wound Classification System

	0	1	2	3
A	Pre- or postulcerative lesion	Superficial, not involving tendon, capsule, or bone	Penetrates to tendon or capsule	Penetrates to bone
B	Infection	Infection	Infection	Infection
C	Ischemia	Ischemia	Ischemia	Ischemia
D	Infection and ischemia	Infection and ischemia	Infection and ischemia	Infection and ischemia

and/or ischemia to grade (depth) when classifying an ulcer with the UT system improves description and adds to the predictive power of a wound classification system, especially for ulcers within the same grade level but at a different stage. Based on this, the UT wound classification showed promise as a more practical system.

As with other classification systems, the UT classification is not void of potential shortcomings. Neuropathy, considered by many to be an important etiological and prognostic factor is not included in the UT classification system. This exclusion may be based on the argument that neuropathy is a preexisting condition in most diabetic foot wounds; however, neuropathy is a component of other classification system. The UT classification system also does not describe the anatomic region of the wound, but it remains to be proven whether anatomic location may potentiate the specificity in grading. Another shortcoming of the UT classification system is that it leaves no room for more specificity or complexity. Simplicity is one of the top reasons why the Meggitt-Wagner classification system has remained so popular, and the UT classification system is already fairly complex with its four-point grading scale subdivisions ranging from 0 to 3 (Table 2).

More recent classification systems that have been proposed include the UT classification modification by Van Acker/Peter *(82)*, the PEDIS system by IWGDF members *(112)* and the S(AD) SAD system proposed by Macfarlane and Jeffcoate *(95,113)*. These systems will require validation and have yet to gain universal acceptance. All the proposed classification systems have attempted to integrate local factors with varying degrees of validated success. These systems might be viewed with the same considerations we use when we think of a language. A universal idiom has dialects, accents, and pragmatic slang. Different exposure and usage of the language will cause it to change over time. These dialects should be judged in light of a progress toward a global lower prevalence of lower extremity amputations. To avoid speaking in tongues we need to continue toward a more descriptive validated and universally accepted diabetic foot wound classification system.

In conclusion, it is observed that many of the most common component causes for neuropathic ulceration, infection, and subsequent amputation may be identified using simple, inexpensive equipment in a primary-care setting and consistent, thoughtful assessment of the diabetic foot is of central importance in identifying risk for both ulceration and amputation. Subsequent to the gathering of clinical data through sequential assessment, appropriate classification of the wound becomes paramount in our efforts to document and communicate the level of risk to all members of the health-care team caring for the person with diabetes. When this is accomplished, we believe that a significant reduction of lower extremity complications can indeed be realized locally. Certainly, with dissemination of the tools and techniques for consistent examination, we believe that a global impact is well within reach.

REFERENCES

1. Boulton AJM, Vileikyte L. Pathogenesis of diabetic foot ulceration and measurements of neuropathy. *Wounds* 2000;12(Suppl B):12B–18B.
2. Reiber GE, Smith DG, Carter J, et al. A comparison of diabetic foot ulcer patients managed in VHA and non-VHA settings. *J Rehabil Res Dev* May–Jun 2001;38(3):309–317.
3. Armstrong DG, Lipsky BA. Advances in the treatment of diabetic foot infections. *Diabetes Technol Ther* 2004;6:167–177.
4. Pecoraro RE, Reiber GE, Burgess EM. Pathways to diabetic limb amputation: basis for prevention. *Diabetes Care* 1990;13:513–521.
5. Armstrong DG, Peters EJ, Athanasiou KA, Lavery LA. Is there a critical level of plantar foot pressure to identify patients at risk for neuropathic foot ulceration? *J Foot Ankle Surg* 1998;37(4):303–307.
6. Cavanagh PR, Ulbrecht JS, Caputo GM. Biomechanical aspects of diabetic foot disease: aetiology, treatment, and prevention. *Diabet Med* 1996;13(Suppl 1):S17–S22.
7. Lavery LA, Vela SA, Lavery DC, Quebedeaux TL. Reducing dynamic foot pressures in high-risk diabetic subjects with foot ulcerations. A comparison of treatments. *Diabetes Care* 1996;19(8):818–821.
8. Lavery LA, Lavery DC, Quebedeax-Farnham TL. Increased foot pressures after great toe amputation in diabetes. *Diabetes Care* 1995;18(11):1460–1462.
9. Brand PW. The diabetic foot, in *Diabetes Mellitus, Theory and Practice* (Ellenberg M, Rifkin H, eds.) 3rd ed. Medical Examination Publishing, New York, 1983, pp. 803–828.
10. King H, Aubert RE, Herman WH. Global burden of diabetes, 1995–2025: prevalence, numerical estimates, and projections [see comments]. *Diabetes Care* 1998;21(9):1414–1431.
11. Singh N, Armstrong DG, Lipsky BA. Preventing foot ulcers in persons with diabetes. *JAMA* 2005;293(2):217–228.
12. Plank J, Haas W, Rakovac I, et al. Evaluation of the impact of chiropodist care in the secondary prevention of foot ulcerations in diabetic subjects. *Diabetes Care* 2003;26(6):1691–1695.
13. Ronnemaa T, Hamalainen H, Toikka T, Liukkonen I. Evaluation of the impact of podiatrist care in the primary prevention of foot problems in diabetic subjects. *Diabetes Care* 1997;20(12):1833–1837.
14. Lavery LA, Armstrong DG, Vela SA, Quebedeaux TL, Fleischli JG. Practical criteria for screening patients at high risk for diabetic foot ulceration. *Arch Intern Med* 1998;158:158–162.
15. Boyko EJ, Ahroni JH, Stensel V, Forsberg RC, Davignon DR, Smith DG. A prospective study of risk factors for diabetic foot ulcer. The Seattle Diabetic Foot Study. *Diabetes Care* 1999;22(7):1036–1042.
16. Abbott CA, Carrington AL, Ashe H, et al. The north-west diabetes foot care study: incidence of, and risk factors for, new diabetic foot ulceration in a community-based patient cohort. *Diabet Med* 2002;19(5):377–384.
17. Peters EJ, Lavery LA. Effectiveness of the diabetic foot risk classification system of the International Working Group on the Diabetic Foot. *Diabetes Care* 2001;24(8):1442–1447.

18. Goldner MG. The fate of the second leg in the diabetic amputee. *Diabetes* 1960;9:100–103.
19. Armstrong DG, Lavery LA, Vela SA, Quebedeaux TL, Fleischli JG. Choosing a practical screening instrument to identify patients at risk for diabetic foot ulceration. *Arch Int Med* 1998;158:289–292.
20. Quebedeaux TL, Lavery LA, Lavery DC. The development of foot deformities and ulcers after great toe amputation in diabetes. *Diabetes Care* 1996;19(2):165–167.
21. Murdoch DP, Armstrong DG, Dacus JB, Laughlin TJ, Morgan CB, Lavery LA. The natural history of great toe amputations. *J Foot Ankle Surg* 1997;36(3):204–208.
22. Uccioli L, Faglia E, Monticone G, et al. Manufactured shoes in the prevention of diabetic foot ulcers. *Diabetes Care* 1995;18(10):1376–1378.
23. Helm PA, Walker SC, Pulliam GF. Recurrence of neuropathic ulcerations following healing in a total contact cast. *Arch Phys Med Rehabil* 1991;72(12):967–970.
24. Reiber GE, Vileikyte L, Boyko EJ, et al. Causal pathways for incident lower-extremity ulcers in patients with diabetes from two settings. *Diabetes Care* 1999;22(1):157–162.
25. Olaleye D, Perkins BA, Bril V. Evaluation of three screening tests and a risk assessment model for diagnosing peripheral neuropathy in the diabetes clinic. *Diabetes Res Clin Pract* 2001;54(2):115–128.
26. Liniger C, Albeanu A, Bloise D, Assal JP. The tuning fork revisited. *Diabet Med* 1990;7(10):859–864.
27. Kastenbauer T, Sauseng S, Brath H, Abrahamian H, Irsigler K. The value of the Rydel-Seiffer tuning fork as a predictor of diabetic polyneuropathy compared with a neurothesiometer. *Diabet Med* 2004;21(6):563–567.
28. Thivolet C, el Farkh J, Petiot A, Simonet C, Tourniaire J. Measuring vibration sensations with graduated tuning fork. Simple and reliable means to detect diabetic patients at risk of neuropathic foot ulceration. *Diabetes Care* 1990;13(10):1077–1080.
29. Armstrong DG. The 10-g monofilament: the diagnostic divining rod for the diabetic foot? (editorial) (in process citation). *Diabetes Care* 2000;23(7):887.
30. Sorman E, Edwall LL. (Examination of peripheral sensibility. Vibration test is more sensitive than monofilament test). *Lakartidningen* 2002;99(12):1339–1340.
31. Gin H, Rigalleau V, Baillet L, Rabemanantsoa C. Comparison between monofilament, tuning fork and vibration perception tests for screening patients at risk of foot complication. *Diabetes Metab* 2002;28(6 Pt 1):457–461.
32. Rith-Najarian SJ, Stolusky T, Gohdes DM. Identifying diabetic patients at risk for lower extremity amputation in a primary health care setting. *Diabetes Care* 1992;15(10):1386–1389.
33. Pham HT, Armstrong DG, Harvey C, Harkless LB, Giurini JM, Veves A. Screening techniques to identify the at risk patients for developing diabetic foot ulcers in a prospective multicenter trial. *Diabetes Care* 2000;23:606–611.
34. Yong R, Karas TJ, Smith KD, Petrov O. The durability of the Semmes-Weinstein 5.07 monofilament. *J Foot Ankle Surg* 2000;39(1):34–38.
35. Booth J, Young MJ. Differences in the performance of commercially available 10-g monofilaments. *Diabetes Care* 2000;23(7):984–988.
36. Ulbrecht JS, Cavanagh PR, Caputo GM. Foot problems in diabetes: an overview. *Clin Infect Dis* 2004;39(Suppl 2):S73–S82.
37. Mueller MJ. Identifying patients with diabetes who are at risk for lower extremity complications: use of Semmes-Weinstein monofilaments. *Phys Ther* 1996;76(1):68–71.
38. Smieja M, Hunt DL, Edelman D, Etchells E, Cornuz J, Simel DL. Clinical examination for the detection of protective sensation in the feet of diabetic patients. International Cooperative Group for Clinical Examination Research. *J Gen Intern Med* 1999;14(7):418–424.
39. Armstrong DG. Loss of protective sensation: a practical evidence-based definition. *J Foot Ankle Surg* 1999;38(1):79–80.

40. Mason J, O'Keeffe C, Hutchinson A, McIntosh A, Young R, Booth A. A systematic review of foot ulcer in patients with Type 2 diabetes mellitus. II: treatment. *Diabet Med* 1999;16(11):889–909.

41. Young MJ, Breddy JL, Veves A, Boulton AJ. The prediction of diabetic neuropathic foot ulceration using vibration perception thresholds. A prospective study. *Diabetes Care* 1994;17(6):557–560.

42. Boulton AJM. The importance of abnormal foot pressure and gait in causation of foot ulcers, in *The Foot in Diabetes* (Connor H, Boulton AJM, Ward JD, eds.) 1st ed. John Wiley and Sons, Chilchester, 1987, pp. 11–26.

43. Duckworth T, Betts RP, Franks CI, Burke J. The measurement of pressure under the foot. *Foot Ankle* 1982;3:130.

44. Birke JA, Novick A, Graham SL, Coleman WC, Brasseaux DM. Methods of treating plantar ulcers. *Phys Ther* 1991;71(2):116–122.

45. Veves A, Murray HJ, Young MJ, Boulton AJM. The risk of foot ulceration in diabetic patients with high foot pressure: a prospective study. *Diabetolgica* 1992;35:660–663.

46. Grant WP, Sullivan R, Sonenshine DE, et al. Electron microscopic investigation of the effects of diabetes mellitus on the Achilles tendon. *J Foot Ankle Surg* 1997;36(4):272–278; discussion 330.

47. Rosenbloom AL, Silverstein JH, Lezotte DC, Riley WJ, Maclaren NK. Limited joint mobility in diabetes mellitus of childhood: natural history and relationship to growth impairment. *J Pediatr* 1982;101(5):874–878.

48. Rosenbloom AL. Skeletal and joint manifestations of childhood diabetes. *Pediatr Clin North Am* 1984;31:569–589.

49. Birke JA, Franks D, Foto JG. First ray joint limitation, pressure, and ulceration of the first metatarsal head in diabetes mellitus. *Foot Ankle* 1995;16(5):277–284.

50. Frykberg RG, Lavery LA, Pham H, Harvey C, Harkless L, Veves A. Role of neuropathy and high foot pressures in diabetic foot ulceration [In Process Citation]. *Diabetes Care* 1998;21(10):1714–1719.

51. Fernando DJS, Masson EA, Veves A, Boulton AJM. Relationship of limited joint mobility to abnormal foot pressures and diabetic foot ulceration. *Diabetes Care* 1991;14:8–11.

52. Armstrong DG, Stacpoole-Shea S, Nguyen HC, Harkless LB. Lengthening of the Achilles tendon in diabetic patients who are at high risk for ulceration of the foot. *J Bone Joint Surg Am* 1999;81A:535–538.

53. Birke J, Cornwall MA, Jackson M. Relationship between hallux limitus and ulceration of the great toe. *Sports Phys Ther J Orthop* 1988;10:172–176.

54. International working group on the diabetic foot. *International Consensus on the Diabetic Foot.* International Working Group on the Diabetic Foot, Maastricht, 1999.

55. Rith-Najarian S, Branchaud C, Beaulieu O, Gohdes D, Simonson G, Mazze R. Reducing lower-extremity amputations due to diabetes. Application of the staged diabetes management approach in a primary care setting. *J Fam Pract* 1998;47(2):127–132.

56. Armstrong DG, Lavery LA, Harkless LB. Who's at risk for diabetic foot ulceration? *Clin Podiatr Med Surg* 1998;15:11–19.

57. Mayfield JA, Reiber GE, Nelson RG, Greene T. A foot risk classification system to predict diabetic amputation in pima indians. *Diabetes Care* 1996;19(7):704–709.

58. Altman MI, Altman KS. The podiatric assessment of the diabetic lower extremity: special considerations. *Wounds* 2000;12(Suppl B):64B–71B.

59. Boike AM, Hall JO. A practical guide for examining and treating the diabetic foot. *Cleve Clin J Med* 2002;69(4):342–348.

60. Macfarlane RM, Jeffcoate WJ. Factors contributing to the presentation of diabetic foot ulcers. *Diabet Med* 1997;14(10):867–870.

61. Murray HJ, Young MJ, Hollis S, Boulton AJ. The association between callus formation, high pressures and neuropathy in diabetic foot ulceration. *Diabetic Med* 1996;13(11):979–982.
62. Young MJ, Cavanagh PR, Thomas G, Johnson MM, Murray H, Boulton AJ. The effect of callus removal on dynamic plantar foot pressures in diabetic patients. *Diabet Med* 1992;9(1):55–57.
63. Pitei DL, Foster A, Edmonds M. The effect of regular callus removal on foot pressures. *J Foot Ankle Surg* 1999;38(4):251–255; discussion 306.
64. Collier JH, Brodbeck CA. Assessing the diabetic foot: plantar callus and pressure sensation. *Diabetes Educ* 1993;19(6):503–508.
65. Rosen RC, Davids MS, Bohanske LM, Lemont H. Hemorrhage into plantar callus and diabetes mellitus. *Cutis* 1985;35(4):339–341.
66. Ahroni JH, Boyko EJ, Forsberg RC. Clinical correlates of plantar pressure among diabetic veterans. *Diabetes Care* 1999;22(6):965–972.
67. Armstrong DG, Lavery LA, Harkless LB. Validation of a diabetic wound classification system. The contribution of depth, infection, and ischemia to risk of amputation (see comments). *Diabetes Care* 1998;21(5):855–859.
68. Reiber GE, Pecoraro RE, Koepsell TD. Risk factors for amputation in patients with diabetes mellitus: a case control study. *Ann Intern Med* 1992;117(2):97–105.
69. Peripheral arterial disease in people with diabetes. *Diabetes Care* 2003;26(12):3333–3341.
70. Gregg EW, Sorlie P, Paulose-Ram R, et al. Prevalence of lower-extremity disease in the US adult population ≥40 years of age with and without diabetes: 1999–2000 national health and nutrition examination survey. *Diabetes Care* 2004;27(7):1591–1597.
71. Edmonds ME. Experience in a multidisciplinary diabetic foot clinic, in *The Foot in Diabetes* (Connor H, Boulton AJM, Ward JD, eds.). John Wiley and Sons, Chichester, 1987, pp. 121–131.
72. Thompson FJ, Veves A, Ashe H, et al. A team approach to diabetic foot care—the Manchester experience. *Foot* 1991;1:75–82.
73. American Diabetes Association. Consensus Development Conference on Diabetic Foot Wound Care. *Diabetes Care* 1999;22(8):1354.
74. Weitz JI, Byrne J, Clagett GP, et al. Diagnosis and treatment of chronic arterial insufficiency of the lower extremities: a critical review. *Circulation* 1996;94(11):3026–3049.
75. Holstein P, Lassen NA. Healing of ulcers on the feet correlated with distal blood pressure measurements in occlusive arterial disease. *Acta Orthop Scand* 1980;51(6):995–1006.
76. Orchard TJ, Strandness DE. Assessment of peripheral vascular disease in diabetes: report and recommendation of an international workshop. *Diabetes Care* 1993;83(12):685–695.
77. Franzeck UK, Talke P, Bernstein EF, Golbranson FL, Fronek A. Transcutaneous PO2 measurements in health and peripheral arterial occlusive disease. *Surgery* 1982;91(2):156–163.
78. Grayson ML, Balaugh K, Levin E, Karchmer AW. Probing to bone in infected pedal ulcers. A clinical sign of underlying osteomyelitis in diabetic patients. *J Am Med Assoc* 1995;273(9):721–723.
79. Birke JA, Novick A, Patout CA, Coleman WC. Healing rates of plantar ulcers in leprosy and diabetes. *Lepr Rev* 1992;63(4):365–374.
80. Wunderlich RP, Peters EJ, Armstrong DG, Lavery LA. Reliability of digital videometry and acetate tracing in measuring the surface area of cutaneous wounds. *Diabetes Res Clin Pract* 2000;49(2–3):87–92.
81. Oyibo SO, Jude EB, Tarawneh I, et al. A comparison of two diabetic foot ulcer classification systems. *Diabetes* 2000;49 (Suppl 1):A33.
82. Armstrong DG, Peters EJ. Classification of wounds of the diabetic foot 2001;1:233–238.
83. Shea JD. Pressure sores: classification and management. *Clin Orthop Relat Res* 1975;112: 89–100.

84. Doughty D. Management of pressure sores. *J Enterostomal Ther* 1984;15(1):39–44.
85. Yarkony GM, Kirk PM, Carlson C, et al. Classification of pressure ulcers. *Arch Dermatol* 1990;126:1218–1219.
86. Meggitt B. Surgical management of the diabetic foot. *Br J Hosp Med* 1976;16:227–332.
87. Wagner FW. The dysvascular foot: a system for diagnosis and treatment. *Foot Ankle* 1981;2:64–122.
88. Smith RG. Validation of Wagner's classification: a literature review. *Ostomy Wound Manage* 2003;49(1):54–62.
89. Calhoun JH, Cantrell J, Cobos J, et al. Treatment of diabetic foot infections: Wagner classification, therapy, and outcome. *Foot Ankle* 1988;9:101–106.
90. Van Acker K. *The Diabetic Foot. A Challenge for Policy-Makers and Health Care Professionals*. Department of Medicine, University of Antwerp, Antwerp, 2000.
91. Forrest RD, Gamborg-Neilsen P. Wound assessment in clinical practice: a critical review of methods and their application. *Acta Med Scand* 1984;687:69–74.
92. Pecoraro RE, Reiber GE. Classification of wounds in diabetic amputees. *Wounds* 1990;2(2):65–73.
93. Arlt B, Protze J. [Diabetic foot]. *Langenbecks Arch Chir Suppl Kongressbd* 1997;114:528–532.
94. Knighton DR, Ciresi KF, Fiegel VD, Austin LL, Butler EL. Classification and treatment of chronic nonhealing wounds: successful treatment with autologous platelet-derived wound healing factors (PDWHF). *Ann Surg* 1986;204:332–330.
95. Jeffcoate WJ, Macfarlane RM, Fletcher EM. The description and classification of diabetic foot lesions. *Diabetic Med* 1993;10:676–679.
96. Pratt TC. Gangrene and infection in the diabetic. *Med Clin North Am* 1965;40:987–992.
97. LoGerfo FW, Coffman JD. Vascular and microvascular disease of the foot in diabetes. *N Engl J Med* 1984;311:1615–1619.
98. Bacharach J, Rooke T, Osmundson P, Glovizzki P. Predictive value of trascutaneous oxygen pressure and amputation success by use of supine and elevation measurements. *J Vasc Surg* 1992;15:558–563.
99. Caputo GM. Infection: investigation and management, in *The Foot in Diabetes* (Boulton AJM, Connor H, Cavanagh PR, eds.) 2nd ed. Wiley and Sons, Chichester, 1994.
100. Carter S. Elective foot surgery in limbs with arterial disease. *Clin Orthop* 1993;289:228–236.
101. Apelqvist J, Castenfors J, Larsson J. Prognostic value of ankle and toe blood pressure levels in outcome of diabetic foot ulcers. *Diabetes Care* 1989;12:373–378.
102. Joseph WS. *Handbook of Lower Extremity Infections*. 1st ed. Churchill Livingston, New York, 1990.
103. Lavery LA, Armstrong DG, Quebedeaux TL, Walker SC. Puncture wounds: the frequency of normal laboratory values in the face of severe foot infections of the foot in diabetic and non-diabetic adults. *Am J Med* 1996;101:521–525.
104. Molinar DM, Palumbo PH, Wilson WR, Ritts RE. Leukocyte chemotaxis in diabetic patients and their first degree relatives. *Diabetes* 1976;25:880–889.
105. Bagdade JD, Root RK, Bulger RJ. Impaired leukocyte function in patients with poorly controlled diabetes. *Diabetes* 1974;23:9–17.
106. Tan JS, Anderson JL, Watanakunakorn C, Phair JP. Neutrophil dysfunction in diabetes mellitus. *J Lab Clin Med* 1975;85:26–33.
107. Armstrong DG, Lavery LA, Sariaya M, Ashry H. Leukocytosis is a poor indicator of acute osteomyelitis of the foot in diabetes mellitus. *J Foot Ankle Surg* 1996;35(4):280–283.
108. Armstrong DG, Perales TA, Murff RT, Edelson GW, Welchon JG. Value of white blood cell count with differential in the acute diabetic foot infection. *J Am Podiatr Med Assoc* 1996;86(5):224–227.

109. Armstrong DG, Lavery LA, Liswood PJ, Todd WF, Tredwell JA. Infrared dermal ther-mometry for the high-risk diabetic foot. *Phys Ther* 1997;77(2):169–175; discussion 176–167.
110. Armstrong DG, Liswood PJ, Todd WF, William J. Stickel Bronze Award. Prevalence of mixed infections in the diabetic pedal wound. A retrospective review of 112 infections. *J Am Podiatr Med Assoc* 1995;85(10):533–537.
111. Oyibo SO, Jude EB, Tarawneh I, Nguyen HC, Harkless LB, Boulton AJ. A comparison of two diabetic foot ulcer classification systems: the Wagner and the University of Texas wound classification systems. *Diabetes Care* 2001;24(1):84–88.
112. Schaper NC. Diabetic foot ulcer classification system for research purposes: a progress report on criteria for including patients in research studies. *Diabetes Metab Res Rev* 2004;20(Suppl 1):S90–S95.
113. Macfarlane RM, Jeffcoate WJ. Classification of diabetic foot ulcers: the S(AD) SAD sys-tem. *Diabetic Foot* 1999;2(4):123–131.

Mary G. Hochman, MD, Yvonne Cheung, MD,
David P. Brophy, MD, FFRRCSI, FRCR, MSCVIR,
and J. Anthony Parker, MD

INTRODUCTION

Foot infections are among the most common causes of hospitalization in the diabetic population, accounting for 20% of all diabetes-related admissions. Complicated foot infections may require treatment by amputation—as many as 6–10% of all patients with diabetes will undergo amputation for treatment of infection *(1–3)*, accounting for 57% of nontraumatic lower extremity amputations *(4–6)*. The scope of the problem is compelling. Infections and complicated vascular diabetic foot problems result in 50,000 amputations a year in the United States *(7)*. The Centers for Disease Control and Prevention estimated the annual treatment cost of amputees within this group at $1.2 billion for the year 1997. However, this figure does not include the cost of rehabilitation, prosthetic devices, or lost income. These treatment costs are likely to escalate as the prevalence of diabetes is on the rise. A recent epidemiology study shows an increase of the overall prevalence of diabetes from 4.9% in 1990 to 6.5% in 1998 *(8)*.

Information derived from imaging studies can play an important role in management of complicated foot problems in the patient with diabetes. Soft tissue abnormalities such as abscesses and cellulitis can be identified, osteomyelitis can be detected, the extent of abnormal marrow can be depicted, neuroarthropathic chances can be diagnosed and followed over time, distribution of atherosclerotic lesions can be noninvasively mapped, and the effectiveness of revascularizaton procedures can be evaluated. A variety of studies are currently available for imaging the diabetic foot. In order to use these imaging studies effectively, it is important to understand the specific strengths and weaknesses of each modality, as they apply to the particular clinical problem in question. The goal of this chapter will be to review the modalities available for imaging of diabetic foot infection and to highlight their relative utilities in the context of clinical problem solving.

INFECTION IN THE DIABETIC FOOT

Risk Factors

Many factors contribute to infection in the diabetic foot including peripheral neuropathy *(9)* and vascular insufficiency *(10)*. Repetitive minor trauma to an insensitive neuropathic foot, exacerbated by abnormal biomechanics or ill-fitting shoes, causes

From: *The Diabetic Foot, Second Edition*
Edited by: A. Veves, J. M. Giurini, and F. W. LoGerfo © Humana Press Inc., Totowa, NJ

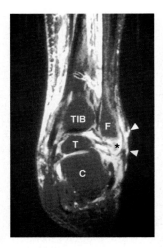

Fig. 1. Osteomyelitis deep to ulcer on MRI. Coronal STIR image of the left foot of a patient with diabetes shows an area of marrow edema (*) at the tip of the fibula. Overlying this focus of abnormal marrow is an ulcer surrounded by diffuse soft tissue swelling (arrowheads). These findings represent osteomyelitis of the distal fibula. F, fibula; C, calcaneus; TIB, tibia; T, talus.

areas of increased plantar pressure to develop callus that predispose to ulcer development. Deep to the callus and clinically occult, an ulcer forms insidiously *(11,12)*. Direct extension of infected ulcers or soft tissue infection leads to osteomyelitis *(13)* (Fig. 1). These infections are usually polymicrobial and involve both anaerobic and aerobic pathogens.

Soft Tissue Abnormalities

Soft tissue abnormalities associated with the diabetic foot include soft tissue edema, cellulitis, soft tissue abscess, ulcers, sinus tracts, tenosynovitis, joint effusions, and arthritis *(14–16)*. The importance of differentiating these conditions lies in their differing management: abscess necessitates prompt surgical drainage, septic arthritis requires surgical debridement, and cellulitis generally entails antibiotic therapy.

Soft tissue edema and swelling is a common finding in the patient with diabetes. Soft tissue swelling can occur in the absence of infection, because of vascular insufficiency or peripheral neuropathy (Fig. 2) *(16)*. However, soft tissue swelling can also reflect the presence of cellulitis, that is, soft tissue infection of the superficial soft tissues. Cellulitis along the dorsum of the foot usually occurs secondary to surface infections in the nails, toes, or web spaces. Simple cellulitis is generally diagnosed clinically, without the need for imaging. The major indication for imaging of patients with cellulitis is suspected underlying deep infection, such as soft tissue abscess, osteomyelitis, or septic arthritis.

Osteomyelitis

Osteomyelitis of the foot occurs in up to 15% of patients with diabetes *(15)*. Bone infection results from local extension of soft tissue infection (Fig. 1). Callus and ulcers serve as the conduit for infection to spread to deep soft tissue compartments, bones, and

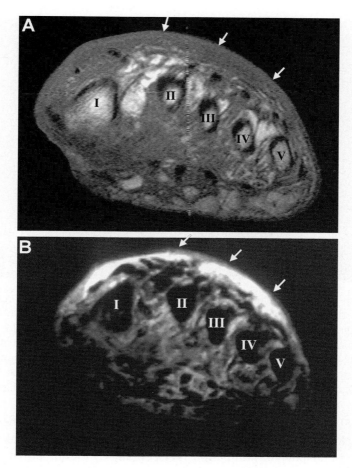

Fig. 2. Dorsal soft tissue swelling on MRI. **(A)** (T1-weighted image) and **(B)** (STIR image) are coronal or short axis images acquired at the level of the mid-metatarsal shafts. This patient with diabetes has diffuse dorsal soft tissue swelling (small arrows). The subcutaneous edema is dark on the T1-weighted image (image A) and bright on STIR (image B). Note the presence of normal marrow signal in the metatarsal bones—high signal (bright) fatty marrow on T1, which is dark on STIR. I–V, first to fifth metatarsals.

joints. The most common sites of soft tissue infection and secondary osteomyelitis are foci of increased plantar pressure, such as the metatarsal heads and the calcaneus (Fig. 3). Evaluation of foot ulcers is important because more than 90% of osteomyelitis cases result from contiguous spread of infection from soft tissue to bone *(7)*. Newman et al. further demonstrate a clear relationship between ulcer depth and osteomyelitis: 100% of ulcers exposing bone and 82% of moderately deep ulcers have osteomyelitis on bone biopsy *(2)* (Fig. 1).

Identification of osteomyelitis in the diabetic foot is difficult both clinically and radiographically. Ability to probe through a pedal ulcer to bone (Fig. 4) has been reported as a useful index of underlying osteomyelitis in a patient with diabetes *(17)* and is commonly used to guide decisions regarding treatment. Nonetheless, clinical judgment was shown to be a poor indicator of infection. The technique of probing to

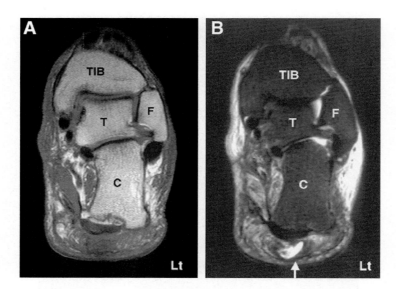

Fig. 3. Deep ulcer or inflammation beneath a focus of high plantar pressure on MRI. A patient with diabetes presented with soft tissue swelling and inflammation of the left foot. Coronal T1-weighted **(A)** and STIR **(B)** images of the left ankle show a fluid collection and an area of inflammation (arrow) in the plantar fat pad. Both the inflammation and fluid collection are dark on T1-weighted (A) and bright on STIR (B) images. Findings depict deep ulcer formation in the heel pad, a common focus of high plantar pressure. The overlying skin appears intact. Normal marrow signal in the calcaneus excludes osteomyelitis. F, fibula; TIB, tibia; T, talus; C, calcaneus.

bone, only 68% sensitive, may underestimate the incidence of bone involvement, according to Newman et al. *(2)*. In the same study, 18 out of 19 pedal ulcers did not expose bone nor display inflammation, yet contained osteomyelitis. Other clinical parameters such as fever and leukocytosis are unreliable in the patient with diabetes. For example, in a study by Bamberger et al. *(13)*, only 18% of patients with clinically severe osteomyelitis were febrile. Neither fever nor leukocytosis predicts the necessity for surgical exploration *(18)*.

IMAGING MODALITIES

Accurate diagnosis in the patient with diabetes translates to differentiation between bone and soft tissue infection, characterization of soft tissue abnormalities and mapping of atherosclerotic disease for surgical intervention. The imaging modalities that are useful in the evaluation of diabetic foot infections include radiography, computed tomography (CT), ultrasound, skeletal scintigraphy, magnetic resonance imaging (MRI), and angiography. Imaging techniques vary in their sensitivity for detection of osteomyelitis, with specificity limited in the presence of cellulitis, peripheral ischemia, and diabetic neuroarthropathy (Table 1). In the appropriate setting, however, noninvasive imaging can aid in diagnosis and treatment planning.

Radiography

Radiography ("X-ray") remains the first screening examination in any patient with suspected infection. Calcification in the interdigital arteries identifies an unsuspected

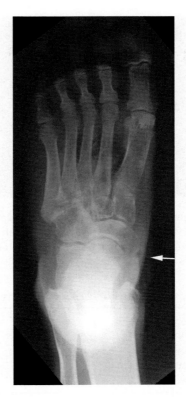

Fig. 4. Osteomyelitis of the navicular bone on radiography. AP view of the right foot shows a deep ulcer (arrow) overlying the navicular bone. The medial cortex of the navicular is destroyed, representing osteomyelitis. On clinical exam, exposed bone was evident at the ulcer.

Table 1
Compilation of Sensitivity and Specificity of Various Imaging Modalities in the Diagnosis of Osteomyelitis

	Range of sensitivity (%)	Range of specificity(%)	Compiled sensitivity/ specificity (%/%)	References
Radiography	52–93	33–92	61/72	*2,24,25, 50–52,62–65*
Three-phase bone scan in patients without bone complications			94/95	*20* Review of 20 published reports
Three-phase bone scan in patients with bone complications			95/33	*20*
In-111-labeled WBC	75–100	69–100	93/80	*8,24–26,29*
Combined gallium and bone scan			81/69	*20*
MRI	29–100	67–95	96/87	*8,50–54*

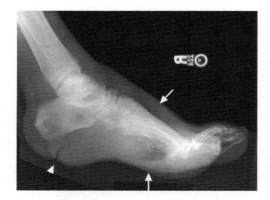

Fig. 5. Soft tissue air and deep ulcers on radiography. The lateral view of the right foot from a patient with diabetes shows subcutaneous air (arrows) in both dorsal and plantar soft tissues surrounding the metatarsals. A deep ulcer dissects into the heel fat pad (arrowhead).

Table 2
Radiographic Findings of Acute Osteomyelitis (19)

Cortical bone destruction
Permeative radiolucency
Focal osteopenia or focal osteolytic lesion
Periosteal new bone formation
Soft tissue swelling

patient with diabetes because these vessels rarely calcify in a patient without diabetes. Gas is readily detected on radiographs (Fig. 5). Denser foreign bodies, such as metal and lead-containing glass, are radio-opaque and generally are visible on X-ray. Detection of nonmetallic foreign bodies and subtle soft tissue calcifications may entail radiographs acquired with a soft tissue technique (i.e., using low kV).

Both soft tissue edema and cellulitis display increased density and thickening of the subcutaneous fat. Infection may result in blurring of the usually visible fat planes. Focal fluid and callus will both demonstrate local increased density in the soft tissues. Ulcers may or may not be visible depending on their size and orientation. In general, all of these soft tissue abnormalities are more clearly evident at physical exam.

The presence of soft tissue swelling, periosteal new bone formation, cortical bone destruction, focal osteopenia, and permeative radiolucency are diagnostic for osteomyelitis (Table 2, Fig. 4). These osseous changes only become evident after osteomyelitis has been present for 10–14 days and require up to a 50% bone loss before becoming evident on a radiograph *(19)*. Thus, radiography is less sensitive compared with other imaging modalities. In the majority of studies, sensitivity ranges between 52% and 93% and specificity ranges between 33% and 92% for detection of osteomyelitis (Table 1).

Not restricted to documentation of osteomyelitis, soft tissue abnormalities, and subcutaneous air (Fig. 5), radiographs can demonstrate bone and soft tissue changes associated with neuroarthropathy and can help assess its progression. Radiographs can also be used as road maps for other imaging exams, by documenting the presence of postsurgical changes, fractures, foreign bodies, gas, foot deformities, and bony variants.

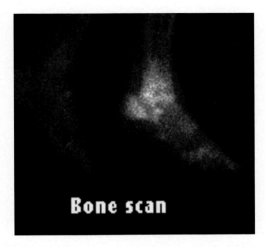

Fig. 6. Osteomyelitis of left ankle—delayed phase of a three-phase bone scan. This lateral view shows diffuse tracer activity about the ankle joint of a febrile patient with diabetes. Similar increase tracer activity is noted on both the first and second phases (not shown) of the three-phase bone scan. Findings represent osteomyelitis.

In the absence of correlative radiographs, these findings can cause unnecessary confusion on MRI or nuclear medicine exams.

Nuclear Medicine Studies

The three most commonly employed nuclear medicine tests are bone, gallium, and labeled leukocyte studies. FDG has recently gained prominence as an infection imaging agent, but it is not yet reimbursed for this indication (*see* Section 3.2.4). Bone, gallium, and labeled leukocyte scans are all considered highly sensitive to the presence of both soft tissue infection and osteomyelitis (Table 1). When preexisting bone changes (i.e., neuroarthropathy, trauma, degenerative changes) are present, labeled leukocyte scan provides the best overall sensitivity and specificity (Table 1).

Three-Phase Technetium-99m Bone Scan

Traditionally, triple-phase bone scan has been the test used for the workup of suspected osteomyelitis in patients with negative radiographs. A three-phase bone scan involves intravenous injection of radioactive technetium-99m methylene diphosphonate, followed by imaging with a γ-camera at three distinct time points. Images acquired every 2–5 seconds immediately following injection provide a radionuclide angiogram (the flow phase) and may demonstrate asymmetrically increased blood flow to the region of interest. The tissue or blood pool phase is obtained within 10 minutes and reveals increased extracellular fluid seen in conjunction with soft tissue inflammation. A delayed, skeletal phase is acquired 2–4 hours after the injection. The skeletal phase demonstrates areas of active bone turnover, which have incorporated the radionuclide tracer, and are seen as focal "hot spots" of increased tracer activity. The tracer is taken up by bone in an amount dependent on the degree of osteoblastic activity.

Osteomyelitis results in increased uptake in all three phases, whereas simple cellulitis demonstrates increased uptake in the first two phases only (Fig. 6). In cellulitis, there may be mild diffuse increased uptake in the bone resulting from inflammation, but this

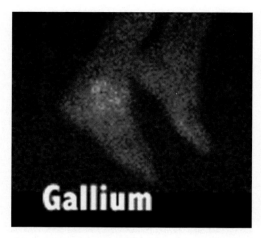

Fig. 7. Osteomyelitis of left ankle—gallium scan. The increased gallium activity in the distal tibia of a patient with diabetes suggests osteomyelitis. However, the lack of resolution of the image precludes distinction of bone vs soft tissue inflammation.

is distinct from the more focal, intense increased uptake seen with osteomyelitis. There are many causes of positive bone scans. In general, a positive delayed phase scan is seen when there is an underlying process that promotes bone remodeling, for example, healing fracture, neuropathic osteoarthropathy, or recent surgery. False-negatives may occur when the radiotracer fails to reach the foot because of diminished vascular flow. This is of particular concern in patients with diabetes who have atherosclerotic disease.

Schauwecker's review of 20 published reports shows a compiled mean sensitivity and specificity of 94% and 95%, respectively *(20)*. Unfortunately, the data apply only to patients without underlying bone deformities. In the diabetic patient with complicated bone conditions, a common clinical presentation, the sensitivity remains at 95%, but the specificity declines to 33% *(20)*. Thus, the American College of Radiology-sponsored appropriateness criteria for detection of osteomyelitis recommends a three-phase bone scan only when radiographic findings of bone complications are absent *(21)*. When radiographic findings of bone complications are absent and the bone scan is normal, there is little likelihood of osteomyelitis and the investigation can be considered complete. However, when the radiograph reveals an underlying focal bony abnormality, then a bone scan is unlikely to be definitive and, therefore, labeled leukocyte study or MRI is recommended instead. If a labeled leukocyte scan or MRI is not available, a gallium scan may provide a useful alternative.

Gallium Scan

Gallium-67 citrate localizes in areas of infection. If the gallium scan is normal, osteomyelitis can be excluded. By itself, gallium is not very specific for the diagnosis of osteomyelitis, because gallium accumulates not only at sites of bone infection, but also at sites of soft tissue infection and at sites of increased bone remodeling, as seen in trauma *(22)*. Gallium scan images frequently lack spatial resolution, which precludes separation of bone from soft tissue uptake (Fig. 7) *(22)*. If there is any bony abnormality, then a bone scan should be obtained prior to obtaining the gallium scan, in order to improve the specificity of diagnosis. (The long half-life of gallium-67 makes it

Table 3
Criteria for Diagnosis of Osteomyelitis Using
Combined Bone and Gallium Exams *(22)*

Gallium uptake exceeds bone scan uptake
Gallium and bone scan uptake are spatially incongruent

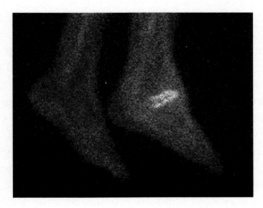

Fig. 8. Osteomyelitis—indium-labeled leukocyte scan. Increased indium accumulation about the ankle represents a focus of osteomyelitis in a patient with swelling and fever. *Staphylococcus aureus* grew from the marrow aspirate.

prudent to acquire the bone scan first.) In that case, if the gallium scan is positive, then the uptake on the bone scan can be used to account for the gallium uptake that is occurring because of bony remodeling *(23)*. The diagnosis of osteomyelitis is made when the gallium and bone scan are incongruent, as summarized in Table 3.

Schauwecker showed the sensitivity and specificity of this technique to be 81% and 69%, respectively *(20)*. However, the author also observed that more than half of the combined bone and gallium exams were equivocal. This technique, therefore, is only helpful when the study is positive or negative. Although the relatively high number of equivocal exams makes this modality less advantageous, gallium scan remains a useful alternative if labeled leukocyte scan or MRI is not available.

Labeled Leukocyte Scan

Labeled leukocyte scans, also known as labeled white blood cell scans, are performed by extracting a patient's blood, fractionating the leukocytes from blood, incubating the white blood cells with the either indium 111-oxine or technetium-99m-hexamethylpropylene amine oxime (Tc-HMPAO) in order to label them, and then reinjecting the labeled white blood cells into the same patient. Imaging is performed 16–24 hours later, using a standard γ-camera. Theoretically, labeled white blood cells only accumulate at sites of infection and not at sites of increased osteoblastic activity and should be extremely useful in the diagnosis of complicated osteomyelitis (Fig. 8).

Indium-labeled leukocyte scan offers the best sensitivity and specificity among the three readily available scintigraphic techniques (Table 1). A compilation of seven studies yielded a sensitivity of 93% and specificity of 89% *(8,24–29)*. In addition, Newman suggested that indium-labeled leukocyte imaging could be used to monitor response to therapy, with images reverting to normal 2–8 weeks after commencement of antibiotic therapy *(8)*.

Despite their potential advantages and reported high sensitivity and specificity, indium-labeled leukocyte scans have not completely displaced other imaging modalities. Recent data show uptake of indium-labeled leukocytes in as many as 31% of noninfected neuropathic joints *(30)*. These false positive exams stem from the inability to determine whether labeled leukocyte located outside the typical marrow distribution represents infection or merely an atypical site of hematopoietic activity *(31)*. Atypical patterns of marrow distribution may accompany fractures, orthopedic hardware, infarctions, and tumors. At sites where bone marrow may be present, it is very helpful to compare the leukocyte scan with a bone marrow scan obtained with technetium-99m-macroaggregated albumin. False negative examinations may occur when the procedure for labeling the leukocytes is inadequate *(32)*. Detection of osteomyelitis is rarely a problem in the forefoot *(2)* in which the osseous structures are equidistant from both dorsal and plantar skin surfaces, but may be compromised in the midfoot and hindfoot because of anatomic complexity in these areas *(31)*. Interpreting the labeled leukocyte study in conjunction with the anatomic localizing information available from a simultaneously acquired bone scan can help to improve accuracy *(29)*.

Tc-HMPAO-labeled leukocyte scans are reported to be as accurate as indium-labeled leukocyte studies in the diagnosis of osteomyelitis. This technique of labeling has the advantage of providing the results on the same day and depositing a much lower radiation dose. Its major drawback is that it does not permit simultaneous acquisition with bone or bone marrow scans.

Other disadvantages associated with both indium- and Tc-HMPAO-labeled leukocyte scans include the complexity of the labeling process, high costs, limited availability of the test, and the risks inherent in handling of blood products.

Newer Radiopharmaceuticals

Newer radioactive agents for imaging osteomyelitis are undergoing trials with favorable results. Flourine-18-labeled fluorodeoxyglucose (FDG) imaging using positron emission tomography (PET) often shows increased activity in areas of inflammation or infection. PET has higher resolution and, especially combined with CT, this improved resolution can help distinguish between osteomyelitis and soft tissue inflammation or infection *(33)*. FDG-PET has shown good sensitivity *(34)*, but is not yet reimbursed for this indication *(35,36)*. Antigranulocyte antibodies labeled with technetium-99-m are considered advantageous because white blood cells do not need to be reinjected into the patient. Some success with this agent has been reported in Charcot joints *(37)*; however, technetium-99-m-labeled antigranulocyte antibodies have only been approved for imaging appendicitis. Polyclonal immunoglobulins labeled with indium and radiolabeled peptides have been used experimentally, but these agents are not commercially available *(38–40)*. These newer radiopharmaceuticals may hold promise for detecting osteomyelitis in the patient with diabetes.

Computed Tomography

CT scan is useful for detection of radiographically occult foreign bodies, even those that are not traditionally considered radio-opaque (e.g., wood). It is superior to radiography

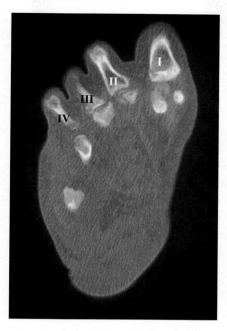

Fig. 9. Metatarsal osteonecrosis on CT. The second and third metatarsal heads are flattened. The radiolucencies beneath the deformed metatarsal heads represent subchondral fractures. CT exquisitely demonstrates these cortical abnormalities.

in detection of cortical destruction (Fig. 9), periostitis, and soft tissue or intraosseous gas *(41,42)*. During early stages, these findings of acute osteomyelitis may be difficult to detect on radiography, but frequently can be documented on CT. The bony sequestrum (a focus of necrotic bone insulated from living bone by granulation tissue), a finding in chronic osteomyelitis, is exquisitely displayed on CT images. This necrotic bone focus is associated with a characteristic CT finding of a dense bone spicule in the medullary cavity surrounded by soft tissue density *(7,43)*. Although CT scans performed with intravenous iodinated contrast material can demonstrate soft tissue abscesses, MRI, and ultrasound, imaging modalities that possess superior intrinsic soft tissue contrast resolution are better suited to imaging of abscess collections and can be performed in the absence of intravenous contrast. Thus, use of CT for detection of soft tissue abscess should be weighed against the risk of contrast-induced complications. Overall, the data on sensitivity or specificity of CT for diagnosis of diabetic pedal osteomyelitis are scant. In light of concerns regarding risks of ionizing radiation, allergic reaction to contrast, and, in particular, contrast-induced nephropathy, there appears to be little enthusiasm for using CT as a routine diagnostic test for osteomyelitis.

Ultrasound

Ultrasound is well suited for evaluation of superficial soft tissues and for guiding aspiration of fluid collections. Imaging of superficial soft tissues requires use of a high-frequency transducer, often in conjunction with a standoff pad. Abscesses are seen as hypoechoic collections with increased through-transmission (i.e., tissue deep to the abscess appears more echogenic than expected because the sound waves are attenuated

Table 4
Indications for MRI in Detection of Infection

Characterize soft tissue abnormalities
Exclude osteomyelitis
Preoperative assessment

to a lesser degree by the fluid in the abscess than by the soft tissue surrounding the abscess). However, an abscess may be difficult to identify on ultrasound when its contents become proteinaceous, because it can then become isoechoic to the surrounding tissues and may fail to demonstrate enhanced signal in the tissues deep to the abscess. Similarly, joint effusions are often visible as hypoechoic on ultrasound, but may be less evident when their contents are complex. Even when sonography demonstrates a fluid collection, the presence or absence of infection within the fluid cannot be established by imaging. Thus, ultrasound is often employed for guiding aspiration of the suspect fluid collection.

Magnetic Resonance Imaging

MRI is notable for its high intrinsic soft tissue contrast, i.e., it depicts the full spectrum of soft tissues without the use of intravenous contrast. It readily delineates an infection's extent, helps guide surgery, characterizes soft tissue abnormalities, and excludes osteomyelitis *(10)* (Table 4). Its advantages over scintigraphy are precise anatomic definition and improved lesion characterization *(44,45)*. The range of available MR techniques is expansive. A brief review of pulse sequences, the MRI contrast agent gadolinium, imaging planes, and optimization of techniques will be presented.

Pulse Sequences

The sequences frequently employed in MRI for detection of bone and soft tissue abnormalities include T1-weighted, STIR (short-tau inversion recovery), T2-weighted, and T1-weighted with fat saturation.

T1-WEIGHTED SEQUENCE (SHORT TE/SHORT TR)

This sequence depicts anatomic detail. Normal fatty marrow is bright or hyperintense on T1-weighted images and is readily distinguished from abnormal marrow that is dark or hypointense (Fig. 10).

STIR SEQUENCE

Normal marrow is dark or low signal on STIR images. Edema and fluid collections become bright or high signal. Thus, the STIR sequence is a very sensitive sequence to screen for fluid collections and for areas of infection or inflammation associated with edema. Uniform suppression of fat signal is readily obtained. Its disadvantage is that anatomic detail is not well depicted on this pulse sequence (Fig. 10).

T2-WEIGHTED SEQUENCE (LONG TE/LONG TR)

This commonly employed sequence highlights the presence of fluid, which is bright or hyperintense on T2-weighted images, but this sequence is less sensitive than STIR in

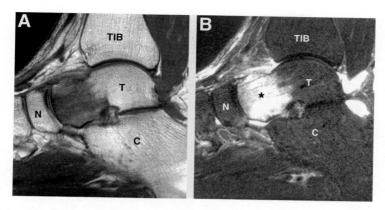

Fig. 10. Marrow edema on MRI. Sagittal images of the ankle show marrow edema (*) which is dark on T1-weighted image **(A)** and bright on STIR **(B)** images. This marrow edema pattern is nonspecific and is similar to the marrow changes in osteomyelitis. However, this patient sustained trauma to the anterior talus and, here, the marrow edema represents a bone bruise. Specificity and accuracy can be improved by administration of gadolinium, as osteomyelitis frequently shows marrow enhancement. C, calcaneus; N, navicula; T, talus; TIB, tibia.

the detection of marrow abnormality. Abnormal edema in marrow, fluid collections, and cellulitis are bright or hyperintense on this sequence. Depending on the precise technique, fat will be of intermediate to relative high (bright) signal intensity, but will not be as bright as fluid.

T1-WEIGHTED WITH FAT SATURATION ("FAT SAT") SEQUENCE

This sequence best documents enhancement following injection of intravenous gadolinium contrast. When fat signal is suppressed, both normal fatty marrow and pathology are generally dark or low in signal. Any bright or high signal seen following administration of intravenous gadolinium contrast represents an area of enhancement. The drawback of this sequence is the potential pitfall of inhomogeneous fat suppression generating signal abnormalities that can lead to erroneous diagnoses. This is a common problem in the foot, in which uniform fat suppression is difficult to achieve. Comparing the postcontrast images to an additional set of precontrast fat suppressed images or using subtraction images can help to minimize this problem (Fig. 11).

Gadolinium Contrast

Intravenous injection of gadolinium-based contrast agent improves sensitivity for the diagnosis of osteomyelitis (Fig. 11). Gadolinium concentrates in areas of infectious or noninfectious inflammation and produces hyperintense (bright) signal on T1 images. As fat is also hyperintense on T1 sequence, contrast-enhanced images are often acquired using a fat suppression technique. Normal marrow in the foot comprises predominantly fat and is hypointense on this pulse sequence. This overall dark background highlights enhancement in inflamed tissues. The accuracy for diagnosis of osteomyelitis is higher in contrast-enhanced studies (89%) than in noncontrast-enhanced studies (78%) *(46)*. The nephrotoxicity of gadolinium contrast is significantly less than that of the iodinated forms of contrast used for CT scans and conventional angiography and is generally

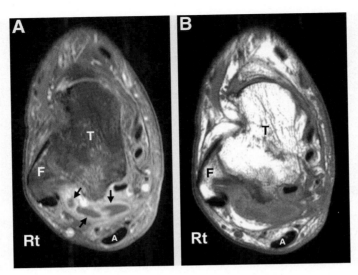

Fig. 11. Soft tissue abscess on MRI. Axial images of the ankle in a patient with diabetes who presented with a posterior abscess. The T1-weighted image with fat suppression and gadolinium **(A)** is more specific than T1 without contrast or fat suppression **(B)** in detection of the abscess. Administration of contrast results in peripheral rim enhancement (black arrows, A) of the abscess that is dark on T1-weighted (B) image. The suppression of surrounding fat signal further highlights the contrast enhancement. (A). A, achilles; F, fibula; T, talus.

Table 5
Optimization of MRI Techniques

MR markers denoting ulcers and inflammation
Dedicated extremity coil or small surface coil
High spatial resolution—small field of view, high resolution matrix
Optimized imaging planes—oblique when necessary

safe when used in diabetic patients with elevated renal function. Marrow enhancement, however, is nonspecific and can also be seen in osteonecrosis, fracture, and reactive hyperemia, as well as in osteomyelitis.

Imaging Planes

It is helpful to acquire MR images in all three planes (sagittal, coronal, and axial). When foot deformities are present, oblique imaging planes may be warranted. Careful attention to imaging planes minimizes volume-averaging artifacts and improves diagnostic accuracy.

Optimization of Technique

Acquisition of high-resolution images requires meticulous technique (Table 5). MR-sensitive markers may be used to denote the area of interest and ulceration. In general, small fields of view and high image matrices result in high image resolution. Use of a dedicated receiver coil, commonly a knee or extremity coil, can aid in improving image resolution. On the other hand, imaging both feet in a head coil and/or utilizing a large field of view significantly degrades image quality and is not recommended.

MRI is contraindicated in patients who have pacemakers and other electronic implants, ferromagnetic cranial aneurysm clips, and intraocular metal. Most claustrophobic patients can be imaged with sedation or with the use of an open architecture magnet. Weight limitations for obese patients currently range from 300 to 450 pounds, depending on the magnet. Although patients with orthopedic hardware can usually be imaged, assessment of the area immediately surrounding the hardware is frequently limited by distortion of the local magnetic field.

Imaging Features

Cellulitis manifests as an ill-defined area in the subcutaneous fat that is of low signal on T1-weighted and high signal on STIR and T2-weighted sequences (Fig. 2) *(16)*. This signal pattern is nonspecific and is common to both cellulitis and noninfected edema. Gadolinium administration may identify uncomplicated cellulitis, which typically shows uniform enhancement of subcutaneous edema *(15)*.

Abscess presents as a focal lesion, which is low signal on T1-weighted images and high signal on T2-weighted and STIR images. Without intravenous gadolinium, an abscess may not be distinguishable from dense soft tissue edema seen in severe cellulitis or from soft tissue phlegmon (Fig. 2) *(46)*. Following administration of intravenous gadolinium, an abscess demonstrates peripheral or rim enhancement, demarcating the fluid collection within (Fig. 11). The enhancing rim is believed to correspond to granulation tissue in the pseudocapsule *(47)* (Fig. 11). However, rim enhancement is a sensitive but nonspecific sign for abscess and has been described in necrotic tumors, seromas, ruptured popliteal cysts, and hematomas *(46)*.

The center of the abscess comprised of pus may present with variable signal intensity depending on its contents. T1 shortening resulting from proteinaceous material may produce intermediate to hyperintense T1 signal, thus comparison to a precontrast fat-suppressed image becomes essential. The diagnosis of septic arthritis is generally made clinically and confirmed by percutaneous joint aspiration or surgery *(15)*. The MR appearance of septic arthritis consists of joint effusion, often with intra-articular debris. Following administration of intravenous gadolinium, there is intense synovial enhancement. Periarticular reactive marrow edema, occasionally seen in the bone marrow surrounding an infected joint, may demonstrate gadolinium enhancement without the presence of osteomyelitis *(15)*. This constellation of findings is suggestive, but not specific for infection and can also be seen in inflammatory conditions such as rheumatoid arthritis and seronegative arthropathies.

The primary MRI finding in osteomyelitis is abnormal marrow signal that enhances *(46)*. The abnormal marrow is low signal (dark) T1-weighted images and high signal (bright) STIR images (Fig. 1, Table 6). Following intravenous administration of gadolinium contrast, the abnormal marrow enhances and is seen as a bright focus on the fat-suppressed T1-weighted images. Secondary signs of osteomyelitis include cortical interruption, periostitis (seen as enhancement at the margins of the periosteum) *(15,48)* and cutaneous ulcer or sinus tract in contiguity with the abnormal marrow. A negative MRI effectively excludes osteomyelitis (Fig. 3) *(49)*. The sensitivity and specificity of MRI for detection of osteomyelitis compiled from seven studies is 96% and 87%, respectively *(8,50–54)*.

Table 6
MRI Findings of Osteomyelitis

Primary signs
    Hyperintense (bright) marrow signal on STIR sequence
    Hypointense (dark) marrow signal on T1-weighted sequence
    Enhancing marrow on postcontrast T1-weighted sequence
Secondary MR signs
    Periosteal reaction
    Subperiosteal abscess
    Periostitis, manifested by periosteal enhancement
    Cortical destruction
    Ulcer
    Sinus tract

Another important use of MRI is surgical planning. As foot-sparing surgical procedures are increasingly performed in the ambulatory patient, accurate depiction of the extent of marrow involvement becomes paramount (Fig. 10) *(46)*. Marrow involvement is best depicted on either T1-weighted or STIR images. Its advantages notwithstanding, MRI has several important limitations. MRI of the infected diabetic foot yields a significant number of false positive diagnoses. The kind of abnormal marrow signal associated with osteomyelitis can also be seen with neuroarthropathy, fractures (Fig. 12), and, occasionally, osteonecrosis. The hyperemic phase of neuroosteoarthropathy may display enhancing marrow edema indistinguishable from osteomyelitis. Use of MRI for following response to treatment of osteomyelitis is limited and remains to be defined.

Angiography

Angiography is indicated in diabetic patients with nonhealing ulcers or osteomyelitis requiring endovascular and surgical planning. Almost without exception, these patients with nonhealing foot ulcers will have severe stenoocclusive disease involving all three runoff vessels of the calf (anterior tibial, posterior tibial, and peroneal arteries) (Fig. 14). In this patient population, 20% of peripheral bypass grafts will have to extend to a pedal artery. The distal anastomosis is either to the dorsalis pedis artery or the proximal common plantar artery trunk *(55)*. Thus, detailed mapping of arterial disease from the abdominal aorta to the pedal vessels is necessary.

Traditionally, vascular imaging has been performed using conventional angiography. Conventional angiography is an invasive procedure, performed in the angiographic suite under fluoroscopic (real-time X-ray imaging) guidance. A thin, flexible catheter is inserted into the aorta or arteries, usually via a femoral artery approach. A relatively large bolus of iodinated contrast is injected into the intraluminal catheter and rapid sequence radiographs are exposed. Although examination of the abdominal aorta and iliac vessels can readily be performed with a multisidehole catheter in the abdominal aorta, examination of the femoral, popliteal, tibioperoneal, and pedal arteries entails placement of an ipsilateral external iliac artery catheter. Selective catheter placement has the advantage of limiting contrast burden in a patient group predisposed to renal insufficiency.

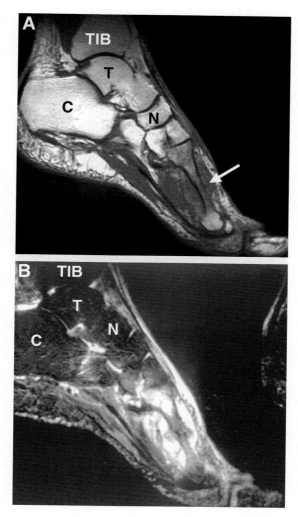

Fig. 12. Stress fracture on MRI. Sagittal T1-weighted **(A)** and STIR **(B)** MR images of the foot demonstrate cortical irregularity of the mid-third metatarsal shaft. The marrow beneath the cortical irregularity shows low T1 signal **(A)** of marrow edema. On the STIR image **(B)**, the marrow of the entire metatarsal shaft becomes bright or hyperintense. The fracture line remains dark and is highlighted by bright edematous marrow. Marked soft tissue swelling is also better seen on the STIR images **(B)**. C, calcaneus, N, navicular, TIB, tibia; T, talus.

The risks of the procedure include radiation exposure, potential for bleeding, and injury to the vessel wall with or without dislodgment of embolic material, and risk of renal failure or allergic reaction from the iodinated contrast. Not infrequently, vascular disease and slow flow can disrupt the timing of the exam with resultant failure to demonstrate the distal vessels. This is especially problematic when demonstration of distal vessels is the key to planning a bypass graft procedure. The major advantage of conventional angiography is that it provides access to perform not only diagnostic, but also therapeutic, vascular procedures, including angioplasty, atherectomy, stenting, and thrombolysis.

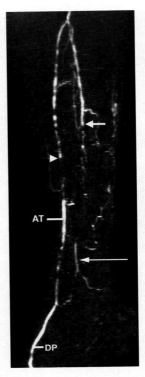

Fig. 13. Time-of-flight MR angiogram of the leg and foot from beneath the knee to the foot in a diabetic patient with ischemic foot ulcer demonstrates occlusion of the peroneal and both anterior (arrowhead) and posterior tibial (arrow) arteries. There is reconstitution of a small distal peroneal artery (long arrow) and of the anterior tibial artery, which, although severely diseased distally, continues as a good caliber dorsalis pedis artery. Bypass to the dorsalis pedis artery with vein graft allowed ulcer healing to occur and ultimately resulted in resumption of normal weight bearing. AT, anterior tibial artery; DP, dorsalis pedis artery.

MR Angiography

More recently, MRI has come to play a role in the imaging of arterial disease, in the form of MR angiography (MRA). MRA has the benefit of providing detailed anatomy of arterial disease. At the same time, it obviates the need for arterial catheter placement and associated complications and the need for nephrotoxic contrast material administration. Time-of-flight (TOF) and gadolinium-enhanced MRA are the preferred techniques for MRA of the lower extremity *(56,57)* (Fig. 13).

TOF MRA relies on a noncontrast-enhanced, flow-sensitive MR sequence. Computer postprocessing of the MR data generates coronal, sagittal, or oblique reconstructions that mimic the appearance of conventional angiograms. TOF MRA can be particularly time consuming, lasting 1–2 hours, in order to cover the distance from the aortic bifurcation to the distal lower extremity. Cardiac gating of the MR images improves image quality but significantly lengthens exam time, especially when the patient has cardiac arrhythmia or is on β-blocker medication. TOF MRA images exaggerate the degree of stenoocclusive disease and are prone to motion and metallic susceptibility artifact.

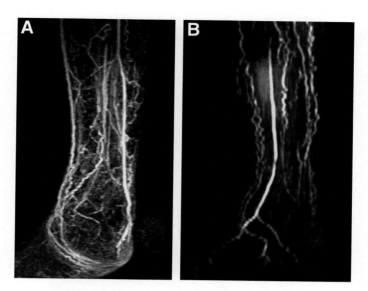

Fig. 14. MRA. **(A)** Gadolinium-enhanced MR angiogram demonstrates a pitfall of contrast-enhanced MRA: inaccurate timing of the contrast bolus. In this instance, the arterial and venous phases are not successfully resolved into separate images. With both arterial and venous enhancement on the same image, the ability to detect arterial pathology is limited. **(B)** Two-dimensional time of flight MRA in the same patient selectively depicts the arterial flow and demonstrates typical severe occlusive disease of all three tibioperoneal arteries, with distal reconstitution of a mildly diseased anterior tibial artery which continues as a good caliber dorsalis pedis artery.

Gadolinium-enhanced MRA relies on intravenous injection of a small volume of gadolinium contrast and fast imaging that is timed to optimally follow the passage of the contrast bolus through the arteries. This technique has the advantage of short scan time, reduced motion, and reduced susceptibility artifacts. It is more accurate than TOF MRA exam in depiction of the grade of stenoocclusive disease. It uses a much smaller volume of contrast than conventional angiography and therefore generates a smaller osmotic load and subsequently a lower incidence of nephrotoxicity. However, visualization of the arteries may be limited by venous enhancement (Fig. 14) or by suboptimal arterial filling related to inaccurate timing of data acquisition.

OSTEOMYELITIS VS NEUROARTHROPATHY

Differentiation between osteomyelitis and neuroarthropathy is often difficult. Certain neuroarthropathic changes resemble osteomyelitis. In order to better understand the similarities and differences, imaging characteristics of neuroarthropathy will be presented here. Frykberg provides an extensive discussion of Charcot changes in another chapter of this book.

Neuroarthropathy

Loss of both pain and proprioceptive sensation is believed to predispose to repetitive trauma leading to diabetic neuroarthropathy *(15)*. Though potentially devastating, the incidence of neuropathic joints in the patient with diabetes is surprisingly low, reported to be 0.1–0.5%. The joints of the forefoot and midfoot are commonly involved. The distribution

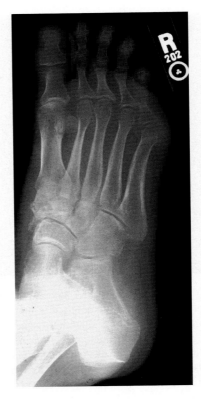

Fig. 15. Neuroarthropathy of the midfoot on radiography. Oblique image of the foot demonstrates diffuse osteopenia of the forefoot. The first and second cuneiform bones are fragmented and are surrounded by osseous debris.

of neuroarthropathy in patients with diabetes is 24% in the intertarsal region, 30% in the tarsometatarsal region (Fig. 15), and 30% in the metatarsophalangeal joints. Abnormalities of the ankle (11%) and interphalangeal (4%) joints are less frequent *(47)*.

Two classic forms of neuroarthropathy, atrophic and hypertrophic, have been described *(58)*. The atrophic form, representing the acute resorptive or hyperemic phase, is characterized by osseous resorption and osteopenia (Fig. 15). This form frequently appears in the forefoot and the metatarsophalangeal joints, leading to partial or complete disappearance of the metatarsal heads and proximal phalanges. Osteolytic changes produce tapering or "pencil-pointing" of phalangeal and metatarsal shafts. Marrow changes in the atrophic or hyperemic form show hypointense T1 and hyperintense STIR and mimic the changes seen in osteomyelitis. The hypertrophic form, representing the healing or reparative phase, is characterized by sclerosis, osteophytosis, and radiographic appearance of extreme degenerative change (Fig. 16). In its early phase, the hypertrophic form of neuroarthropathy may be confused with osteoarthritis. Concurrent osseous fragmentation, subluxation, or dislocation predominates in the intertarsal and tarsometatarsal joints. Ruptured ligaments in the mid- and forefoot cause dorso-lateral displacement of the metatarsals in relation to the tarsal bones. This classic finding resembles an acute Lisfranc fracture-dislocation.

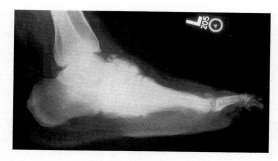

Fig. 16. Hypertrophic form of neuroarthropathy on radiography. Lateral image of the foot shows the hypertrophic form of neuroarthropathy, characterized by sclerosis, osteophytosis, and radiographic appearance of extreme degenerative change. In its early phase, it may be confused with osteoarthritis.

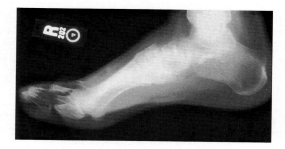

Fig. 17. Midfoot deformity related to neuroarthropathy on radiography. Lateral radiograph demonstrates dorsal dislocation of the tarsometatarsal joints leading to reversal of the normal arch of the foot. The metatarsal bases are superiorly subluxed. Progression of the subluxation will eventually result in "rocker bottom deformity."

Disruption of the talonavicular and calcaneocuboid joints causes collapse of the longitudinal arch with subsequent plantar displacement of the talus (Fig. 17). These changes produce the classic "rocker bottom" deformity *(59)*. Recognition of this deformity is important because it creates new pressure points that lead to callus formation and ulceration (Fig. 18). Attempts to classify neuropathic joints into the two classic forms may be difficult, as a mixed pattern, composed of both forms, occurs in 40% of neuropathic joints *(60)*.

Osteomyelitis vs Neuroarthropathy

Other than the characteristic findings of diffuse dark marrow signal on T1-, STIR, and T2-weighted MR images associated with hypertrophic neuroarthropathy (vs high T2 and STIR signal seen in osteomyelitis), there is no easy method of distinguishing between osteomyelitis and neuroarthropathy. Secondary findings such as involvement of the midfoot and multiple joints, absence of cortical destruction, presence of small cyst-like lesions, and distance between soft tissue infection and bone changes favor a diagnosis of neuroarthropathy (Table 7) *(15)*. In contrast, osteomyelitis favors the toes or metatarsal heads, and is associated with focal cortical lesions and close proximity to the ulcer.

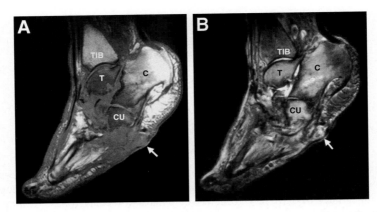

Fig. 18. Rocker bottom deformity and ulceration at focus of high plantar pressure on MRI. **(A)** Sagittal T1-weighted and **(B)** STIR images show disruption of the talonavicular joint causing collapse of the longitudinal arch. These changes produce the classic "rocker bottom" deformity. This deformity is important because it creates new pressure points that lead to callus and ulcer formation (arrow). The diffuse marrow edema associated with neuroarthropathy of the tarsal bones mimics osteomyelitis. T, talus; CU, cuboid; C, calcaneus; TIB, tibia.

Table 7
Osteomyelitis vs Neuroarthropathy

	Favors osteomyelitis	Favors neuroarthropathy
Radiography		
Location	Forefoot, metatarsal heads and toes	Midfoot
Cortical destruction	Discrete cortical lesion	Absent
Proximity to soft tissue ulcer	Beneath or close to the ulcer or soft tissue infection	Some distance from soft tissue infection or ulcer
MR		
Signal characteristics of the abnormal marrow	Hyperintense STIR or T2 marrow signal. (This signal pattern is nonspecific and overlaps the hyperemic form of neuroarthropathy and acute fracture.)	Hypointense marrow signal on all T1, T2 and STIR sequences. (This signal pattern corresponds to the hypertrophic form of neuroarthropathy.)
Cysts	Not common in osteomyelitis	Well marginated cyst-like lesions, hypointense on T1 and hyperintense on T2

IMAGING ALGORITHM: APPROACHES TO DIAGNOSIS OF PEDAL OSTEOMYELITIS IN THE PATIENT WITH DIABETES

A suggested algorithm for imaging pedal osteomyelitis in the patient with diabetes is presented in Fig. 19.

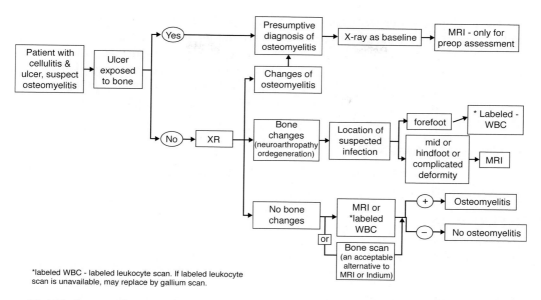

Fig. 19. Suggested approach to diagnosis of osteomyelitis in diabetic foot infection. * labeled-WBC refers to a labeled leukocyte scan. If labeled leukocyte scan is unavailable, may replace with gallium scan.

Soft Tissue Ulceration Exposing Bone

When the soft tissue ulcer exposes bone, no imaging is needed to confirm the diagnosis of osteomyelitis. Radiography is appropriate to provide a baseline and to document bone complications.

Soft Tissue Inflammation (Ulcers and/or Cellulitis) With No Exposed Bone

Radiographic findings are used to further separate the patients into two groups. If the radiographs are normal and the clinical suspicion for osteomyelitis is high, a three-phase bone scan can effectively detect or exclude osteomyelitis. MRI or labeled leukocyte study is an acceptable alternative *(21)*. A gallium scan may replace labeled leukocyte study if the latter is not available *(61)*. Unlike plain radiographs, these modalities should become positive in the first few days of infection. In light of their high sensitivity, these studies provide a high negative predictive value for osteomyelitis. If the bone scan is equivocal, supplementary imaging with either MRI or labeled leukocyte scans is required.

When the radiographs are abnormal, showing neuroarthropathic, degenerative, or traumatic changes, either labeled leukocyte scan or MRI is acceptable. The choice depends on the location of the suspected osteomyelitis. If the inflammation is in the forefoot, an indium leukocyte study efficiently identifies osteomyelitis. In contrast, when the infection is in the mid- or hindfoot, MRI adequately separates bone from soft tissue inflammation.

CONCLUSION

Imaging plays an important role in the assessment of the diabetic patient with foot problems. Nuclear medicine and MRI techniques detect osteomyelitis, characterize various soft tissue abnormalities and depict the extent of bone involvement. MR angiographic studies assess foot vessel runoff when conventional angiography fails to detect distal lesions because of proximal obstruction. Nevertheless, distinguishing osteomyelitis from coincident neuropathic change remains a challenge. Only with an understanding of the specific strengths and weaknesses of each modality, as they apply to the particular clinical problem in question, can this wide variety of imaging studies be utilized in an effective and efficient manner.

ACKNOWLEDGMENTS

Special thanks to Clotell Forde and Ron Kukla for their assistance in the preparation of this manuscript.

REFERENCES

1. Scher KS, Steele FJ. The septic foot in patients with diabetes. *Surgery* 1988;104:661–666.
2. Newman LG, Waller J, Palestro CJ, et al. Unsuspected osteomyelitis in diabetic foot ulcers. Diagnosis and monitoring by leukocyte scanning with indium in 111 oxyquinoline [see comments]. *JAMA* 1991;266:1246–1251.
3. Kaufman M, Bowsher JE. Preventing diabetic foot ulcers. *Med Surg Nurs* 1994;3:204.
4. Bild DE, Selby JV, Sinnock P, Browner WS, Braveman P, Showstack JA. Lower-extremity amputation in people with diabetes. Epidemiology and prevention. *Diabetes Care* 1989;12:24–31.
5. Ecker ML, Jacobs BS. Lower extremity amputation in diabetic patients. *Diabetes* 1970;19:189–195.
6. Penn I. Infections in the diabetic foot, in *The Foot in Diabetes* (Sammarco GJ, ed.). Lea & Febiger, Philadelphia, 1991, pp. 106–123.
7. Gold RH, Tong DJ, Crim JR, Seeger LL. Imaging the diabetic foot. *Skeletal Radiol* 1995; 24:563–571.
8. Mokdad A, Ford E, Bowman B, et al. Diabetes trends in the US: 1990–1998. *Diabetes Care* 2000;23:1278–1283.
9. Horowitz JD, Durham JR, Nease DB, Lukens ML, Wright JG, Smead WL. Prospective evaluation of magnetic resonance imaging in the management of acute diabetic foot infections. *Ann Vasc Surg* 1993;7:44–50.
10. Edmonds ME, Roberts VC, Watkins PJ. Blood flow in the diabetic neuropathic foot. *Diabetologia* 1982;22:9–15.
11. Murray HJ, Young MJ, Hollis S, Boulton AJ. The association between callus formation, high pressures and neuropathy in diabetic foot ulceration. *Diabet Med* 1996;13:979–982.
12. Gooding GA, Stess RM, Graf PM, Moss KM, Louie KS, Grunfeld C. Sonography of the sole of the foot. Evidence for loss of foot pad thickness in diabetes and its relationship to ulceration of the foot. *Invest Radiol* 1986;21:45–48.
13. Bamberger DM, Daus GP, Gerding DN. Osteomyelitis in the feet of diabetic patients. Long-term results, prognostic factors, and the role of antimicrobial and surgical therapy. *Am J Med* 1987;83:653–660.
14. Linklater J, Potter HG. Emergent musculoskeletal magnetic resonance imaging. *Top Magn Reson Imaging* 1998;9:238–260.
15. Marcus CD, Ladam-Marcus VJ, Leone J, Malgrange D, Bonnet-Gausserand FM, Menanteau BP. MR imaging of osteomyelitis and neuropathic osteoarthropathy in the feet of diabetics. *Radiographics* 1996;16:1337–1348.
16. Moore TE, Yuh WT, Kathol MH, El-Khoury GY, Corson JD. Abnormalities of the foot in patients with diabetes mellitus: findings on MR imaging. *AJR Am J Roentgenol* 1991;157: 813–816.

17. Grayson ML, Gibbons GW, Balogh K, Levin E, Karchmer AW. Probing to bone in infected pedal ulcers. A clinical sign of underlying osteomyelitis in diabetic patients (see comments). *JAMA* 1995;273:721–723.

18. Cook TA, Rahim N, Simpson HC, Galland RB. Magnetic resonance imaging in the management of diabetic foot infection. *Br J Surg* 1996;83:245–248.

19. Bonakdar-pour A, Gaines VD. The radiology of osteomyelitis. *Orthop Clin North Am* 1983;14: 21–37.

20. Schauwecker DS. The scintigraphic diagnosis of osteomyelitis. *AJR Am J Roentgenol* 1992; 158:9–18.

21. Alazraki N, Dalinka M, Berquist T, et al. Imaging diagnosis of osteomyelitis in patients with diabetes mellitus, in *American College of Radiology ACR Appropriateness Criteria*. Reston: American College of Radiology, 2000, 303–310.

22. Losbona R, Rosenthall L. Observations on the sequential use of 99mTc-phosphate complex and 67Ga imaging in osteomyelitis, cellulitis, and septic arthritis. *Radiology* 1977;123: 123–129.

23. Tumeh SS, Aliabadi P, Weissman BN, McNeil BJ. Chronic osteomyelitis: bone and gallium scan patterns associated with active disease. *Radiology* 1986;158:685–688.

24. Keenan AM, Tindel NL, Alavi A. Diagnosis of pedal osteomyelitis in diabetic patients using current scintigraphic techniques. *Arch Intern Med* 1989;149:2262–2266.

25. Larcos G, Brown ML, Sutton RT. Diagnosis of osteomyelitis of the foot in diabetic patients: value of 111In-leukocyte scintigraphy. *AJR Am J Roentgenol* 1991;157:527–531.

26. McCarthy K, Velchik MG, Alavi A, Mandell GA, Esterhai JL, Goll S. Indium-111-labeled white blood cells in the detection of osteomyelitis complicated by a pre-existing condition. *J Nucl Med* 1988;29:1015–1021.

27. Maurer A, Millmond S, Knight L, et al. Infection in diabetic osteoarthropahty: use of indium-labeled leukocytes for dianosis. *Radiology* 1986;161:221–225.

28. Splittgerber GF, Spiegelhoff DR, Buggy BP. Combined leukocyte and bone imaging used to evaluate diabetic osteoarthropathy and osteomyelitis. *Clin Nucl Med* 1989;14:156–160.

29. Schauwecker DS, Park HM, Burt RW, Mock BH, Wellman HN. Combined bone scintigraphy and indium-111 leukocyte scans in neuropathic foot disease. *J Nucl Med* 1988;29: 1651–1655.

30. Seabold JE, Flickinger FW, Kao SC, et al. Indium-111-leukocyte/technetium-99m-MDP bone and magnetic resonance imaging: difficulty of diagnosing osteomyelitis in patients with neuropathic osteoarthropathy. *J Nucl Med* 1990;31:549–556.

31. Palestro CJ, Torres MA. Radionuclide imaging in orthopedic infections. *Semin Nucl Med* 1997;27:334–345.

32. Abreu SH. Skeletal uptake of indium 111-labeled white blood cells. *Semin Nucl Med* 1989;19:152–155.

33. Keidar Z, Militianu D, Melamed E, Bar-Shalom R, Israel O. The diabetic foot: initial experience with 18F-FDG PET/CT. *J Nucl Med* 2005;46:444–449.

34. Hopfner S, Krolak C, Kessler S, et al. Preoperative imaging of Charcot neuroarthropathy in diabetic patients: comparison of ring PET, hybrid PET, and magnetic resonance imaging. *Foot Ankle Int* 2004;25:890–895.

35. Zhuang H, Duarte PS, Pourdehand M, Shnier D, Alavi A. Exclusion of chronic osteomyelitis with F-18 fluorodeoxyglucose positron emission tomographic imaging. *Clin Nucl Med* 2000;25:281–284.

36. Zhuang H, Yu JQ, Alavi A. Applications of fluorodeoxyglucose-PET imaging in the detection of infection and inflammation and other benign disorders. *Radiol Clin North Am* 2005;43:121–134.

37. Hakki S, Harwood SJ, Morrissey MA, Camblin JG, Laven DL, Webster WB, Jr. Comparative study of monoclonal antibody scan in diagnosing orthopaedic infection. *Clin Orthop Relat Res* 1997:275–285.

8. Babich JW, Graham W, Barrow SA, Fischman AJ. Comparison of the infection imaging properties of a 99mTc labeled chemotactic peptide with 111In IgG. *Nucl Med Biol* 1995;22: 643–648.

39. Fischman AJ, Babich JW, Barrow SA, et al. Detection of acute bacterial infection within soft tissue injuries using a 99mTc-labeled chemotactic peptide. *J Trauma* 1995;38:223–227.

40. Rubin RH, Fischman AJ. The use of radiolabeled nonspecific immunoglobulin in the detection of focal inflammation. *Semin Nucl Med* 1994;24:169–179.

41. Sartoris DJ. Cross-sectional imaging of the diabetic foot. *J Foot Ankle Surg* 1994;33: 531–545.

42. Sartoris DJ, Devine S, Resnick D, et al. Plantar compartmental infection in the diabetic foot. The role of computed tomography. *Invest Radiol* 1985;20:772–784.

43. Magid D, Fishman EK. Musculoskeletal infections in patients with AIDS: CT findings. *AJR Am J Roentgenol* 1992;158:603–607.

44. Chandnani VP, Beltran J, Morris CS, et al. Acute experimental osteomyelitis and abscesses: detection with MR imaging versus CT. *Radiology* 1990;174:233–236.

45. Beltran J, McGhee RB, Shaffer PB, et al. Experimental infections of the musculoskeletal system: evaluation with MR imaging and Tc-99m MDP and Ga-67 scintigraphy. *Radiology* 1988;167:167–172.

46. Morrison WB, Schweitzer ME, Wapner KL, Hecht PJ, Gannon FH, Behm WR. Osteomyelitis in feet of diabetics: clinical accuracy, surgical utility, and cost-effectiveness of MR imaging. *Radiology* 1995;196:557–564.

47. Beltran J. MR imaging of soft-tissue infection. *Magn Reson Imaging Clin N Am* 1995;3:743–751.

48. Morrison WB, Schweitzer ME, Batte WG, Radack DP, Russel KM. Osteomyelitis of the foot: relative importance of primary and secondary MR imaging signs. *Radiology* 1998;207: 625–632.

49. Horowitz SH. Diabetic neuropathy. *Clin Orthop* 1993:78–85.

50. Nigro ND, Bartynski WS, Grossman SJ, Kruljac S. Clinical impact of magnetic resonance imaging in foot osteomyelitis (published erratum appears in J Am Podiatr Med Assoc 1993 Feb;83(2):86). *J Am Podiatr Med Assoc* 1992;82:603–615.

51. Weinstein D, Wang A, Chambers R, Stewart CA, Motz HA. Evaluation of magnetic resonance imaging in the diagnosis of osteomyelitis in diabetic foot infections. *Foot Ankle* 1993;14:18–22.

52. Yu JS. Diabetic foot and neuroarthropathy: magnetic resonance imaging evaluation. *Top Magn Reson Imaging* 1998;9:295–310.

53. Wang A, Weinstein D, Greenfield L, et al. MRI and diabetic foot infections. *Magn Reson Imaging* 1990;8:805–809.

54. Beltran J, Campanini DS, Knight C, McCalla M. The diabetic foot: magnetic resonance imaging evaluation. *Skeletal Radiol* 1990;19:37–41.

55. Pomposelli FB Jr, Marcaccio EJ, Gibbons GW, et al. Dorsalis pedis arterial bypass: durable limb salvage for foot ischemia in patients with diabetes mellitus. *J Vasc Surg* 1995;21: 375–384.

56. Cotroneo AR, Manfredi R, Settecasi C, Prudenzano R, Di Stasi C. Angiography and MR-angiography in the diagnosis of peripheral arterial occlusive disease in diabetic patients. *Rays* 1997;22:579–590.

57. Kreitner KF, Kalden P, Neufang A, et al. Diabetes and peripheral arterial occlusive disease: prospective comparison of contrast-enhanced three-dimensional MR angiography with conventional digital subtraction angiography. *AJR Am J Roentgenol* 2000;174:171–179.

58. Sequeira W. The neuropathic joint. *Clin Exp Rheumatol* 1994;12:325–337.

59. Zlatkin MB, Pathria M, Sartoris DJ, Resnick D. The diabetic foot. *Radiol Clin North Am* 1987;25:1095–1105.

60. Brower A, Allman R. Pathogenesis of the neuropathic joint:Neurotraumatic versus neurovascular. *Radiology* 1981;139:349–354.
61. Donohoe KJ. Selected topics in orthopedic nuclear medicine. *Orthop Clin North Am* 1998; 29:85–101.
62. Park HM, Wheat LJ, Siddiqui AR, et al. Scintigraphic evaluation of diabetic osteomyelitis: concise communication. *J Nucl Med* 1982;23:569–573.
63. Segall GM, Nino-Murcia M, Jacobs T, Chang K. The role of bone scan and radiography in the diagnostic evaluation of suspected pedal osteomyelitis. *Clin Nucl Med* 1989;14:255–260.
64. Seldin DW, Heiken JP, Feldman F, Alderson PO. Effect of soft-tissue pathology on detection of pedal osteomyelitis in diabetics. *J Nucl Med* 1985;26:988–993.
65. Oyen WJ, Netten PM, Lemmens JA, et al. Evaluation of infectious diabetic foot complications with indium-111-labeled human nonspecific immunoglobulin G. *J Nucl Med* 1992;33: 1330–1336.

13
Microbiology and Treatment of Diabetic Foot Infections

Adolf W. Karchmer, MD

INTRODUCTION

The foot of patients with diabetes mellitus is affected by several processes which not only contribute to the development and progression of infection but on occasion alter the appearance of the foot in ways, which may obscure the clinical features of local infection. Neuropathy involving the motor fibers supplying muscles of the foot causes asymmetric muscle weakness, atrophy, and paresis which in turn result in foot deformities and maldistribution of weight (or pressure) on the foot surface. Dysfunction of the sensory fibers supplying the skin and deeper structural elements of the foot allows minor and major injury to these tissues to proceed without appreciation by the patient. As a result of neuropathy, the foot may be dramatically deformed, ulcerate in areas of unperceived trauma (mal perforans), and on occasion be warm and hyperemic in response to deep structural injury (acute Charcot's disease). This warmth and hyperemia may be misinterpreted as cellulitis and ulceration, whereas a major portal of entry for infection may be uninfected. In the patient with diabetes, peripheral neuropathy may develop in isolation or commonly in parallel with atherosclerotic peripheral vascular disease. The latter involves major inflow vessels to the lower extremity but commonly is associated with occlusive lesions of the tibial and peroneal arteries between the knee and ankle. The resulting arterial insufficiency can alter the appearance of the foot and obscure infection. Rubor may reflect vascular insufficiency rather than inflammation and conversely pallor may mute the erythema of acute infection. Gangrene and necrosis may be primarily ischemic or may reflect accelerated ischemia in the setting of infection. In sum, the diagnosis of infection involving the foot in patients with diabetes requires a careful detailed examination of the lower extremity and its blood supply.

THE DIAGNOSIS OF FOOT INFECTIONS

Infection involving the foot is diagnosed clinically and to varying degrees supported by test results. Finding purulent drainage (pus) or two or more signs or symptoms of inflammation (erythema, induration, pain, tenderness, or warmth) is indicative of infection. Clinical signs on occasion belie the significance and severity of infection. A minimally inflamed but deep ulceration may be associated with underlying osteomyelitis (1). Serious limb-threatening infection may not result in systemic toxicity. For example, among patients hospitalized for limb-threatening infection only 12–35% have significant

From: *The Diabetic Foot, Second Edition*
Edited by: A. Veves, J. M. Giurini, and F. W. LoGerfo © Humana Press Inc., Totowa, NJ

fever *(2–4)*. In fact, fever in excess of 102°F suggests infection involving deeper spaces in the foot with tissue necrosis and undrained pus, extensive cellulitis, or bacteremia with hematogenous seeding of remote sites. Laboratory studies are neither sensitive nor specific in the diagnosis of these infections but must be interpreted in the context of clinical findings. Thus, the erythrocyte sedimentation rate and C-reactive protein concentration may be normal in infected patients and in up to 50% of patients with deep foot infection the white blood cell count may be normal *(5)*. Open skin wounds and ulcerations are often contaminated or colonized by commensal organisms that on occasion become pathogens. As a consequence, cultures essential in the assessment of the microbiology of foot infections, do not in isolation establish the presence of infection. Unless the cultured material is obtained from deep tissue planes by percutaneous aspiration, the results of cultures must be interpreted in the clinical context.

THE SEVERITY OF FOOT INFECTIONS

Multiple classification schema have been designed to define the severity of foot wounds or infection. The Wagner system has been used commonly but only one of six grades includes infection *(6)*. The University of Texas classification of foot wounds uses four grades each of which can be modified by the presence of ischemia, infection, or both *(7)*. Grade 0 is a previously ulcerated lesion which is completely epithelialized; Grade 1 is a superficial wound not involving tendon or joint capsule; Grade 2 wounds penetrate to tendon or joint capsule; and Grade 3 wounds penetrate to bone or joint. Increasing depth of the wounds and complications of ischemia or infection in this classification has been associated with increased likelihood of amputation *(7)*. The Infectious Diseases Society of America (IDSA), in recently published guidelines for the diagnosis and treatment of diabetic foot infection, has proposed a classification that utilizes depth of a wound, presence of ischemia, presence and extent of infection, and systemic toxicity to designate the severity of foot infection. This schema classifies wounds from having no infection to being severely infected (Table 1) *(8)*.

A simple practical classification of foot infection into limb threatening or nonlimb threatening has also been described *(9)*. In this schema, infection is categorized primarily based on depth of the tissues involved, this being largely function of depth of a predisposing ulceration, and the presence or absence of significant ischemia. Patients with non-limb-threatening infection have superficial infection involving the skin, lack major systemic toxicity, and do not have significant ischemia. What might have been a nonlimb-threatening infection becomes limb threatening in the face of severe ischemia. If ulceration is present in a nonlimb-threatening infection, it does not penetrate fully through skin. Limb-threatening infection, which is not categorized as such based on severe ischemia, involves deeper tissue planes with the portal of entry being an ulcer which has penetrated into subcutaneous tissue or potentially to tendon, joint, or bone. Although limb-threatening infections may be dramatic with extensive tissue necrosis, purulent drainage, edema, and erythema, they may be cryptic as well. Thus, an infected deep ulcer with a rim of cellulitis which is ≥2 cm in width is considered limb threatening. Of note, hyperglycemia occurs almost universally in patients with nonlimb-threatening and limb-threatening infections. In contrast, significant fever occurs in only 12–35% of patients with limb-threatening infection *(2–4)*. Fever is

Table 1
Classification of Severity of Diabetic Foot Infection

Clinical manifestation of infection	Infection severity[a]
Wound lacking purulence of any manifestations of inflammation	Uninfected
Presence of ≤2 cm manifestations of inflammation (purulence, or erythema, pain, tenderness, warmth, or induration), but any cellulitis/erythema extends ≤2 cm around the ulcer, and infection is limited to the skin or superficial subcutaneous tissues; no other local complications or systemic illness	Mild
Infection (as above) in a patient who is systemically well and metabolically stable but which has ≥1 of the following characteristics: cellulitis extending >2 cm, lymphangitic streaking, spread beneath the superficial fascia, deep-tissue abscess, gangrene, and involvement of muscle, tendon, joint, or bone	Moderate
Infection in a patient with systemic toxicity or metabolic instability (e.g., fever, chills, tachycardia, hypotension, confusion, vomiting, leukocytosis, acidosis, severe hyperglycemia, or azotemia)	Severe

Adapted from ref. *8* with permission.
[a]In the setting of severe ischemia all infections are considered severe.

found primarily in these patients with extensive cellulitis and lymphangitis, infection (abscesses) loculated in the deep spaces of the foot, bacteremia, or hematogenously seeded remote sites of infection.

This simplified schema accommodates the more complex University of Texas wound classification and that proposed in the IDSA guidelines. Unless the foot is compromised by severe ischemia, patients with foot infections categorized as University of Texas Grade 0, or those with mild or less extensive moderate infection by the IDSA guidelines would be considered to have nonlimb-threatening infection. Those with infection categorized as University of Texas Grades 1–3 or by the IDSA schema as more extensive moderate to severe would have limb-threatening infection. In contrast to the University of Texas schema, the classification of foot infection into nonlimb-threatening and limb-threatening groups has not been demonstrated to correlate with the risk of amputation *(7)*. Nevertheless, this simple classification, when adjusted for prior medical therapy and antibiotic exposure which is likely to have resulted in infection by resistant organisms, allows one to anticipate the organisms causing wound infections and thus is an excellent point of departure from which to plan empiric antimicrobial therapy.

MICROBIOLOGY

Cultures of open foot ulcers cannot be used to establish the presence of infection. Foot ulcers whether infected or not will contain multiple comensal or colonizing bacteria, some of which have the potential to become invasive pathogens. As a foot ulcer transitions from uninfected to infected, organisms isolated from the ulcer cavity include both colonizing flora and invasive pathogens. Assigning specific significance to organisms isolated from ulcers may be difficult and has resulted in some investigators designating cultures from specimens obtained through the ulcer as unreliable. In contrast, reliable specimens are those obtained aseptically at surgery, by aspiration of pus, or by biopsy of the infected tissue across intact skin. Although the organisms recovered from reliable specimens are likely to be invasive pathogens, it is unlikely that cultures of reliable specimens yield all of the pathogens present and the obtaining of these specimens is often impractical. Sapico and colleagues demonstrated that the organism cultured from specimens obtained by aspiration or by curettage of the cleansed ulcer base was most concordant with those isolated from necrotic infected tissue excised from adjacent to the ulcer base *(10,11)*. Of note, cultures of aspirated material failed to yield pathogens recovered from curettage or excised tissue in 20% of patients. Wheat et al. *(12)* found poor concordance between organisms isolated from specimens obtained through ulceration and those recovered from specimens obtained without traversing the ulceration. Cultures obtained through the ulcers were more likely to yield comensals and antibiotic resistant Gram-negative bacilli than were the more reliable specimens. In contrast, Slater et al. *(13)* found that in wounds, which did not extend to bone, essentially the same organisms were recovered from cultures of swab specimens and deep tissue specimens. When wounds extended to bone, swab cultures recovered only 65% of organisms cultured from deep tissues. Pellizzer et al. *(14)* also found that on initial wound cultures swab specimens taken from deep in the ulcer yielded the same bacterial species as did cultures of deep tissue biopsies, with the exception that *Corynebacterium* species, likely colonizers or contaminants, were isolated from swab cultures.

As a consequence of the variable specimens examined as well as the microbiological techniques used to culture specimens, i.e., inconsistent and incomplete efforts to recover anaerobic bacteria, the precise microbiology of foot infections is not established. Although the microbiology from clinical reports, wherein most specimens are obtained through the ulceration, requires interpretation to adjust for the inclusion of organisms of known low invasive potential and likely to be comensals or colonizers, it is possible to sense the major pathogens causing nonlimb-threatening and limb-threatening foot infections. Similarly, when surgical or aspiration specimens are not readily available for culture, antibiotic therapy can be designed with reasonable confidence based on the culture results from specimens obtained by curettage of the ulcer base. The exception to the utility of ulcer cultures is in the design of antimicrobial therapy for osteomyelitis when the infected bone is to be debrided piecemeal, as opposed to resected en bloc. In this situation, more precise biopsy based culture information is highly desirable *(8,15)*.

In nonlimb-threatening infections, particularly those occurring in patients who have not previously received antimicrobial therapy, *Staphylococcus aureus* and streptococci, particularly Group B Streptococci, are the predominant pathogens *(8,15–19)*. *S. aureus* has been isolated from more than 50% of these patients and in more than 30% *S. aureus* is the only bacteria isolated *(17)*.

Limb-threatening foot infections are generally polymicrobial. Cultures from these infections yield on average 4.1–5.8 bacterial species per culture. Both Gram-positive cocci and Gram-negative rods are commonly isolated from a single lesion and in 40% of infections both aerobic and anaerobic organisms are recovered *(2,8,10–12,15,16,18,20)* (Table 2). Individual cultures have yielded on average 2.9–3.5 aerobes and 1.2–2.6 anaerobes *(21)*. *S. aureus*, streptococci, and facultative Gram-negative bacilli (*Proteus* species, *Enterobacter* spp, *Escherichia coli*, and *Klebsiella* spp) are the predominant

Table 2
Microbiology of Limb-Threatening Infections in Patients with Diabetes[a]

Organisms	Percent of patients (number of patients)					
	Gibbons et al. (N = 50)	Wheat et al. (N = 54)	Hughes et al. (N = 42)	Bamberger et al. (N = 51)	Scher et al. (N = 65)	Grayson et al. (N = 96)
Aerobic						
S. aureus	22	20	25	22	23	54
S. epidermidis	12	17	14	19	18	12
Enterococcus spp	16	15	17			28
Streptococcus spp	13	23	20	41	54	55
Corynebacterium spp	7	11		8		
E. coli	7	5	3	1	19	6
Klebsiella spp	4	6	7	4	10	5
Proteus mirabilis	11	9	11	5	36	9
Enterobacter spp	3	4	7	7		9
Other						
Enterobacteriaceae	2	15	5	7	50	17
P. aeruginosa	3	4	0	5	15	8
Acinetobacter spp	1	0	0	0		7
Anaerobic						
Gram-positive cocci	21	30	40	14	52	12
Bacteroides fragilis		2	5	4		
Bacteroides melaninogenicus		3	11			
Other						
Bacteroides spp	6	12	2	5	55	30
Clostridium spp	2	3	1	3	23	
Other anaerobes			13	2	20	14
Number isolates/ infection	2.76	3.31	3.62	2.88	5.76	2.77

Data from refs. *2,12,20,42,47,50* with permission.

[a]Specimens obtained by various routes, including deep ulcer swabs, curettage of the ulcer base, aspiration or tissue biopsy, except Wheat et al., who excluded specimens obtained through the ulcer cavity.

aerobic pathogens in these infections. Among the anaerobes, *Peptostreptococcus* species, *Prevotella* spp, and *Bacteroides* spp, including those of the *Bacteroides fragilis* group, are recovered frequently *(21,22)*. Of note, *Clostridium* spp are recovered infrequently. Although anaerobes are recovered from 41% to 53% of limb-threatening infections in clinical trials, with optimal methods these organisms can be recovered from 74% to 95% of these infections *(21)*. The frequency of isolating anaerobic bacteria is greatest in those patients with the most severe infections, particularly those in which infection involves necrotic gangrenous tissue and amputation is often required. Nevertheless, the clinical features of foot infections beyond those, which allow categorization as nonlimb threatening or limb threatening, are not sufficiently sensitive clues to the microbiology of these infections. Fetid infections suggest infection with anaerobes; however, anaerobes including *B. fragilis* may be recovered from infections that are not particularly foul-smelling.

Hence, clinical clues beyond the major categorization of infections are not sufficient to predict the microbiology of foot infections.

The spectrum of bacterial species recovered from foot infections, especially those that are limb threatening, can be dramatically altered by prior failed antimicrobial therapy or contact with the health care system. Although *Pseudomonas aeruginosa*, *Acinetobacter* species, *Enterobacter* spp, and other antibiotic-resistant facultative Gram-negative bacilli are uncommon in previously untreated infections, these organisms are not infrequent isolates from infected chronic ulcers *(2)*. Similarly, methicillin-resistant *S. aureus* may be encountered commonly in patients with chronically infected foot ulcers, which have persisted in spite of multiple prior courses of antimicrobial therapy or in patients with extensive health care requirements, for example, chronic dialysis, hospitalization for comorbid conditions, or residence in skilled nursing facilities. These resistant bacteria are probably acquired nosocomially or alternatively emerge from endogenous flora during hospitalization or repetitive antibiotic treatment of patients with nonhealing foot ulcers. Accordingly, when selecting an antimicrobial regimen to treat a foot infection in a patient who has had contact with the health care system or prior courses of antibiotics, physicians should anticipate the presence of antibiotic-resistant pathogens.

The role of relatively avirulent bacteria, many of which are part of skin flora that are often isolated from cultures of specimens obtained through an ulcer, is uncertain. *Staphylococcus epidermidis* has been recovered, usually in conjunction with other bacteria, from 15% to 35% of these infections and may reflect ulcer colonization. On the other hand, *S. epidermidis* has been isolated from reliable foot specimens with similar frequency to *S. aureus* suggesting these organisms may be pathogens in some patients *(12)*. Enterococci, *viridans streptococci*, and *Corynebacterium* spp, organisms that are often considered contaminants and not pathogens when isolated from skin and soft tissue infections, are among the isolates recovered frequently from polymicrobial limb-threatening foot infections. When recovered from specimens in conjunction with typical pathogens, these organisms are often disregarded as contaminants *(8,15)*. Often, foot infections respond to therapy with antimicrobials which are active in vitro against the pathogens but not against these presumed contaminants *(21,23)*. Although these observations support the designation of these organisms as contaminants, they could also indicate that with the eradication of major pathogens, host defenses, and surgical debridement can control these less virulent organisms. On occasion *Enterococci*, *viridans streptococci*, or *Corynebacterium* spp are isolated from uncontaminated specimens and may even be the sole bacterial isolate from an infection *(17,24)*. Thus, these organisms should not be routinely disregarded but rather interpreted in the clinical context.

MICROBIOLOGICAL ASSESSMENT

Clinically uninfected ulcers should not be cultured. When infection is present, a microbiological diagnosis will usually facilitate subsequent therapy, particularly in the setting of limb-threatening infection or failure of prior antimicrobial therapy *(3,9,19)*. Although cultures of tissue obtained aseptically at surgery or purulent specimens aspirated percutaneously are more likely to contain only true pathogens, obtaining these specimens before initiating therapy is often either impractical or not feasible (no abscess present). Accordingly, after cleansing the skin and debriding any overlying eschar, specimens for culture should be obtained before initiating therapy by curettage of the necrotic base of the ulcer. Specimens should be handled and processed as both routine wound cultures and primary anaerobic cultures. As noted, specimens obtained by swabbing deep in the ulcer or from curretted tissue in the base of the ulcer provide reasonable assessment of infecting organisms *(13,14,25)*. If patients have been febrile recently, blood cultures should also be obtained before initiating antimicrobial therapy. During the initial days of therapy and with debridement, specimens from necrotic purulent tissue or exposed bone should be recultured. Concurrent antimicrobial therapy may preclude isolation of susceptible organisms during effective therapy; however, resistant organisms missed on the initial cultures can be recovered from these debridement specimens *(14)*. Osteomyelytic bone in the forefoot (visible or detectable on probing) and that will be totally resected does not require specific cultures. If *en bloc* resection of the involved bone, i.e., foot sparing amputation, was not planned, more precise microbiological data from bone biopsy would be desirable to allow optimal antibiotic selection *(8,15,26)*. Biopsy of abnormal bone underlying infected ulcers is generally safe and in severely neuropathic patients may not require anesthesia. Infected bone in the midfoot or posterior foot that can be probed or that lies beneath an ulcer and appears infected on imaging studies should be biopsied for culture and histopathology, ideally using fluoroscopic guidance and through a route other than the ulcer *(8,15,26)*. Here where debridement is likely to be piecemeal, rather than *en bloc* resection of all involved bone, precise microbiological data from bone are required so that optimal antimicrobial therapy can be selected. Alternatively, bone that remains unexposed after debridement and wherein osteomyelitis is not strongly suspected based on radiological findings may not be biopsied but rather the infection treated as if it is limited to soft tissue. Careful clinical and radiological follow-up of this bone in 2–4 weeks will often resolve the question of osteomyelitis without the potential hazards of an invasive procedure.

TREATMENT

Debridement and Surgery

With the exception of cellulitis or lymphangitis arising from an unrecognized (or microscopic) portal of entry, infected foot lesions generally require debridement. Debridement should be done surgically rather than by chemical or enzymatic agents *(27)*. For apparent nonlimb-threatening infections, debridement may be limited but nevertheless allows full evaluation of the portal of entry and prepares the site for culture. Occasionally, what appeared to be a nonlimb-threatening infection is discovered on debridement to actually be limb threatening with extension of infection to deep tissue plane. Limb-threatening infection by virtue of extension to deep tissue planes requires surgical debridement *(3,9)*. Early surgical intervention can reduce the duration of hospitalization and the need for major amputations *(28)*. Failure to decompress involved compartments and debride necrotic tissue and drain purulent collections increases the risk of amputation *(3,9,28,29)*. Percutaneously placed drains or aspiration drainage is inadequate; rather devitalized tissue must be resected and purulent collections drained by incision. Uncertainty about the patient's arterial circulation status should not delay initial debridement. Effective debridement may require multiple procedures as the extent of tissue destruction becomes progressively more apparent. Optimal surgical treatment, which minimizes tissue loss initially and subsequently, requires a thorough understanding of resulting foot function, avoidance of subsequent deformities that will predispose to recurrent ulceration, and recognition of the potential need for revascularization to ensure healing *(29)*. The experience of the surgeon in this area and the availability of vascular surgery support are important in achieving optimal results *(29)*. If the infection has destroyed the function of the foot or if it threatens the patient's life, a guillotine amputation to allow prompt control of the infection with a subsequent definitive closure is advised *(30)*.

Antibiotic Therapy

Antimicrobial treatment of foot infections in patients with diabetes is begun empirically and thereafter revised based on the results of cultures, which were obtained before therapy and on occasion during therapy, and the clinical response of the infection. Knowledge of the spectrum of bacteria which cause nonlimb-threatening infection and limb-threatening infection, as well as the changes in these organisms, which might have been induced by selected circumstances, for example, prior antimicrobial treatment, serves as the basis for selecting effective empiric therapy. The potential toxicity of various antibiotics for individual patients and the unique vulnerability of patients with diabetes as a group must be considered. Thus, for this population with an increased frequency of renal disease, the availability of nonnephrotoxic antimicrobials with potent activity against Gram-negative bacilli renders the aminoglycosides relatively undesirable and unnecessary. Antibiotic therapy is administered intravenously when patients are systemically ill, have severe local infection, are unable to tolerate oral therapy, or are infected by bacteria that are not susceptible to available oral antimicrobials. Some antimicrobials are fully bioavailable after oral administration, for example, selected fluoroquinolones, clindamycin, and metronidazole, and, when appropriate microbiologically, could often be used in lieu of parenteral therapy initially. After control of infection, continued therapy commonly can be affected with oral agents. For patients who require prolonged courses of parenteral therapy, for example, for osteomyelitis, generally treatment can be provided in an outpatient setting *(31)*.

Topical antimicrobials, including silver sulfadiazine, polymixin, gentamicin, and mupirocin have been used to treat selected soft tissue infections; however, this approach has not been studied in foot infections. In randomized trials, a cationic peptide antimicrobial, pexiganin acetate (not yet approved by the Food and Drug Administration) was used as a 1% cream, topical application was nearly as effective (85–90%) as oral ofloxacin in treating mildly infected foot ulcers *(32)*. Although antimicrobials have been applied topically to foot infections, it seems unlikely that the topical route would result in effective tissue concentrations of the antimicrobial. Accordingly, topical therapy should only be used to supplement effective systemic therapy and then with the realization that its efficacy is not established.

The potential therapeutic or prophylactic benefits of systemic antibiotic therapy in patients with uninfected neuropathic ulcer, is a subject of debate. One controlled trial showed no benefit from antibiotic therapy *(33)*. In view of the potential adverse consequences, including colonization with resistant bacteria, antibiotic therapy is not recommended for clinically uninfected neuropathic ulcer *(27)*. Similarly, continuation of antibiotics beyond a limited course that was sufficient to eradicate infection has not been required to accomplish the healing of ulcers that remain open *(17,34)*.

Table 3
Selected Antibiotic Regimens for Initial Empiric Therapy of Foot Infections in Patients With Diabetes Mellitus

Infection	Antimicrobial regimen[a]
Nonlimb threatening[b]	Cephalexin 500 mg p.o. q 6 hour
	Clindamycin 300 mg p.o. q 8 hour
	Amoxicillin–clavulanate (875/125 mg) one q 12 hour
	Dicloxacillin 500 mg p.o. q 6 hour
	Levofloxacin 500–750 mg p.o. q day
	Moxifloxacin 400 mg p.o. q day
Limb threatening[b]	Ceftriaxone[c] 1 gm iv daily plus clindamycin 450–600 mg iv q 8 hour
	Ciprofloxacin 400 mg iv q 12 hour plus clindamycin 450–600 mg iv q 8 hour
	Ampicillin/sulbactam 3 g iv q 6 hour
	Linezolid 600 mg q 12 hour iv or p.o. plus a fluoroquinolone
	Piperacillin/tazobactam 3.375 g iv q 4 hour or 4.5 g iv q 6 hour
	Fluoroquinolone[d] iv plus metronidazole 500 mg iv q 6 hour
	Ertapenem 1 gm iv daily
Life threatening	Imipenem cilastatin 500 mg iv q 6 hour[b]
	Piperacillin/tazobactam 4.5 g iv q 6 hour plus gentamicin[e] 1.5 mg/kg iv q 8 hour[b]
	Vancomycin 1 g iv q 12 hour plus gentamicin plus metronidazole

[a]Doses for patients with normal renal function.
[b]If clinical information suggests possible methicillin resistant *S. aureus* infection, include vancomycin, daptomycin, linezolid, or quinupristin/dalfopristin.
[c]An alternative is cefotaxime 2 g iv q 8 hour.
[d]Fluoroquinolone with increased activity against Gram-positive cocci, for example, levofloxacin 500–750 mg iv q day.
[e]Can be given as single daily dose 5.1 mg/kg/day.

Empiric therapy for patients with nonlimb-threatening infection, many of whom can be treated as outpatients, is directed primarily at *Staphylococci* and *Streptococci* (Table 3) *(8,15,16,27)*. Lipsky et al. *(17)* demonstrated that oral therapy with clindamycin or cephalexin for 2 weeks in patients with previously untreated nonlimb-threatening foot infection resulted in satisfactory clinical outcome in 96 and 86%, respectively. Caputo et al. *(19)* in a retrospective study reported that 54 of 55 patients with nonlimb-threatening infections were improved or cured with oral therapy, primarily first generation cephalosporins or dicloxacillin, directed at staphylococci and streptococci. If patients with superficial ulcers present with more extensive cellulitis, which warrants hospitalization and parenteral antimicrobial treatment, cefazolin should be effective. However, if prior microbiological data or exposure to the health care system suggests that infection might be caused by methicillin-resistant *S. aureus,* therapy should be initiated with vancomycin. Quinupristin/dalfopristin, daptomycin, and linezolid, which can be administered intravenously or orally, have provided effective treatment of skin–soft tissue infection caused by methicillin-resistant *S. aureus* and could be considered alternatives to vancomycin *(35–40)*. The duration of treatment, which in the final analysis is determined by the time-course of the clinical response, is usually 1–2 weeks.

Multiple antibiotics have been demonstrated to be effective therapy in prospective treatment trials of complicated skin and soft tissue infections, many of which were foot infections. Additionally, some of these antimicrobials have been proven effective in prospective studies of foot infections, many of which have been limb threatening: amoxicillin-clavulanate, ampicillin-sulbactam, piperacillin-tazobactam, ticarcillin-clavulanate, cefoxitin, ceftizoxime, ciprofloxacin, ofloxacin, trovafloxacin, imipenem/cilastatin, linezolid, daptomycin, and ertapenem *(2,23,37,39,41–44)*. In comparative prospective (sometimes blinded) trials of treatment for limb-threatening foot infections, the clinical and microbiological response rates for the studied agents have been similar and no single agent has been proven superior to all others *(8,15,16)*.

In selecting empiric therapy for limb-threatening foot infections, reasonable principles emerge from clinical trials and other published studies *(3,8,9,15,16,27)*. The choice of agents used empirically should be based on the known polymicrobial nature of these infections with modification, where appropriate, to address anticipated highly resistant pathogens that might have been selected in the process of prior hospitalizations and treatment. Although empiric therapy should be effective against an array of Enterobacteriaceae and anaerobes, including *B. fragilis*, especially in the more severe infection in which there is tissue necrosis and gangrene, therapy should always be effective against *S. aureus* and Group B streptococci. When a patient has previously been infected by methicillin-resistant *S. aureus*, or the medical history suggests an increased risk of infection by this organism, empiric therapy should be effective against that staphylococcus also. Drug selection should attempt to minimize toxicity and be cost effective. Glucose metabolism (control of blood sugar) should be pursued aggressively. In limb-threatening infection (but not in life-threatening infection) initial empiric therapy does not have to be effective in vitro for all potential pathogens. Broad spectrum therapy which is active against many, but not necessarily all, Gram-negative bacilli, and against anaerobes, *S. aureus* and streptococci when combined with good wound care is as effective as even broader spectrum antimicrobial therapy. Thus, in a randomized blinded trial ampicillin-sulbactam therapy was not only as effective as imipenem–cilastatin at the end of treatment, but on initial evaluation of responses on day 5 the two regimens also performed comparably *(2)*. Thus, in infections wherein initial cultures yielded organisms resistant to ampicillin-sulbactam but susceptible to imipenem–cilastatin, patients with limb-threatening infections treated with ampicillin-sulbactam responded as well as those treated with imipenem-cilastatin. Adequate debridement not only shortens required duration of therapy but is required for effective therapy.

Empiric antimicrobial treatment should be reassessed between days 3 and 5 of treatment in the light of culture results and clinical response. When therapy is unnecessarily broad spectrum (effective therapy for the bacteria isolated could be achieved by less broad spectrum antimicrobials with possible cost savings, avoidance of toxicity, or a reduction in selective pressure for emergence of antimicrobial resistance) and patients have responded clinically, treatment regimens should be simplified based on culture data *(8,15)*. If a bacteria which is resistant to the current therapy has been recovered and yet the clinical response is satisfactory, treatment need not be expanded. Alternatively, if in the face of an isolate resistant to treatment the response to therapy is unsatisfactory, the wound should be examined for necrotic tissue that has not been debrided, the adequacy of arterial circulation must be assessed, and because the resistant organism might be a pathogen (rather than colonizing flora), antimicrobial therapy should be expanded to treat this isolate as well as others.

A number of regimens have been recommended as reasonable initial empiric therapy of limb-threatening infections (Table 3) *(8,9,15,16,27)*. Some antimicrobials that have been used to treat these infections in the past are, because of gaps in their spectrum of activity vs the typically anticipated pathogens, are no longer considered ideal when used alone: cefuroxime, cefamandole, cefoxitin, cefotetan, ceftazidime, or ciprofloxacin. Trovafloxacin, which possesses an appropriate spectrum of activity for this infection and was effective in early trials, is not advocated for routine therapy because of potential hepatotoxicity *(45)*. It is likely that new fluoroquinolones with a spectrum of activity similar to trovafloxacin will be studied as single agents for treatment of these infections. If patients with limb-threatening infections have had extensive prior antimicrobial therapy or medical care, highly antibiotic resistant pathogens should be anticipated and empiric therapy must be expanded, perhaps using regimens similar to those advocated for life-threatening foot infections.

Patients with life-threatening infections, for example, those with hypotension or severe ketoacidosis, should be treated with maximal regimens (Table 3). If highly resistant Gram-negative bacilli are anticipated, gentamicin or another aminoglycoside is advocated. Similarly, if infection with methicillin resistant *S. aureus* is suspected, vancomycin, linezolid, daptomycin, or quinupristin/dalfopristin should be utilized.

The duration of antimicrobial therapy for severe soft tissue foot infection is based on the temporal response to wound care and antimicrobial therapy. Two weeks of therapy is often effective; however, some recalcitrant infections will require longer courses of treatment *(2)*. After acute infection has been controlled, antimicrobial therapy that was begun parenterally should be changed to oral therapy with comparable orally bioavailable antibiotics. Even if the ulcer has not fully healed, antibiotics can in general be discontinued when evidence of infection has resolved *(8,15)*. Persistent ulcers must be managed with wound care, including avoidance of weight bearing, so that healing can be achieved and the ulcer eliminated as a portal for later infection. The occurrence of bacteremia, especially if remote sites are seeded, may require extended therapy. Of note, *S. aureus* bacteremia entails a distinct risk for secondary endocarditis *(46)*. These patients should be evaluated carefully including an assessment for endocarditis with a transesophageal echocardiogram.

The antibiotic therapy of osteomyelitis must be coordinated with the surgical debridement of the involved bone. Several reports have suggested that osteomyelitis of bones in the foot can be cured or at least arrested for extended periods with minimal debridement and prolonged courses of antimicrobial therapy *(4,8,15,26,43,47)*. Others have suggested that cure rates for osteomyelitis (in which bone destruction is evident or bone is visible or detectable by probing) will be enhanced by aggressive debridement, and even excision of all infected bone when feasible in the fore foot *(3,9,48)*. If all infected bone is resected *en bloc*, for example, amputation of a phalanges or phalanges and the related distal metatarsal, the residual infection has in essence been converted to a soft tissue process and can be treated accordingly *(8)*. The bacteriology defined by wound cultures can be used to guide therapy and antibiotic treatment can often be abbreviated, i.e., 2–3 weeks *(2,3,9,49)*. In contrast, if osteomyelitis involves bones that cannot be resected *en bloc* without disruption of the functional integrity of the foot, debridement must be done in a piecemeal fashion. As a result, the adequacy of the debridement cannot be assured and the management strategy must be altered. In this setting, bone cultures to allow precise targeting of antimicrobial therapy are necessary, antimicrobial therapy must be administered in a manner that results in adequate serum concentration (intravenously or orally) for a prolonged period (at least 6 weeks) and adequate blood supply to infected tissues must be assured *(3,8,15,26,49)*.

OUTCOME

The effective treatment of foot infection is far more than the administration of antibiotics that are active in vitro against the implicated pathogens. Optimal therapy involves the integration of wound care, control of glucose metabolism, antibiotic therapy, debridement and possibly reconstructive foot surgery, and when ischemia is a limiting factor vascular reconstruction *(27)*. The knowledge and skills to achieve an optimal outcome often require the collaboration of multiple care providers, including diabetologists, infectious disease specialists, podiatrists, and vascular surgeons. With appropriate care a satisfactory clinical response can be anticipated in 90% of patients with nonlimb-threatening infection and at least 60% of those with limb-threatening infection. Limb-threatening infections may require foot-sparing amputations but salvage of a weight bearing foot is usually achievable. Vascular reconstruction, especially bypass grafts to pedal arteries which restore pulsable flow to the foot, decrease major amputations and enable foot-sparing/foot-salvage surgery.

REFERENCES

1. Newman LG, Waller J, Palestro CJ, et al. Unsuspected osteomyelitis in diabetic foot ulcers: diagnosis and monitoring by leukocyte scanning with indium and 111 oxyquinoline. *JAMA* 1991;266:1246–1251.
2. Grayson ML, Gibbons GW, Habershaw GM, et al. Use of ampicillin/sulbactam versus imipenem/cilastatin in the treatment of limb-threatening foot infections in diabetic patients. *Clin Infect Dis* 1994;18:683–693.
3. Karchmer AW, Gibbons GW. Foot infections in diabetes: evaluation and management, in *Current Clinical Topics in Infectious Diseases* (Remington JS, Swartz MN, eds.), 14 ed., Blackwell Scientific Publications, Boston, 1994, pp. 1–22.
4. Pittet D, Wyssa B, Herter-Clavel C, Kursteiner K, Vaucher J, Lew PD. Outcome of diabetic foot infections treated conservatively. *Arch Intern Med* 1999;159:851–856.
5. Williams DT, Hilton JR, Harding KG. Diagnosing foot infections in diabetes. *Clin Infect Dis* 2004;39:S83–S86.
6. Wagner FW Jr. The diabetic foot and amputation of the foot, in *Surgery of the Foot* (Mann RA, ed.), 5th ed., CV Mosby, St. Louis, 1986, pp. 421–455.
7. Armstrong DG, Lavery LA, Harkless LB. Validation of a diabetic wound classification system. The contribution of depth, infection, and ischemia to risk of amputation. *Diabetes Care* 1998;21:855–859.
8. Lipsky BA, Berendt AR, Deery HG, et al. Diagnosis and treatment of diabetic foot infections. *Clin Infect Dis* 2004;39:885–910.
9. Caputo GM, Cavanagh PR, Ulbrecht JS, Gibbons GW, Karchmer AW. Assessment and management of foot disease in patients with diabetes. *N Engl J Med* 1994;331: 854–860.

10. Sapico FL, Witte JL, Canawati HN, Montgomerie JE, Bessman AN. The infected foot of the diabetic patient: quantitative microbiology and analysis of clinical features. *Rev Infect Dis* 1984;6:S171–S176.

11. Sapico FL, Canawah HN, Witte JL, Montgomerie JZ, Wagner FW, Bessman AN. Quantitative aerobic and anaerobic bacteriology of infected feet. *J Clin Microbiol* 1980;12:413–420.

12. Wheat LJ, Allen SD, Henry M, et al. Diabetic foot infections: bacteriologic analysis. *Arch Intern Med* 1986;146:1935–1940.

13. Slater RA, Lazarovitch T, Boldur I, et al. Swab cultures accurately identify bacterial pathogens in diabetic foot wounds not involving bone. *Diabet Med* 2004;21:705–709.

14. Pellizzer G, Strazzabosco M, Presi S, et al. Deep tissue biopsy vs. superficial swab culture monitoring in the microbiological assessment of limb-threatening diabetic foot infection. *Diabet Med* 2001;18:822–827.

15. Lipsky BA. Medical treatment of diabetic foot infections. *Clin Infect Dis* 2004;39:S104–S114.

16. Lipsky BA. Evidence-based antibiotic therapy of diabetic foot infections. *FEMS Immunol Med Microbiol* 1999;26:267–276.

17. Lipsky BA, Pecoraro RE, Larson SA, Hanley ME, Ahroni JH. Outpatient management of uncomplicated lower-extremity infections in diabetic patients. *Arch Intern Med* 1990;150: 790–797.

18. Lipsky BA, Pecoraro RE, Wheat LJ. The diabetic foot: soft tissue and bone infection. *Infect Dis Clin North Am* 1990;4:409–432.

19. Caputo GM, Ulbrecht JS, Cavanagh PR, Juliano PJ. The role of cultures in mild diabetic foot cellulitis. *Infect Dis Clin Pract* 2000;9:241–243.

20. Scher KS, Steele FJ. The septic foot in patients with diabetes. *Surgery* 1988;104:661–666.

21. Gerding DN. Foot infections in diabetic patients: the role of anaerobes. *Clin Infect Dis* 1995;20(Suppl 2):S283–S288.

22. Johnson S, Lebahn F, Peterson LP, Gerding DN. Use of an anaerobic collection and transport swab device to recover anaerobic bacteria from infected foot ulcers in diabetics. *Clin Infect Dis* 1995;20(Suppl 2):S289, S290.

23. Lipsky BA, Baker PD, Landon GC, Fernau R. Antibiotic therapy for diabetic foot infections: comparison of two parenteral-to-oral regimens. *Clin Infect Dis* 1997;24:643–648.

24. Watanakunakorn C, Burkert T. Infective endocarditis at a large community teaching hospital, 1980–1990: a review of 210 episodes. *Medicine* 1993;72:90–102.

25. National Diabetes Advisory Board. *The National Long-Range Plan to Combat Diabetes*, 9 ed., US Government Printing Office, Washington, 1987.

26. Jeffcoate WJ, Lipsky BA. Controversies in diagnosing and managing osteomyelitis of the foot in diabetes. *Clin Infect Dis* 2004;39:S115–S122.

27. American Diabetes Association. Consensus development conference on diabetic foot wound care, April 7–8, 1999, Boston, Massachusetts. *Diabetes Care* 1999;22:1354–1360.

28. Tan JS, Friedman NM, Hazelton-Miller C, Flanagan JP, File TM Jr. Can aggressive treatment of diabetic foot infections reduce the need for above-ankle amputation? *Clin Infect Dis* 1996;23:286–291.

29. van Baal JG. Surgical treatment of the infected diabetic foot. *Clin Infect Dis* 2004;39: S123–S128.

30. McIntyre KE Jr, Bailey SA, Malone JM, Goldstone J. Guillotine amputation in the treatment of non-salvageable lower extremity infections. *Arch Surg* 1984;119:450–453.

31. Fox HR, Karchmer AW. Management of diabetic foot infections, including the use of home intravenous antibiotic therapy. *Clin Podiatr Med Surg* 1996;13:671–682.

32. Lipsky BA, McDonald D, Litka PA. Treatment of infected diabetic foot ulcers: topical MSI-78 vs. oral ofloxacin. *Diabetologia* 1997;40(Suppl 1):A482.

33. Chantelan E, Tanudjaja T, Altenhofer F, Ersuli Z, Lacigova S, Metzger C. Antibiotic treatment for uncomplicated neuropathic forefoot ulcers in diabetes: a controlled trial. *Diabet Med* 1996;13:156–159.

34. Jones EW, Edwards R, Finch R, Jaffcoate WJ. A microbiologic study of diabetic foot lesions. *Diabet Med* 1984;2:213–215.
35. Drew RH, Perfect JR, Srinath L, et al. Treatment of methicillin-resistant *Staphylococcus aureus* infections with quinupristin-dalfopristin in patients intolerant of or failing prior therapy. *J Antimicrob Chemother* 2000;46:775–784.
36. Nichols RL, Graham DR, Barriere SL, et al. Treatment of hospitalized patients with complicated gram-positive skin and skin structure infections: two randomized, multicentre studies of quinupristin/dalfopristin versus cefazolin, oxacillin or vancomycin. *J Antimicrob Chemother* 1999;44:263–273.
37. Lipsky BA, Itani K, Norden C, The Linezolid Diabetic Foot Infections Study Group. Treating foot infections in diabetic patients: a randomized, multicenter, open-label trial of linezolid versus ampicillin-sulbactam/amoxicillin-clavulanate. *Clin Infect Dis* 2004;38:17–24.
38. Stevens DL, Herr D, Lampiris H, et al. Linezolid versus vancomycin for the treatment of methicillin-resistant *Staphylococcus aureus* infections. *Clin Infect Dis* 2002;34:1481–1490.
39. Lipsky BA, Stoutenburgh U. Daptomycin for treating infected diabetic foot ulcers: evidence from a randomized, controlled trial comparing daptomycin with vancomycin or semi-synthetic penicillins for complicated skin and skin-structure infections. *J Antimicrob Chemother* 2005;55:240–245.
40. Arbeit RD, Maki D, Tally FP, Campanaro E, Eisenstein BI, The Daptomycin 98-01 and 99-01 Investigators. The safety and efficacy of daptomycin for the treatment of complicated skin and skin-structure infections. *Clin Infect Dis* 2004;38:1673–1681.
41. Beam TR Jr, Gutierrez I, Powell S, et al. Prospective study of the efficacy and safety of oral and intravenous ciprofloxacin in the treatment of diabetic foot infections. *Rev Infect Dis* 1989;11(Suppl 5):S1163–S1163.
42. Hughes CE, Johnson CC, Bamberger DM, et al. Treatment and long-term follow-up of foot infections in patients with diabetes or ischemia: a randomized, prospective, double-blind comparison of cefoxitin and ceftizoxime. *Clin Ther* 1987;10(Suppl A):36–49.
43. Peterson LR, Lissack LM, Canter K, Fasching CE, Clabots C, Gerding DN. Therapy of lower extremity infections with ciprofloxacin in patients with diabetes mellitus, peripheral vascular disease, or both. *Am J Med* 1989;86:801–808.
44. Lipsky BA, Armstrong D, Citron D, et al. Study of infections in diabetic feet comparing the efficacy, safety, and tolerability of ertapenem vs. piperacillin-tazobactam. Lancet 2005; 366:1695–1703.
45. Anonymous. Unpublished data. Pfizer, Inc., 2001.
46. Cooper G, Platt R. *Staphylococcus aureus* bacteremia in diabetic patients: endocarditis and mortality. *Am J Med* 1982;73:658–662.
47. Bamberger DM, Daus GP, Gerding DN. Osteomyelitis in the feet of diabetic patients: long-term results, prognostic factors and the role of antimicrobial and surgical therapy. *Am J Med* 1987;83:653–660.
48. Van GH, Siney H, Danan JP, Sachon C, Grimaldi A. Treatment of osteomyelitis in the diabetic foot. *Diabetes Care* 1996;19:1257–1260.
49. Lipsky BA. Osteomyelitis of the foot in diabetic patients. *Clin Infect Dis* 1997;25:1318–1326.
50. Gibbons GW, Eliopoulos GM. Infections of the diabetic foot, in *Management of Diabetic Foot Problems* (Kozak GP, Hoar CS, Jr, Rowbotham RL, eds.), WB Saunders, Philadelphia, 1984, pp. 97–102.

14

Charcot Arthropathy in the Diabetic Foot

Robert G. Frykberg, DPM, MPH

INTRODUCTION

Charcot's classic work on the "arthropathies of locomotor ataxia" was first published in 1868 while he was the chief physician at the Salpetriere in Paris *(1,2)*. In describing the joint affectations of patients with tabes dorsalis, he noted severe deformities, crepitations, and instability with gradual degrees of healing over time. Of primary importance, he believed these changes to be secondary to the underlying disease in which there was an associated nutritive deficiency in the spinal cord. Although lesions in this structure are far less frequently involved in the pathogenesis of neuroarthropathy than peripheral nerve lesions, Charcot was certainly intuitive in this regard. In his own words,

> "How often have not I seen persons, not yet familiar with this arthropathy, misunderstand its real nature, and, wholly preoccupied with the local affection, even absolutely forget that behind the disease of the joint there was a disease far more important in character, and which in reality dominated the situation. . . ." *(1)*

Although Musgrave in 1703 and later Mitchell in 1831 ostensibly described osteoarthropathy associated with venereal disease and spinal cord lesions respectively, Charcot's name remains synonymous with neuropathic arthropathies of multiple etiologies *(2–5)*.

In 1936, Jordan was the first to fully recognize and report on the association of neuropathic arthropathy with diabetes mellitus *(6)*. In that rather comprehensive review of the neuritic manifestations of diabetes, Jordan described a 56-year-old woman with diabetes duration of approx 14 years who presented with "a rather typical, painless Charcot joint of the ankle." His description typifies the classic presentation we now commonly recognize in patients with long standing diabetes and neuropathy. Subsequently, Bailey and Root, in their 1947 series, noted that 1 in 1100 patients with diabetes mellitus developed neurogenic osteoarthropathy *(7)*. In the classic 1972 Joslin Clinic review of 68,000 patients by Sinha et al. *(8)*, 101 patients were encountered with diabetic Charcot feet. This ratio of 1 case in 680 patients with diabetes brought greater attention to this disorder and characterized the affected patients' clinical and radiographic presentations. In the subsequent 30 years, there has been a significant increase in the number of reports on diabetic osteoarthropathy, its complications, and management *(6–10)*. The prevalence of this condition is highly variable, ranging from 0.15% of all patients with diabetes to as high as 29% in a population of only neuropathic diabetic subjects *(2,8,10,11)*.

Recently, a prospective study of a large group of diabetic patients from Texas reported an incidence of 8.5/1000 per year. Neuroarthropathy was significantly more common in Caucasians than in Mexican Americans. (11.7/1000 vs 6.4/1000) *(12)*. Although this study may give us better insight into the true frequency of osteoarthropathy in diabetes, much of the data we currently rely on are based on retrospective studies of small single center cohorts. Nonetheless, the incidence of Charcot cases reported is very likely an underestimation because many cases go undetected, especially in the early states *(2,11,13)*. The frequency of diagnosis of the diabetic Charcot foot appears to be increasing as a result of increased awareness of its signs and symptoms *(14)*. Although the original descriptions of neuropathic osteoarthropathy were attributed to patients with tertiary syphilis, diabetes mellitus has now become the disease most often associated with this severe foot disorder. Not only are diabetic patients with Charcot foot deformities at greater risk of amputation than those with neuropathic ulcers without osteoarthropathy, a study from the United Kingdom has also found them to have a higher mortality *(15)*. Although the power of this study did not allow for significant differences to emerge, it does confirm the need for larger population-based studies to fully elucidate the epidemiology of this limb-threatening complication.

Etiology

Charcot foot (neuropathic osteoarthropathy) can be defined as a noninfectious and progressive condition of single or multiple joints characterized by joint dislocation, pathological fractures, and severe destruction of the pedal architecture which is closely associated with peripheral neuropathy *(2,9,16)*. Almost uniformly, trauma of some degree when superimposed on the neuropathic extremity precipitates the cascade of events leading to the joint destruction. Osteoarthropathy, therefore, may result in debilitating deformity with subsequent ulceration and even amputation *(4,13,17)*. Neuroarthropathy can result from various disorders which have the potential to cause a peripheral neuropathy. With the decline in numbers of patients with tertiary syphilis since Charcot's time and the concomitant rise in prevalence of diabetes mellitus, the latter disease has now become the primary condition associated with Charcot joints. Table 1 lists the various neuropathic disorders which can compromise joint mechanisms including their predilection for sites of involvement *(2,8,9,14)*.

There are several conditions producing radiographic changes similar to Charcot joints. These include acute arthritides, psoriatic arthritis, osteoarthritis, osteomyelitis, osseous tumors, and gout. These joint affectations in the presence of neuropathy make the correct diagnosis even more difficult to ascertain *(8)*. Nonetheless, the characteristics of the joint changes, site for predilection, and even age of the patient assist in determining the true underlying diagnosis.

The primary risk factors for this potentially limb threatening deformity are the presence of dense peripheral neuropathy, normal circulation and a history of preceding trauma, often minor in nature *(4,13,18)*. There is no apparent predilection for either sex *(2)*. Trauma is not necessarily limited to typical injuries such as sprains, contusions, or fractures. Foot deformities, prior amputations, joint infections, or surgical trauma may result in sufficient stress that can lead to Charcot joint disease. The other factors possibly implicated in the etiology of osteoarthropathy are metabolic abnormalities, renal transplantation, immunosuppressive/steroid therapy, impaired cartilage growth, and nonenzymatic glycosylation *(2)*.

Table 1
Diseases With Potential for Causing Neuropathic Osteoarthropathy

Disorder	Predilection site
Diabetes mellitus	Foot and ankle
Tabes dorsalis	Knee, shoulder, hip, ankle, and spine
Syringomyelia	Shoulder, elbow, and cervical spine
Leprosy (Hansen's disease)	Foot, ankle, and hand
Spina bifida	Hip and knee
Meningomyelocele	Foot and ankle
Congenital insensitivity to pain	Ankle and foot
Chronic alcoholism	Foot
Peripheral nerve injury	Ankle and knee
Sciatic nerve severance	Ankle and knee
Spinal cord injury	Varies with level of injury
Hysterical insensitivity to pain	Variable
Myelodysplasia	Variable
Multiple sclerosis	Variable
Riley-day syndrome	Variable
Intra-articular injections	Variable
Paraplegia	Variable

Although the exact pathogenesis may vary from patient to patient, it is undoubtedly multifactorial in nature *(2,10,14,18)*. The neurotraumatic (German) theory has traditionally been proposed as the primary etiology of osteoarthropathy in which neuropathy and repeated trauma produce eventual joint destruction. The loss or diminution of protective sensation allows repetitive micro or macrotrauma producing intracapsular effusions, ligamentous laxity, and joint instability. With continued use of the injured extremity further degeneration ensues and eventually results in a Charcot joint. Underlying sensory neuropathy resulting from any disorder, is therefore a prerequisite under this theory of pathogenesis. However, the neurotraumatic theory does not explain all accounts of Charcot arthropathy, especially its occurrence in bedridden patients *(2,4,9–11,13)*.

The neurovascular reflex (French) theory, in contrast, proposes that increased peripheral blood flow owing to autonomic neuropathy that leads to hyperemic bone resorption *(19)*. This theory might indeed correspond to Charcot's original hypothesis of a central "nutritional" defect, although we now recognize this process as a peripheral nerve disorder. Autonomic neuropathy (and endothelial dysfunction) results in an impairment of vascular smooth muscle tone and consequently produces a vasodilatory condition in the small arteries of the distal extremities *(20,21)*. Impairment of neurogenic vascular responses in patients with diabetic neuropathy has been supported by one study that consequently also showed preserved maximal hyperemic responses to skin heating in patients with Charcot arthropathy *(22)*. In concert with associated arteriovenous shunting there is a demonstrable increase in bone blood flow in the neuropathic limb. The resultant osteolysis, demineralization, and weakening of bone can predispose to the development of neuro-osteoarthropathy *(2,18–20,23,24)*. Several studies have demonstrated reduced bone

Pathogenesis of the Charcot Foot

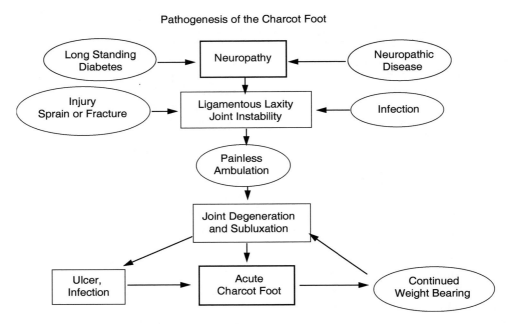

Fig. 1. Pathogenesis of diabetic neuropathic osteoarthropathy.

mineral density with an apparent imbalance between the normally linked bone resorption and production in patients with osteoarthropathy *(25–27)*. Specifically, greater osteoclastic than osteoblastic activity has been noted in acute neuroarthropathy, suggesting an explanation for the excessive bone resorption during the acute stage *(20,25)*.

The actual pathogenesis of Charcot arthropathy most likely is a combined effect of both the neurovascular and neurotraumatic theories *(14,18,28,29,23)*. It is generally accepted that trauma superimposed on a well perfused but severely neuropathic extremity can precipitate the development of an acute Charcot foot. The presence of sensory neuropathy renders the patient unaware of the initial precipitating trauma and often profound osseous destruction taking place during ambulation. The concomitant autonomic neuropathy with its associated osteopenia and relative weakness of the bone predisposes it to fracture *(20,26)*. A vicious cycle then ensues in which the insensate patient continues to walk on the injured foot, thereby allowing further damage to occur *(9,13,14)*. With added trauma and fractures in the face of an abundant hyperemic response to injury, marked swelling soon follows. Capsular and ligamentous distension or rupture is also a part of this process and leads to the typical joint subluxations and loss of normal pedal architecture culminating in the classic rocker-bottom Charcot foot. The amount of joint destruction and deformity which results is highly dependent on the time at which the proper diagnosis is made and when nonweight-bearing immobilization is begun *(9)*. A simplified cycle of the pathogenesis of Charcot joints is illustrated in Fig. 1.

Often it is a fracture, either intra-articular or extra-articular, which initiates the destructive process. This had not been fully appreciated until Johnson presented a series of cases in which patients with diabetes developed typical Charcot joints after sustaining

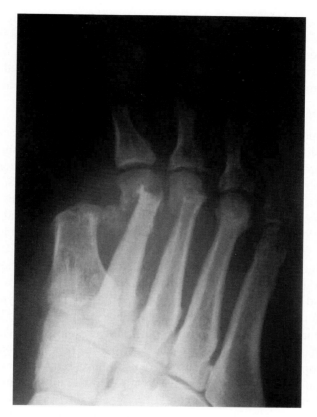

Fig. 2. Neuropathic changes (fractures) in the lesser metatarsal heads after undergoing a first ray amputation. Biomechanical imbalances and increased stress presumably lead to these changes.

neuropathic fractures *(30)*. Additionally, amputation of the great toe or first ray, often a consequence of infection or gangrene in the patient with diabetes, may lead to neuropathic joint changes in the lesser metatarsophalangeal joints (Fig. 2). Presumably, this is a stress related factor secondary to an acquired biomechanical imbalance. Intra-articular infection can also be implicated as an inciting event leading to this endpoint. In effect, almost any inflammatory or destructive process introduced to a neuropathic joint has the potential for creating a Charcot joint. Herbst et al. *(31)* have recently reported their findings concerning the type of presentation as related to patients' bone mineral density (BMD). They found that patients with normal BMD had typical changes in the midfoot primarily made up of joint dislocations. However, in those patients with reduced BMD, fracture patterns predominated in the ankle and forefoot.

Several authors have noted the similarities between the acute destructive phase in Charcot arthropathy and reflex sympathetic dystrophy (complex regional pain syndrome) *(20,21)*. Both conditions are associated with an exaggerated vascular response as well as with the development of osteopenia. Both can also be related to previous acute trauma. Although the underlying pathophysiological processes are not yet firmly established, both are marked by excessive osteoclastic activity and seem to respond well to treatment with bisphosphonates *(20,21,32)*. Jeffcoate has also suggested that a dysregulation of the receptor activator of nuclear factor-κB ligand/osteoprotegerin signaling pathway and attendant affects on blood flow and bone turnover might also play a role in this regard *(33)*. Further study is required, however, to determine how these pathways interact in patients with neuropathy to cause increased vascularity and subsequent osteopenia.

Classification of Charcot Arthropathy

The most common classification system of Charcot arthropathy is based on radiographic appearance as well as physiological stages of the process. The Eichenholtz classification divides osteoarthropathy into developmental, coalescence, and reconstructive stages *(34)*. Several other authors have subsequently proposed an earlier Stage 0 that corresponds to the initial inflammatory period following injury but prior to the development of characteristic bony radiographic changes *(35–37)*. This prodromal period might be considered as an "osteoarthropathy *in situ*" stage. The traditional developmental stage is characterized by fractures, debris formation, and fragmentation of cartilage and subchondral bone. This is followed by capsular distension, ligamentous laxity, and varying degrees of subluxation and marked soft tissue swelling. Synovial biopsy at this time will show osseous and cartilaginous debris embedded in a thickened synovium, which is pathognomonic for the disease *(34)*. The coalescence stage is marked by the absorption of much of the fine debris, a reduction in soft tissue swelling, bone callus proliferation and consolidation of fractures. Finally, the reconstructive stage is denoted by bony ankylosis and hypertrophic proliferation with some restoration of stability when this stage is reached. In certain cases, however, severe osseous disintegration occurs because of prolonged activity. In these situations the condition may be referred to as chronically active and little healing, if any, takes place. Although the system is radiologically very descriptive and useful, its practical clinical applicability is less so. In clinical practice, the initial developmental stage is considered active or acute, whereas the coalescent and reconstructive stages are considered to be the quiescent or reparative stages *(2,10)*. Other classification systems have been described based on anatomic sites of involvement but do not describe the activity of the disease *(2,36,38–40)*. Several systems primarily focus on disorders of the midfoot and/or hindfoot *(38–40)*, whereas Sanders and Frykberg's classification includes involvement of the forefoot, midfoot, and rearfoot *(2,10)*.

Radiographic Findings

Radiographically, osteoarthropathy takes on the appearance of a severely destructive form of degenerative arthritis. Serial X-rays will customarily demonstrate multiple changes occurring throughout the process and can assist in monitoring disease activity *(10)*. Rarely will nucleotide scanning, computed tomography (CT), or magnetic resonance imaging (MRI) be necessary to establish the diagnosis. The acute or developmental stage is marked by an abundance of soft tissue edema, osteopenia, multiple fractures, loose bodies, dislocations, or subluxations *(28,29,41)*. These radiographic findings are fairly typical of noninfective bone changes associated with diabetes and have been described well by Newman *(42)*. In addition to alterations in the normal pedal architecture, the metatarsal heads and phalanges will frequently demonstrate atrophic changes often called diabetic osteolysis *(13)*. Synonyms for this phenomenon include a "sucked candy" appearance, "pencil pointing," "hour glass" deformities of the phalanges, or mortar and pestle deformity

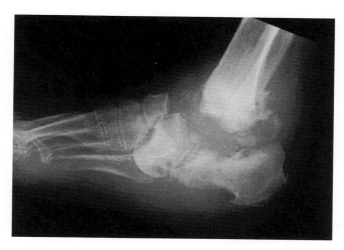

Fig. 3. Osteolysis of the talus and disintegration of the ankle and subtalar joints.

Table 2
Radiographic Changes in Osteoarthropathy

Stage	Atrophic changes	Hypertrophic changes	Miscellaneous

Acute	Osteolysis
	Resorption of bone
	Metatarsal heads,
	  Phalangeal diaphyses,
	  MTP, Subtalar, Ankle
	Osteopenia
		Periosteal new bone
		Intra-articular debris,
		  Joint mice, fragments
		Osteophytes,
		  Architectural collapse,
		  Deformity
			Joint effusions
			Subluxations
			Fractures
			Soft tissue edema
			Medial arterial
			  calcification
			Ulceration

Quiescent	Distal metatarsal
	  and rearfoot osteolysis,
	Bone loss
		Periosteal new bone,
		  Marginal osteophytes,
		  Fracture bone callus
		Rocker bottom, midfoot
		  or ankle deformity
		Ankylosis
			Resorption of
			  debris
			Diminished edema
			Sclerosis
			Ulceration

of the metatarsophalangeal joints. Massive osteolysis can also occur in the rearfoot during the acute stage, especially in the ankle and subtalar joints (Fig. 3). These changes will often coexist with the obvious ankle fractures that initiated the destructive process. Medial arterial calcification is another associated, but unrelated finding frequently observed in these patients *(20)*.

Chronic reparative or quiescent radiographic changes include hypertrophic changes such as periosteal new bone formation, coalescence of fractures and bony fragments, sclerosis, remineralization, and a reduction in soft tissue edema *(2,13,30,41,42)*. Rocker-bottom deformities, calcaneal equinus, dropped cuboid, or other deformities not previously appreciated may also become visible, especially when taking weight-bearing images. Table 2 summarizes the varieties of radiographic changes found in osteoarthropathy.

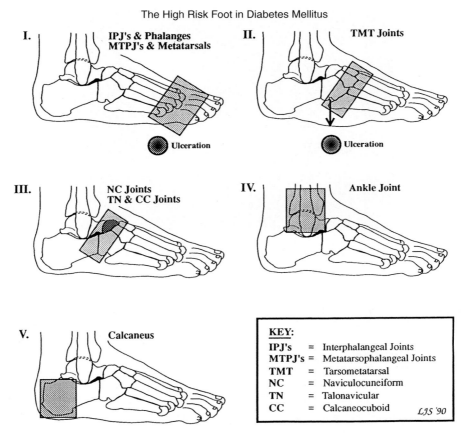

Fig. 4. Patterns of diabetic osteoarthropathy based on anatomic sites of involvement. (From ref. *2* with permission.)

Sanders and Frykberg describe typical neuropathic osteoarthropathy patterns of joint involvement based on joint location in patients with diabetes *(2,10)*. These patterns may exist independently or in combination with each other as determined through clinical and radiographic findings. They are illustrated in Fig. 4 and described as follows: pattern I—forefoot—metatarsal–phalangeal joints, pattern II—tarsometatarsal (Lisfranc's) joint, pattern III—midtarsal and navicular-cuneiform joints, pattern IV—ankle and subtalar joints, and pattern V—calcaneus (calcaneal insufficiency avulsion fracture) *(2,28)*.

Pattern I: Forefoot

Pattern I encompasses atrophic changes or osteolysis of the metatarsophalangeal and interphalangeal joints with the characteristic sucked candy appearance of the distal metatarsals *(24)* (Fig. 5). Frequently, atrophic bone resorption of the distal metatarsals and phalanges accompanies other changes found in the midfoot and rearfoot. An infectious etiology has been proposed for these findings although osteolysis can occur without any prior history of joint sepsis. Reports of 10–30% of the neuropathic osteoarthropathies have been categorized as pattern I *(2,8)*.

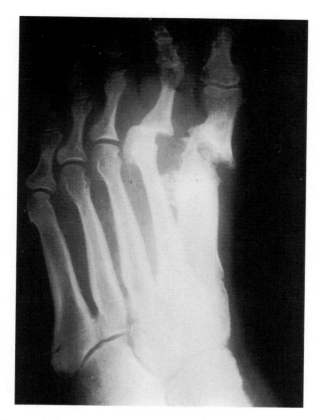

Fig. 5. Pattern I: osteolytic changes involving the first metatarsals and phalanx are evident without any current infection documented.

Pattern II: Tarsometatarsal (Lisfranc's) Joint

Pattern II involves Lisfranc's joint, typically with the earliest clue being a very subtle lateral deviation of the base of the second metatarsal at the cuneiform joint. Once the stability of this "keystone" is lost, the Lisfranc joint complex will often subluxate dorsolaterally.

Fracture of the second metatarsal base allows for greater mobility in which subluxation of the metatarsal bases will occur. The rupture of intermetatarsal and tarsometatarsal ligaments plantarly will also allow a collapse of the arch during normal weight bearing, leading to the classic rocker-bottom deformity. Compensatory contracture of the gastrocnemius muscle will frequently follow and create a further plantarflexory moment to accentuate the inverted arch. This pattern also is commonly associated with plantar ulcerations at the apex of the collapse, which typically involves the cuboid or cuneiforms *(2,18,24)*. This was the most frequent pattern of presentation for diabetic Charcot feet in the Sinha series and represents the most common presentation in clinical practice *(8)* (Fig. 6).

Pattern III: Midtarsal and Naviculocuneiform Joints

Pattern III incorporates changes within the midtarsal (Chopart's) joint with the frequent addition of the naviculo-cuneiform joint. As described by Newman *(43)* and

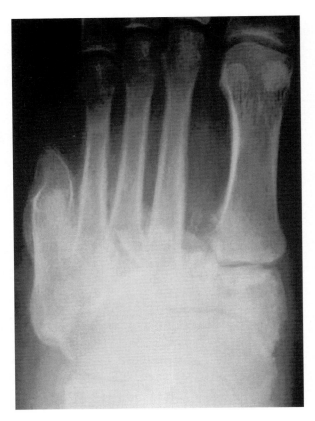

Fig. 6. Pattern II: Lisfranc's joint dislocation with associated fractures are evident in this common presentation of the Charcot foot (Fifth ray had previously been amputated.)

Lesko and Maurer *(44)*, spontaneous dislocation of the talonavicular joint with or without fragmentation characterize this pattern. Newman further suggests that isolated talonavicular joint subluxation might even be considered as an entity separate from osteoarthropathy, although still an important element of noninfective neuropathic bone disease *(43)*. Lisfranc's joint changes (pattern II) are often seen in combination with pattern III deformities of the lesser tarsus (Fig. 7).

Pattern IV: Ankle and Subtalar Joint

Pattern IV involves the ankle joint, including the subtalar joint and body of the talus (Fig. 8). Disintegration of the talar body is equivalent to the central tarsal disintegration of Harris and Brand *(38)*. The destructive forces are created by joint incongruity and continued mechanical stress which eventually erodes the talus. Massive osteolysis is frequently observed in this pattern with attendant ankle or subtalar subluxation and angular deformity. As noted, tibial or fibular malleolar fractures frequently are seen in association with osteoarthropathy in this location and most likely precipitated the development of the joint dissolution. Pattern IV Charcot is found in approx 10% of reported cases *(2,8,10,45)*.

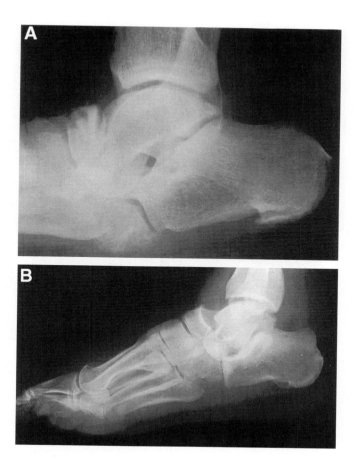

Fig. 7. Pattern III: **(A)** Talonavicular dislocation with "dropped cuboid" and plantarflexed calcaneus. **(B)** Talonavicular dislocation with early subtalar and calcaneal-cuboid subluxation. Note absence of fractures or osteochondral defects.

Pattern V: Calcaneus (Calcaneal Insufficiency Avulsion Fracture)

Pattern V, the least common presentation (approx 2%), is characterized by extra-articular fractures of the calcaneus (posterior pillar). This osteopathy is usually included in the neuropathic osteoarthropathy classification, however, there is no joint involvement (Fig. 9). This is more appropriately considered as a neuropathic fracture of the body or, more commonly, the posterior tuberosity of the calcaneus. El-Khoury *(46)* and Kathol *(47)* have termed this entity the "calcaneal insufficiency avulsion fracture."

CLINICAL PRESENTATION

The classic presentation for acute osteoarthropathy includes several characteristic clinical findings (Table 3). Typically, the patient with a Charcot foot will have had a long duration of diabetes, usually in excess of 12 years. Although all age groups can be affected, a review of the literature in this regard indicates that the majority of patients are in their sixth decade (mid-50s) *(2,18)*. A recent report, however, indicates that there is an

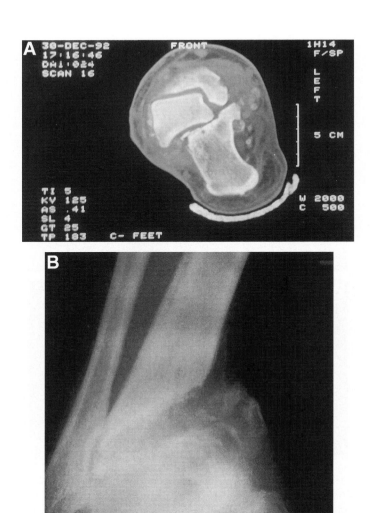

Fig. 8. Pattern IV **(A)** Subtalar joint dislocation diagnosed on CT Scan. **(B)** Acute ankle Charcot with medial malleolar fracture and medial displacement of foot.

apparent age difference in onset between patients with type 1 and patients with type 2 diabetes *(48)*. Whereas the average age at presentation for the entire cohort and patients with type 2 is indeed in the sixth decade, for patients with type 1 the age at onset was in the fifth decade (40s). Patients with type 1 diabetes also demonstrated a longer duration of the disease than in patients with type 2 diabetes who have osteoarthropathy (24 vs 13 years) *(48)*. This has also been corroborated by an earlier report from Finland *(49)*. There does not appear to be a predilection for either sex. Although unilateral involvement is the most frequent presentation, bilateral Charcot feet can be found in 9–18% of patients *(4,8)*.

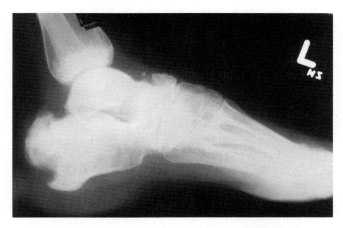

Fig. 9. Pattern V: calcaneal insufficiency avulsion fracture of the calcaneus.

Table 3
Clinical Features of Acute Charcot Joint

Vascular	Neuropathic	Skeletal	Cutaneous
Bounding pedal pulse	Absent or diminished: Pain	Rocker bottom deformity	Neuropathic ulcer
Erythema	Vibration	Medial tarsal subluxation	Hyperkeratoses
Edema	Deep tendon reflexes	Digital subluxation	Infection
Warmth	Light touch	Rearfoot equinovarus	Gangrene
	Anhidrosis	Hypermobility, crepitus	

The initial presentation for acute Charcot arthropathy is usually quite distinct in which a patient with diabetes will seek attention for a profoundly swollen foot that is difficult to fit into a shoe (Fig. 10). Although classically described as painless, 75% of these patients will complain of pain or aching in an otherwise insensate foot *(4)*. Almost uniformly, an antecedent history of some type of injury can be elicited from the patient. When no such history is available, the precipitating event might simply have gone unrecognized in the neuropathic limb.

On examination, the pulses will be characteristically bounding even through the grossly edematous foot *(13,18)*. Occasionally, however, the swelling will obscure one or both pedal pulses. In concert with the hyperemic response to injury, the foot will also be somewhat erythematous and warm. The skin temperature elevation can be ascertained by dermal infrared thermometry and will contrast with the unaffected side by 3–8°C *(2,4,45,49,50)*. There is always some degree of sensory neuropathy in which reflexes, vibratory sense, proprioception, light touch, and/or pain (pin prick) are either diminished or absent *(9)*. As mentioned, the patients will most often relate some localized pain although often mild in comparison to the deformity present *(11,13)*. Motor neuropathy can present as a foot drop deformity or with intrinsic muscle atrophy. Triceps surae equinus can sometimes be ascertained initially, but cannot at this time be considered a precipitating or causal factor for osteoarthropathy. Autonomic neuropathy,

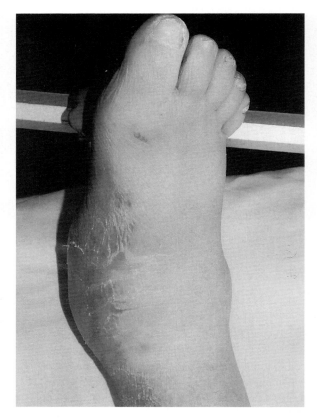

Fig. 10. Acute Charcot ankle with profound foot and leg edema.

which coexists with somatosensory neuropathy, can be clinically appreciated by the presence of anhidrosis with very dry skin and/or thick callus *(20,21)*. Another fairly frequent cutaneous finding is a plantar neuropathic ulceration, especially in chronic or chronically active Charcot feet. A concomitant ulceration will therefore raise questions of potential contiguous osteomyelitis *(10,18,24,28)*.

The skeletal changes frequently manifest as obvious deformity of the medial midfoot with collapse of the arch and/or rocker-bottom deformity *(2,10,28)* (Fig. 11). Associated findings might often include hypermobility with crepitus, significant instability, and ankle deformity.

CLINICAL DIAGNOSIS OF ACUTE CHARCOT ARTHROPATHY

When presented with a warm, swollen, insensate foot, plain radiographs are invaluable in ascertaining the presence of osteoarthropathy *(18,28,29,51)*. In most cases, no further imaging studies will be required to make the correct diagnosis. However, in the prodromal stage 0 there may be primarily soft tissue changes noted without evidence of distinct bone or joint pathology *(52)*. Further investigation with scintigraphy, MRI, or serial radiographs should be considered when suspicion is high for osteoarthropathy *(28,52–55)*. With a concomitant wound, it may initially be difficult to differentiate between acute Charcot arthropathy and osteomyelitis solely based on plain radiographs

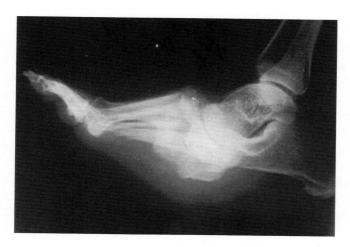

Fig. 11. Radiograph of rocker bottom Charcot foot with collapse of the midfoot.

(10,17). Additional laboratory studies may prove useful in determining the appropriate diagnosis. Leukocytosis can often suggest acute osteomyelitis, however, this normal response to infection can be blunted in persons with diabetes *(56).* Although the erythrocyte sedimentation rate may also be elevated in the case of acute infection, it often responds similarly to any inflammatory process and is therefore nonspecific. When the ulcer probes to bone, a bone biopsy is indicated and should be considered as the most specific method of distinguishing between osteomyelitis and osteoarthropathy in these circumstances *(18).* A biopsy consisting of multiple shards of bone and soft tissue embedded in the deep layers of synovium is pathognomonic for neuropathic osteoarthropathy *(34).*

Technetium bone scans are exquisitely sensitive for detecting Charcot arthropathy but nonetheless are generally nonspecific in assisting in the differentiation between osteomyelitis and acute Charcot arthropathy *(52,53,57).* Indium scanning, although still expensive, has been shown to be more specific for infection *(55,57–59).* However, false-positive scans can frequently be found in a rapidly evolving acute osteoarthropathy without associated osteomyelitis. Additional studies helpful in differentiating Charcot arthropathy from osteomyelitis include Tc-HMPAO labeled white blood cell scans and magnetic resonance imaging *(52,54,60,61).* MRI examination can also be very sensitive to the earliest changes in neuroarthropathy, but again it is difficult to reliably detect bone infection superimposed on the gross changes noted surrounding a Charcot joint *(28,52,54,62).* Another imaging modality that may show some promise in this regard is positron emission tomography. Hopfner and colleagues recently reported that this modality could not only detect early osteoarthropathy with 95% sensitivity, but could also reliably distinguish between Charcot lesions and osteomyelitis even in the presence of implanted hardware *(62).* However, no study is 100% accurate in distinguishing neuropathic bone lesions from infectious entities. In as much as clinical acumen is necessary for detecting Charcot arthropathy at its onset, clinical judgment remains of paramount importance in properly assessing and managing these patients.

CONSERVATIVE MANAGEMENT

Immobilization and reduction of stress are considered the mainstays of treatment for acute Charcot arthropathy *(4,10,13,14,16,18,28,29,45,63)*. Nonweight bearing on the affected limb for 8–12 weeks removes the continual trauma and should promote conversion of the active Charcot joint to the quiescent phase *(18,41,49)*. This author advocates complete nonweight bearing through the use of crutches, wheelchair or other assistive modalities during the initial acute period. Although it is an accepted form of treatment, three point crutch gait may in fact increase pressure to the contralateral limb, thereby predisposing it to repetitive stress and ulceration or neuroarthropathy *(44)*. A short leg plaster or fiberglass nonweight-bearing cast can additionally be used for acute Charcot events even in those patients with superficial noninfected ulcerations *(2,4,9)*. A soft compressive dressing or Unna's Boot in concert with a removable cast walker or pneumatic walking brace can also be used effectively in this regard *(28)*. Following a relatively brief period of complete off-loading, a rapid reduction in edema and pain will occur. Although there is no uniform consensus, some centers advocate the initial use of a weight bearing total contact cast in the management of acute osteoarthropathy *(4,29,51,64–66)*. Such casts need to be changed at least weekly to adjust to the changes in limb volume as the edema decreases. When deeper or infected ulcerations are present, frequent debridements and careful observation are required. These patients will therefore benefit from removable immobilization devices or bivalved casts.

Off-loading with or without immobilization should be anticipated for approx 3–6 months, depending on the severity of joint destruction *(4,10,18,45,49)*. Conversion to the reparative phase is indicated by a reduction in pedal temperature toward that of the unaffected side, and a sustained reduction in edema *(2,4,10,16,18,21,45,50)*. This should be corroborated with serial radiographs indicating consolidation of osseous debris, union of fractures, and a reduction in soft tissue edema *(13)*. McGill et al. *(50)* have found a reduction in skin temperature and bone scan activity that mirrors activity of Charcot neuroarthropathy, both of which improve as the condition achieves quiescence.

When the patient enters the quiescent phase, management is directed at a gradual resumption of weight bearing with prolonged or permanent bracing *(4,14,18,41,64–67)*. Care must be taken to gradually wean the patient from nonweight bearing to partial to full weight bearing with the use of assistive devices (i.e., crutches, cane, or walker). Progression to protected weight bearing is permitted, usually with the aid of some type of ambulatory immobilizing device *(67)*. Through the use of appropriately applied total contact casts or other immobilizing ambulatory modalities (i.e., fixed ankle walker, bivalved casts, total contact prosthetic walkers, patellar tendon-bearing braces, and so on), most patients may safely ambulate although bony consolidation of fractures progresses *(10,18,51,68,69)* (Table 4). Charcot restraint orthotic walkers or other similar total contact prosthetic walkers have gained acceptance as useful protective modalities for the initial period of weight bearing *(68–70)*. These custom made braces usually incorporate some degree of patellar tendon bearing as well as a custom foot bed with a rocker sole. A more readily available option is a pneumatic walking brace or similar removable cast walker that might incorporate a cushioned foot bed or insole. These can be made nonremovable by simply applying adhesive tape or cast bandaging around the body of the walker to help encourage compliance *(21,71)* (Fig. 12).

Table 4
**Off-Loading/Immobilizing Devices Used
in the Management of Charcot Feet**

Wheelchair
Crutches
Walker
Elastic bandage or Jones dressing
Unna's Boot
Total contact cast
Bivalved cast
Posterior splint
Fixed ankle walking brace
Patellar tendon-bearing brace
Charcot restraint orthotic walker (CROW)
Surgical shoe with custom inlay

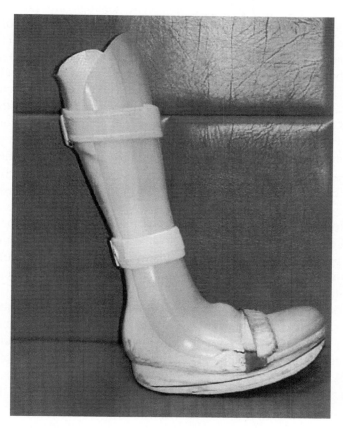

Fig. 12. Total contact custom orthosis with rocker sole.

The mean time of rest and immobilization (casting followed by removable cast walker) before return to permanent footwear is approx 4–6 months *(2,4,13,14,17,29,45,49)*. Feet must be closely monitored during the time of transition to permanent footwear to insure that the acute inflammatory process does not recur. Forefoot and midfoot deformities (patterns I–III) often do well with custom full length inserts and comfort or extra depth shoes once bracing is no longer required *(18)*. Healing sandals made from full length custom inserts placed into a surgical shoe often serve as interim footwear before wearing permanent footwear *(13)*. Severe midfoot deformities will often require the fabrication of custom shoes to accommodate the misshapen foot. Rearfoot osteoarthropathy with minimal deformity may require only a deep, well cushioned shoe with a full length orthotic device. For mildly unstable ankles without severe deformity or joint dissolution, high top custom shoes can sometimes provide adequate stability against transverse plane rotational forces. The moderately unstable ankle will benefit from an ankle foot orthosis and a high top therapeutic shoe. The severely unstable or maligned rearfoot will require a patellar tendon bearing brace incorporated into a custom shoe *(51,72,73)*. The patellar tendon bearing brace has reportedly decreased the rearfoot mean peak forces by at least 32% *(73)*.

In the setting of altered BMD in patients with diabetes and neuropathy, there has been recent interest in the adjunctive use of bisphosphonate therapy in acute Charcot arthropathy *(20,26,74–76)*. These pyrophosphate analogs are potent inhibitors of osteoclastic bone resorption and are widely used in the treatment of osteoporosis, Paget's disease, and reflex sympathetic dystrophy syndrome *(20,21)*. Although one uncontrolled study of six patients found significant reductions in foot temperature and alkaline phosphatase levels as compared with baseline, its small size and lack of a control group preclude making any meaningful conclusions from the treatment *(74)*. A subsequent multicenter randomized trial in the United Kingdom from this same group was performed using a single intravenous infusion of pamidronate compared to saline infusion *(75)*. The treatment group had significant falls in temperature and markers of bone turnover (deoxypyridinoline crosslinks and bone specific alkaline phosphatase) in subsequent weeks as contrasted to the control subjects. However, no differences in clinical or radiographic outcomes were reported. Trials of oral bisphosphonates with alendronate are currently being conducted and are expected to have similar results *(21)*. Until definitive controlled outcome studies are performed that concurrently measure serum markers of osteoclastic activity and attempt to assess improvements in clinical and radiological healing, bisphosphonate therapy should be considered as simply an adjunctive therapy in acute osteoarthropathy that could possibly expedite conversion to the quiescent stage.

Another modality that has been applied to the management of acute neuroarthropathy is the use of electrical bone stimulation *(77–79)*. In one study of 31 subjects randomized to either casting alone or cast with combined magnetic field electrical bone stimulation, there was a significant reduction in time to consolidation of the Charcot joints in the study group (11 vs 24 weeks) *(78)*. Low intensity pulsed ultrasound has also been suggested as a useful adjunct in promoting healing of Charcot fractures, although this report only presented two cases of patients successfully treated after undergoing revisional surgery for recalcitrant deformities *(80)*. Although both types of modalities have been proven successful in healing chronic nonunions, or even fresh fractures (in the case of low intensity pulsed ultrasound), their efficacy in promoting prompt healing of acute Charcot fractures or union of surgical arthrodeses has yet to be proven by large, well controlled randomized clinical trials.

SURGICAL THERAPY

Neuropathic arthropathy should not be considered as primarily a surgical disorder. To the contrary, there is an abundance of support in the literature confirming the need for initial attempts at conservative therapy to arrest the destructive process by converting the active Charcot joint to its quiescent, reparative stage *(2,4,10,17,18,45,49,51,66)*. As indicated by Johnson in 1967, the three keys to treatment of this disorder should be prevention first, followed by early recognition, and once diagnosed, protection from further injury until all signs of "reaction" have subsided *(30)*. Surgery should be contemplated when attempts at conservative care as previously outlined have failed to provide a stable, plantigrade foot. Additionally, when uncontrollable shearing forces result in recurrent plantar ulcerations or in those unusual cases that demonstrate continued destruction despite nonweight bearing, procedures such as simple bone resections, osteotomies, midfoot or major tarsal reconstruction, and ankle arthrodeses might become necessary *(29,30,40,64–66,81–83)*. However, a recent review of one center's experience with midfoot neuroarthropathy in 198 patients (201 ft) indicated that more than half of these patients could be successfully managed without the need for surgery *(66)*.

Although becoming more common in clinical practice, surgery on the Charcot foot is not a new concept. Steindler, in 1931, first reviewed his series of operative results in tabetic patients including one subtalar arthrodesis *(84)*. He, like Samilson *(85)*, Harris and Brand *(38)* and Johnson *(30)* many years later, recommended early recognition of the arthropathy, immediate protection from external deforming forces, and early operative stabilization when significant malalignment and instability precluded further conservative treatment. Samilson in 1959 *(85)* and Heiple in 1966 *(86)* were early to recognize the necessity for compressive internal fixation and prolonged immobilization in effectuating a solid bony fusion.

Harris and Brand in 1966 provided insight into this disorder associated with leprosy and described their five patterns of "disintegration of the tarsus" *(38)*. Full immobilization was always deemed imperative as an initial treatment, however, when progression continued or an unsatisfactory result was obtained, early surgical fusion was advocated. One year later Johnson published his large series which established the need for early recognition and protection to allow the acute inflammatory response to subside before surgical intervention *(30)*. As he stated, "Appropriate surgery on neuropathic joints, performed according to these principles, should be undertaken with great respect for the magnitude of the problem but not with dread." Johnson clearly favored osteotomy or arthrodesis in selected patients with quiescent Charcot joints and deformity in order to restore more normal alignment. Because the trauma of surgery could result in further absorption of bone during the acute stage, great emphasis was placed on resting the part until there was clinical and radiographic evidence of repair. Only then could surgery be attempted with a favorable chance for success *(30)*.

INDICATIONS AND CRITERIA

Instability, gross deformity, and progressive destruction despite immobilization are the primary indications for surgical intervention in neuroarthropathy *(2,10,18,41,82,87)*. Additionally, recurrent ulceration overlying resultant bony prominences of the collapsed rear, mid, and forefoot may require partial ostectomy to effect final healing when performed in

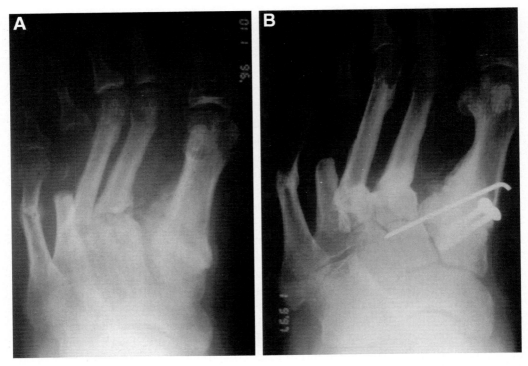

Fig. 13. (A) Preoperative X-ray of patient with dorsally dislocated first metatarsal-cuneiform joint and several metatarsal fractures. **(B)** Stability, resolution of symptoms, and complete healing was achieved with a limited arthrodesis of the first ray.

conjunction with appropriate footwear therapy *(64,88,89)*. Pain or varying degrees of discomfort will frequently accompany the deformity and may be refractory to conservative care in some patients. Attributable to chronic instability, this can be effectively eliminated by limited arthrodeses at the primary focus of the neuroarthropathy (Fig. 13).

Lesko and Maurer *(44)* and Newman *(42,43)* in their considerations of spontaneous peritalar dislocations advocate primary arthrodesis in those acute cases in which there is a reducible luxation in the absence of significant osseous destruction. Because these luxations may be the initial event in the sequence leading to typical osteoarthropathy, early intervention following a period of nonweight bearing has been recommended to counteract forces which would most likely lead to further progression of the deformity.

Age and overall medical status should also weigh heavily in the decision regarding suitability for surgery. Recognizing that arthrodeses and major reconstructions will require cast immobilization and nonweight bearing for 6 months or more, selection of the appropriate patient is critical to a successful outcome *(4,82,83)*. Because the majority of patients with osteoarthropathy are in their sixth to seventh decades and may likely have coexistent cardiovascular or renal disease *(2,10)*, careful consideration must be given to the risk vs benefit of lengthy operative procedures and the attendant prolonged recuperation *(45)*. As mentioned, a simple bone resection or limited arthrodesis might suffice in an older patient with a rocker-bottom deformity prone to ulceration as opposed to a complete reconstruction of the midfoot *(24,29,88–90)*. The former procedures can be done under local anesthesia relatively quickly, require a shorter convalescence, are prone to fewer complications, and can provide a stable, ulcer free foot when maintained in protective footwear. Nevertheless, major foot reconstructions and arthrodeses are certainly indicated in those healthier patients with severe deformity, instability, or recurrent ulcerations who have not satisfactorily responded to conservative efforts *(29,66,81–83,87)*. In all cases, however, the patient must be well educated as to the necessity for strict compliance with post operative immobilization and nonweight bearing for as long as 6–12 months.

An acute deformity, either a spontaneous dislocation or the more advanced fracture—dislocation paradigmatic of osteoarthropathy, must be rested and immobilized prior to any attempted surgery. Surgery during the active stage has the potential to compound and exacerbate the bone atrophy indicative of this inflammatory stage of destruction. Hence, it is often counterproductive as well as detrimental to operate on these feet until they have been converted to the quiescent, reparative stage. One small series, however, indicates successful arthrodeses rates with preserved foot function in patients with acute arthropathy of the midfoot *(91)*. Others have also advocated early operative repair with arthrodesis during stage 0 or stage 1, especially when nonoperative treatment has failed to prevent further deformity or arrest the destructive process *(35,87,92,93)*. Notwithstanding, this aggressive surgical approach needs confirmation through larger comparative trials prior to its adoption in the routine management of the acute Charcot foot. Overall, however, surgery performed primarily on chronic Charcot feet has met with increased success in recent years as experience develops. With an average union rate of 70% and improved alignment with stability, surgery on the neuroarthropathic foot has the potential not only to save limbs, but improve quality of life *(29,94)*.

Ostectomy of plantar prominences in the face of recalcitrant or recurrent neuropathic ulceration is perhaps the most frequent procedure performed on Charcot feet *(2,17,64,65,88–90)*. Such operations are fairly easy to perform and do not generally require lengthy periods of immobilization beyond attaining wound closure. Surgical approaches are varied, with direct excision of ulcers by ellipse or rotational local flaps predominating *(88–90)*. Alternative incisions are performed adjacent to ulcers or prominences, either through a medial or lateral approach. One report suggests that excision of medial plantar prominences fare better and with fewer complications than those under the lateral midfoot *(89)*. However, an earlier study reviewing experience with only lateral column ulcers reported an 89% overall healing rate *(90)*. A flexible approach to both incision and soft tissue coverage, including tissue transfer, is therefore required for optimal outcomes in cases of midfoot plantar ulceration *(89,90)*.

Arthrodesis of unstable Charcot joints of the midfoot and rearfoot frequently becomes necessary to provide a useful, plantigrade foot in those situations in which bracing or footwear therapy have been unsuccessful *(18,30,35,64–66,82,83,95)*. Major foot reconstruction is also an attractive alternative to amputation in patients with chronic or recurrent ulceration. Thompson et al. *(96)* recommend reconstructive surgery for Charcot deformities unable to function with load sharing orthoses. Commonly a tendoachilles lengthening precedes the fusion to ultimately diminish the plantarflexory forces contributing to pedal destruction *(18,29,65)*. The traditional method for arthrodesis

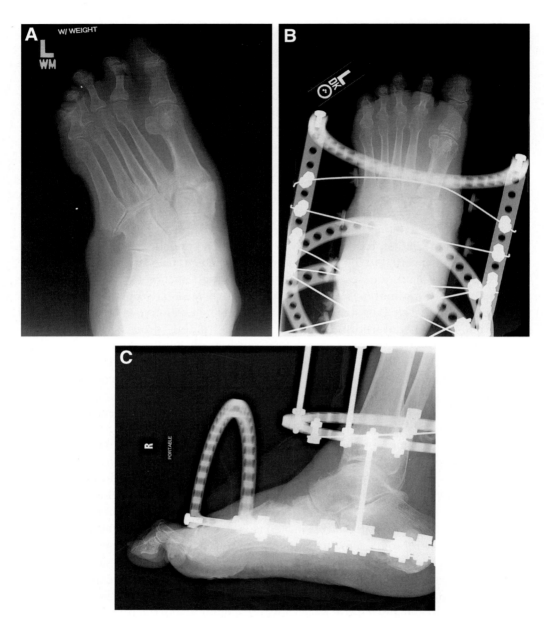

Fig. 14. Midfoot Charcot deformity corrected with circular external fixation. **(A)** Preoperative AP view showing midfoot deformity. **(B)** Postoperative AP view showing correction and frame in place. **(C)** Lateral postoperative X-ray with circular frame in place.

has been open reduction with solid internal fixation for noninfected Charcot joints, whereas external fixation is utilized when there is suspected infection of the joint fusion site *(18,30,35,81,97)*. In recent years, however, there has been greater interest in using external fixation and circular (Ilizarov) frames for stabilization in the acute stage as well as chronic stage and maintenance of correction for major reconstructions *(87,92,93,98)* (Fig. 14). Proposed benefits of circular frames include their ability to maintain fixation even in osteopenic bone, early weight-bearing ability, avoidance of fixation devices at sites of ulceration and potential bone infection, the ability to correct severe deformities, and the capability for gradual adjustments in position and compression throughout the reparative process *(93,98)*. For ankle deformities requiring arthrodesis, some prefer to use retrograde intramedullary nails alone or in concert with external fixators to provide stability and enhanced rates of fusion *(29,99–101)*.

Operative fusion techniques vary by site, but generally require meticulous excision of the synovium, resection of sclerotic bone down to a healthy bleeding bed, open manipulation, and precise osteotomies prior to rigid fixation *(30,35,38)*. Tissue handling must be gentle to avoid undue trauma and dissection must be mindful of underlying neurovascular structures. After reduction of deformity temporary fixation is achieved with large Steinman pins, K-wires, or guidepins when cannulated screw systems are to be used. After copious lavage, a surgical drain is placed before primary wound closure. External circular frames are generally constructed preoperatively and then applied with appropriate technique after wound closure *(93,98)*.

Postoperative to internal fixation procedures, the patient immediately undergoes immobilization of the foot with a posterior splint or bivalve cast. The patient must adhere to strict bedrest and prevent lower extremity dependency for several days until the soft tissue swelling subsides and serial below knee casting begins. The patient will remain nonweight bearing for a minimum of 2–3 months prior to considering partial weight bearing *(4,81)*. In general, protected weight bearing should be the rule for 6–12 months in order to avoid nonunion or late deformity in these difficult patients *(29,35)*. After external fixation weight-bearing status is variable—some surgeons allow limited or full weight bearing whereas others choose to keep patients nonweight bearing while the frame is in place *(92,98)*. Advancement to weight-bearing cast, total contact cast, or walking brace will follow after evidence of consolidation. One reasonable approach is to remove the fixator after 2 months with subsequent application of an ambulatory total contact cast for several more months until there is evidence of radiographic consolidation *(95)*. Once healed, therapeutic footwear with or without bracing is necessary to prevent recurrent foot lesions.

COMPLICATIONS

Traditionally, surgery on neuropathic joints met with a good deal of failure including high rates of nonunion, pseudoarthrosis, and infection *(2)*. Most such occurrences can now be attributed to a failure of appreciation of the natural history of osteoarthropathy and lack of attention to the necessary criteria and the basic tenets of surgery on Charcot joints as previously discussed. Even with this knowledge, however, complications can ensue in these high risk feet during the immediate postoperative period and beyond.

Infection can be a major sequel of surgery and of course can threaten the success of an attempted arthrodesis site as well as the limb itself. Most longitudinal studies and reports of surgery on Charcot joints indicate a certain percentage of patients in whom osteomyelitis or severe infection developed that necessitated major amputation *(30,45,65,66,81)*. Therefore, caution must constantly be exercised in these patients to ensure that infection or osteomyelitis is controlled and eradicated prior to reconstructive

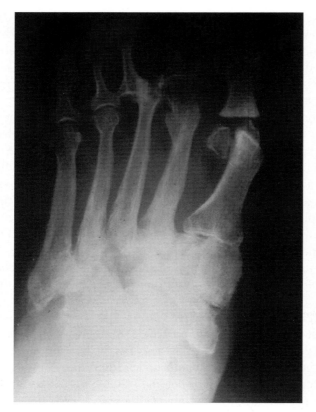

Fig. 15. Resection of the first MTP joint in this neuropathic patient eventually lead to the development of patterns I, II, and III changes presumably owing to biomechanical alterations.

surgery. Perioperative antibiotic therapy is certainly indicated in these compromised patients and once present, infection must be aggressively treated.

Pseudoarthrosis and nonunion are very troublesome complications in non-neuropathic patients undergoing arthrodesis or osteotomy. However, this is not always the case in neuropathic patients undergoing the same type of reconstructive procedures. As long as stability and satisfactory alignment are achieved, a failure of complete arthrodesis or union is not necessarily considered to be a failure of surgery *(29,30,98)*. Just as they will not sense the discomfort of post-traumatic arthritis in unreduced fracture-dislocations, these patients will have no symptoms from a stable, well aligned nonunion. Nonetheless, the surgical principles for achieving solid union as previously discussed must always be followed when operating on these patients.

Because the trauma of surgery in itself can potentially incite an acute reaction in a chronic neuropathic joint, one must always treat the newly operated foot as an active Charcot joint. Furthermore, Clohisy makes a strong argument for prophylactic immobilization of the contralateral extremity to prevent the development of an acute deformity on the supporting foot *(102)*. Ablative or corrective procedures of the forefoot can also have detrimental effects on adjacent structures as well as on the midfoot and rearfoot *(2)*. Biomechanical alterations will result in increased areas of vertical and shear stress in new sites which will then be predisposed to ulceration and osteoarthropathy (Fig. 15).

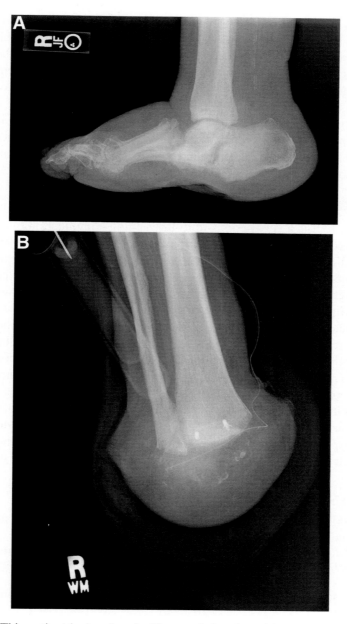

Fig. 16. (A) This patient had a chronic Charcot deformity with ulceration and recalcitrant osteomyelitis of the rearfoot for several years. **(B)** Postoperative X-ray of Syme amputation performed on same patient.

Therefore, surgery of any kind on the neuropathic foot must be performed with discretion and with attention to proper postoperative care to obviate the occurrence of these potentially destructive sequelae.

Amputation should usually be regarded as a procedure of last resort in neuropathic patients and not as a normal consequence of osteoarthropathy. Although this outcome can sometimes represent a failure in early recognition and management, amputation usually results from overwhelming postoperative infection or late stage ulcerations. Unfortunately, amputation will always be a necessary consideration in this complicated group of patients *(66,103)*. In certain situations, amputation might be the best alternative to a difficult reconstruction in an unstable patient or in those patients who do not wish to engage in the lengthy recuperative period that follows major arthrodeses. However, this must be reserved for those extremities beyond salvage after all other attempts at conservative and reconstructive care have failed. The Syme amputation can effectively be performed as a limb salvage measure in such patients when the heel pad is preserved (Fig. 16). This operation can result in a fully ambulatory patient with very rapid accommodation to the full length prosthesis *(103)*.

CONCLUSION

The Charcot foot is a very serious limb-threatening complication of diabetes, which can be attributed to preexisting peripheral neuropathy compounded by trauma of some degree. With the attendant hypervascular response coupled with osteopenia, fractures, and dislocations can rapidly evolve into severe foot deformities as a consequence of continued weight bearing. It is therefore incumbent on the practitioner to diagnose this process early in order to arrest the progression of the destructive phase and institute appropriate treatment. Although nonweight bearing and immobilization remain the mainstays of treatment in the acute stage, over the last decade there has been greater interest in surgical solutions for the severe deformities, recurrent ulcers, or instability that frequently results in later stages. As our knowledge and experience have grown, long term outcomes have improved. As of yet, however, many questions remain unanswered pertaining to the precise mechanisms involved in the etiology of osteoarthropathy as well as those concerning optimal early and late stage treatments. With a heightened suspicion for the disorder, further prospective research, and an evidence-based approach to treatment, the future holds even greater promise for these patients.

REFERENCES

1. Charcot JM. Sur quelques arthropathies qui paraissent dependre d'une lesion du cerveau ou de la moelle epiniere. *Arch Physiol Norm et Pathol* 1968;1:161.
2. Sanders LJ, Frykberg RG. "Diabetic neuropathic osteoarthropathy: charcot foot," in *The High Risk Foot in Diabetes Mellitus*. (Frykberg RG. ed.), Churchill Livingstone, New York, 1991.
3. Kelly M. John Kearsley Mitchell and the neurogenic theory of arthritis. *J Hist Med* 1965;20:151–157.
4. Armstrong DG, Todd WF, Lavery LA, Harkless LB, Bushman TR. The natural history of acute Charcot's arthropathy in a diabetic foot specialty clinic. *Diabet Med* 1997;14:357–363.
5. Mitchell JK. On a new practice in acute and chronic rheumatism. *Am J Med Sci* 1831;8:55.
6. Jordan WR. Neuritic manifestations in diabetes mellitus. *Arch Intern Med* 1936;57:307.
7. Bailey CC, Root HF. Neuropathic foot lesions in diabetes mellitus. *N Engl J Med* 1947;236:397.
8. Sinha S, Munichoodappa G, Kozak GP. Neuroarthropathy (Charcot Joints) in diabetes mellitus. Clinical study of 101 cases. *Medicine* 1972;52:191.
9. Frykberg RG, Kozak GP. Neuropathic arthropathy in the diabetic foot. *Am Fam Physician* 1978;17:105.

10. Sanders LJ, Frykberg RG. Charcot neuroarthropathy of the Foot, in *Levin and O'Neals The Diabetic Foot*. (Bowker JH, Pfeiffer MA eds.), 6th ed. Mosby, St. Louis, 2001, p. 439.

11. Cofield RH, Morrison MJ, Beabout JW. Diabetic neuroarthropathy in the foot:patient characteristics and patterns of radiographic change. *Foot Ankle* 1983;4:15.

12. Lavery LA, Armstrong DG, Wunderlich RP, Tredwell J, Boulton AJM. Diabetic foot syndrome: evaluating the prevalence and incidence of foot pathology in Mexican Americans and non-Hispanic whites from a diabetes disease management cohort. *Diabetes care* 2003; 26:1435–1438.

13. Frykberg RG, Kozak GP. The diabetic Charcot foot, in *Management of Diabetic Foot Problems*. (Kozak GP, Campbell DR, Frykberg RG, Habershaw GM eds.), 2nd ed. WB Saunders, Philadelphia, 1995, pp. 88–97.

14. Frykberg RG. Charcot foot: an update on pathogenesis and management, in *The Foot in Diabetes*. (Boulton AJM, Connor H, Cavanagh PR eds.), 3rd ed. John Wiley and Sons, Chichester, UK, 2000, pp. 235–260.

15. Gazis A, Pound N, MacFarlane R, Treece K, Game F, Jeffcoate W. Mortality in patients with diabetic neuropathic osteoarthropathy (Charcot foot). *Diabet Med* 2004;21:1243–1246.

16. International Working Group on the Diabetic Foot: International Consensus on the Diabetic Foot. Amsterdam, The Netherlands, 1999.

17. Banks AS. A clinical guide to the Charcot foot, in *Medical and Surgical Management of the Diabetic Foot*. (Kominsky SJ ed.), Mosby Yearbook, St Louis, 1994, pp. 115–143.

18. Frykberg RG, Armstrong DG, Giurini J, et al. Diabetic foot disorders: a clinical practice guideline. *J Foot Ankle Surg* 2000;39(Suppl 1):2–60.

19. Brower AC, Allman RM. Pathogenesis of the neuropathic joint: neurotraumatic vs neurovascular. *Radiology* 1981;139:349.

20. Jeffcoate W, Lima J, Nobrega L. The Charcot foot. *Diabet Med* 2000;17:253–258.

21. Boulton AJM. The diabetic foot: from art to science. The 18th Camillo Golgi lecture. *Diabetologia* 2004;47:1343–1353.

22. Veves A, Akbari CM, Primavera J, et al. Endothelial dysfunction and the expression of endothelial nitric oxide synthetase in diabetic neuropathy, vascular disease, and foot ulceration. Diabetes 1998;47:457–463.

23. Edelman SV, Kosofsky EM, Paul RA, et al. Neuro-osteoarthropathy (Charcot's Joint) in diabetes mellitus following revascularization surgery. *Arch Intern Med* 1987;147:1504.

24. Banks AS, McGlamry ED. Charcot foot. *J Am Podiatr Med Assoc* 1989;79:213.

25. Gough A, Abraha H, Li F, et al. Measurement of markers of osteoclast and osteoblast activity in patients with acute and chronic diabetic Charcot neuroarthropathy. *Diabet Med* 1997;14:527–531.

26. Young MJ, Marshall A, Adams JE, Selby PL, Boulton AJM. Osteopenia, neurological dysfunction, and the development of Charcot neuroarthropathy. *Diabetes Care* 1995;18:34–38.

27. Jirkovska A, Kasalicky P, Boucek P, Hosova J, Skibova J. Calcaneal ultrasonometry in patients with Charcot osteoarthropathy and its relationship with densitometry in the lumbar spine and femoral neck and with markers of bone turnover. *Diabet Med* 2001;18: 495–500.

28. Rajbhandari SM, Jenkins RC, Davies C, Tesfaye S. Charcot neuroarthropathy in diabetes mellitus. *Diabetologia* 2002;45:1085–1096.

29. Trepman E, Nihal A, Pinzur MS. Charcot neuroarthropathy. *Foot Ankle Int* 2005;26:46–63.

30. Johnson JTH. Neuropathic fractures of joint injuries. Pathogenesis and rationale of prevention and treatment. *J Bone Joint Surg* 1967;49A:1.

31. Herbst SA, Jones KB, Saltzman CL. Pattern of diabetic neuropathic arthropathy associated with peripheral bone mineral density. *J Bone Joint Surg* 2004;86-B:378–383.

32. Jude EB, Selby P, Burgess J, et al. Bisphosphonates in the treatment of Charcot neuroarthropathy: a double-blind randomised controlled trial. *Diabetologia* 2001;44:2032–2037.

33. Jeffcoate W. Vascular calcification and osteolysis in diabetic neuropathy—is RANK-L the missing link? *Diabetologia* 2004;47:1488–1492.
34. Eichenholtz SN. *Charcot Joints*. Charles C Thomas, Springfield, IL, 1966.
35. Schon LC, Marks RM. The management of neuroarthropathic fracture-dislocations in the diabetic patient. *Ortho Clin N Am* 1995;26:375–392.
36. Sella EJ, Barrette C. Staging of Charcot neuroarthropathy along the medial column of the foot in the diabetic patient. *J Foot Ankle Surg* 1999;38:34–40.
37. Yu GV, Hudson JR. Evaluation and treatment of Stage 0 Charcot's neuroarthropathy of the foot and ankle. *J Am Pod Med Assoc* 2002;92:210–220.
38. Harris JR, Brand PW. Patterns of disintegration of the tarsus in the anaesthetic foot. *J Bone Joint Surg* 1966;48B:4.
39. Brodsky JW, Rouse AM. Exostectomy for symptomatic bony prominences in diabetic Charcot feet. *Clin Orth Rel Res* 1993;296:21–26.
40. Schon LC, Weinfeld SB, Horton GA, Resch S. Radiographic and clinical classification of acquired midtarsus deformities. *Foot Ankle Int* 1998;19:394–404.
41. Frykberg RG, Mendeszoon ER. Charcot arthropathy: pathogenesis and management. *Wounds* 2000;12(Suppl B):35B–42B.
42. Newman JH. Non-infective disease of the diabetic foot. *J Bone Joint Surg* 1981;63B:593.
43. Newman JH. Spontaneous dislocation in diabetic neuropathy: a report of six cases. *J Bone Joint Surg* 1979;61B:484.
44. Lesko P, Maurer RC. Talonavicular dislocations and midfoot arthropathy in neuropathic diabetic feet: natural course and principles of treatment. *Clin Orthop* 1989;240:226.
45. Fabrin J, Larsen K, Holstein PE. Long-term follow-up in diabetic Charcot feet with spontaneous onset. *Diabet Care* 2000;23:796–800.
46. El-Khoury GY, Kathol MH. Neuropathic fractures in patients with diabetes mellitus. *Radiology* 1980;134:313.
47. Kathol MH, El-Khoury GY, Moore TE, et al. Calcaneal insufficiency avulsion fractures in patients with diabetes mellitus. *Radiology* 1991;180:725.
48. Petrova NL, Foster AVM, Edmonds ME. Difference in presentation of Charcot osteoarthropathy in type 1 compared with type 2 diabetes. *Diabet Care* 2004;27:1235, 1236.
49. Pakarinen T-K, Laine H-J, Honkonen SE, Peltonen J, Oksala H, Lahtela J. Charcot arthropathy of the diabetic foot. Current concepts and review of 36 cases. *Scand J Surgery* 2002;91:195–201.
50. McGill M, Molyneaux L, Ioannou K, Uren R, Yue DK. Response of Charcot's arthropathy to contact casting: assessment by quantitative techniques. *Diabetologia* 2000;43:481–484.
51. Caputo GM, Ulbrecht J, Cavanagh PR, Juliano P. The Charcot foot in diabetes: six key points. *Am Fam Phys* 1998;57:2705–2710.
52. Sella EJ, Grosser DM. Imaging modalities of the diabetic foot. *Clin Podiatr Med Surg* 2003;20:729–740.
53. Keenan AM, Tindel NL, Alavi A. Diagnosis of pedal osteomyelitis in diabetic patients using current scintigraphic techniques. *Arch Intern Med* 1989;149:2262–2266.
54. Schweitzer ME, Morrison WB. MR imaging in the diabetic foot. *Radiol Clin N Am* 2004;42:61–71.
55. Palestro CJ, Mehta HH, Patel M. Marrow versus infection in Charcot joint: indium-111 leukocyte and technetium-99m sulphur colloid scintigraphy. *J Nucl Med* 1998;39:346–350.
56. Armstrong DG, Lavery LA, Sariaya M, Ashry H. Leukocytosis is a poor indicator of acute osteomyelitis of the foot in diabetes mellitus. *J Foot Ankle Surgery* 1996;35:280–283.
57. Seabold JE, Flickinger FW, Kao S, et al. Indium-111 leukocyte/technetium-99m-MDP bone and magnetic resonance imaging: difficulty of diagnosing osteomyelitis in patients with neuropathic osteoarthropathy. *J Nucl Med* 1990;31:549–556.

58. Schauwecker DS, Park HM, Burt RW, Mock BH, Wellman HN. Combined bone scintigraphy and Indium-111 leukocyte scans in neuropathic foot disease. *J Nucl Med* 1988;29:1651–1655.
59. Johnson JE, Kennedy EJ, Shereff MJ, Patel NC, Collier BD. Prospective study of bone, indium-111-labeled white blood cell, and gallium-67 scanning for the evaluation of osteomyelitis in the diabetic foot. *Foot Ankle Int* 1996;17:10–16.
60. Blume PA, Dey HM, Daley LJ, Arrighi JA, Soufer R, Gorecki GA. Diagnosis of pedal osteomyelitis with Tc-99m HMPAO labeled leukocytes. *J Foot Ankle Surg* 1997;36: 120–126.
61. Croll SD, Nicholas GG, Osborne MA, Wasser TE, Jones S. Role of magnetic resonance imaging in the diagnosis of osteomyelitis in diabetic foot infection. *J Vasc Surg* 1996;24: 266–270.
62. Hopfner S, Krolak C, Kessler S, Tiling R, Brinkbaumer K, Hahn K, et al. Preoperative imaging of Charcot neuroarthropathy in diabetic patients: comparison of ring PET, hybrid PET, and magnetic resonance imaging. *Foot Ankle Int* 2004;25:890–895.
63. Pinzur MS, Shields N, Trepman E, Dawson P, Evans A. Current practice patterns in the treatment of Charcot foot. *Foot Ankle Int* 2000;21:916–920.
64. Pinzur MS, Sage R, Stuck R, Kaminsky S, Zmuda A. A treatment algorithm for neuropathic (Charcot) midfoot deformity. *Foot and Ankle* 1993;14:189–197.
65. Myerson MS, Henderson MR, Saxby T, Short KW. Management of midfoot diabetic neuroarthropathy. *Foot Ankle Int* 1994;15:233–241.
66. Pinzur M. Surgical versus accommodative treatment for Charcot arthropathy of the midfoot. *Foot Ankle Int* 2004;25:545–549.
67. Armstrong DG, Peters EJG. Charcot's arthropathy of the foot. *J Am Pod Med Assoc* 2002;92:390–394.
68. Giurini JM. Applications and use of in-shoe orthoses in the conservative management of Charcot foot deformity. *Clin Podiatr Med* 1994;11(2):271.
69. Morgan JM, Biehl WC, Wagner FW. Management of neuropathic neuropathy with the Charcot restraint orthotic walker. *Clin Orthop* 1993;296:58.
70. Mehta JA, Brown C, Sargeant N. Charcot restraint orthotic walker. *Foot Ankle* Int 1998; 19:619–623.
71. Armstrong DG, Short B, Espensen EH, Abu-Rumman PL, Nixon BP, Boulton AJM. Technique for fabrication of an "instant total-contact cast" for treatment of neuropathic diabetic foot ulcers. *J Am Pod Med Assoc* 2002;92:405–408.
72. Guse ST, Alvine FG. Treatment of diabetic foot ulcers and Charcot neuroarthropathy using the patellar tendon-bearing brace. *Foot Ankle* 1997;18(10):675.
73. Saltzman CL, et al. The patellar tendon-bearing brace as treatment for neuropathic arthropathy: a dynamic force monitoring study. *Foot Ankle* 1992;13(1):14.
74. Selby PL, Young MJ, Boulton AJM. Bisphosphonates: a new treatment for diabetic charcot neuroarthropathy? *Diabetic Med* 1994;11(1):28.
75. Jude EB, Selby P, Burgess J, et al. Bisphosphonates in the treatment of Charcot neuroarthropathy: a double-blind randomised controlled trial. *Diabetologia* 2001;44:2032–2037.
76. Anderson JJ, Woelffer KE, Holtzman JJ, Jacobs AM. Bisphosphonates for the treatment of Charcot neuroarthropathy. *J Foot Ankle Surg* 2004;43:285–289.
77. Beir RR, Estersohn HS. A new treatment for Charcot joint in the diabetic foot. *J Am Pod Med Assoc* 1987;77(2):63.
78. Hanft JR, Goggin JP, Landsman A, et al. The role of combined magnetic field bone growth stimulation as an adjunct in the treatment of neuroarthropathy/Charcot Joint: an expanded pilot study. *J Foot Ankle Surg* 1998;37:510–515.
79. Grady JF, O'Connor KJ, Axe T, Zager EJ, Dennis LM, Brenner LA. Use of electrostimulation in the treatment of diabetic neuroarthropathy. *J Am Pod Med Assoc* 2000;90: 287–294.

80. Strauss E, Gonya G. Adjunct low intensity ultrasound in Charcot neuroarthropathy. *Clin Ortho Related Res* 1998;349:132–138.
81. Papa J, Myerson M, Girard P. Salvage, with arthrodesis, in intractable diabetic neuropathic arthropathy of the foot and ankle. *J Bone Joint Surg* 1993;75A(12):1056.
82. Pinzur MS. Benchmark analysis of diabetic patients with neuropathic (Charcot) foot deformity. *Foot Ankle Int* 1999;20:564–567.
83. Myerson MS, Alvarez RG, Lam PW. Tibiocalcaneal arthrodesis for the management of severe ankle and hindfoot deformities. *Foot Ankle Int* 2000;21:643–650.
84. Steindler A. The tabetic arthropathies. *JAMA* 1931;96:250.
85. Samilson RL, Sankaran B, Bersani FA, Smith AD. Orthopedic management of neuropathic joints. *Arch Surg* 1959;78:115.
86. Heiple KG, Cammarn MR. Diabetic neuroarthropathy with spontaneous peritalar fracture-dislocation. *JBJS* 1966;48A:1177.
87. Baravarian B, Van Gils CC. Arthrodesis of the Charcot foot and ankle. *Clin Podiatr Med Surg* 2004;21:271–289.
88. Leventen EO. Charcot Foot—a technique for treatment of chronic plantar ulcer by saucerization and primary closure. *Foot and Ankle* 1986;6:295.
89. Catanzariti AR, Mendocino R, Haverstock B. Ostectomy for diabetic neuroarthropathy involving the midfoot. *J Foot Ankle Surg* 2000;39:291–300.
90. Rosenblum BI, Giuini JM, Miller LB, Chrzan JS, Habershaw GM. Neuropathic ulcerations plantar to the lateral column in patients with Charcot foot deformity: a flexible approach to limb salvage. *J Foot Ankle Surg* 1997;36:360–363.
91. Simon SR, Tejwani SG, Wilson DL, Santner TJ, Denniston NL. Arthrodesis as an early alternative to nonoperative management of Charcot arthropathy of the diabetic foot. *J Bone Joint Surg* 2000;82-A:939–950.
92. Wang JC, Le AW, Tsukuda RK. A new technique for Charcot's foot reconstruction. *J Am Pod Med Assoc* 2002;92:429–436.
93. Jolly GP, Zgonis T, Polyzois V. External fixation in the management of Charcot neuroarthropathy. *Clin Podiatr Med Surg* 2003;20:741–756.
94. Johnson JE. Operative treatment of neuropathic arthropathy of the foot and ankle. *J Bone Joint Surg* 1998;80-A:1700–1709.
95. Farber DC, Juliano PJ, Cavanagh PR, Ulbrecht J, Caputo G. Single stage correction with external fixation of the ulcerated foot in individuals with Charcot neuroarthropathy. *Foot Ankle Int* 2002;23:130–134.
96. Thompson RC, Clohisy DR. Deformity following fracture in diabetic neuropathic osteoarthropathy: operative management of adults who have type-I diabetes. *J Bone Joint Surg* 1993;75A(12):1765.
97. Marks RM, Parks BG, Schon LC. Midfoot fusion technique for neuroarthropathic feet: biomechanical analysis and rationale. *Foot Ankle Int* 1998;19:507–510.
98. Cooper PS. Application of external fixators for management of Charcot deformities of the foot and ankle. *Seminars Vasc Surg* 2003;16:67–78.
99. Medicino RW, Catanzariti AR, Saltrick KR, et al. Tibiotalocalcaneal arthrodesis with retrograde intramedullary nailing. *J Foot Ankle Surg* 2004;43:82–86.
100. Pinzur MS, Kelikian A. Charcot ankle fusion with a retrograde locked intramedullary nail. *Foot Ankle Int* 1997;18:699–704.
101. Moore TJ, Prince R, Pochatko D, Smith JW, Fleming S. Retrograde intramedullary nailing for ankle arthrodesis. *Foot Ankle Int* 1995;16:433–436.
102. Clohisy DR, Thompson RC. Fractures associated with neuropathic arthropathy in adults who have juvenile-onset diabetes. *J Bone Joint Surg* 1988;70A:1192.
103. Eckardt A, Schollner C, Decking J, et al. The impact of Syme amputation in surgical treatment of patients with diabetic foot syndrome and Charcot neuro-osteoarthropathy. *Arch Orthop Trauma Surg* 2004;124:145–150.

15

Preparation of the Wound Bed of the Diabetic Foot Ulcer

Vincent Falanga, MD, FACP

INTRODUCTION

Over the last few years, substantial advances have been made in our understanding of diabetic foot ulcers, the importance of thorough surgical debridement, and how this standard therapeutic modality impacts on wound bed preparation. Importantly, wound bed preparation is revolutionizing the way we approach nonhealing or difficult to heal wounds. Much of what we do clinically, from elimination of bacterial burden, to debridement, and to the use of new technologies to heal diabetic foot ulcers, can now be seen as helping wound bed preparation and facilitating the process of healing. From a therapeutic standpoint, at least in the United States, large multicenter clinical trials have led to the regulatory approval of topically applied platelet-derived growth factor (PDGF)-BB (Regranex, Ortho McNeill, NJ) and bioengineered skin (Apligraf, Organogenesis, Canton, MA; Dermagraft, Smith & Nephew, Largo, FL), and have dramatically increased the number of available therapeutic options. However, not to be forgotten are advances that these and other clinical trials have brought to the standard of care for treating neuropathic diabetic foot ulcers. Indeed, these improvements in standards of care for diabetic foot ulcers have raised the bar for proving the effectiveness of new treatments. Stated differently, it has become harder to prove the effectiveness of new therapeutic agents. Thus, from now on we may be looking for "quantum" jumps in therapeutic efficacy in the treatment of diabetic foot ulcers.

The aim of this review is to examine certain basic science factors involved in the development of diabetic foot ulcers, critical therapeutic advances, such as topically applied growth factors and dermal (Dermagraft) or bilayered (Apligraf) bioengineered skin, and to discuss these topics in the context of wound bed preparation (discussed later). We will focus on the role of debridement, how it affects wound bed preparation, and how the two are intimately linked.

OVERVIEW OF DEBRIDEMENT AND WOUND BED PREPARATION

It was always assumed that clinicians would uniformly perform surgical debridement as part of a unified approach to the care of chronic wounds. However, this assumption may have been wrong, and the meaning of debridement was variable. The extent of

From: *The Diabetic Foot, Second Edition*
Edited by: A. Veves, J. M. Giurini, and F. W. LoGerfo © Humana Press Inc., Totowa, NJ

debridement, too, did not reflect the reality of office practice and clinical trials. This is not to say that competent clinicians did not perform debridement of eschars and frankly necrotic tissue in compromised diabetic foot ulcers. However, it has become increasingly clear that regular debridement, to remove the callus surrounding the wound and the fibrinous wound bed (not necessarily frankly necrotic), may not have been widely practiced *(1,2)*. We have called this more thorough and regular approach "maintenance debridement" for diabetic foot ulcers, in the context of wound bed preparation *(3–5)*. To what extent not following this "standard of care" may have played a role in the failure of showing effectiveness of certain therapeutic products in the past is unclear. The initial pilot study of topically applied PDGF changed the way we conduct clinical trials for diabetic foot ulcers. Indeed, the effectiveness of PDGF in those trials seems to have been highly dependent on concomitant and thorough maintenance debridement, and actually worked synergistically with it. This important relationship between debridement and efficacy of and advanced therapeutic product has been discussed elsewhere, and is part of this review in the way it affects the way we view wound bed preparation. It should be noted here that subsequent trials in diabetic ulcers adopted maintenance debridement of the wound bed and callus, to the point that maintenance debridement is now considered the standard of care. In this review, we will discuss certain abnormalities involved in the pathogenesis of diabetic foot ulcers and their failure to heal and which have a great impact on wound bed preparation. Traditionally, these cellular and molecular abnormalities have been wrongly considered separately from the clinical approach, with debridement being seen mostly as a mundane clinical procedure. However, as we shall see, close interactions are emerging between molecular events and certain critical aspects of wound care. Wound bed preparation is a unifying concept, which embodies many of these interactions. Figure 1 illustrates this important concept.

OVERVIEW OF DIABETIC FOOT ULCERS
AND PATHOPHYSIOLOGICAL PRINCIPLES

Recent publications provide reviews of diabetic ulcers, their basic pathophysiology, and appropriate treatments *(6,7)*. Besides arterial insufficiency, neuropathy plays a major role in the development of ulceration in patients with diabetes. It is important to realize that our concepts of pathophysiology have important consequences on treatment. For example, for decades it was thought that the main problem in diabetes was "small vessel disease," a rather poorly defined term that was offered as an explanation for many of the complications of this disease, including foot ulcers. It is likely that much needed surgical revascularizing procedures were not performed because of the notion of small vessel disease. Therefore, the realization a few years ago that the concept of a true occlusive microangiopathy in the lower extremities of patients with diabetes is incorrect or not specific for patients with diabetes has brought about a dramatic benefit in how revascularization of the diabetic foot is viewed and practiced *(8)*.

Particularly in the context of diabetic ulcers, in the past clinicians and scientists have talked about "failure to heal" *(9)*. However, this term does not accurately describe what is observed clinically, and it may be preferable to use the term "impaired healing." The fact is that many chronic wounds, including those resulting from diabetic complication, do heal in an appropriate time frame. For example, with uncomplicated diabetic

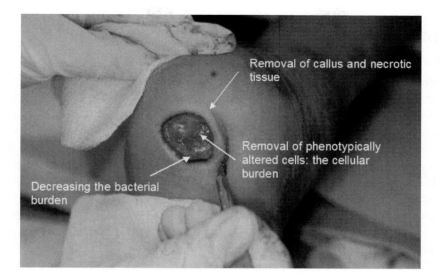

Removal of callus and necrotic tissue

Removal of phenotypically altered cells: the cellular burden

Decreasing the bacterial burden

Fig. 1. Clinical photograph showing surgical debridement of the callus and wound bed in a diabetic neuropathic foot ulcer. The photograph also indicates how the surgical debridement may remove the necrotic tissue, bacterial burden and, possibly, phenotypically altered cells that may interfere with healing.

neuropathic foot ulcers, healing should occur relatively unimpeded once off-loading is appropriately practiced *(10)*. However, truly prospective studies are required to answer the question of whether relatively simple measures, such as contact casting, can greatly improve ulcer healing.

A typical feature of diabetic ulcers is their propensity to become heavily colonized with bacterial and, less commonly, fungal organisms. These factors play a major role in the failure to heal. Bacterial colonization has also been called bioburden or bacterial burden. There remain questions regarding what constitutes an unacceptable level of organisms in the tissues and one that would disrupt the healing process. This has been discussed extensively in other publications *(11)*. However, there is evidence that, regardless of the type of bacteria present, a level greater than or equal to 10^6 organisms per gram of tissue is associated with serious healing impairment. Federal guidelines developed for the treatment of pressure (decubitus) ulcers (pressure plays a major role diabetic neuropathic foot ulcers) recommend quantitative bacteriology, requiring a wound biopsy, if there is continued healing impairment. In practical terms, it makes theoretic and clinical sense to decrease the bacterial burden of wounds. Nevertheless, we know very little about the mechanisms underlying impaired healing in the presence of large number of organisms. More recently, there has been increasing interest in the possible presence of biofilms in chronic wounds and their role in impaired healing or even ulcer recurrence. Biofilms represent bacterial colonies surrounded by a protective coat of polysaccharides; such colonies become more easily resistant to the action of antimicrobials *(12)*. At the moment, there is no hard evidence for what role biofilms play in diabetic foot ulcers. Debridement can remove the bacterial burden and "reset" the diabetic foot ulcer in a mode that is more conducive to healing.

OTHER PATHOPHYSIOLOGICAL FACTORS INTERACTING WITH DEBRIDEMENT AND WOUND BED PREPARATION

Growth Factor "Trapping"

Debridement has other important impacts on basic pathophysiological abnormalities. Thus, removing the callus and the fibrinous wound bed can have consequences on growth factor availability. The concept of growth factor trapping was first developed in the context of venous ulcers *(13)*, but has applicability to a variety of chronic wounds, including diabetic neuropathic foot ulcers. The hypothesis is that certain macromolecules and even growth factors are bound or "trapped" in the tissues, which could result in unavailability or maldistribution of critical mediators, including cytokines *(13,14)*. Even topically applied growth factors can suffer the same fate of becoming bound to leaked macromolecules and altered matrix components. Trapping of growth factors and cytokines, as well as matrix material, however limited, has the potential to cause a cascade of pathogenic abnormalities. For example, in the well-coordinated process of wound healing, disruption of some key mediators could have adverse consequences well downstream. Binding of growth factors by macromolecules that leak into the dermis, such as albumin, fibrinogen, and α-2-macroglobulin may disrupt the healing process. α,-2-macroglobulin is an established scavenger for growth factors. There is also evidence that transforming growth factor-β_1, a critical multifunctional polypeptide, is bound within the pericapillary fibrin cuffs in the dermis *(13,14)*.

Wound Fluid and Metalloproteinases

The bacterial burden, the inflammatory process developing in diabetic foot ulcers, alter the balance between appropriate moisture levels in the wound, matrix deposition and remodeling, and the levels of tissue metalloproteinases. A major breakthrough of the last 50 years, in terms of how we manage wounds, was the experimental evidence by George Winter indicating that re-epithelization is accelerated when wounds are kept moist *(15)*. This advance has led to the development of a vast array of moisture-retentive dressings that promote "moist wound healing" *(16,17)*. The experimental evidence for moist wound healing was mainly developed in acute wounds, and its lessons were quickly extrapolated to chronic wounds. Contrary to what had always been conventional wisdom, keeping the wound moist has not resulted in increased infection rates *(18–20)*. However, that remains a fear of many clinicians. It is not entirely clear whether moisture-retentive dressings work mainly by keeping the wound fluid in contact with the wound. One of the reasons for this uncertainty is that wound fluid appears to have distinctly different properties in acute and chronic wounds. For example, it has been shown that fluid collected from acute wounds will stimulate the in vitro proliferation of fibroblasts, keratinocytes, and endothelial cells *(21–23)* Conversely, fluid obtained from chronic wounds will block cellular proliferation and angiogenesis *(24)* and contains excessive amounts of matrix metalloproteinases (MMPs) capable of breaking down critical extracellular matrix proteins, including fibronectin and vitronectin *(25–27)*. Undoubtedly, MMPs play a key role in the wound healing *(28)*. For example, interstitial collagenase (MMP-1) is important for keratinocyte migration *(29)*. In contrast, it has been suggested that excessive activity (or maldistribution) of other enzymes (MMP-2, MMP-8, MMP-9) contribute to healing impairment *(30,31)*. Taken together, however, the emerging evidence is that control of MMPs and their localization could have important therapeutic implications, including the enhanced survival of topically applied growth factors.

Impaired Blood Flow and Hypoxia

Of particular importance in diabetic ulcers is the level of oxygen tension at the wound site. In the case of ulcers because of poor tissue perfusion and consequent hypoxia, revascularization is required. However, in ulcers whose pathogenesis is mainly pressure in the presence of adequate blood flow, hypoxia may be playing some interesting roles. Ischemia will lead to tissue necrosis, and that will often result in wounds that are more easily compromised by infection. There is a substantial body of data indicating that low levels of oxygen tension as measured at the skin surface (transcutaneous oxygen measurements or $TcPO_2$) correlate with inability to heal *(32)*. These data are most relevant in the treatment of diabetic ulcers, and can often guide therapy and even the level of amputation. However, it should be noted that ischemia is not the same as hypoxia. Interestingly, from a biological standpoint, low levels of oxygen tension can stimulate fibroblast proliferation and clonal growth *(33)* and can actually enhance the transcription and synthesis of a number of growth factors *(34–36)*. However, there is also evidence that exposure to hyperbaric oxygen can increase the production of vascular endothelial growth factor *(37)*. It is possible that low oxygen tension can serve as a potent initial stimulus after injury but that prolonged hypoxia, as seen in chronic wounds, can lead to a number of abnormalities including scarring and fibrosis.

The Pathophysiological Status of the Wound and Phenotypic Alteration of Wound Cells

Another critical relationship can be established between the value of maintenance debridement and the removal of resident wound cells that have become phenotypically abnormal. The normal process of wound repair goes through well-defined stages that are well studied. However, as stated, chronic wounds do not seem to have defined time frames for healing. This is apparent both clinical and from the pathophysiological standpoint. It has been stated that the diabetic ulcers is "stuck" in the proliferative phase of wound repair. Indeed, there is evidence that the accumulation and remodeling of diabetic foot ulcers are impaired with respect to certain matrix protein, including fibronectin *(38–40)*. There is also increasing evidence that the resident cells of chronic wounds have undergone phenotypic changes that impair their capacity for proliferation and movement *(38–40)*. To what extent this is because of cellular senescence is unknown, but the response of diabetic ulcer fibroblasts to growth factors seems to be either impaired or requiring a sequence of growth factors. Similar observations have been made in other types of chronic wounds. For example, it has been reported that fibroblasts from venous and pressure ulcers are senescent, show diminished ability to proliferate *(41–44)*, and that their decreased proliferative capacity correlates with failure to heal and lack of response to PDGF *(45,46)*. There is also substantial evidence that ulcer fibroblasts are insensitive to the action of transforming growth factor-β_1, and that this is the result of decreased receptor expression *(47)* and phosphorylation of key signaling proteins, including Smads and MAPK *(48)*. At the moment, it is not known whether this phenotypic abnormality of wound cells is only observed in vitro and whether it plays a role in impaired healing.

WOUND BED PREPARATION AS A NEW PARADIGM
FOR DIABETIC FOOT ULCERS

Advances in the treatment of diabetic foot ulcers have relied heavily on the concepts developed for acute wounds. In the last few years, however, a new paradigm for addressing chronic wounds, including diabetic foot ulcers, is emerging. We have applied the term "wound bed preparation" to this paradigm, trying to emphasize the importance of optimizing the appearance and readiness of the wound bed *(3)*. The main point, however, is that this approach represents a way for us to emphasize that and their way to achieve complete closure is different than from acute wounds *(4,5)*. As new insights and therapeutic modalities become available, for example, stem cells, we may be talking more about "wound bed reconstitution." The critical concept is that, once appropriate steps have been taken to optimize the wound bed, then the normal endogenous process of wound healing is going to be facilitated *(5)*. It is important to note that wound bed preparation is more than surgical debridement alone, but rather a very comprehensive approach aimed at reducing edema and exudate, eliminating or reducing the bacterial burden and, importantly, correcting the abnormalities discussed earlier as contributing to impaired healing. There are both basic and more advanced approaches to wound bed preparation/optimization. Basic aspects, as with compromised acute wounds, include debridement, infection control, edema removal, and surgical correction of underlying defect. More advanced aspects, for which we may not have all the answers yet, include attempts at wound bed reconstitution, as with the use of biological agents.

THERAPEUTIC ADVANCES INTERACTING
WITH WOUND BED PREPARATION

As stated throughout this review, important and intimate links exist between debridement, wound bed preparation and reconstitution, and therapeutic advances. In the last few years, we have seen the development and marketing of very sophisticated products for impaired healing. These products, whether they are growth factors or tissue engineering constructs, represent the culmination of decades of basic research. As we have already mentioned, the efficacy of many advanced therapeutic agents has not matched the expectations, partly because the standards of care for some chronic wounds, including diabetic foot ulcers, were not adequate. In a way, wound bed preparation was not born yet. For example, the process of surgical debridement of diabetic foot ulcers becomes more than simply removing necrotic tissue; at the same time one is also removing the excessive bacterial burden and, possibly, the phenotypically abnormal cells that may be present in and around the wound (Fig. 1). Another example is the removal of edema, which is also critical in the management of diabetic ulcers. Edema removal decreases the chronic wound fluid that has been shown to be deleterious to resident cells and which may enhance bacterial colonization. Therefore, existing therapies can be integrated better with pathophysiological principles *(3–5)*.

Moreover, we have now found that even advanced therapies may be thought of as methods for improving wound bed preparation, because ultimately we are accelerating the endogenous process of wound healing. There are many examples of this. Over the last two decades, several recombinant growth factors have been tested for their ability to accelerate the healing of chronic wounds. Among others, some promising results have been obtained with the use of epidermal growth factor for venous ulcers *(49)*, fibroblast growth factor *(50)*, and PDGF for pressure ulcers *(51)*. However, at least in the United States, the only topically applied growth factor that is commercially approved for use is PDGF. In randomized controlled clinical studies, PDGF has been shown to accelerate the healing of neuropathic diabetic foot ulcers by approx 15% *(1,52)*.

One may wonder why we do not have a greater number of growth factors approved for clinical use, and why the results of clinical trials have not been of greater magnitude, as we might have predicted from preclinical data. A number of explanations can be given for this, and perhaps all of them apply. Inadequate dosage, mode of delivery of the peptide, and possibly the need for combinations of growth factors are some of the problems hypothesized to explain the lack of more dramatic clinical effects. It is also possible however, that closer attention should have been paid to appropriately preparing the chronic wound before treatment with the growth factor being tested in clinical trials. Notably, there is evidence that the aggressive approach to surgical debridement in the initial PDGF trial for diabetic neuropathic ulcers seems to have worked synergistically with the application of the growth factor *(2)*. It is important to note that the treatment of chronic wounds has been evolving in the last few years, and it might be argued that the increased number of randomized clinical trials for chronic wounds has improved standard wound care. If this is so, it is expected that in the future new products will need to perform much better than control to show efficacy.

Bioengineered Skin

Another major advanced treatment that can improve wound bed preparation is cell therapy, such as with the use of bioengineered skin. A number of bioengineered skin products or skin equivalents have become available for the treatment of acute and chronic wounds, as well as for burns. Since the initial use of keratinocyte sheets *(53,54)*, several more complex constructs have been developed and tested in human wounds. Skin equivalents may contain living cells, such as fibroblasts or keratinocytes or both *(55–59)*, whereas others are made of acellular materials or extracts of living cells. Some allogeneic constructs consisting of living cells derived from neonatal foreskin have been shown to accelerate the healing of neuropathic diabetic foot ulcers in randomized controlled trials, and are available for clinical use *(60,61)*. The clinical effect of these constructs is between 15% and 20% over conventional "control" therapy. One of the important arguments relates to what constitutes an appropriate control. In the US trials, saline soaked gauze and off-loading have been accepted by the Food and Drug Administration as the control. However, the methods for off-loading differ in many countries, and the wound dressings to be used are also subject to controversy *(10)*. Truly prospective trials need to be done to determine the contribution of off-loading done with contact casting and how this approach can improve the outcome in patients treated with advanced biological products.

Bioengineered skin may work by delivering living cells, which are said to be "smart" in engineering terms, and thus capable of adapting to their environment. There is evidence that some of the living constructs are able to release growth factors and cytokines, but this cannot yet be interpreted as being their mechanism of action *(62)*. It should be noted that some of these allogeneic constructs do not survive for more than a few weeks when placed in a chronic wound.

Gene Therapy and Stem Cells

At the forefront of advanced treatments, stand gene therapy and the use of stem cells. As we have discussed, a spectrum is likely to evolve, going from wound bed preparation to wound bed reconstitution. Gene therapy and stem cells have the potential to drastically alter the wound bed and may thus be at the right end of the spectrum, toward wound bed reconstitution. For some time now, there has been ample technology for introducing certain genes into wounds by a variety of physical means or biological vectors, including viruses. There are ex vivo approaches, in which cells may be manipulated before reintroduction into the wound, to more direct in vivo techniques, which may rely on simple injection or the use of the gene gun *(63)*. Inability to achieve stable and prolonged expression of a gene product, which has been a problem in the gene therapy treatment of systemic conditions, can actually be an advantage in the context of nonhealing wounds, in which only transient expression may be required. Most of the work with gene therapy of wounds has been done in experimental animal models. However, there are promising indications that certain approaches may work in human wounds. For example, the introduction of naked plasmid DNA encoding the gene for vascular endothelial growth factor has been reported to enhance healing and angiogenesis in selected patients with ulcers from arterial insufficiency *(64)*. Undoubtedly, the area of gene therapy for chronic human wounds will become very active in the next few years. The introduction of the gene, rather than its product, i.e., a growth factor, is seen as a less expensive and potentially more efficient delivery method.

An extension of the hypothesis that cell therapy may be required to recondition chronic wounds and to accelerate their healing is the notion that stem cells might perhaps offer greater advantages. Pluripotential stem cells are capable of differentiating into a variety of cell types, including fibroblasts, endothelial cells, and keratinocytes, which are critical cellular components required for healing. Although the subject of some controversy, pluripotential mesenchymal stem cells may be present in the bone marrow *(65–67)*. A recent uncontrolled report suggests that direct application of autologous bone marrow and its cultured cells may accelerate the healing of nonhealing chronic wounds *(68)*. This type of report needs to be confirmed in a larger controlled trial. Nevertheless, when considering the pathophysiological abnormalities present in chronic wounds, there is the potential that stem cells may reconstitute dermal, vascular, and other components required for optimal healing.

SUMMARY

A rational strategy for addressing diabetic foot ulcers will likely require greater understanding of the clinical factors involved as well as the pathophysiological components that underlie their impaired healing. Greater therapeutic aggressiveness is required as well. For example, existing advanced therapeutic products tested in diabetic foot ulcers, such as growth factors and skin equivalents, have focused entirely on neuropathic ulcers of the metatarsal heads; arterial insufficiency, and the more complex heel ulcers have been exclusion criteria in those trials. Such purely neuropathic ulcers are relatively straightforward, and many clinicians believe that they can be effectively treated with sound surgical debridement and off-loading. Although it may be argued that accelerating the healing of even these relatively simple ulcers may prevent complications from infection, more needs to be done to show cost-effectiveness to our society as a whole. Still, considerable progress has been made, and a number of therapeutic approaches, including improved standard care, are now available. It is hoped that continued advances will come about which, when combined with basic medical and surgical approaches will accelerate healing of chronic wounds to an extent that is still not possible with present therapeutic agents. Wound bed preparation is changing the approach to diabetic foot ulcers and other types of chronic wounds. Debridement is seen as more than removal of unwanted necrotic tissue and callus. As illustrated in Fig. 1, surgical debridement may be a way to also decrease the bacterial burden and to remove phenotypically altered cells that may be interfering with the healing process. As stated earlier, debridement in diabetic foot ulcers is preferably done by surgical means, although there is a need for better topical debriding agents. Presently, there is also reliance on slow release antiseptics (silver or iodine based) and, to a lesser extent, on autolytic debridement with occlusive dressings. The emphasis by regulatory agency to determine the efficacy of debriding agents in terms of healing endpoints has not helped; industry has been reluctant to embark on such expensive studies, and patients may be suffering from this regulatory link between debridement and healing outcome. Hopefully, this regulatory policy will change in the future. What has also become clear is that therapeutic agents may actually work by improving wound bed preparation, thus allowing the endogenous process of wound healing to move forward. As a result of many advances, including the concepts of maintenance debridement and wound bed preparation, the standards of care for diabetic foot ulcers have improved. As stated earlier, because the control group will receive better care in therapeutic trials, it will become more difficult to prove the effectiveness of novel therapeutic agents. However, we should strive for a "quantum" jump in the way we deal with diabetic foot ulcers and other chronic wounds. Perhaps, the use of gene therapy, stem cells, may provide a quantum advance in accelerating diabetic foot ulcer healing. With the acceptance of wound bed preparation of which debridement is an integral part, we will move toward wound bed reconstitution, which will require more active and innovative therapeutic approaches.

ACKNOWLEDGMENT

This work was supported by NIH grants AR42936, AR46557, and DK067836.

REFERENCES

1. Steed DL. Clinical evaluation of recombinant human platelet-derived growth factor for the treatment of lower extremity diabetic ulcers. Diabetic Ulcer Study Group. *J Vasc Surg* 1995;21(1):71–78 (Discussion 79–81).
2. Steed DL, et al. Effect of extensive debridement and treatment on the healing of diabetic foot ulcers. Diabetic Ulcer Study Group. *J Am Coll Surg* 1996;183(1):61–64.
3. Falanga V. Classifications for wound bed preparation and stimulation of chronic wounds. *Wound Repair Regen* 2000;8(5):347–352.
4. Falanga V. Wound bed preparation: future approaches. *Ostomy Wound Manage* 2003;49(5A Suppl):30–33.
5. Saap LJ, Falanga V. Debridement performance index and its correlation with complete closure of diabetic foot ulcers. *Wound Repair Regen* 2002;10(6):354–359.
6. Jeffcoate WJ, Price P, Harding KG. Wound healing and treatments for people with diabetic foot ulcers. Diabetes Metab Res Rev 2004;20(Suppl 1):S78–S89.

7. Boulton AJ, Kirsner RS, Vileikyte L. Clinical practice. Neuropathic diabetic foot ulcers. N Engl J Med 2004;351(1):48–55.
8. LoGerfo FW, Coffman JD. Current concepts. Vascular and microvascular disease of the foot in diabetes. Implications for foot care. *N Engl J Med* 1984;311(25):1615–1619.
9. Pecoraro RE, et al. Chronology and determinants of tissue repair in diabetic lower-extremity ulcers. *Diabetes* 1991;40(10):1305–1313.
10. Armstrong DG, et al. Off-loading the diabetic foot wound: a randomized clinical trial. *Diabetes Care* 2001;24(6):1019–1022.
11. Robson MC, et al. Maintenance of wound bacterial balance. *Am J Surg* 1999;178(5):399–402.
12. Edwards R, Harding KG. Bacteria and wound healing. *Curr Opin Infect Dis* 2004;17(2):91–96.
13. Falanga V, Eaglstein WH. The "trap" hypothesis of venous ulceration. *Lancet* 1993; 341(8851):1006–1008.
14. Higley HR, et al. Extravasation of macromolecules and possible trapping of transforming growth factor-beta in venous ulceration. *Br J Dermatol* 1995;132(1):79–85.
15. Falanga V. Occlusive wound dressings. Why, when, which?. *Arch Dermatol* 1988; 124(6): 872–877.
16. Helfman T, Ovington L, Falanga, V. Occlusive dressings and wound healing. *Clin Dermatol* 1994;12(1):121–127.
17. Ovington LG. The evolution of wound management: ancient origins and advances of the past 20 years. *Home Healthc Nurse* 2002;20(10):652–656.
18. Hutchinson JJ. Infection under occlusion. *Ostomy Wound Manage* 1994;40(3):28–30, 32, 33.
19. Hutchinson JJ, Lawrence JC. Wound infection under occlusive dressings. *J Hosp Infect* 1991;17(2):83–94.
20. Smith DJ, Jr, et al. Microbiology and healing of the occluded skin-graft donor site. *Plast Reconstr Surg* 1993;91(6):1094–1097.
21. Katz MH, et al. Human wound fluid from acute wounds stimulates fibroblast and endothelial cell growth. *J Am Acad Dermatol* 1991;25(6 Pt 1):1054–1058.
22. Drinkwater SL, et al. Effect of venous ulcer exudates on angiogenesis in vitro. *Br J Surg* 2002;89(6):709–713.
23. Schaffer MR, et al. Stimulation of fibroblast proliferation and matrix contraction by wound fluid. *Int J Biochem Cell Biol* 1997;29(1):231–239.
24. Falanga V, et al. Workshop on the pathogenesis of chronic wounds. *J Invest Dermatol* 1994;102(1):125–127.
25. Wysocki AB, Staiano-Coico L, Grinnell, F. Wound fluid from chronic leg ulcers contains elevated levels of metalloproteinases MMP-2 and MMP-9. *J Invest Dermatol* 1993;101(1):64–68.
26. Trengove NJ, Bielefeldt-Ohmann H, Stacey MC. Mitogenic activity and cytokine levels in non-healing and healing chronic leg ulcers. *Wound Repair Regen* 2000;8(1):13–25.
27. Trengove NJ, et al. Analysis of the acute and chronic wound environments: the role of proteases and their inhibitors. *Wound Repair Regen* 1999;7(6):442–452.
28. Madlener M, Parks WC, Werner S. Matrix metalloproteinases (MMPs) and their physiological inhibitors (TIMPs) are differentially expressed during excisional skin wound repair. *Exp Cell Res* 1998;242(1):201–210.
29. Pilcher BK, et al. The activity of collagenase-1 is required for keratinocyte migration on a type I collagen matrix. *J Cell Biol* 1997;137(6):1445–1457.
30. Weckroth M, et al. Matrix metalloproteinases, gelatinase and collagenase, in chronic leg ulcers. *J Invest Dermatol* 1996;106(5):1119–1124.
31. Nwomeh BC, et al. MMP-8 is the predominant collagenase in healing wounds and non-healing ulcers. *J Surg Res* 1999;81(2):189–195.
32. Fife CE, et al. The predictive value of transcutaneous oxygen tension measurement in diabetic lower extremity ulcers treated with hyperbaric oxygen therapy: a retrospective analysis of 1,144 patients. *Wound Repair Regen* 2002;10(4):198–207.

33. Falanga V, Kirsner RS. Low oxygen stimulates proliferation of fibroblasts seeded as single cells. *J Cell Physiol* 1993;154(3):506–510.
34. Kourembanas S, Hannan RL, Faller DV. Oxygen tension regulates the expression of the platelet-derived growth factor-B chain gene in human endothelial cells. *J Clin Invest* 1990;86(2):670–674.
35. Kourembanas S, et al. Hypoxia induces endothelin gene expression and secretion in cultured human endothelium. *J Clin Invest* 1991;88(3):1054–1057.
36. Helfman T, Falanga V. Gene expression in low oxygen tension. *Am J Med Sci* 1993;306(1):37–41.
37. Sheikh AY, et al. Effect of hyperoxia on vascular endothelial growth factor levels in a wound model. *Arch Surg* 2000;135(11):1293–1297.
38. Loot MA, et al. Fibroblasts derived from chronic diabetic ulcers differ in their response to stimulation with EGF, IGF-I, bFGF and PDGF-AB compared to controls. *Eur J Cell Biol* 2002;81(3):153–160.
39. Loots MA, et al. Cultured fibroblasts from chronic diabetic wounds on the lower extremity (non-insulin-dependent diabetes mellitus) show disturbed proliferation. *Arch Dermatol Res* 1999;291(2–3):93–99.
40. Loots MA, et al. Differences in cellular infiltrate and extracellular matrix of chronic diabetic and venous ulcers versus acute wounds. *J Invest Dermatol* 1998;111(5):850–857.
41. Bruce SA, Deamond SF. Longitudinal study of in vivo wound repair and in vitro cellular senescence of dermal fibroblasts. *Exp Gerontol* 1991;26(1):17–27.
42. Hehenberger K, et al. Inhibited proliferation of fibroblasts derived from chronic diabetic wounds and normal dermal fibroblasts treated with high glucose is associated with increased formation of l-lactate. *Wound Repair Regen* 1998;6(2):135–141.
43. Hehenberger K, et al. Fibroblasts derived from human chronic diabetic wounds have a decreased proliferation rate, which is recovered by the addition of heparin. *J Dermatol Sci* 1998;16(2):144–151.
44. Mendez MV, et al. Fibroblasts cultured from distal lower extremities in patients with venous reflux display cellular characteristics of senescence. *J Vasc Surg* 1998;28(6):1040–1050.
45. Stanley A, Osler, T, Senescence and the healing rates of venous ulcers. *J Vasc Surg* 2001;33(6):1206–1211.
46. Agren MS, et al. Proliferation and mitogenic response to PDGF-BB of fibroblasts isolated from chronic venous leg ulcers is ulcer-age dependent. *J Invest Dermatol* 1999;112(4):463–469.
47. Hasan A, et al. Dermal fibroblasts from venous ulcers are unresponsive to the action of transforming growth factor-beta 1. *J Dermatol Sci* 1997;16(1):59–66.
48. Kim BC, et al. Fibroblasts from chronic wounds show altered TGF-beta-signaling and decreased TGF-beta type II receptor expression. *J Cell Physiol* 2003;195(3):331–336.
49. Falanga V, et al. Topical use of human recombinant epidermal growth factor (h-EGF) in venous ulcers. *J Dermatol Surg Oncol* 1992;18(7):604–606.
50. Robson MC, et al. The safety and effect of topically applied recombinant basic fibroblast growth factor on the healing of chronic pressure sores. *Ann Surg* 1992;216(4):401–406 (Discussion 406–408).
51. Robson MC, et al. Platelet-derived growth factor BB for the treatment of chronic pressure ulcers. *Lancet* 1992;339(8784):23–25.
52. Smiell JM, et al. Efficacy and safety of becaplermin (recombinant human platelet-derived growth factor-BB) in patients with nonhealing, lower extremity diabetic ulcers: a combined analysis of four randomized studies. *Wound Repair Regen* 1999;7(5):335–346.
53. Gallico GG, 3rd. Biologic skin substitutes. *Clin Plast Surg* 1990;17(3):519–526.
54. Phillips TJ, Gilchrest BA. Clinical applications of cultured epithelium. *Epithelial Cell Biol* 1992;1(1):39–46.
55. Bell E, et al. Living tissue formed in vitro and accepted as skin-equivalent tissue of full thickness. *Science* 1981;211(4486):1052–1054.

56. Sabolinski ML, et al. Cultured skin as a 'smart material' for healing wounds: experience in venous ulcers. *Biomaterials* 1996;17(3):311–320.

57. Boyce ST. Design principles for composition and performance of cultured skin substitutes. *Burns* 2001;27(5):523–533.

58. Falanga V, et al. Rapid healing of venous ulcers and lack of clinical rejection with an allogeneic cultured human skin equivalent. Human Skin Equivalent Investigators Group. *Arch Dermatol* 1998;134(3):293–300.

59. Hansbrough JF, et al. Clinical trials of a biosynthetic temporary skin replacement, Dermagraft-transitional covering, compared with cryopreserved human cadaver skin for temporary coverage of excised burn wounds. *J Burn Care Rehabil* 1997;18(1 Pt 1):43–51.

60. Marston WA, et al. The efficacy and safety of Dermagraft in improving the healing of chronic diabetic foot ulcers: results of a prospective randomized trial. *Diabetes Care* 2003;26(6):1701–1705.

61. Veves A, et al. Graftskin, a human skin equivalent, is effective in the management of non-infected neuropathic diabetic foot ulcers: a prospective randomized multicenter clinical trial. *Diabetes Care* 2001;24(2):290–295.

62. Falanga V, et al. Wounding of bioengineered skin: cellular and molecular aspects after injury. *J Invest Dermatol* 2002;119(3):653–660.

63. Badiavas EV, Falanga V. Gene therapy. *J Dermatol* 2001;28(4):175–192.

64. Comerota AJ, et al. Naked plasmid DNA encoding fibroblast growth factor type 1 for the treatment of end-stage unreconstructible lower extremity ischemia: preliminary results of a phase I trial. *J Vasc Surg* 2002;35(5):930–936.

65. Badiavas EV, et al. Participation of bone marrow derived cells in cutaneous wound healing. *J Cell Physiol* 2003;196(2):245–250.

66. Quesenberry, PJ, et al. Stem cell plasticity: an overview. *Blood Cells Mol Dis* 2004;32(1):1–4.

67. Quesenberry, PJ, et al. Developmental biology: Ignoratio elenchi: red herrings in stem cell research. *Science* 2005;308(5725):1121, 1122.

68. Badiavas EV, Falanga V. Treatment of chronic wounds with bone marrow-derived cells. *Arch Dermatol* 2003;139(4):510–516.

16

Local Care of Diabetic Foot Ulcers

Assessment, Dressings, and Topical Treatments

Oscar M. Alvarez, PhD, Lee Markowitz, DPM,
and Martin Wendelken, DPM, RN

INTRODUCTION

The ideal wound environment can be described as moist, warm, and clean. There is no single dressing that is suitable for all wounds or even for the same wound at different stages in the healing process. Successful wound management involves the use of dressing or agents to control moisture content, insulate the wound from its surroundings, and provide an environment that reduces inflammation and bacterial burden without harming the cells involved in the repair process. Therefore, wound-dressing functions will vary depending on the type of wound and the particular stage of repair. For example, during the inflammatory phase of wound healing, the ideal dressing should provide an environment that would limit or control vascular leakage, proteolytic degradation of the provisional matrix, free radical generation, oxygen consumption, and breakdown products of nonviable tissue *(1)*. All of these are disruptive to the wound and any measure that limits or controls inflammation should promote wound healing, provided that it does not compromise the ability to resist infection nor leukocyte and macrophage function. Throughout the inflammatory phase wounds are most vulnerable to infection, especially in the patient with diabetes *(2)*. Therefore, the goals are to control infection, and reduce bacterial burden by the removal of nonviable tissues and the use of antibacterial agents. During the regenerative phase (granulation and re-epithelialization) the environment should be moist, warm and protective to endothelium, fibroblasts, and keratinocytes. After the wound has resurfaced (and for a period of weeks thereafter), the wound is particularly vulnerable to reinjury because the epithelium is thin and immature. During this last phase of tissue remodeling the wound dressing environment should provide protection from pressure and friction while controlling edema. During this third phase, the clinician should begin to plan for prevention of ulcer recurrence.

In this chapter we will discuss the following:

1. Ulcer assessment and measurement;
2. Wound-dressing function;
3. Traditional and advanced wound dressings;

From: *The Diabetic Foot, Second Edition*
Edited by: A. Veves, J. M. Giurini, and F. W. LoGerfo © Humana Press Inc., Totowa, NJ

4. Biological dressings and skin equivalents;
5. Medicated dressings;
6. Antiseptic cleansers;
7. The effect of wound temperature;
8. Negative pressure, electric stimulation, and low-frequency ultrasound; and
9. When to perform wound cultures.

ULCER ASSESSMENT AND MEASUREMENT

A thorough assessment of the patient and the foot ulcer is essential in the design of an effective standardized program for local wound management. Ulcer assessment should guide management principles by helping to determine whether the wound is infected, whether light or heavy sharp debridement is indicated, what type of supportive care may be needed, approximately how long it will take to heal, and what types of dressings should be used as healing progresses.

A physical exam, detailed history and diagnostic procedures designed to rule out osteomyelitis and ischemia will help to determine the etiology of the ulcer. The most common ulcer etiology in the patient with diabetes is neuropathy *(3)*. Diabetic neuropathy (not peripheral vascular disease) accounts for approx 60% of all foot ulcerations. Therefore, the majority has adequate circulation and heals with sensible local management coupled with effective off-loading to reduce pressure and friction. At times diabetic foot ulcers (initially caused by neuropathy) are complicated by other disease conditions that affect the healing process. Most common complications in the patient with diabetes include peripheral vascular disease and chronic venous (or lymphatic) insufficiency *(4)*. Less common complications include inflammatory conditions of the skin such as vasculitis, pyoderma gangrenosum, necrobiosis, and rheumatoid arthritis. With this patient population, it is important to realize right away that successful local wound care greatly depends on effective supportive strategies that specifically address the cause of the wound and additional complications.

Each ulcer should be classified by wound morphology, severity, and location. In Table 1 a format for ulcer assessment is presented which incorporates steps that correspond with all levels of the widely used (but less comprehensive) Wagner *(5)* and Pecoraro et al. *(6)* wound classifications. A description of wound and limb appearance, including edema, erythema, exudate, granulation, and the presence of fibrin or nonviable tissues should be recorded. An accurate history of the wound such as duration of nonhealing and previous (local and supportive) treatments should also be included. Ulcer area, depth, and degree of undermining should be recorded at weekly intervals and compared in order to evaluate compliance and the treatment approach. Thorough surgical debridement should be performed at the initial visit *(7)*. This initial (heavy) debridement includes the removal of all nonviable tissues, elimination of undermining, and cutting back to bleeding at the wound margin. Following initial debridement the wound should be re-examined to accurately determine depth and tissue involvement. At each follow-up visit, additional light debridement should be performed to remove callousity surrounding the ulcer, eliminate any undermining and entirely exposing the wound margins.

With the ability to accurately predict healing outcomes *(8–11)*, accurate and reproducible wound measurements have become increasingly important. Most clinician

Table 1
Diabetic Foot Ulcer Assessment

Wound parameters	Severity/descriptions		
Periwound erythema	None: blanches on digital pressure	Mild: nonblanching, may or may not be warm	Marked: nonblanching, warm to touch, with edema
Periwound edema	None	Mild	Marked
Wound purulence	None: exudate is clear, no odor, no pain	Mild: slightly viscous exudates, may be some odor, there could be pain with pressure	Marked: viscous, exudates, heavy drainage, odor, pain with pressure
Wound fibrin: nonviable tissue	None	Mild: covering <50% of the wound bed	Marked: covering >50% of the wound bed
Lower leg edema: localized, pitting, accumulation of interstitial fluid	None	Mild: pretibial digital pressure leaves small but rebounding depression	Marked: pretibial pressure leaves persistant depression
Brawny edema: hemosiderosis, CVI	None	Mild: appears in a limited area, no lipodermatosclerosis	Marked: involving ankle and calf with lipodermatosclerosis
Wound granulation	None	Mild: beginning to fill in, covering <50%, no epithelialization	Marked: covering most of the wound >50% showing signs of epithelialization
Pedal pulses (using hand held Doppler)	Monophasic sounds, ABI < 0.70	Biphasic sounds, ABI > 0.70	Three pulse sounds, ABI > 0.80
Wound measurement	Surface area obtained by tracing the perimeter	Depth: measure with probe at 90° to normal skin	Undermining: measure with probe the deepest part of any tunneling or shearing

Adapted from refs. *4–6* with permission.

measure wound length and width with a ruler whereas depth is usually measured with a probe. Those more specialized, measure wounds by tracing the perimeter to determine surface area. Most techniques work well if the wounds are measured by the same individual, using the same measurement parameters. However, if wound measurements are performed by different clinicians the interrater reliability can vary as much as 50% *(12)*. More recently, more objective noninvasive wound measurement systems have become available. These include high-resolution ultrasound, digital photo software programs and tracing programs that simultaneously measure wound surface area *(12,13)*. Examples of wound measurements obtained with high-resolution ultrasound (Wound Mapping™), digital photography software (PicZar™), are presented in Fig. 1.

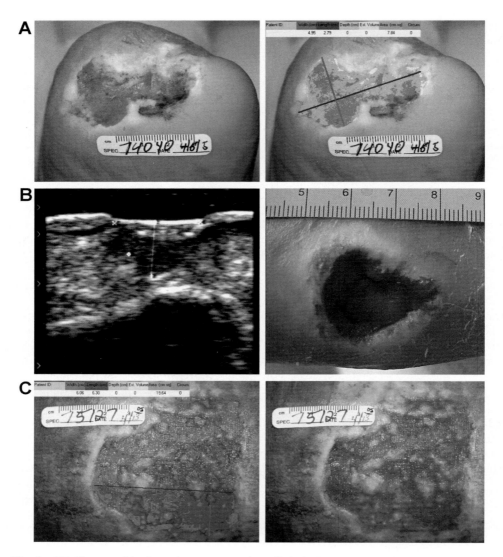

Fig. 1. (A) Neuropathic foot ulcer measured on digital photographs using digital planimetry software. **(B)** High-resolution ultrasonography provides noninvasive, objective, and accurate measurements for deeper wounds and allows for examination of undermining and tunneling *(13)*. **(C)** For partial thickness wounds like this healing venous ulcer traditional measurements such as tracings are problematic and inaccurate. With digital planimetry software the epithelial islands can be easily seen and traced to obtain accurate and reproducible serial measurements of surface area.

WOUND-DRESSING FUNCTION

Until the mid-1900s wound dressings were basically all the same. They consisted of woven textile fibers whose primary function was to cover the wound, contain (staunch) bleeding, and conceal the wound from the outside environment. The first published scientific confirmation that wounds healed faster in an environment in which moisture was retained and crust formation prevented was in 1948. A Norwegian dermatologist, Oscar Gilje noticed that if he covered venous ulcers with strips of adhesive tape spaced apart by 3 mm, the portion of the ulcer covered by the tape epithelialized faster. He replicated these tests in a clinical study involving 23 patients with venous ulcers. Fifteen patients (65%) healed in 12 week *(14)*. These first scientifically controlled studies of moist wound healing beneath occlusive adhesive tape ushered in the age of scientific exploration of wound dressings. In the early 1960s research by George Winter initiated the concept of an optimal local environment for wound healing and an awareness that the wound dressing could have an interactive role in healing by creating and maintaining such an environment *(15)*. Winter's studies in 1962 compared the effects of a moist wound environment (with an occlusive dressing) to a dry wound environment (by air exposure) on the epidermal resurfacing of shallow wounds in domestic pigs. His studies demonstrated that re-epithelialization occurred twice as fast under a moist environment in which a crust (scab) was unable to form. Although at first skeptical of Winter's findings, thinking that an occlusive environment would result in infection, Himman and Maibach, replicated Winter's studies in human subjects. Their studies published in the journal *Nature* in 1963 confirmed Winter's results *(16)*. This awareness precipitated an evolution of wound dressings to interact with the wound to provide an ideal environment for repair.

Despite the many years of favorable results with moist dressings, much work in wound care practice is still not evidence-based. Taking the research and putting it into practice is a goal that still needs to be filled. Even with the tremendous number of new wound care products on the market today gauze continues to be the *de facto* wound dressing. Studies over many years clearly show that a dressing that retains moisture (enough to prevent crust formation) allows wounds to heal faster, are at less risk for infection, require fewer dressing changes and is also associated with less pain *(17,18)*. Contrary to concerns, the moist (occlusive) environment created by occlusive dressings does not lead to increased infection rates. In fact, a retrospective analysis of the literature found a decrease in the incidence of wound infection (on both acute and chronic wounds) with the use of occlusive dressings *(19)*.

TRADITIONAL AND ADVANCED WOUND DRESSINGS

Today there are nearly 200 product manufacturers marketing hundreds of brands of traditional (woven and nonwoven) and advanced wound dressings *(20)*. Combined there are thousands of wound dressings available today. For purposes of reimbursement, dressings have been positioned in several product categories (generally based on the structure or composition of the dressing). Dressing categories include: gauze, impregnated gauze, nonwoven sleeve dressings, transparent films, foams, hydrogels, hydrocolloids, alginates, collagen or extracellular matrix type, superabsorbents, hydrofibers, hydropolymers, medicated dressings, and combination products. The following section describes the category and our experience with use in diabetic foot ulcers.

"Moist gauze" has traditionally been used as the control arm in most diabetic foot ulcer healing trials. Moist to moist gauze dressings and effective off-loading is considered standard care for diabetic (neuropathic) foot ulcers *(21)*. The dressing regimen consists of daily dressing changes with dry gauze as the secondary dressing and anchored with an adhesive tape or bulky rolled gauze bandage. This dressing regimen is useful for uncomplicated superficial ulcers that can be off-loaded easily with a healing sandal and the use of crutches. It should be avoided in large exudative ulcers, if it affects the fit of the treatment shoe and with the use of a total contact cast.

"Nonwoven dressings" such as sleeve dressings or Telfa® nonadherent brand dressings can serve the role of gauze. Because these dressings are not very absorptive the same rules apply as when using gauze. Nonwoven island dressings with an adhesive border are useful for very superficial minimally draining wounds. Be sure that the adhesive is safe for use with diabetic skin and does not reinjure on removal.

"Transparent film dressings" were first introduced as IV site dressings or surgical incise drapes. They were used as wound dressings in the late 1970s and have been shown to promote the healing of partial thickness minimally draining wounds *(22)*. We find that transparent film dressings are not useful for the treatment of diabetic foot ulcers mainly because they do not have any absorptive capacity. The exudates tend to remain in contact with the wound and surrounding skin causing maceration. In addition, frequent strike-through eliminates the edge seal and exogenous bacteria can gain entry. For superficial abrasions, skin tears, and diabetic bullae, transparent films are useful when used together with a topical antibiotic agent.

"Foam dressings" combine occlusion and moist wound healing with some degree of absorption. These wound dressings are made from foamed urethane or another polymer creating open compartments (open cell foam) that house the exudates. To a certain degree, absorption by a foam dressing depends on the size and number of open cells generated during the foaming process. Most foam dressings are between 0.5 and 1 cm thick. Foams have a thin urethane film covering the outer surface. This polymeric film over the top maintains the moist environment by regulating the moisture vapor transmission rate. The film covering also provides a seal to water and exogenous bacteria. Foam dressings may have an adhesive coating over the wound contact layer or may have an island configuration in which the foam is at the center and the perimeter provides the adhesive contact layer. Foam dressings may also contain additives such as surfactants, glycerin or superabsorbents aimed at improving the function of the foam. There are also foam dressings that are impregnated with antibacterial agents such as silver or polyhexamethylene biguanide (PHMB). Foam dressings are appropriate for diabetic ulcers with moderate to heavy drainage, or for ulcers with minimal drainage in which the dressing can remain in place for 3–7 days. Unless the foam is an island dressing in which adhesive covers the perimeter, a secondary dressing, adhesive tape or a bandage will be necessary to anchor the product. The foam design will imbibe wound fluid and keep it away from the wound. For chronic wounds (or wounds that are >2 months old) this is a desirable attribute as it has been shown that chronic wound fluid may be harmful to cells and provisional matrix *(23)*. Foam dressings also provide a cushion that may be helpful to protect the wound from friction or trauma.

"Hydrocolloid dressings" are the direct descendants of ostomy devices and barrier products. Hydrocolloid dressings are completely air-tight and do not allow the transport of oxygen or other gases. In the 1970s, wound healing research with hydrocolloids dispelled the old notion that "the wound should be allowed to breathe" *(24)*. From these studies it became obvious that the oxygen necessary for wound repair came from the blood and that atmospheric oxygen often harmed or delayed the healing process *(25)*. These dressings are created by mixing a hydrocolloid such as carboxy methyl cellulose (CMC) with gelling agents such as gelatin and combining them with an adhesive elastomer such as isobutylene. Hydrocolloids are dispersions of discrete particles around which water molecules and solvated ions form a shell-like structure. Fluid absorption occurs principally by particle swelling and enlargement of this structure. The hydrocolloid mass of these dressings consists of gum-like materials such as guar or karaya, sodium CMC, and pectin bound by an adhesive such as polyisobutylene. Certain hydrocolloid formulations can adhere to wet surfaces (wet-tack) because of particle swelling and phase inversion. When placed over a moist wound the immediate wound contact area dissolves in time to form a semisolid gel that allows for dressing removal without reinjury. Exudate absorption by most hydrocolloid dressings results in the formation of a yellow/light brown gelatinous mass that remains covering the wound on dressing removal. This may be irrigated from the wound and should not be confused with pus. As hydrocolloids and gelatin decompose over the wound there may be a characteristic odor that resolves once the wound has been cleansed. Hydrocolloid dressings are particularly useful when autolytic debridement is desirable *(17,25)*. The wound environment created under a hydrocolloid dressing is acidic (pH 5.0) and has been shown to inhibit the growth of pathogens such as *Pseudomonas aeruginosa* and *Staphylococcus aureus* *(26)*. Although hydrocolloid dressings are absorbent they do not absorb wound fluid at the same rate as traditional dressings (made with gauze or nonwoven), foams, biocellulose dressings, or alginates.

"Hydrogel sheets" are three-dimensional lattices made up of a hydrophilic polymer such as polyvinylpyrollidone. Hydrogel dressings are nonadherent and have high water content. Hydrogels allow a high rate of evaporation without compromising wound hydration. This property makes them useful for burn treatment or large superficial abrasions. Compared with untreated, hydrogel as well as hydrocolloid dressings have been reported to increase epidermal healing by about 40% *(31)*. Hydrogel dressings are soothing and have been shown to cool the skin by as much as 5°C *(17,27)*. Hydrogel dressings are not very useful for diabetic (neuropathic) foot ulcers unless the wound is very shallow and only drains minimally. However, they are useful for excoriation or cracking caused by dry skin in this patient population. Hydrogel dressings are also useful to treat painful inflammatory ulcers and other superficial wounds caused by trauma.

Included in this category, though not true hydrogel sheets are biocellulose wound dressings. A biocellulose wound dressing made from purified bacterial cellulose has been introduced that can both deliver or absorb moisture. This dressing accelerates autolytic debridement while it provides a protective seal over the wound similar to a blister roof *(28)*.

"Amorphous hydrogels" come packaged in tubes, spray bottles or foil packets, and they may also be impregnated into gauze. In the amorphous hydrogel the hydrophilic polymer has not been crosslinked and therefore remains in a more aqueous (gel-like) state. The primary ingredient is water and can dry rather quickly if not covered with a semiocclusive or occlusive dressing. Several amorphous hydrogels contain additives such as collagen, calcium alginate, or CMC in order to be more absorptive. Like a moisturizing agent, amorphous hydrogels will donate moisture and can be useful to soften dry eschar or callous.

"Alginate dressings" are the calcium salts of alginic acid (derived from brown seaweed) which have been spun into a fiber. These dressings are available as compressed nonwoven sheets or bound into ropes. When wound fluid contacts the calcium alginate, the sodium in the fluid replaces the calcium in the alginate increasing the viscosity of the fluid producing a gel (sodium alginate). Alginates are emulsifiers and serve as thickening agents that are frequently used in prepared foods. Alginates are bioerodible and will gradually dissolve with moisture over time. The greatest advantage of the alginate dressings is their absorptive capacity. Alginates are ideal for heavily draining wounds. If used appropriately, they can significantly reduce the number of dressing changes required. If used in wounds that drain minimally, the fibers will dry out and will adhere to the wound bed. The secondary dressing is important and one should be chosen that helps to keep the gel moist. Alginates have been reported to have hemostatic and bacteriostatic properties *(29)*. Alginate dressings are also available with the topical antibacterial silver.

"Hydrofibers" are fibers of CMC. Hydrofiber dressings rapidly absorb exudates and have a large absorptive capacity (approximately two to three times greater than alginates *[30]*). Obviously, they are indicated for heavily draining wounds or when extended wear is required. Hydrofibers can also contain silver with the intent to reduce the wound's bacterial burden. In patients with neuropathic ulcers that are being treated with a total contact cast the hydrofiber dressing can be kept on for 7 days. It has been our experience that the hydrofiber containing silver helps to reduces wound odor.

"Hydropolymers" are foamed gels that wicks exudates away from the wound to the upper layers of the pad. The backing material has a very high moisture vapor transmission rate and allows for the evaporation of excess fluid. Hydropolymer dressings are available with silver as well. These dressings are useful for moderate and heavily draining wounds or when the dressing needs to remain in place for an extended period of time.

"Medicated dressings" are devices that contain an agent (usually an antimicrobial) in order to supplement its function. Recently there has been great interest in the use of silver-containing dressings. The antimicrobial properties of metallic silver have been used empirically for thousands of years and a great deal has been published regarding its mechanism of action, toxicity, and historical background *(31)*. Many dressings have been introduced that contain silver in a variety of different forms. There are dressings that contain a silver coated polyethylene membrane, ones that contain silver-impregnated activated charcoal cloth, alginates, foams and hydrocolloids containing silver, microcrystalline silver on the adhesive portion of a transparent film, silver powders, and even an amorphous hydrogel containing silver. The antimicrobial properties of several of these silver-containing dressings have been studied previously *(32)*. Interestingly the silver content and antimicrobial activity of the various dressings varies considerably. PHMB has been used as an antimicrobial agent by the contact lens industry for years. Recently, several manufacturers have incorporated this antimicrobial agent into their wound dressings. A biocellulose wound dressing containing PHMB has recently been introduced and PHMB has also been impregnated into gauze and nonwoven.

Iodine preparations have been criticized in the past because of their cytotoxicity. However, in cadexomer iodine formulations the iodine is released in quantities that are not harmful to cells. Cadexomer iodine is available in an absorbent gel and also as a paste dressing. Cadexomer iodine has been studied in both venous ulcers *(33)* and diabetic foot ulcers *(34)* with favorable results, but these studies had relatively small sample populations. A randomized controlled clinical trial of cadexomer iodine for the treatment of diabetic foot ulcers has not been done to date.

"Combination products/impregnated gauze dressings" are gauzes and nonwovens that are incorporated with agents that affect their function. Dressings have long been used as drug delivery devices. Agents most commonly used include saline, oil, zinc salts, or petrolatum, Vaseline®, Aquaphor®, or (bismuthtribromophenate) bacteriostatic agents. Gauze or polyethylene may also be impregnated with salts and inorganic ions that are appear to decrease the harmful effects of matrix metalloproteases in chronic wounds.

"Collagen and extracellular matrix" materials are available for the treatment of acute and chronic wounds. For the most part, these devices consist of purified collagen extracted from rat tendon, bovine skin, or pig intestine. The renatured-purified collagen is lyophilized to form a sheet or a wafer and packaged for application onto an acute or chronic wound. The matrix material is thought to provide a temporary provisional matrix or scaffold for anchorage-dependent cells involved in the repair process *(35)*. Also, it is thought that the collagen matrix may provide a substrate for the proteolytic enzymes present in chronic wounds thereby causing less destruction to the wound matrix *in situ (23)*. There are a variety of matrix materials available: collagen sheets (consisting of collagen type I), collagen matrix composites (consisting of collagen types I and types I and III), combinations of collagen and other connective tissues, combinations of collagen with calcium alginate and or oxidized cellulose, and cryopreserved human acellular dermis. One collagen-containing product has been evaluated in a randomized controlled clinical trial for the treatment of diabetic foot ulcers *(36)*. In this study ulcers receiving treatment with Promogran® (a collagen/oxidized regenerated cellulose dressing) had better healing (45%) than those receiving standard care (33%). Although better healing was observed with collagen-ORC wound dressing the study sample size was too small to reach statistical significance ($p = 0.056$). AlloDerm® is a human cadaveric skin product that is processed to remove the epidermis and all cellular elements. This acellular dermal matrix is nonimmunogenic and still contains an intact basement membrane. It has been mostly used as a dermal graft for the treatment of burn wounds. A study is under way to evaluate the effectiveness of GraftJacket®, (an orthopedic version of AlloDerm) on the healing of diabetic foot ulcers. Preliminary results show faster healing with a one-time application of acellular human dermal matrix when compared to conventional treatment consisting of moist gauze *(37)*.

Table 2 lists the category type, characteristics and clinical evidence of available wound dressings. "Skin equivalents and tissue engineered skin products" is the newest category of FDA-approved medical devices that provide active therapy to chronic wounds. It is also the category in which the greatest amount of reliable scientific evidence may be found. The term tissue engineered skin refers to skin products produced from cells, extracellular matrix materials, or a combination, and in some cases includes cells impregnated in nonbiological materials. There are four products that combine a matrix material with cultured cells.

Apligraf® (Graftskin) is a bilayered skin construct with a dermis (collagen gel seeded with neonatal fibroblasts) and an epidermis (neonatal keratinocytes layered on top and grown in an air–liquid interface culture). The end product is a sophisticated

Table 2
Wound-Dressing Category, Type, and Clinical Evidence

Category	Characteristics	Advantages/disadvantages	Product examples	Evidence/research support
Moist gauze	Saline moist gauze is applied damp and overlapped with dry gauze. It maintains a moist environment depending on the secondary dressings and tape used	Can cause maceration, does not provide a barrier to exogenous bacteria	Gauze sponges 2 × 2 and 4 × 4	Moist to moist saline gauze has been used as the control regimen in most clinical trials. The mean incidence of healing in a 12-week period for the control patients (treated with moist gauze) in these studies was 30% (21,36,41,70). Of 127 patients treated with moist gauze and placebo gel, 35% healed in 20 weeks (52). Of 21 patients treated with saline gauze, 29% healed in 20 weeks (53,54). From a retrospective analysis, the probability of developing an infection was 6% (71,72)
Nonwoven/ absorptive/ composites	Multilayer wound covers that provide semiadherent or nonadherent layer, combined with absorbent fibers such as cellulose cotton or rayon	Designed to minimize adherence and manage slight amounts of exudates, can cause maceration, is not a barrier to exogenous bacteria	Curad® Telfa® pads Curity® abdominal pads (Tyco/Kendall) Primapore® Coversite® (Smith & Nephew) Tenderwet® (Medline) Medipore® (3-M) Coverlet® (BSN-Jobst)	There are no published studies using this category on diabetic foot ulcers. In one clinical study (not published) with 302 patients, Telfa with a placebo gel was used as the control arm. Thirty percent healed in 12 weeks
Transparent films	Provide moist environment, transparent, waterproof, adhesive	Good for very superficial wounds that do not drain much, can cause maceration, if strike through occurs can allow bacteria in	OpSite® (Smith & Nephew) Tegaderm® (3-M) BlisterFilm® Polyskin® (Tyco/Kendall) Suresite® (Medline)	There are no published studies available on diabetic foot ulcers. Up to 50% enhanced healing in superficial wounds when compared with air-exposed wounds (27)

Foam dressing	Foamed polymer solutions, absorption generally depends on thickness, contact layer is nonadherent	Provides good absorption for partial thickness and moderately draining full-thickness wounds, foams can be treated with agents to enhance absorption, most are coated with thin film that serves as a barrier	Allevyn® (Smith & Nephew) Biatain® (Coloplast) 3M Foam (3-M) Curafoam® Hydrasorb® (Tyco/Kendall) Polymem® Polymax® (Ferris) Tielle® (J & J) Lyofoam® (Convatec) Optifoam® (Medline)	There are no published studies available for diabetic foot ulcers. In venous ulcers with 50 patients, 34% healed in 13 weeks (73). In pressure ulcers with 50 patients 20% of stage II-III healed in 6 weeks (74). Of 24 stage II-III patients, 42% healed in 12 weeks (74)
Hydrocolloid dressing	Wafers made up of gelatin, pectin and CMC. Absorption is slower and generally depends on thickness. They are self adhering, impervious to air, and gases	Provides excellent seal from the outside environment. Moldable, contours well to heels, good for superficial, and full-thickness wounds with mild to moderate exudation, provides excellent autolytic debridement	Exuderm® XCell® (Medline) Comfeel® (Coloplast) DuoDerm® (Convatec) Tegasorb® (3-M) Nu-Derm® (J & J) RepliCare® (Smith & Nephew) Restore® (Hollister) Ultec® (Tyco/Kendall)	Of 36 diabetic and Hansen's disease patients, 80% healed in 10 weeks with a hydro-colloid dressing and total contact cast (75,76). Of 84 ulcers in 45 patients, 88% healed in 14 weeks (72). Probability of infection (measured retrospectively) was 2.5% (72). Of 164 patients with long-standing venous ulcers, 55% healed in 12 weeks when used with graduated compression (73). A biocellulose dressing XCell® was reported to be more effective ($p = 0.0094$) than standard care for autolytic debridement of venous ulcers (28)
Hydrogel sheets	Crosslinked hydrophilic polymers insoluble in water interact with exudates by swelling	Conformable, permeable, absorbancy is based on composition, must use a secondary dressing to anchor	Nu-Gel® (J & J) Curagel® Aquaflo® (Tyco/ Kendall) Derma-Gel® (Medline) Elasto-Gel® (Southwest) FlexiGel® (Smith-Nephew) CaraDres® (Carrington)	There are no published studies available on diabetic foot ulcers. In partial thickness and full-thicknesss acute wounds, hydrogels increase healing by 30–36% (17,18,27)

(Continued)

Table 2 (Continued)

Category	Characteristics	Advantages/disadvantages	Product examples	Evidence/research support
Amorphous hydrogels	Water, polymers, and other ingredients combined into a topical that donates moisture, when combined with CMC can provide absorption as well	Helps to rehydrate and soften wound tissues, good for superficial wounds such as cracks because of dry skin	Curasol® (Tyco/Kendall) IntraSite® SoloSite® (Smith-Nephew) Dermagran® (Derma Sciences) WounDress® (Coloplast) DuoDerm® Hydroactive (Convatec)	There are no published studies available in diabetic foot ulcers. In acute partial thickness wounds, healing was accelerated by 28% compared with untreated wounds (18,27)
Alginates	Nonwoven pads and ropes of natural polysaccharide fibers derived from seaweed. On contact with wound, fluid alginates gel	Indicated for wound with moderate to heavy exudates, they require a secondary dressing to anchor	AlgiSite® (Smith-Nephew) AlgiCell® (Derma Sciences) Maxorb (Medline) Kaltostat® (Convatec) SeaSorb® (Coloplast) Sorbsan® (Bertek)	There are no published studies available on diabetic foot ulcers. Favorable healing compared with standard care has been reported in pressure ulcers (77), venous ulcers (78), and dehisced wounds (79)
Hydrofibers/hydropolymers	Consist of foamed gels or highly absorbent fibers, wick exudates away from the wound	Useful for heavily draining ulcers or when extended use is desirable	Aquacel® (Convatec) Exu-Dry® Allevyn® Plus Smith-Nephew Tielle® Plus (J & J)	There are no published studies available on diabetic foot ulcers. In preclinical animal models, this dressing category speeds healing by approx 30% compared with untreated (80)
Medicated/antimicrobial dressing	Dressings that deliver the effects of agents such as cadexomer iodine, silver and PHMB	Useful when localized minor wound infection is present and to lower bacterial bioburden, some provide odor control	Acticoat® (Smith-Nephew) Contreet® Ag foam, hydrocolloid (Coloplast) Actisorb® Silvercel® (J & J)	Cadexomer iodine was shown to improve the healing of foot ulcers in patients with diabetes (34). In venous ulcers, Iodosorb significantly improved wound closure in a 12-week study with standard compression (33). Acticoat® effective in lowering bacterial counts in

Category	Description	Products	Notes
		Aquacel® Ag (Convatec) Arglaes® SilvaSorb® XCell® AM Maxorb® Ag (Medline) Silverlon® (Argentum) Telfa® AMD (Tyco/Kendall) Iodosorb® Iodoflex® (Healthpoint)	burns (81). There are many in vitro studies reporting bacterial kill when using silver or PHMB
Combination/ impregnated dressing	Gauzes and nonwovens saturated with an agent or compound	Adaptic® (J & J) Aquaphor (Smith-Nephew) Curasalt® Xeroform® Xeroflo® (Tyco/Kendall) EpiMax® (Dermagenics) Mesalt® (Molnlycke)	There are no published studies available on diabetic foot ulcers. Impregnated gauze has been reported to only slightly enhance healing (5%) compared with air exposure in superficial wounds (27)
	Good for providing a nonadherent surface to the wound, some dressings may deliver zinc salts, mild antibacterial agents, or a moist soothing occlusive such as petrolatum		
Collagens and dermal matrix materials	Gel pads, particles, pastes, powder, sheets derived from human, porcine, bovine or avian collagen. Some are combined with oxidized cellulose, silver, or alginate	Promogran® Prisma® Fibracol® (J & J) Biobrane® (Bertek) Oasis® (Healthpoint) Stimulen® (Southwest) Primatrix® (TEI Biosciences) GraftJacket®, AlloDerm (Life Sciences) Integra® (Integra Life Sciences)	Of the 95 patients treated with promogran, 45% healed compared with 33% of 89 treated with moist gauze (35). Statistical significance was not reached ($p = 0.056$) in this trial. Of 37 diabetic foot ulcer patients treated with small intestine submucosa (SIS Oasis®), 49% healed in 12 weeks compared with 28% treated with beclapermin (the difference was not statistically significant [81]). Preliminary results of a randomized controlled trial show faster healing with acellular human dermal matrix (GraftJacket) vs moist gauze (37)
These dressings should be used in clean wounds. The collagen bioerodes and may provide a temporary provisional matrix to protect the wound from harmful proteases			

(Continued)

323

Table 2 (Continued)

Category	Characteristics	Advantages/disadvantages	Product examples	Evidence/research support
Skin equivalents and tissue engineered skin products cell therapy	Living human skin cells incorporated in a matrix usually consisting of collagen. This cell therapy provides growth factors and cytokines to the wounds	Only Apligraf and Dermagraf® are approved by FDA for treatment of diabetic foot ulcers. Most beneficial when the wound bed is healthy without the presence of nonviable tissue.	Apligraf (Organogenesis) Dermagraft Transcyte® (Smith-Nephew) OrCel® (Ortec) Epicel (Genzyme)	In a diabetic foot ulcer study of 208 patients, 75% healed in the group treated with Apligraf compared with 41% in the control group ($p < 0.05$). In the same study, the time to healing in the Apligraf group was 38.5 days compared with 91 days for the control group (40). Diabetic foot ulcer patients treated with Dermagraft had a statistically significant higher percent wound closure by week 12 than patients treated with moist gauze (68). The percentage of patients who experienced wound infection was less in the Dermagraft treatment group

skin equivalent that histologically resembles human skin. Apligraf has been shown to make matrix proteins and growth factors and has the capacity to heal itself *(38,39)*. Although the exact mechanisms of efficacy in chronic wounds are not known, improved healing is probably the result of cell or matrix therapy (because there is no permanent take *[39,40]*). The release of growth factors and cytokines, combined with matrix-induced cell migration are likely responsible *(40)*. In a prospective, randomized, controlled, multicenter trial, 208 patients with diabetic ulcers were treated with either Graftskin plus standard care or diabetic foot standard care alone. Treatment with Graftskin once a week for a maximum of 4 week reduced the median time to healing to 38.5 days from 91 days in the control group *(41)*. This difference was statistically significant ($p = 0.01$). Seventy-five percent of the Graftskin treated group achieved complete healing vs 41% for the control group ($p < 0.05$). A statistically significant improvement in time to healing was also demonstrated in a prospective randomized controlled multicenter clinical trial for venous ulcer patients *(42)*.

OrCel® (Composite Cultured Skin) is also a living skin equivalent consisting of allogeneic fibroblasts and keratinocytes grown in vitro and attached to opposing sides of a bilayered matrix of bovine collagen *(43)*. The matrix is made up of a cross-linked collagen sponge that is covered with a layer of pepsinized insoluble collagen gel. Keratinocytes are seeded over the one side of the nonporous collagen gel and the fibroblasts on the opposing aspect of the porous collagen sponge. After seeding, it is cultured for 10–15 days, producing a thin, 2–3-cell layer thick "epidermis" overlying the fibroblast imbedded collagen sponge. At present OrCel is FDA-approved for use over donor sites and in the surgical repair of digits of children with dystrophic epidermolysis bullosa *(44)*. Data from a recently completed randomized clinical trial on venous ulcers is currently being analyzed *(43)*. As with all tissue engineered skin products, the exact mode of action of composite cultured skin is not known but probably involves the aforementioned delivery of growth factors and cytokines (cell therapy).

Epicel® (Cultured Autologous Keratinocyte Construct) is a confluent sheet of autologous epidermal cells grown in culture. The clonal growth of human keratinocytes was first described by Rheinwald and Green in 1975 *(45)*. This technique permits the growth of keratinocytes to form a multilayered stratified sheet of epidermis that is used autologously. Application of autologous epidermal sheets to speed or stimulate wound healing has been described in leg ulcers *(46)*, burns *(47)*, excisions *(47)*, and pressure ulcers *(48)*. The preparation of a healthy dermal substrate (wound bed) is important when planning to use autologous keratinocyte sheets. The use of autologous cultured epidermal sheets has many advantages including pain relief, rapid coverage of the wound and decreased requirement for split thickness grafts (donor sites). However, cultured autologous epithelium is expensive to produce and can take as much as 3 week to manufacture. Because the epithelial cell sheet is very thin, a high level of skill is required for proper application.

Dermagraft® (Living Allogeneic Dermal Construct) is a cryopreserved living dermal equivalent made from neonatal foreskin fibroblasts cultured on a bioabsorbable polyglactin (Vycril®) or polyglycolic acid (Dexon®) polymer matrix. The dermal fibroblasts are grown in the bioerodible mesh along with circulating nutrients *(49)*. It has been shown that the fibroblast in Dermagraft produce growth factors that are thought to aid wound healing *(50)* such as: vascular endothelial growth factor (VEGF), and hepatocyte growth factor/scatter factor. Dermagraft has been shown to be effective for the treatment of diabetic (neuropathic) ulcers when compared to moist gauze in a large multicenter randomized clinical trial *(21)* and is FDA approved for that indication.

Transcyte® (Extracellular Matrix with Allogeneic Human Dermal Fibroblasts) is a temporary skin cover made up of a collagen-coated nylon mesh seeded with neonatal fibroblasts. The mesh is not biodegradable and must eventually be removed. In vitro studies have demonstrated that the Transcyte fibroblasts synthesize fibronectin and proteoglycans to provide a provisional matrix for subsequent grafting *(51)*. Transcyte® has been shown to be as effective as allograft for the treatment of excised burn wounds in a controlled randomized clinical trial and is approved by FDA for the treatment of burn wounds *(51)*.

GROWTH FACTORS

The results of clinical trials investigating the topical application of growth factors to chronic wounds have not been as impressive as initially expected. More than likely this can be explained by the complex nature of the wound healing process and by our lack of understanding about wound chronicity. Also, it is possible that, because growth factors are pleiotrophic (influence a wide range of cellular behavior), it may be difficult to gauge their efficacy using the chronic wound model. To date, only platelet-derived growth factor (PDGF) has been approved by FDA. Topical PDGF gel is commercially available as Regranex® (Beclapermin) indicated for use in neuropathic diabetic foot ulcers. In one prospective randomized double blind clinical trial of 118 patients, beclapermin gel (30 µg/g) was shown to be significantly better than the placebo gel in the treatment of diabetic foot ulcers *(52)*. In another placebo-controlled clinical trial with 379 patients daily applications of beclapermin gel at 30 µg/g had no effect on wound healing, but 100 µg/g did *(53)*. Combined analyses of these and other studies suggest that daily application of beclapermin (100 µg/g) combined with aggressive surgical debridement is effective in improving diabetic foot ulcer healing *(54)*.

ANTISEPTIC WOUND CLEANSERS

Antiseptics are agents that kill or inhibit microorganisms on living tissue. Providone-iodine, 70% alcohol and hydrogen peroxide are still very commonly used today by both the public and health professionals. However, all three agents have been found to have only limited value in wound care today. Seventy percent isopropyl alcohol only shows limited effect against microorganisms and for only short amounts of time. It can be a strong irritant to an open wound and draws away moisture from the wound as it evaporates *(55)*. Providone-iodine is very widely used in wound care. It is, however, not recommended for use in open wounds. In vitro studies have shown that povidone-iodine, unless highly diluted, is toxic to most cell types implicated in the healing process *(56)*. Because povidone-iodine is water soluble, diluting it actually releases free iodine into the tissue *(57)*. In certain patients in which the primary goal is not wound closure (palliative wound care), povidone-iodine can be very effective at drying the eschar thus inhibiting the development of wet gangrene. Hydrogen peroxide 3% solution is also commonly used today. It cleanses the wound through its release of oxygen. It has been shown to delay wound healing by 8%

compared with untreated *(17,27)*. However, in patients who require at home wound care and hygiene is a concern it may be worthwhile to give in to the slight delay and use 3% hydrogen peroxide to cleanse the wound before dressing application. If hydrogen peroxide is diluted to 0.3% its effectiveness against microorganisms is reduced *(57–59)*.

"Negative pressure wound therapy" (Vacuum Assisted Closure, VAC Therapy) consists of a sterile foam cell dressing that is applied directly over a wound and sealed from above with an adhesive film. An evacuation tube is placed into the foam which is attached to a pump. The pumping action creates subatmospheric or negative pressure uniformly to all tissues within the wound *(60)* causing a gentle compression over the wound surface. VAC has been tremendously helpful for heavily draining wounds and when dressing changes are difficult for the patient. To date there is no reliable evidence (results from a randomized controlled clinical trial) that demonstrates that negative pressure improves chronic wound healing. In one evaluation involving six patients (with diabetic foot ulcers) VAC appeared to decrease ulcer depth when compared with with moist gauze dressings *(60)*.

LOW-FREQUENCY ULTRASOUND

Mist ultrasound therapy resulted in improved healing rates in a double blind, controlled, diabetic foot ulcer study of 63 patients *(61)*. The group treated with the ultrasound device had greater healing (41%) compared with sham control (14.3%).

WOUND AND SKIN TEMPERATURE

The warming of wounds to aid healing has been practiced since the time of Hippocrates (460–380 BC). Warmth around the wound is thought to cause dialation of the local blood vessels and thus improve the delivery of oxygen, growth factors and other nutrients to the wound *(62)*. A wound healing therapy system has been developed that provides a warm and moist environment to the wound. This therapy is known as noncontact normothermic wound therapy (NNWT) or Warm Up®. In a randomized clinical trial of 20 patients NNWT was found to improve the rate of wound healing when compared to standard care *(63)*. After 12 weeks, 70% of the wounds treated with NNWT had healed compared with 40% for the control group (treated with moist gauze). Patients in both groups received the same off-loading and supportive therapies. One advantage of NNWT to traditional warming systems is that the temperature is set not to exceed 37°C. It is not known whether other methods of warming the skin such as a warm water bottle, or a heating pad would provide the same benefits.

ELECTRICAL STIMULATION

Electric current has been shown to facilitate fracture healing, enhance fibroblast and epidermal migration, and provide antibacterial effects *(64,65)*. One randomized controlled double blind clinical trial of 40 patients studied the effectiveness of high-volt (50 V with 80 twin peak monophasic pulsees), pulse galvanic electric stimulation on diabetic foot ulcer healing *(66,67)*. Sixty-five percent of the patients healed in the group treated with electric stimulation, whereas 35% healed with placebo ($p = 0.058$).

Table 3
Diabetic Foot Ulcer Treatments That Have Been Studied in Randomized Clinical Trials

Treatments	Description/significance	References
Bilayered skin construct (Apligraf)	Or the group treated with Apligraf, 75% healed compared with 41% in the control group ($p < 0.05$)	*(41)*
Dermal construct (Dermagraft)	Patients treated with Dermagraft had a statistically significant ($p < 0.05$) higher percent wound closure by week 12 than patients treated with control	*(21,70)*
PDGF-BB Beclapermin (Regranex)	Beclapermin (100 μg/g) combined with aggressive surgical debridement was effective in improving diabetic foot ulcer healing ($p = 0.007$)	*(53,54)*
Collagen-ORC wound dressing (Promogran), small intestine submucosa (SIS, Oasis® Wound Matrix)	Of 95 patients treated with Promogran, 45% healed compared with 33% of 89 treated with moist gauze. Statistical significance was not reached ($p = 0.056$) in this trial. In a 73-patient diabetic foot ulcer trial, 49% of 37 in the Oasis® group healed after 12 weeks. Statistical significance was not reached ($p = 0.055$)	*(36,82)*
Hydrocolloid dressing (DuoDerm®)	Of 36 diabetic and Hansen's disease patients, 80% healed in 10 weeks with a hydrocolloid dressing and total contact cast Of 84 ulcers in 45 patients, 88% healed in 14 weeks	*(72,75)*
Moist saline gauze	Moist to moist saline gauze has been considered standard care and therefore has been used as the control regimen in most clinical trials. Combined results show that 29–33% of ulcers treated with moist gauze heal within 12 weeks	*(21,36,41,70)*

WHEN TO PERFORM A WOUND CULTURE

Routine culturing of wounds is not indicated. Wound cultures should only be taken when the wound has the clinical signs of infection or those that have no clinical signs of infection but are deteriorating or have failed to heal. For those wounds that have the clinical signs of infection swab cultures can provide useful data regarding the presence of potential pathogens and the diversity of microorganisms present as well as antimicrobial sensitivity. A swab sample can also provide a semiquantitative estimation of the microbial load ($>10^5$ CFU/mL). A correlation between semiquantitative swab data and quantitative biopsy data has previously been demonstrated *(68,69)*. For deteriorating wounds or wounds failing to improve, a tissue biopsy culture for quantitative and qualitative analysis should be obtained.

CONCLUSION

Local care for diabetic foot ulcers should commence with a complete history and physical examination. Diagnostic procedures should be aimed at exclusion of osteomyelitis, dysvascular problems, extent of neuropathy, electrolyte imbalance, high or low blood glucose levels, nutritional defects and the use of agents that impede wound healing such as corticosteroids, chemotherapeutic agents, and topical cytotoxic agents. Oral antibiotics should be prescribed if a wound infection is present. Topical antibiotics are helpful for localized minor infections combined with frequent examination until resolution. An ulcer care strategy combining frequent debridement, moist wound care, and effective off-loading should be developed for each patient. The patient should be followed and wounds measured regularly for 4 weeks. If (after 4 weeks) the wound has healed by 50% or more continue with the same treatments until healing. If the wound has not healed by 50% in 4 weeks then an alternative (more aggressive approach) such as an active modality should be considered. A list of agents that have been studied in randomized clinical trials for the treatment of diabetic foot ulcers is presented in Table 3.

REFERENCES

1. Clark RAF. Wound repair: overview and general considerations, in *The Molecular and Cellular Biology of Wound Repair* (Clark RAF, ed.), Plennum Press, New York, 1996, pp. 3–35.
2. Little JR, Vobayashi GS. Infection in the diabetic foot, in *The Diabetic Foot* (Levin ME, O'Neil LW, eds.), 4th ed, Mosby Yearbook, St Louis MO, 1988, pp. 104–118.
3. Reiber GE. Epidemiology of the diabetic foot, in *The Diabetic Foot*, (Levin ME, O'Neil LW, Bowker JH, eds.), 5th ed., Mosby Yearbook, St. Louis, MO, 1993, pp. 1–15.
4. Alvarez OM, Gilson G, Auletta M. Local aspects of diabetic foot ulcer care: assessment, dressings, and topical agents, in *The Diabetic Foot* (Levin ME, O'Neil LW, Bowker JH, eds.), 5th ed., Mosby Yearbook, St. Louis, MO, 1993, pp. 259–281.
5. Wagner FW Jr. A classification and treatment program for diabetic neuropathic and dysvascular foot problems, in *American Academy of Orthopedic surgeons: Instructional Course Lectures,* Volume 28, Mosby Yearbook, St Louis, MO, 1979.
6. Pecoraro RE, Reiber GE. Classification of wounds in diabetic amputees. *Wounds,* 1990;2:65–73.
7. Laing P. Diabetic foot ulcers. *Am J Surg* 1994;167(Suppl 1A):31S–36S.
8. Sheehan P, Caselli A, Giurini J, Veves A. Percent change in wound area of diabetic foot ulcers over a 4-week period is arobust predictor of complete healing in a 12 week prospective trial. *Diabetes Care* 2003;26(6):1879–1882.
9. van Rijswijk L, Polansky M. Predictors of time to healing deep pressure ulcers. *Wounds* 1994;6(5):159–165.
10. van Rijswijk L. Multi-center leg ulcer study group. Full thickness leg ulcers: patient demographics and predictors of healing. *J Fam Pract* 1993;36(6):625–632.
11. Alvarez OM, Markowitz L, Rogers R, Booker J, Waltrous L. Effectiveness of 4-layer compression and the modified unna's boot for the treatment of lower leg ulcers in ambulatory patients with chronic venous disease: a crossover study of 80 patients. Abstract presented at the 18th annual SAWC San Diego, CA 2005.
12. Wendelken M, Markowitz L, Alvarez OM. Wound mapping with high resolution ultrasound provides objective, accurate and reproducible wound measurements for clinical trials. *Wounds* 2005;17(3);A40.
13. Wendelken M, Markowitz L, Patel M, Alvarez OM. Objective, noninvasive wound assessment using b-mode ultrasonography. *Wounds* 2003;15(11)1–10.

14. Gilje O. On taping (adhesive tape treatment) of leg ulcers. *Acta Dermatol Venereol* 1948;28:454–467.

15. Winter GD. Formation of the scab and the rate of epithelialization of superficial wounds in the skin of the young domestic pig. *Nature (London)* 1962;193:293, 294.

16. Hinman CD, Maibach H. Effect of air exposure and occlusion on experimental human skin wounds. *Nature (London)* 1963;200:377–379.

17. Alvarez OM, Rozint J, Wiseman D. Moist environment for healing: matching the dressing to the wound. *Wounds* 1989 Premier Issue;1(1);35–50.

18. Eaglstein WH, Mertz PM, Falanga V. Occlusive Dressings. *Am Fam Phys* 1987; 35:211–216.

19. Hutchinson JJ, McGuckin M. Influence of occlusive dressings: a microbiological and clinical review. *Am J Infect Control* 1990;18:257–268.

20. Motta G (ed.). *Wound Source; The Kestrel Wound Product sourcebook* 8th ed. Kestrel health Information Inc. Toronto Canada, 2005. (http://www.woundsource.com). Date accessed: 01/23/06.

21. Gentzkow GD, Iwasaki SD, Hershon KS, et al. Use of dermagraft a cultured human dermis, to treat diabetic foot ulcers. *Diabetes Care* 1992;19:350–354.

22. Alvarez OM, Mertz PM, Eaglstein WH. The effect of occlusive dressings on collagen synthesis and re-epithelialization in superficial wounds. *J Surg Res* 1983;35:142–148.

23. Tomic-Canic M, Agren MS, Alvarez OM. Epidermal repair and the chronic wound, in *The Epidermis in Wound Healing* (Rovee DT, Maibach H, eds.), CRC Press, Boca Raton, FL, 2004, pp. 25–57.

24. Alvarez OM, Hefton JM, Eaglstein WE. Healing wound:occlusion or exposure. *Infect Surg* 1984;3:173–181.

25. Burton CS. Management of chronic and problem lower extremity wounds. *Dermatol Clin* 1993;11:767–773.

26. Varghese MC, Balin AK, Carter M, et al. Local environment of chronic wounds under synthetic dressings. *Arch Dermatol* 1986;122:52–57.

27. Alvarez OM. Pharmacological and environmental modulation of wound healing, in *Connective Tissue Disease. Molecular Pathology of the Extracellular Matrix* (Uitto J, Parejda AJ, eds.), New York, Marcel Dekker, 1987, pp. 367–384.

28. Alvarez OM, Patel M, Booker J, Markowitz L. Effectiveness of a biocellulose wounddressing for the treatment of chronic venous leg ulcers: results of a single center randomized study involving 24 patients, *Wounds* 2004;16(7):224–233.

29. Thomas S. Alginate dressings in surgery and wound management-part 3 *J Wound Care* 2000;9:163–166.

30. Ovington LG. The well dressed wound: an overview of dressing types. *Wounds* 1998;10 (Suppl A):1A–11A.

31. Klasen HJ. A historical review of the use of silver in the treatment of burns. II. Renewed interest for silver. *Burns* 2000;26:131–138.

32. Kucan JO, Robson MC, Heggers JP, et al. Comparison of silver sulfadiazine, povidone iodine and physiologic saline in the treatment of pressure ulcers. *J Am Geriatr Soc* 1981; 29:232–235.

33. Holloway GA, Johansen KH, Barnes RW, Pierce GE. Multicenter trial of cadexomer iodine to treat venous stasis ulcers. *West J Med* 1989;151:35–38.

34. Apelqvist J, Ragnarson Tennvall G. Cavity foot ulcers in diabetic patients: a comparative study of cadexomer iodine and standard treatment. An economic analysis alongside a clinical trial. *Acta Dermatol Venereol* 1996;76:231–235.

35. Leipziger LS, Glushko V, DiBernardo B, Shafaie F, Noble J, Alvarez OM. Dermal wound repair: role of collagen matrix implants and synthetic polymer dressings. *J Am Acad Dermatol* 1985;12(2):409–419.

36. Veves A, Sheehan P, Pham HT, et al. A randomized controlled trial of promogran (a collagen/oxidized regenerated cellulose dressing) vs standard treatment in the management of diabetic foot ulcers. *Arch Surg* 2002;137:822–827.
37. Brigido SA, Boc SF, Lopez RC. Effective management of major lower extremity wounds using an acellular regenerative tissue matrix: a pilot study. *Orthopedics* 2004;27(1 Suppl): s145–s149.
38. Falanga V. How to use Apligraf to treat venous ulcers. *Skin Aging* 1999;7:30–36.
39. Sabolinski ML, Alvarez OM, Auletta M, Mulder G, Parentau NL. Cultured skin as a smart material for healing wounds: experience in venous ulcers. *Biomaterials* 1996;17:311–320.
40. Falanga V. Tissue engineering in wound repair. *Adv Skin Wound Care* 2000;13(2 Suppl);15–19.
41. Veves A, Falanga V, Armstrong DG, et al. Graftskin a human skin equivalent, is effective in the management of noninfected neuropathic diabetic foot ulcers: a prospective randomized multicenter clinical trial. *Diabetes Care* 2001;24(2);290–295.
42. Falanga V, Margolis D, Alvarez OM, et al. (The human skin equivalent investigators group), Rapid healing of venous ulcers and lack of clinical rejection with an allogeneic cultured human skin equivalent. *Arch Dermatol* 1998;134:293–300.
43. Charles C, Eaglstein WH. Active Treatments for acute and chronic wound, in *Wound Healing* (Rovee DT, Maibach H, eds.), CRC Press, Boca Raton, FL, 2004, pp. 351–373.
44. Eisenberg M, Llewellen D. Surgical management of hands in children with recessive dystrophic epidermolysis bullosa: use of allogeneic composite cultured skin grafts. *Br J Plat Surg* 1998;51:608–613.
45. Rheinwald JG, Green H. Serial cultivation of strains of human epidermal keratinocytes: the formation of keratinizing colonies from single cells. *Cell* 1975;6:331–343.
46. Leigh IM, Purkis PE, Navasaria HA, Phillips TJ. Treatment of chronic venous ulcers with sheets of cultured allogeneic keratinocytes. *Br J Dermatol* 1987;117:591–597.
47. Carsin H, Ainaud P, Le Bever H, Rives J, et al. Cultured epithelial autografts in extensive burn coverage of severely traumatized patients: a five year single center experience with 30 patients. *Burns* 2000;26:379–387.
48. Phillips TJ, Pachas W. Clinical trial of cultured autologous keratinocyte grafts in the treatment of long standing pressure ulcers. *Wounds* 1994;6:133–139.
49. Cooper M, Hansbrough J, Spielvogel R, et al. In vivo optimization of a living dermal substitute employing cultured human fibroblasts on a biodegradable polyglycolic acid or polyglactin mesh. *Biomaterials* 1991;12:243–248.
50. Jiang WG, Harding KG. Enhancement of wound tissue expansion and angiogenesis by matrix-embedded fibroblast (Dermagraft), a role for hepatocyte growth factor/scatter factor. *Int J Mol Med* 1998;2:203–210.
51. Purdue GF, Hunt JL, Still JM, et al. A multicenter clinical trial of biosynthetic skin replacement, Dermagraft-TC, compared with cryopreserved human cadaver skin for temporary coverage of excised burn wounds. *J Burn Care Rehabil* 1997;18 (1 Pt1), 52–57.
52. Steed DL. Clinical evaluation of recombinant human platelet-derived growth factor for the treatment of lower extremity diabetic ulcers. Diabetic Ulcer Study Group. *J Vasc Surg* 1995;21:71–78.
53. Weiman TJ, Smiel JM, Su Y. Efficacy and safety of a topical gel formulation of recombinant human platelet-derived growth factor-BB (beclapermin) in patients with chronic neuropathic ulcers. A phase III randomized placebo-controlled double blind study. *Diabetes Care* 1998;21:822–837.
54. Smiel JM, Wieman TJ, Steed DL, et al. Efficacy and safety of beclapermin (recombinant human platelet derived growth factor-BB) in patients with nonhealing, lower extremity diabetic ulcers: a combined analysis of four randomized studies. *Wound Repair Regen* 1999; 7:335–346.

55. Mertz PM, Alvarez OM, Smerbeck RV, Eaglstein WH. A new in vivo model for the evaluation of topical antiseptics on superficial wounds: the effect of 70% alcohol and povidoneiodine solution. *Arch Dermatol* 1984;120:58–62.

56. Van Den Broek PJ, Buys LMF, Van Furth R. Interaction of povidone-iodine compounds, phagocytic cells, and microorganisms. *Antimicrob Agents Chemother* 1982;22:593–597.

57. Lineaweaver W, Howard R, Soucy D, et al. Topical antimicrobial toxicity. *Arch Surg* 1985; 120:267–270.

58. Doughty D. A rational approach to the use of topical antiseptics. *J Wound Ostomy Continence Nurs* 1994;21:224–231.

59. Gruber RP, Vistnes L, Pardoe R. The effect of commonly used antiseptics on wound healing. *Plast Reconstr Surg* 1975;55:472–476.

60. Armstrong DG, Attinger CE, Boulton, AJM, et al. Guidelines regarding negative pressure wound therapy (NPWT) in the diabetic foot: Results of the Tucson Expert Concensus Conference (TECC) on V.A.C. Therapy *Ostomy Wound Manage* 2004;50(4 Suppl B): 3s–27s.

61. Ennis WJ, Meneses P. MIST ultrasound: the results of a multicenter randomized, double blind sham controlled trial of the healing of diabetic foot ulcers. *Wounds* 2005;17(3):A43.

62. Cope Z. The treatment of wounds through the ages. *Med Hist* 1958;2:163–174.

63. Alvarez OM, Rogers RS, Booker J, Patel M. Effect of noncontact normothermic wound therapy on the healing of neuropathic (diabetic) foot ulcers: an interim analysis of 20 patients. *J Foot Ankle Surg* 2003;42:30–35.

64. Carley PJ. Electrotherapy for acceleration of wound healing: low density direct current. *Arch Phys Med Rehabil* 1985;66:443–446.

65. Spadaro JA. Electrically stimulated bone growth in animals and man: review of the literature. *Clin Orthop* 1977;122:325–332.

66. Peters EJG, Armstrong DG, Wunderlich RP, et al. The benefit of electric stimulation to enhance perfusion in persons with diabetes mellitus. *J Foot Ankle Surg* 1998;37(5): 396–400.

67. Peters EJ, Lavery LA, Armstrong DG, Fleischli JG. Electric stimulation as an adjunct to heal diabetic foot ulcers: a randomized clinical trial. *Arch Phys Med Rehabil* 2001;82:721–724.

68. Levine NS, Lindberg RB, Mason AD, Pruitt BA. The quantitative swab culture and smear: a quick simple method for determining the number of viable bacteria in open wounds. *J Trauma* 1976;16:89–94.

69. Bornside GH, Bornside BB. Comparison between moist swab and tissue biopsy methods for quantitation of bacteria in experimental incisional wounds. *J Trauma* 1979;19:103–106.

70. Gentzkow GD, Jensen JL, Pollack RA, et al. Improved healing of diabetic foot ulcers after grafting with a living human dermal replacement. *Wounds* 1999;11:77–84.

71. Bentkover JD, Champpion AH. Economic evaluation of alternative methods of treatment for diabetic foot ulcer patients: cost effectiveness of platelet realesate and wound care clinics. *Wounds* 1993;5:207–215.

72. Boulton AJ, Meneses P, Ennis WJ. Diabetic foot ulcers: a framework for prevention and care. *Wound Rep Regen* 1999;7:7–17.

73. Thomas S, Banks V, Bale S, et al. A comparison of two dressings in the management of chronic wounds. *J Wound Care* 1997;6:383–386.

74. Kraft MR, Lawson L, Pohlman B, et al. A comparison of Epi-Lock and saline dressings in the management of pressure ulcers. *Decubitus* 1993;48:42–44.

75. Laing PW, Cogley DI, Klenerman L. Neuropathic foot ulceration treated by total contact casts. *J Bone Joint Surg* 1991;74:133–136.

76. Lyon RT, Veith FJ, Bolton L, Machado F. Clinical benchmark for healing of chronic venous ulcers. *Am J Surg* 1998;176:172–175.

77. Berry DP, Bale S, Harding KG. Dressings for treating cavity wounds. *J Wound Care* 1996;5:10–17.

78. Thomas S, Tucker CA. Sorbsan in the management of leg ulcers. *Pharm J* 1989;243:706–709.
79. Cannavo M, Fairbrother G, Owen D, et al. A comparison of dressings in the management of surgical abdominal wounds. *J Wound Care* 1998;7:57–62.
80. Davis S. Department of Dermatology University of Miami School of Medicine, personal communication.
81. Demling RH, DeSanti L. Effects of silver on wound management. *Wounds* 2001;13:5–15.
82. Niezgoda JA, Van Gils CC, Frykberg RG, et al. Randomized clinical trial comparing Oasis wound matrix to regranex gel for diabetic ulcers. *Skin Wound Care* 2005;18:258–266.

17

Surgical Treatment of the Ulcerated Foot

John M. Giurini, DPM

INTRODUCTION

Foot ulceration with infection is one of the leading causes of hospitalization for patients with diabetes mellitus. Although solid data on the true incidence and prevalence of diabetic foot ulcerations do not exist, it is believed that approx 15% of patients with diabetes will develop a foot or leg ulceration in their lifetime (1). The rate of recidivism is also staggering in this population with 50% of ulcerations recurring within 18 months. The number of lower extremity amputations among patients with diabetes has been well documented for years. Patients with diabetes are 15 times more likely to undergo a major lower extremity amputation than patients without diabetes, with the total number of major limb amputations being more than 50,000 (2).

When one considers there are 16 million people in the United States with diagnosed or undiagnosed diabetes mellitus, this not only places a significant sociological impact on the health care system but an enormous economic impact as well (3). It is estimated that in 1992 in the United States, the direct and indirect cost for care of the patient with diabetes was $91.8 billion. In comparison, $20.4 billion was spent in 1987. Treatment of diabetic foot infections cost $300 million per year and lower extremity amputations $600 million per year (1,3). These numbers are so staggering that the Department of Health and Human Services set as a goal of Healthy People 2000 a 40% reduction in diabetic amputations by the year 2000 (4).

The ability to achieve this goal requires a thorough understanding of the risk factors for ulcerations and amputations. Current algorithms take advantage of recent advances in antimicrobial therapy, wound healing strategies including topical growth factors and surgical intervention. One of the key components in establishing successful outcomes is identifying a dedicated team of healthcare professionals to manage these complex problems (5–8).

GOALS OF SURGERY

There was a time not too long ago when surgery on the patient with diabetes was to be avoided at any cost. In the past 5 years, however, surgical intervention is more readily accepted as a form of treatment and prevention of chronic ulcerations.

As with any surgery, the goals of the procedure must be clearly delineated. This is no different in patients with diabetes. What is different is the goals of surgery in patients with neuropathy as opposed to patients with normal sensation.

From: *The Diabetic Foot, Second Edition*
Edited by: A. Veves, J. M. Giurini, and F. W. LoGerfo © Humana Press Inc., Totowa, NJ

Table 1
Surgical Goals in the Insensate Patient

Reduce risk for ulceration/amputation
Reduce foot deformity
Provide stable foot for ambulation
Reduce pain
Improve appearance of foot

The primary reason for surgical intervention in patients with normal sensation is to reduce a painful condition by correcting an underlying deformity. In the absence of pain as in the neuropathic foot, the primary goal of surgery is to reduce the risk of lower extremity amputation by eliminating a focus of osteomyelitis or correcting those structural factors or deformities which may lead to ulcerations (Table 1).

It is also important to make a distinction between elective surgery, prophylactic surgery and urgent surgery. Elective surgery implies the presence of a deformity that can be corrected surgically but does not put the patient or the limb at risk. Often times, these deformities in the patient with diabetes can be managed noninvasively. There are clearly clinical situations where this type of conservative approach may be in the patient's best interest.

Prophylactic surgery is the surgery performed to prevent a more serious event. In the case of the diabetic patient with neuropathy, this event is most likely some type of amputation. This implies the presence of a deformity and a history of a chronically recurrent ulceration that puts the limb at risk. The goals of surgery in this scenario are to eliminate the deformity, reduce the risk of reulceration, thus reducing the risk of amputation.

Urgent surgery is self-explanatory. These patients commonly present with foul-smelling ulcerations with purulent drainage and cellulitis. Necrosis and abscess formation are not uncommon. These patients require immediate surgical intervention. The ultimate goal of surgery in this scenario is to control the infection, to prevent the patient from becoming septic and to save as much of the foot and/or leg as possible.

PREOPERATIVE EVALUATION

A detailed present and past medical history, past surgical history, list of current medications, and identification of risk factors such as smoking and nephropathy is critical to proper perioperative risk assessment. Patients with long-standing diabetes mellitus will often present with cardiac and renal complications, which must be managed to reduce the morbidity and mortality of the local foot procedure *(9)*. The surgeon would be well advised to obtain consultations with cardiology, nephrology, and endocrinology when appropriate.

A special word about vascular evaluation should be added. Because of the presence of autonomic neuropathy, the patient with diabetes will often present with pink, warm skin on the surface of the foot. This will give the appearance of a well-perfused foot even in the presence of critical ischemia (Fig. 1). Patients who lack palpable pulses at the level of the dorsalis pedis or posterior tibial artery should be evaluated further with noninvasive arterial studies in the form of pulse volume recordings or a formal

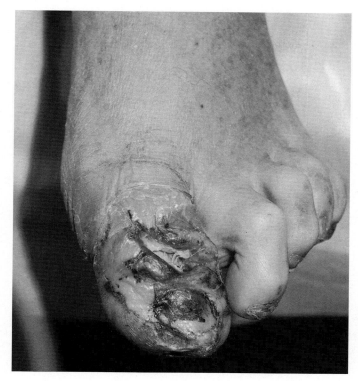

Fig. 1. Failure to recognize critical ischemia resulted in surgical failure in diabetic patient with autonomic neuropathy.

vascular surgery consultation. It is often necessary for patients to undergo lower extremity revascularization prior to limb-sparing foot surgery *(10)*.

A detailed social history has become increasingly important in recent years as more of the burden for a patient's aftercare is placed on the family. Because the majority of patients will require daily dressing changes and will be nonweightbearing for prolonged periods of time, visiting nurses, home health aides and physical therapists have become vital members of the multidisciplinary team. In situations where there is less than adequate support for these services at home, admission to a rehabilitative center or transitional care unit should be considered. These factors should be identified early in the course of the patient's hospitalization so as discharge planning can proceed in a timely and stress-free manner.

ANESTHESIA TECHNIQUES

The presence of profound peripheral sensory neuropathy and the localized nature of many of these procedures make local anesthesia with monitored intravenous sedation ideal. Epidural or general anesthesia should only be contemplated when more extensive surgery is being considered. This includes most major rearfoot procedures. It should be remembered that either of these techniques increases the perioperative morbidity and mortality *(11)*. The final choice of anesthesia should be made following discussion with the anesthesiologist and the patient's primary medical doctor and with a clear understanding of the procedure being performed.

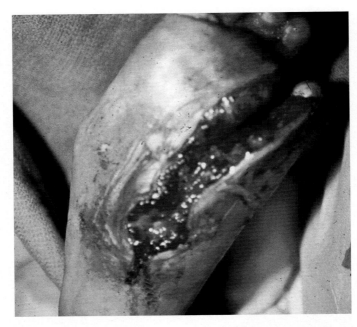

Fig. 2. An appropriate incision and drainage of infection should allow dependent drainage as the patient lies recumbent in bed.

SURGICAL APPROACH

Prior to definitive surgery or correction of an underlying deformity, the foot must be free of any acute infection. This implies that any areas of undrained sepsis be adequately drained and all necrotic tissue debrided to healthy granular tissue. The proper technique for draining wounds is to incise the wound in such a fashion to promote dependent drainage. As the patient lies recumbent in bed with the extremity elevated, this implies the wound will drain from distal to proximal (Fig. 2) *(12)*. Multiple stab incisions with the use of penrose drains should be avoided as they do not promote dependent drainage. Any tissue that appears infected or necrotic should be sharply excised at this time, including any exposed or infected bone. The wound is then packed widely open and inspected daily for the resolution of sepsis, cellulitis, and the development of healthy granulation tissue. The goal of this initial surgical debridement is to convert an acute infection into a chronic wound. Although negative cultures following initial debridement is preferred, it is not a prerequisite for definitive surgery and wound closure as additional surgical debridement is performed at the time of wound closure.

FOREFOOT PROCEDURES

First Ray

Although there are no studies showing the incidence of ulcers and their locations, ulcerations of the first ray (hallux and first metatarsal) are clearly among the most common ulcers treated. Common sites of ulcerations include (1) plantarmedial aspect of the hallux, (2) distal tip of the hallux, (3) directly plantar to the interphalangeal joint

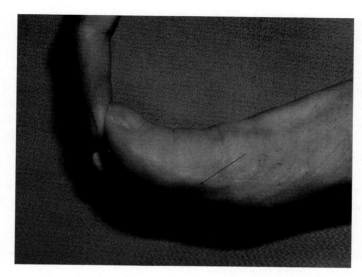

Fig. 3. A common location for ulcerations of the great toe is on the plantarmedial aspect of the interphalangeal joint of the hallux. The most common reason for these ulcerations is a hallux limitus.

of the hallux, (4) directly plantar to the metatarsophalangeal joint (MTPJ), (5) directly plantar to the first metatarsal head, and (6) medial aspect of the first metatarsal head. The primary reason this area is so susceptible is the combination of increased weightbearing forces across this joint and faulty biomechanics leading to excessive pronation *(13–15)*. Excessive pronation leads to a medial transfer of the weightbearing forces through the medial longitudinal arch, the first metatarsal and ultimately the hallux *(16)*.

Any structural deformities such as osteoarthritis, hallux limitus/rigidus, or severe plantarflexion will increase the susceptibility of this joint to ulceration by altering the biomechanics of the joint. Assessing the underlying structural or mechanical cause of the ulceration is vital to selecting the most appropriate procedure.

Ulcerations of the hallux, either plantarmedial or directly plantar to the interphalangeal joint, are most commonly related to abnormal biomechanics of the first ray resulting from excessive pronation. This is often manifested by the development of callus on the medial aspect of the hallux ("medial pinch" callus) or limitation of motion at the first MTPJ (i.e., hallux limitus) (Fig. 3). A resulting hyperextension of the interphalangeal joint occurs to compensate for this lack of motion *(17,18)*. Other less common causes of ulceration are an enlarged medial condyle on the distal phalanx or the presence of an interphalangeal sesamoid bone, in which case the ulceration is typically directly plantar to the interphalangeal joint.

The surgical treatment of this entity clearly depends on the underlying cause. When the cause of the ulceration is related to lack of adequate motion, restoring motion by way of an arthroplasty of the hallux interphalangeal joint or of the first MTPJ can be helpful. By resecting the head of the proximal phalanx, further motion is available to the first ray and the ulceration often resolves *(18)*. This procedure can also be employed when osteomyelitis of the proximal phalanx is suspected. Occasionally, resection of an enlarged medial condyle can be effective in eliminating the callus. This, however, can result in instability of the joint and development of Charcot joint disease. In cases where there are significant degenerative changes at the level of the first MTPJ or complete lack of dorsiflexion, it is best to resect the base of the proximal phalanx and increase motion at this joint.

Surgical treatment of ulcerations directly plantar to the first metatarsal head can be addressed with excision of one or both sesamoid bones. During the propulsive phase of gait, the sesamoids will migrate distally and more plantar thus becoming more prominent. In the intrinsic minus foot this could serve as a potential pressure point and site of ulceration *(19)*.

The basic indication for sesamoidectomy is the presence of a chronically, recurrent ulceration directly plantar to the first metatarsal head without clinical or radiographic evidence of osteomyelitis of the first metatarsal head *(20)*. Contraindications for the procedure is the presence of significant degenerative changes of the first MTPJ or osteomyelitis of the first MTPJ. These are best treated with a Keller or first MPTJ arthroplasty. Additionally, the presence of a rigid plantarflexed first ray may be a relative contraindication to sesamoidectomy.

When the ulceration is found to extend to the level of the joint, osteomyelitis should be clinically suspected. Treatment must involve complete resection of the infected bone and joint. The procedure of choice is resection of the first MTPJ with excision of the ulceration. Although there may be alternate methods for addressing this problem surgically, there are clear advantages to utilizing this approach rather than allowing the ulcer to heal by secondary intention. By excising the ulceration, all infected, nonviable tissue is removed. It also allows for excellent exposure of all potentially infected tissues, such as the flexor hallucis longus tendon and the sesamoids which are commonly involved. Wounds which are closed primarily heal more predictably. As a rule, these wounds will heal in 3–4 weeks. The healing rate of wounds which are allowed to heal by secondary intention are dependent on size and depth. The longer these wounds remain open, the greater the risk of secondary infection as patient compliance often becomes an issue. Although disadvantages exist to closing these wounds primarily, it is our philosophy that the benefits of primary closure outweigh the risks *(21)*.

The indication for the first MTPJ resection with ulcer excision is the presence of an ulcer directly plantar to the first MTPJ with direct extension into the joint. This is best determined by the ability to pass a blunt sterile probe through the ulceration and palpate bone. Additionally, the presence of clear, viscous drainage is indicative of synovial fluid. This is an ominous sign as this can only be coming from the joint itself (suggesting a tear in the joint capsule) or from the sheath of the flexor hallucis longus tendon (Fig. 4). Even in the presence of negative X-rays, this finding is sufficient to make the clinical diagnosis of osteomyelitis *(22)*.

An elliptical incision is made which completely excises the ulceration. It is recommended that the ratio of incision length to incision width is at least 3:1 so that wound closure can be achieved with as little tension as possible. This incision is full-thickness and is carried down to the first metatarsal joint (Fig. 5). This should excise all necrotic, infected tissue. At this point the flexor hallucis longus tendon will be visible. Typically focal necrosis within the body of the tendon will be present, indicating infectious involvement. It is therefore best to sacrifice the tendon in order to prevent recurrence of the infection.

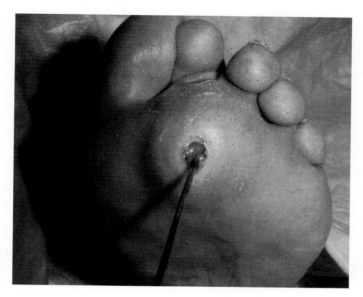

Fig. 4. The presence of synovial drainage from a ulceration is indicative of joint involvement and requires resection of that joint.

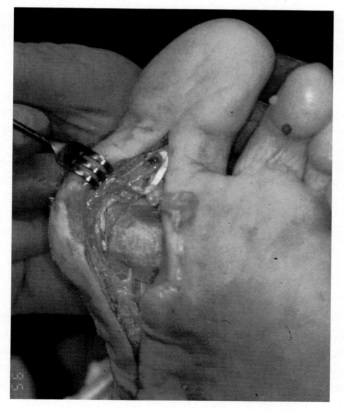

Fig. 5. Osteomyelitis of the first metatarsophalangeal joint is best addressed by elliptical excision of the ulcer with resection of the joint. Adequate resection of the first metatarsal should be performed to assure complete eradication of infected bone.

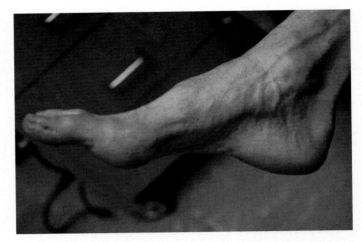

Fig. 6. Motor neuropathy is characterized by wasting of the intrinsic musculature in the arch of the foot. This typically results in deformities such as hammertoes, clawtoes, or plantarflexed metatarsals.

Once the tendon is removed, the sesamoids will be visualized. These should also be sacrificed as these are intra-articular structures and are in direct communication with the first MTPJ. The base of the proximal phalanx and the cartilage of the first metatarsal head are now resected. Although it is preferred to leave as much of the first metatarsal behind as possible to maintain function, enough metatarsal head must be resected so as to remove all focus of osteomyelitis.

The wound is closed by using full-thickness nonabsorbable sutures. Prolene is generally a good choice as it is nonabsorbable and monofilament. Sutures should be placed evenly and used to coapt skin edges with as little tension as possible. It is best to avoid using any deep sutures because these can serve as a potential focus of infection and may be difficult to retrieve at a later date if necessary. It is advisable to pack the proximal 1 cm of the wound with a 2 × 2 gauze sponge to promote drainage and avoid the development of a hematoma. This is usually removed after 24–48 hours and the wound should heal uneventfully. The postoperative care mandates a period of total nonweightbearing of at least 4 weeks. Early ambulation will result in wound dehiscence, persistent drainage, postoperative infection, and possible hypertrophic scar. The sutures are left in place this entire time.

Lesser Digits

Atrophy of the intrinsic muscles of the foot commonly occurs with the development of motor neuropathy. This can result in forefoot deformities such as hammertoes and clawtoes (Fig. 6) *(11,23)*. When sensory neuropathy is also present, ulcerations develop over the proximal interphalangeal joint, at the distal tip of a toe or on adjacent sides of toes. Amputation of a lesser toe rarely results in long-term complications with the exception of loss of the second toe. This can precipitate a hallux valgus deformity. When ulceration is discovered early enough and treated aggressively, amputation of a toe can be avoided, thus maintaining appearance as well as function.

Hammertoes are classified as either reducible or nonreducible. A reducible hammertoe implies the deformity is being held by contractures of the soft tissues, whereas a nonreducible deformity suggests there has been joint adaptation as well as extensive soft-tissue contractures. A reducible deformity is often amenable to correction by a tenotomy of the corresponding flexor tendon, whereas a nonreducible deformity requires resection of the phalangeal head as well as a release of the soft tissue *(23)*. A proximal interphalangeal joint arthroplasty can be combined with excision of the ulcer. In longstanding hammertoe deformities there may be a concomitant contracture at the level of the MTPJ, often indicative of a subluxation or even a dislocation. When dislocated, an area of high focal pressure can develop on the ball of the foot under the corresponding metatarsal head. This is often manifested as callus or even ulceration. Failure to recognize this fact can lead to incomplete correction of the deformity and failure to resolve the ulceration. The contracture at the MTPJ often requires a tenotomy and capsulotomy of the joint. If the joint cannot be relocated following release of the soft tissue alone, a shortening osteotomy of the metatarsal may be necessary to relocate the joint and relieve the plantar pressure.

Osteomyelitis of the tip of the distal phalanx can often be treated by local excision of the distal phalangeal tuft and primary closure of the ulceration. If, however, there is any concern of residual infection the wound may be left open and closed at a later date.

Lesser Metatarsal Procedures

The area under the metatarsal heads represents the next most common location of diabetic foot ulcerations. Common causes of high foot pressures include: abnormal foot mechanics, plantarflexed metatarsals, limited joint mobility, and prior surgical intervention *(23–26)*. There are no definitive studies on ulcer incidence and location. Empirically, however, it appears that the second metatarsal is more susceptible to ulceration. This is most likely because of the second metatarsal's dependence on the mechanics of the first ray. When excessive pronation of the medial column occurs, there is increased weight transfer and pressure to the lateral metatarsals. This is most often manifested by the development of callus under the second metatarsal head *(25)*. After the second metatarsal, the typical order of ulcer development is the third metatarsal then the fifth followed by the fourth.

Selection of surgical procedures for ulcerations under the metatarsal heads requires careful evaluation of the ulcer. A critical determinant in the surgical management of these ulcerations is whether osteomyelitis is present or not.

Lesser Metatarsal Osteotomy

The primary goal of procedures to surgically treat metatarsal head ulcerations is to alleviate areas of high focal pressure. A metatarsal osteotomy can serve as a valuable adjunct in the management and resolution of these ulcerations *(27)*. The primary indication is the presence of a chronically recurrent ulceration under a metatarsal head without direct extension into bone. An incision is made dorsally over the involved metatarsal. Once the surgical neck is identified, a through and through osteotomy is made. Although varying techniques have been described, the preferred technique is a V-type osteotomy with the apex directed toward the joint (Fig. 7). This provides a stable bone-cut resistant to medial or lateral dislocation. A small collar of bone can be resected

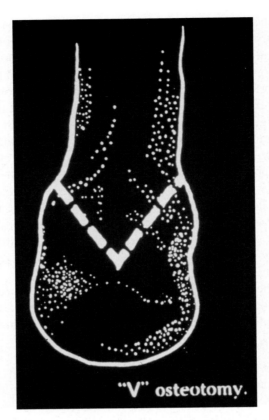

Fig. 7. A dorsal to plantar V-osteotomy through the surgical neck of the lesser metatarsal allows for adequate relief of plantar pressure overlying a ulceration. The medial and lateral wings of the "V" decrease the risk of medial or lateral dislocation of the metatarsal head.

which allows for both shortening as well as elevating the metatarsal. This is often desirable when the metatarsophalangeal joint is either subluxed or dislocated. The metatarsal head is then elevated to the same level of the adjacent metatarsals. Fixation of the osteotomy with a 0.045 Kirschner wire is preferred. However, in the presence of an open ulceration, this is contraindicated. Fixation and stability is achieved by impacting the head onto the shaft. The patient is then maintained nonweightbearing for 4–6 weeks to allow for early bone healing.

Recently, we have been utilizing the Weil osteotomy *(28)*. In this approach, the bone is osteotomized in a dorsal-distal to plantar-proximal direction at the level of the surgical neck. It is then fixated with a single 2.0 cortical screw (Fig. 8A,B). The advantage of this technique is that it allows for both shortening and dorsiflexion of the metatarsal head with little risk of dorsal dislocation. The Weil osteotomy works well in patients with a relatively normal to flatfoot. However, in patients with a rigid anterior cavus foot, the amount of proximal translocation is often not enough to resolve the ulceration. The V-osteotomy is the preferred procedure in this group of patients.

Complications following metatarsal osteotomies include transfer calluses or ulcerations and stress fractures of adjacent metatarsals. These most commonly result when the metatarsal head is elevated above the plane of the adjacent metatarsals. The risk of

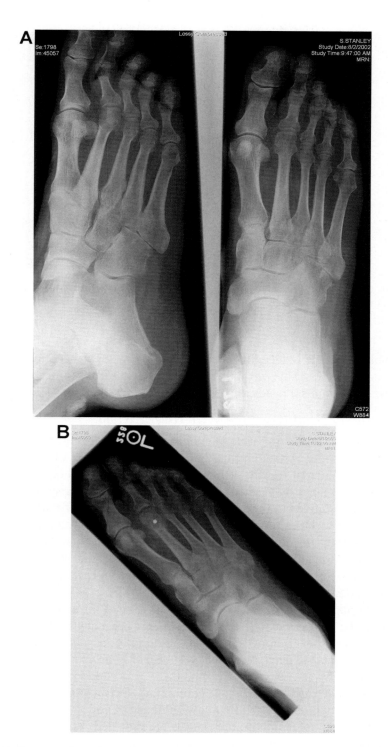

Fig. 8. (A) Preoperative X-ray demonstrating long second metatarsal resulting in plantar ulceration. **(B)** Postoperative X-ray showing corrected metatarsal position following Weil osteotomy fixated with a single 2.0-mm cortical screw.

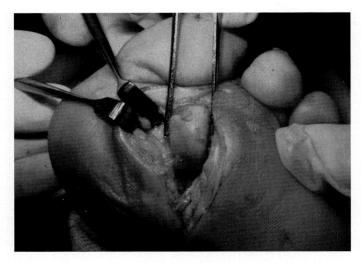

Fig. 9. An osteomyelitic lesser metatarsal head can be resected through a plantar elliptical incision excising the ulceration *in toto.*

transfer problems can be reduced if the patient is fitted with an accommodative custom orthosis postoperatively. This will allow for more even distribution of weightbearing forces across all metatarsal heads. Shoegear modification may also assist in this role.

Lesser Metatarsal Head Resection With Ulcer Excision

An alternative approach for relieving plantar pressure is to resect the offending metatarsal head entirely. Although this will result in resolution of the ulceration, this carries a high incidence of transfer lesion or ulceration. For this reason, it is preferred to perform this procedure only when osteomyelitis of the metatarsal head is suspected and there is no alternative but to resect the offending metatarsal head.

Resection of the metatarsal head can be approached through a dorsal linear incision centered directly over the metatarsal head. It should be remembered that the base of the corresponding proximal phalanx should also be resected as this structure is contiguous with the metatarsal head and is also involved. The ulcer is then allowed to heal by secondary intention.

An alternate approach is to resect the metatarsal head through a plantar approach while excising the ulceration. The advantage of this approach is that all necrotic and infected tissue can be excised and all tissue be directly inspected (Fig. 9). Following resection of the metatarsal head, the wound can be closed primarily as described for first MTPJ resection.

The postoperative care requires that sutures are left in place for a minimum of 3 weeks and the patient is kept totally nonweightbearing for 3–4 weeks. The patient is maintained on oral antibiotics until the sutures are removed. Long-term complications include possible transfer lesions or ulcerations and stress fractures resulting from the altered weightbearing surface. It is therefore recommended that patients be fitted with an appropriate orthotic device to distribute pressures evenly.

Panmetatarsal Head Resection

Weightbearing forces are designed to be evenly dispersed across all metatarsal heads. This weightbearing interdependence between the metatarsal heads has been previously described first by Morton and later by Cavanagh *(13,14)*. Disruption of this relationship will alter normal weight distribution. This can occur from trauma to the metatarsals resulting in dorsiflexed or shortened metatarsals as seen in stress fractures, the atrophic form of Charcot joint resulting in dissolution of metatarsal heads or prior surgical resection of metatarsal heads for osteomyelitis.

The recidivistic nature of diabetic foot disease makes multiple metatarsal procedures common in this patient population. Osteomyelitis of multiple metatarsal heads was previously treated by transmetatarsal amputation. This procedure was popularized by Dr. Leland McKittrick of the New England Deaconess Hospital and was responsible for saving thousands of limbs *(29)*. It is not without its complications. Ulcerations at the distal stump and equinovarus contractures are common long-term complications (Fig. 10A,B). Patients have difficulty psychologically accepting this procedure because it will often require special shoegear that draws attention to the fact they have had an amputation.

The panmetatarsal head resection and its variations were originally described for the treatment of painful lesions in patients with rheumatoid arthritis *(30–33)*. Jacobs first described the use of the panmetatarsal head resection for the successful treatment of chronic neuropathic ulcerations *(34)*. This report was subsequently followed by a report by Giurini et al. in which a larger series of patients was studied and an alternate technique was described *(32)*. Similar success rates were cited. Over the years, the panmetatarsal head resection has replaced the transmetatarsal amputation (TMA) as the procedure of choice in patients with recurrent ulcerations following prior surgical resection of metatarsal heads *(35,36)*.

The primary indication for the panmetatarsal head resection is the presence of chronically recurrent neuropathic ulcerations on the plantar aspect of the foot following prior metatarsal head resections or ray amputations. It is our belief that if two or more metatarsals have already been resected or need to be resected to eliminate osteomyelitis, the patient would then be best served by a panmetatarsal head resection (Fig. 11). At first this may appear to be a drastic, aggressive approach. However, experience has shown that this approach may actually spare patients additional trips to the operating room for transfer ulcerations.

Various surgical approaches have been described for the panmetatarsal head resection. Dorsal approaches, plantar approaches, or a combination of the two have been performed with equal success *(37)*. When possible the preferred approach is the 4 incision dorsal approach: one incision directly over the first metatarsal, one between the second and third metatarsals, one directly over the fourth metatarsal and one directly over the fifth metatarsal. This approach has the advantages of allowing adequate exposure of all metatarsal heads, decreases the potential for retraction injury on the skin edges, and maintains adequate skin islands so as not to affect vascular supply. Because the primary indication for this procedure is the presence of an open ulceration with osteomyelitis, the most common approach is to combine a dorsal incision with a plantar incision which excises the ulceration. The plantar wound and all necrotic tissue can then be excised, the involved metatarsal head(s) can be resected and the wound closed primarily as previously described.

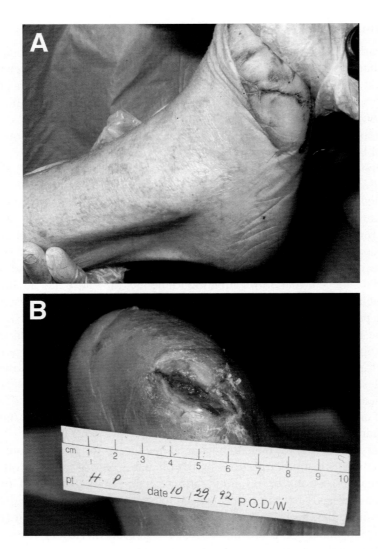

Fig. 10. (A) A common complication following transmetatarsal amputation is contracture of the Achilles tendon and subsequent equinus deformity. This can lead to characteristic lesions at the distal end of the TMA. **(B)** A distal lateral ulceration of a TMA with an underlying equinovarus deformity.

The surgical technique for resection of the metatarsal heads has already been described. The most important technical point to remember in performing this procedure is to maintain the metatarsal parabola. This typically means that the first and second metatarsals are left approximately the same length, whereas the third, fourth, and fifth metatarsals are each successfully shorter. Failure to maintain this relationship can lead to recurrent ulceration and additional surgery. If a prior metatarsal head resection or ray amputation has already been performed, then a perfect parabola may not be achievable. In that case the metatarsal parabola should be recreated with the remaining metatarsals. Additionally, the extensor tendons are identified and are retracted. This will maintain the function of these tendons during the gait cycle affording this procedure the prime advantage over the TMA.

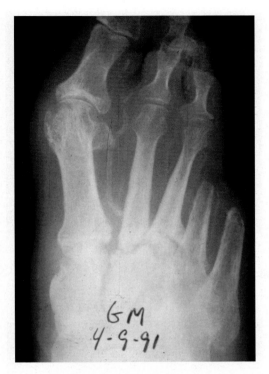

Fig. 11. Prior resection of two metatarsal heads and the presence of osteomyelitis of a remaining metatarsal head is indication for panmetatarsal head resection.

MIDFOOT PROCEDURES

Surgery in this region of the foot is most commonly necessary following foot deformities resulting from neuroarthropathic (Charcot) joint disease. The most common location of Charcot joint involves the tarsometatarsal (Lisfranc's) joints but other joints in the midfoot may also be affected *(38,39)*. Instability of Lisfranc's joint often results in a rockerbottom deformity of the midfoot with plantarmedial ulceration. This is primarily resulting from subluxation of the first metatarsal and medial cuneiform creating a plantar prominence. Ulcerations on the plantar and lateral aspect of the foot are not uncommon. These result from plantar extrusion of the cuboid from a Charcot process at the calcaneocuboid joint *(38)*. These pose a significant management problem as they are typically recalcitrant to conservative measures. There is no one surgical procedure that can be applied to all ulcers in this location. Therefore, a flexible approach to these lesions is required. Surgical approaches may involve simple ostectomy with or without fasciocutaneous flap or primary arthrodesis of unstable joints.

Ostectomy

This is the simplest approach to chronic ulcerations of the midfoot. This is reserved for those deformities that have their apex directly plantar to the first metatarsal–medial cuneiform joint and in which the midfoot is not hypermobile.

The depth of the ulceration will dictate the best surgical approach. A direct medial incision which is centered over the joint is preferred when the ulceration is superficial

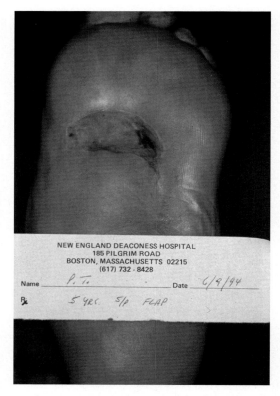

NEW ENGLAND DEACONESS HOSPITAL
185 PILGRIM ROAD
BOSTON, MASSACHUSETTS 02215
(617) 732 - 8428

Name _____ P. T. _____ . Date __6/9/94__

Rx _____ 5 yrs. S/p FLAP ____

Fig. 12. Patient who is 5 years status postcuboid exostectomy with an interpositional muscle flap and a rotational fasciocutaneous flap.

and not involving bone. This will allow for excellent visualization of the joint and the prominent bone. The prominence can then be resected from medial to lateral either with an osteotome or with a saw. The goal should be to remove an adequate amount of bone to alleviate the plantar pressure and not create a new bony prominence which could create a new source of irritation and ulceration, thus negating the benefits of the procedure.

Ulcerations which communicate with bone and show signs of osteomyelitis clinically are best managed by excision of the ulceration with bone resection and primary closure of the ulceration. This is performed as previously described. In addition to removing the infected bone, the ability to close the ulceration without tension is an additional goal. The use of closed suction irrigation is also recommended in order to prevent hematoma formation which can lead to wound dehiscence or infection.

This approach can be used when the ulcer is located either plantar central or plantar lateral in the midfoot. The most likely etiology for these ulcerations is plantar displacement of the cuboid. When the ulceration measures less than 2.5 cm, this surgical approach can be used. For ulcerations greater than 2.5 cm in diameter, an alternate approach should be employed. This will often require some form of rotational or fasciocutaneous flap. The flexor digitorum brevis muscle is well suited for this purpose because of its anatomic location and ease of dissection. The muscle is rotated laterally to cover the cuboid. A full-thickness fasciocutaneous flap which is based on the medial plantar artery is then rotated from medial to lateral to cover the actual ulcer site. A split thickness skin graft is then used to cover the donor site in the medial arch (Fig. 12).

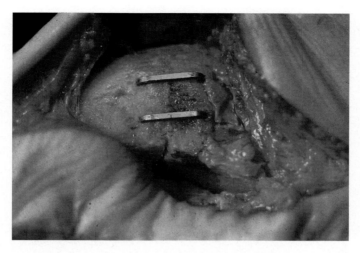

Fig. 13. Fusion of the first metatarsal–medial cuneiform joint for an unstable Charcot joint complicated by recurrent ulceration can be achieved by use of staples.

Six weeks of total nonweightbearing is required for adequate healing and incorporation of the flap. This is followed by an additional 2–4 weeks of protected weightbearing in a healing sandal. Long-term care will require the use of plastizote orthoses and modified shoegear.

Medial Column Fusion

When resolution of the Charcot joint process has resulted in significant bone loss such that there is significant instability at the first metatarsal–medial cuneiform joint, primary fusion of this joint should be considered. Simple exostectomy in the presence of instability will often fail because of continued collapse of this segment, resulting in a new bony prominence. Stabilization of this joint therefore is the better alternative.

The joint can be approached surgically through a direct medial incision. This will afford adequate exposure of the dorsum of the joint as well as the plantar surface. The articular cartilage on both sides of the joint can be resected with a sagittal saw. It is recommended that the bone cut on the first metatarsal side be slightly angulated from dorsal-proximal to plantar-distal. This will plantarflex the first metatarsal slightly, restoring the weightbearing function of the first ray. In addition, it is recommended that any plantar bony prominence also be resected from medial to lateral.

Fixation of the joint can be achieved in a variety of ways. Although crossed 0.062 Kirschner wires and staples are acceptable means of fixation, the authors prefer the use of a medial plate with an interfragmentary screw to provide rigid internal fixation and compression (Figs. 13 and 14A,B). It is advisable to insert a Jackson-Pratt drain to prevent the accumulation of a hematoma.

The postoperative course requires immobilization and nonweightbearing. Although there is no standard length of immobilization and nonweightbearing, the patient can expect to be nonweightbearing on average 3 months. Partial weightbearing may begin when serial X-rays show early trabeculation across the first metatarsal–medial cuneiform joint. Continued resumption of weightbearing is allowed as long as both clinical and radiographic evaluations suggest continued healing of the fusion site.

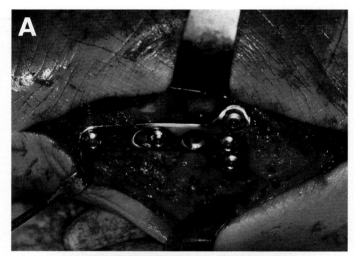

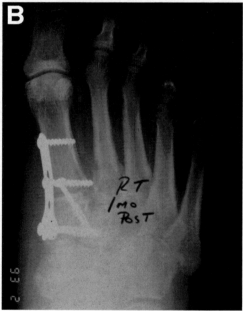

Fig. 14. (A) A T-plate with an interfragmentary screw is another acceptable form of fixation of the first metatarsal–medial cuneiform joint in the presence of unstable Charcot joint. **(B)** Radiograph of patient with T-plate and interfragmentary screw across the first metatarsal–medial cuneiform joint.

Exostectomy With Fasciocutanous Flap

One of the more difficult ulcerations to manage is an ulcer located centrally in the midfoot secondary to plantar subluxation of the cuboid bone. This is the type 5 of the Harris and Brand classification of Charcot joint disruption (pattern II in the Sanders classification) and has been described as being very resistant to conservative care

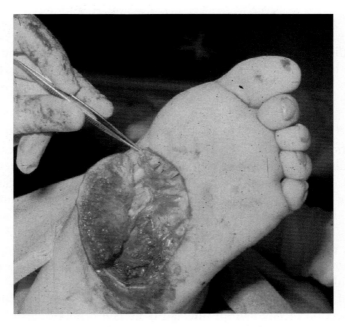

Fig. 15. The flexor digitorum brevis muscle is commonly used for closure in large plantar ulcerations following ulcer excision and exostectomy of the offending bone.

(38,39). Resolution of these ulcerations often require surgical intervention of some type. As previously discussed when ulcerations of this type exceed 2.5 cm in diameter, primary excision with closure is often not possible and an alternate technique must be sought *(40)*.

Ulcerations of this size are typically excised circumferentially to the level of the cuboid bone. This will allow removal of all necrotic, infected tissue as well as any hyperkeratotic margins bordering the ulcer. The joint capsule and periosteum of the cuboid are next encountered which are reflected off the underlying cuboid. This will expose the peroneal groove of the cuboid bone. The peroneus longus will often be found running in the groove. When possible this should be retracted so as to protect it from inadvertent injury. On rare occasions, however, it may be necessary to sacrifice the peroneus longus in order to gain adequate exposure of the bony prominence. The peroneal groove is next resected with the use of an osteotome and mallet. Once completed, the wound should be carefully inspected for any remaining bony prominence or bone spicules which can serve as a new point of pressure and possible ulceration.

This procedure will often leave a relatively large dead space which can serve for the collection of a hematoma. It is best to fill this dead space with a muscle flap which will serve two purposes: (1) it will decrease the dead space following the bony resection and (2) it will provide a layer of soft tissue between the underlying bone and the overlying skin (Fig. 15).

REARFOOT PROCEDURES

Surgical procedures of the rearfoot are most commonly performed for reconstruction of unstable Charcot joint disease and can be truly classified as limb salvage procedures. These include partial or subtotal calcanectomy, triple arthrodesis, and pantalar arthrodesis.

Indications for these reconstructive procedures include chronic, nonhealing ulcerations with underlying rearfoot deformity or instability, severe instability of the rearfoot making ambulation difficult at best or chronic heel ulcerations with underlying osteomyelitis. Because of the high-risk nature of these procedures, all conservative measures should be attempted prior to intervening surgically or when the only alternative is a major limb amputation.

Calcanectomy

Heel ulcerations are not an uncommon event in patients with diabetes. Owing to the comorbid conditions most patients with diabetes display, periods of prolonged bedrest is not unusual. Without proper protection decubitus ulcerations can occur. However, other causes for heel ulcers include blisters from shoe or cast irritation and heel fissures resulting from dry skin or puncture wounds. Regardless of the precipitating cause, the end result is prolonged disability and morbidity. In cases of bone involvement (i.e., osteomyelitis), below knee amputation can be the final outcome. Attempts to save this extremity to provide a limb capable of functional ambulation can involve excision of the ulceration and the calcaneus, either partial or subtotal.

The goals of the calcanectomy should include excision of all necrotic and infected soft tissue, resection of any and all infected bone and primary closure of the wound whenever possible. Additional bone resection may be necessary in order to achieve primary closure. Hindrances to primary closure can include the lack of mobility of the surrounding soft tissue and severe tissue loss from infection. In these cases, a more creative approach may be necessary. This can include rotational skin flaps or free tissue transfers.

The second goal of this procedure is resection of the calcaneus. The majority of times this procedure is being performed for osteomyelitis. It is therefore critical that adequate bone is removed to eliminate the infection. It is also important that no plantar prominence be left behind which could serve as an irritant to the soft tissue and result in ulceration. In resecting the calcaneus the Achilles tendon is often encountered. Depending on the extent of infection, it may need to be debrided or even released. Although one may be tempted to reattach the tendon, it is rarely advisable to do so. Advancement of the Achilles tendon would require the introduction of foreign materials such as screws or anchors which could serve as a possible source of recurrent infection. In those cases in which the Achilles tendon is detached, it will often fibrose to the surrounding tissues and provide some degree of plantarflexion (Fig. 16A,B).

Triple Arthrodesis

The incidence of Charcot joint disease involving the tarsal joints—talonavicular, calcaneocuboid or subtalar—ranges from 1.8% to 37% depending on the reports *(40–44)*. Clinically, these feet may appear with a rockerbottom deformity from plantar subluxation of the talonavicular joint or the calcaneocuboid joint. This can then lead to chronic ulceration. When faced with a significant degree of instability from this destructive process, the approach should include surgical stabilization of the involved joint or joints. This often requires fusion of the talonavicular joint, calcaneocuboid joint, and the subtalar joint, i.e., triple arthrodesis.

The goal of a triple arthrodesis is to stabilize the foot and to reduce the deformity, thereby reducing the risk of recurrent ulceration. While there have been recent publications advocating early rather than late reconstruction, it remains advisable to delay any surgery

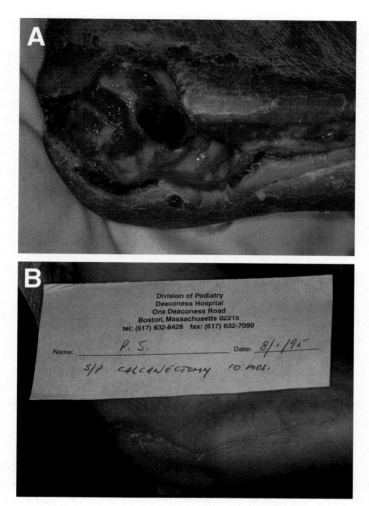

Fig. 16. (A) Osteomyelitis of the calcaneus with resultant soft-tissue loss is a common cause of lower limb amputation. **(B)** Patient in 14A following partial calcanectomy with excision and debridement of infected, necrotic tissue, and primary closure. Successful eradication of infected bone resulted in limb salvage.

until the acute phase has resolved and the Charcot joint has entered the coalescent phase *(45)*. If an open ulceration is present, surgery should be delayed until all acute signs of infection are resolved.

The triple arthrodesis is performed in the standard manner *(46)*. The calcaneocuboid joint is approached through a lateral incision just inferior to the lateral malleolus and extending distally to the base of the fourth and fifth metatarsals. Although it is possible to obtain adequate exposure of the talonavicular joint through this incision, one should not hesitate to make a separate incision medially if this affords better exposure.

The cartilage is resected off all joint surfaces until bleeding bone is exposed. The joints are then reapproximated. If significant deformity exists, wedge resections through the joints may be required to adequately reduce the deformity. Additionally, significant bone resorption may have occurred as a result of the destructive process. In these cases bone graft may be necessary to fill the gaps between joint surfaces. This can be obtained from the iliac crest or from the bone bank.

The method of fixation is the surgeon's choice. Typically, the posterior subtalar joint is fixated with a 6.5 mm cancellous screw. This screw can be introduced from a dorsal approach through the talar neck or a small stab incision can be made on the plantar surface of the heel. The screw is then inserted from plantar to dorsal, across the subtalar joint into the body of the talus. Although screws are preferred for the talonavicular and calcaneocuboid joints, staples can also be used. Adequate apposition of joints and accurate placement of fixation devices is achieved by the use of intraoperative X-rays. The goal of surgery is correction of the deformity with good apposition of all joint surfaces. Minimal to no gapping should be present. This should always be confirmed with a final intraoperative X-ray to confirm the final position of all fixation devices, adequate joint apposition appropriate foot position. The position of the calcaneus should be neutral to slight valgus.

Postoperatively, the patient is initially placed in a posterior splint to immobilize the fusion site. This is replaced with a below-the-knee fiberglass cast usually 4–5 days following surgery. Total nonweightbearing is maintained for a minimum of 3–4 months. Serial X-rays are obtained to evaluate bone healing and maintenance of postoperative correction and alignment. The patient is then advanced to gradual protected weightbearing when X-rays show signs of bony union. Anecdotal reports suggest that the likelihood and rate of fusion may be improved with the use of electrical bone stimulation although prospective, randomized double-blinded trials are needed to determine overall efficacy *(47)*. However, even if primary fusion is not achieved, it has been shown that patients can do well even in the presence of a stable pseudoarthrosis *(48)*. The primary goals in these patients are limb salvage and to convert a nonbraceable extremity to an extremity that can be supported with a brace if necessary.

Pantalar Arthrodesis

The ankle joint that has undergone severe destruction from Charcot joint disease is particularly problematic. This typically will result in an ankle joint so flail that it makes ambulation extremely difficult if not impossible. This deformity may result from total collapse of the talar body, fractures through the medial malleolus, lateral malleolus, or both. Patients with these types of fractures will often be found ambulating directly on either the medial or lateral malleolus. This inherent instability will result in the development of chronic ulcerations and are extremely difficult to control with conservative care alone. The prognosis for these deformities is poor. In order for limb salvage to be achieved, primary fusion of the ankle and subtalar joints is necessary.

The surgical approach depends on the level and degree of destruction. If the primary level of instability and destruction involves the tibiotalar joint, isolated fusion of this joint may be sufficient. However, if destruction of the other rearfoot joints is present, then fusion of the ankle, talonavicular, subtalar, and calcaneocuboid joints (i.e., pantalar fusion) should be performed. All surgical intervention should be delayed until all signs of acute Charcot joint disease have resolved. Attempted fusion during the active, hyperemic phase of this disorder will not only make fusion technically difficult but may also result in failure to fuse.

A lateral incision which begins approximately at the midfibula and extends to the tip of the lateral malleolus offers adequate exposure of the ankle joint. If a pantalar fusion is to be performed, this incision can be extended distally to the calcaneocuboid joint. The fibula is typically osteotomized just proximal to the ankle joint line. The anterior

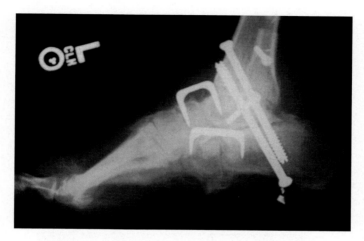

Fig. 17. Severe instability of the rearfoot resulting from Charcot joint often requires major reconstructive surgery of the hindfoot and ankle. A pantalar fusion was performed in this patient for severe cavoadductovarus deformity and chronic ulceration resulting from Charcot joint. Two 7 mm cannulated screws were used to fuse the subtalar and ankle joints.

aspect of the fibula is dissected free and reflected posteriorly. This preserves the vascular supply to the fibula. This will allow the fibula to be used as a vascularized strut graft on the lateral side of the ankle joint. The ankle joint is now well visualized.

The articular cartilage is resected down to bleeding cancellous bone from the inferior surface of the tibia surface and the dome of the talus. The ankle joint is repeatedly reapproximated so as to realign the foot. The joint surfaces are continually remodeled until optimal bone apposition and foot alignment is achieved. Recently, we have used femoral head allograft to fill in any defect or accommodate for any significant bone loss. If a pantalar fusion is being performed, the remaining rearfoot joints can be addressed at this time in the same manner as in a triple arthrodesis.

After all articular surfaces have been resected, the foot should be positioned so that all bone surfaces are in good apposition with minimal to no gapping. Care should also be taken to avoid any interposition of soft tissue. If the foot cannot be aligned properly or bone surfaces do not appose adequately, further remodeling of the bone should be performed. Once optimal alignment has been achieved, the ankle joint is ready for fixation. This can be performed with the introduction of two 7 mm cannulated screws. These are inserted from a plantar to dorsal direction through the body of the calcaneus and across the resected ankle joint. This will also fixate the posterior subtalar joint (Fig. 17). Ideally, the tips of the screw should purchase the cortex of the tibia. When bone quality precludes the use of internal fixation, external devices for fixation are appropriate alternatives. The use of intraoperative imaging is critical in the placement of temporary fixation. This can be achieved with fluoroscopy or intraoperative radiographs. It is critical that the calcaneus be positioned either in neutral or in slight valgus position. Any degree of varus should be avoided. After fixation of the ankle joint, the remaining rearfoot joints can be fixated as previously described.

As with triple arthrodesis, the postoperative care is critical to successful limb salvage. Wound infection, dehiscence, and nonunion are the major complications seen with this procedure. Immobilization of the extremity immediately postoperatively can decrease the risks of these complications. Total nonweightbearing in a fiberglass below the knee

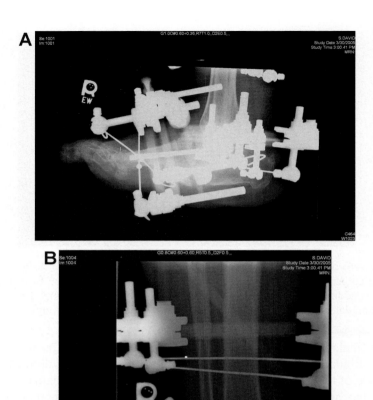

Fig. 18. (A) Charcot reconstruction demonstrating correction with combination of internal and external fixation to address midfoot and hindfoot deformities (Lateral view). **(B)** External ring fixator using thin wire technique (AP view).

cast is required for a minimum of 4–6 months. The fusion site must be protected with cast immobilization and casts must be changed frequently to prevent abrasions or cast irritations. Once it is felt fusion is sufficient to support weightbearing, this should be instituted in a gradual protected manner. A return to protected weightbearing will be dictated by serial X-rays. The use of adjunctive modalities to promote fusion, such as electrical bone stimulation, should be considered in this patient population as these patients and procedures are considered at high risk for nonunion.

The surgical reconstruction of these complex deformities have benefited by recent advances in external fixation. As previously stated, the degree of bone loss in these

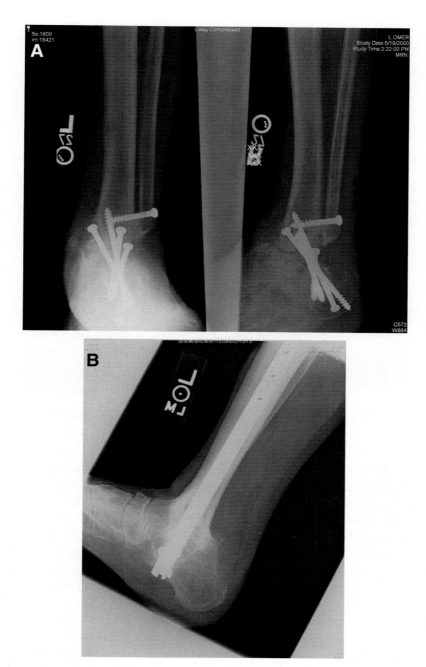

Fig. 19. (A) Failed ankle arthrodesis resulting from lack of bone substance and poor fixation technique. **(B)** Revision of ankle arthrodesis using intramedullary nail (5 years post-operation).

hindfoot deformities will often not allow for dependable use of internal fixation devices. In addition, the presence of an open ulceration and osteomyelitis makes the use of internal fixation contraindicated. It has therefore become necessary to use various external fixation constructs to achieve stabilization of these deformities without the inherent

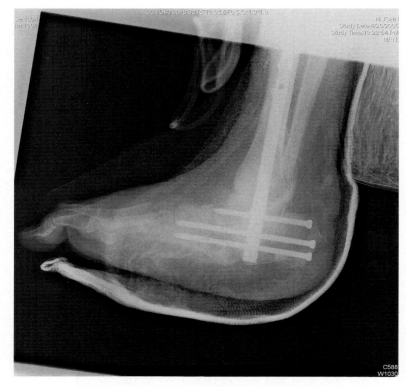

Fig. 20. X-ray showing Charcot ankle reconstruction using an intramedullary nail and femoral head allograft.

risks of internal fixation. The most common construct utilizes a combination of multiplane fine wire ring fixators, half pins, and a foot plate attached to the leg and foot at different levels *(49)*. It was previously felt that external fixation devices were contraindicated in the patients with diabetes for fear of pin tract infections. However, the introduction of fine wires has made the use of external fixation devices feasible in patients with diabetes. Where possible, this can be used in conjunction with internal fixation (Fig. 18A,B). This offers the added advantage that rigid internal fixation remains in place even after the external fixator is removed, typically 8–10 weeks postoperatively. This is often employed when there is a combined midfoot and hindfoot Charcot process.

When faced with the flail Charcot ankle joint, there are limited options. In most circumstances, there is such extensive bone loss that use of internal fixation is bound to fail (Fig. 19A,B). In these cases, we have had success using the intramedullary nail, a technique borrowed from the trauma arena. The ankle joint is exposed through a standard lateral incision over the lateral malleolus. The lateral malleolus is resected distally exposing the Charcot ankle joint. All cartilage and bony debris is resected leaving healthy bleeding bone surfaces behind. The nail is then introduced through an incision plantar to the calcaneal body. A channel is then created over a guide wire through the calcaneus, across the joint and into the distal tibia. The nail is then inserted over the guide wire. It can be secured in place by proximal screws securing the nail to the tibia and a second screw distally through the posterior calcaneus. This will prevent either proximal or distal migration of the nail.

When large amounts of the ankle joint are resected, an allograft fashioned from femoral head can be inserted in the ankle joint (Fig. 20).

REFERENCES

1. Reiber GE, Boyko EJ, Smith DG. Lower extremity foot ulcers and amputations in diabetes. *Diabetes in America*, 2nd ed. Bethesda, Md., National Institutes of Health, NIH Publication No. 95-1468, 1995, pp. 409–428.
2. Centers for Disease Control and Prevention. Diabetes Surveillance, 1993. Atlanta, GA, US Dept. Health and Human Services, 1993, pp.87–93.
3. Jiwa F. Diabetes in the 1990s—An overview. Stat. Bull. Metropolitan Life Insurance Co. 1997;78:2–8.
4. Diabetes and Chronic Disabling Conditions in *Healthy People 2000*. US Department of Health and Human Services, Public Health Service. DHHS publ. No. PHS 91-50212, 1991, p. 442.
5. Edmonds ME, Blundell MP, Morris HE, Maelor-Thomas E, Cotton LT, Watkins PJ. Improved survival of the diabetic foot: the role of the specialist foot clinic. *Q J Med* 1986;232:763–771.
6. Thomson FJ, Veves A, Ashe H, et al. A team approach to diabetic foot care-the Manchester experience. *Foot* 1991;1:75–82.
7. Frykberg RG. Diabetic foot ulcerations, in *The High Risk Foot in Diabetes Mellitus* (Frykberg RG, ed.), Churchill Livingstone, New York, 1991, p. 151.
8. Caputo GM, Cavanagh PR, Ulbrecht JS, Gibbons GW, Karchmer AW. Assessment and management of foot disease in patients with diabetes. *N Engl J Med* 1994;331:854–860.
9. Gibbons GW. Vascular evaluation and long-term results of distal bypass surgery in patients with diabetes. *Clin Podiatr Med Surg* 1995;12:129–140.
10. Rosenblum BI, Pomposelli FB, Giurini JM, et al. Maximizing foot salvage by a combined approach to foot ischemia and neuropathic ulceration in patients with diabetes: a 5-year experience. *Diabetes Care* 1994;17(0):983–987.
11. Young MJ, Coffey J, Taylor PM, Boulton AJM. Weight bearing ultrasound in diabetic and rheumatoid arthritis patients. *Foot* 1995;5:76–79.
12. Gibbons GW. The diabetic foot: amputations and drainage of infection. *J Vasc Surg* 1987;5:791–793.
13. Morton DJ. *The Human Foot*. Columbia University Press, New York, 1935.
14. Cavanagh PR, Rodgers MM, Iiboshi A. Pressure distribution under symptom-free feet during barefoot standing. *Foot Ankle* 1987;7:262–276.
15. Ctercteko GC, Chanendran M, Hutton WC, Lequesne LP. Vertical forces acting on the feet of diabetic patients with neuropathic ulceration. *Br J Surg* 1981;68:608–614.
16. Root M, Weed J, Orien W. *Normal and Abnormal Function of the Foot*. Clinical Biomechanics Corp., Los Angeles, 1977, p. 211.
17. Dannels E. Neuropathic foot ulcer prevention in diabetic American Indians with hallux limitus. *J Am Podiatr Med Assoc* 1989;76:33–37.
18. Downs DM, Jacobs RL. Treatment of resistant ulcers on the plantar surface of the great toe in diabetics. *J Bone Joint Surg Am* 1982;64:930–933.
19. Rosenblum BI, Giurini JM, Chrzan JS, Habershaw GM. Preventing loss of the great toe with the hallux interphalangeal joint arthroplasty. *J Foot Ankle Surg* 1994;33:557–560.
20. Giurini JM, Chrzan JS, Gibbons GW, Habershaw GM. Sesamoidectomy for the treatment of chronic neuropathic ulcerations. *J Am Podiatr Med Assoc* 1991;81:167–173.
21. Frykberg RF, Giurini JM, Habershaw GM, Rosenblum BI, Chrzan JS. Prophylactic surgery in the diabetic foot, in *Medical and Surgical Management of the Diabetic Foot* (Kominsky, SJ. ed.), Mosby – Year Book, St. Louis, 1994, pp. 399–439.
22. Grayson ML, Gibbons GW, Balogh K, Levin E, Karchmer AW. Probing to bone in infected pedal ulcers: a clinical sign of underlying osteomyelitis in diabetic patients. *JAMA* 1995;273:721–723.
23. Masson EA, Hay EM, Stockley I, Veves A, Betts RP, Boulton AJM. Abnormal foot pressures alone may not cause ulceration. *Diabet Med* 1989;6:426–428.

24. Giurini JM, Rosenblum BI. The role of foot surgery in patients with diabetes. *Clin Podiatr Med Surg* 1995;12:119–127.
25. Fernando DJ, Masson EA, Veves A, Boulton AJM. Relationship of limited joint mobility to abnormal foot pressures and diabetic foot ulceration. *Diabetes Care* 1991;14:8–11.
26. Veves A, Sarnow MR, Giurini JM, et al. Differences in joint mobility and foot pressures between black and white diabetic patients. *Diabet Med* 1995;12:585–589.
27. Tillo TH, Giurini JM, Habershaw GM, Chrzan JS, Rowbotham JL. Review of metatarsal osteotomies for the treatment of neuropathic ulcerations. *J Am Podiatr Med Assoc* 1990;80:211–217.
28. Roukis TS. Central metatarsal head-neck osteotomies: indications and operative techniques. *Clin Podiatr Med Surg* 2005;22(2):197–222.
29. McKittrick LS, McKittrick JB, Risley T. Transmetatarsal amputation for infection or gangrene in patients with diabetes mellitus. *Ann Surg* 1949;130:826.
30. Kates A, Kessel L, Kay A. Arthroplasty of the forefoot. *J Bone Joint Surg* 1967;49B:552.
31. Hoffman P. Operation for severe grades of contracted or clawed toes. *Am J Orthop Surg* 1912;9:441–449.
32. Marmor L. Resection of the forefoot in rheumatoid arthritis. *Clin Orthop* 1975;108:223.
33. Clayton ML. Surgery of the forefoot in rheumatoid arthritis. *Clin Orthop* 1960;16:136–140.
34. Jacobs RL. Hoffman procedure in the ulcerated diabetic neuropathic foot. *Foot Ankle* 1982;3:142–149.
35. Giurini JM, Habershaw GM, Chrzan JS. Panmetatarsal head resection in chronic neuropathic ulcerations. *J Foot Surg* 1987;26:249–252.
36. Giurini JM, Basile P, Chrzan JS, Habershaw GM, Rosenblum BI. Panmetatarsal head resection: a viable alternative to the transmetatarsal amputation. *J Am Podiatr Med Assoc* 1993;83:101–107.
37. Hodor L, Dobbs BM. Pan metatarsal head resection: a review and new approach. *J Am Podiatr Assoc* 1983;73(6):287–292.
38. Harris JR, Brand PW. Patterns of disintegration of the tarsus in the anesthetic foot. *J Bone Joint Surg* 1966;48B:4–16.
39. Sanders LJ, Frykberg RG. Diabetic neuropathic osteoarthropathhy: the Charcot Foot, in *The High Risk Foot in Diabetes Mellitus*. (Frykberg RG, ed.), Churchill-Livingstone, New York, 1990, pp. 297–338.
40. Rosenblum BI, Giurini JM, Miller LB, Chrzan JS, Habershaw GM. Neuropathic ulcerations plantar to the lateral column in patients with Charcot foot deformity: a flexible approach to limb salvage. *J Foot Ankle Surg* 1997;36(5):360–363.
41. Miller DS, Lichtman WF. Diabetic neuropathic arthropathy of feet. *Arch Surg* 1955;70:513.
42. Sinha S, Munichoodappa C, Kozak GP. Neuroarthropathy (Charcot Joints) in diabetes mellitus. Clinical study of 101 cases. *Medicine* 1972;52:191.
43. Cofield RH, Morison MJ, Beabout JW. Diabetic neuroarthropathy in the foot: patient characteristic and patterns of radiographic change. *Foot Ankle* 1983;4:15.
44. Sanders LJ, Mrdjenovich D. Diabetic neuropathic osteoarthropathy: an analysis of 28 cases. (in press).
45. Simon S, Tejwani S, Wilson D. Arthrodesis as an early alternative to nonoperative management of Charcot arthropathy of the diabetic foot. *J Bone Joint Surg* 2000;82A(7):939–950.
46. Banks AS, McGlamry ED. Charcot foot. *J Am Podiatr Med Assoc* 1989;79:213–235.
47. Bier RR, Estersohn HS. A new treatment for Charcot joint in the diabetic foot. *J Am Podiatr Med Assoc* 1987;77:63–69.
48. Papa J, Myerson M, Girard P. Salvage, with arthrodesis, in intractable diabetic neuropathic arthropathy of the foot and ankle. *J Bone Joint Surg* 1993;75A(7):1056–1066.
49. Cooper PS. Application of external fixators for management of Charcot deformities of the foot and ankle. *Foot Ankle Clin* 2002;7:207–254.

18

Amputation and Rehabilitation of the Diabetic Foot

Ronald A. Sage, DPM, Michael Pinzur, MD,
Rodney Stuck, DPM, and Coleen Napolitano, DPM

INDICATIONS AND BASIC PRINCIPLES OF AMPUTATION

Amputation of the foot may be indicated when neuropathy, vascular disease, and ulcerative deformity have led to soft tissue necrosis, osteomyelitis, uncontrollable infection, or intractable pain.

Amputations of the lower extremity are often considered either a failure of conservative management or an unpreventable outcome of diabetes. The patient sees amputation as the end of productivity and the start of significant disability. Amputation should be viewed as a procedure leading to rehabilitation and return to productivity for the patient disabled by an ulcerated, infected, or intractably painful extremity. The patient needs assurance, and efforts should be made to follow-up the procedure with efforts to return him or her to productive community activity. This may involve consultation among the specialties of medicine, podiatry, orthopedics, vascular surgery, physiatry, and prosthetics. As the patient is rehabilitated and returns to the activities of daily living, the residual limb and the contralateral limb must be protected. Revision amputation and amputation of the contralateral limb remain a significant problem, occurring in as many as 20% of amputee cases *(1)*.

The goal of any limb salvage effort is to convert all patients' diabetic feet, from Wagner grades 1 through 4, back to grade 0 extremities. Those patients with grade 5 feet will require an appropriate higher level of amputation. If salvage is not feasible, then all efforts are made to return the patient with some functional level of activity after amputation. The more proximal the amputation, the higher the energy cost of walking. This problem is most significant in our patients who have multisystem disease and limited cardiopulmonary function. These factors may negatively impact the patient's postoperative independence.

Patients may require several surgical treatments before definitive amputation. Incision and drainage or open amputation is frequently required to stabilize acute infection. The parameters of healing, to be mentioned later, may not apply at that time. The goal of the first stage of a multistaged procedure is simply to eradicate infection and stabilize the patient. If medical review of the patient suggests an inability to tolerate multiple operations,

From: *The Diabetic Foot, Second Edition*
Edited by: A. Veves, J. M. Giurini, and F. W. LoGerfo © Humana Press Inc., Totowa, NJ

a higher initial level of amputation may be indicated foregoing attempts at distal salvage. However, if salvage is possible, and the patient is medically stable, then a systematic approach to limb salvage should be pursued.

LIMB SALVAGE VS LIMB AMPUTATION

Enlightened orthopedic care of the new millennium has changed focus from results to outcomes. Burgess taught us that amputation surgery is the first step in the rehabilitation of a patient with a nonfunctionally reconstructable limb *(2)*. He taught us to focus on the re-entry of the amputee into their normal activities, setting achievable functional goals.

Lower extremity amputation is performed for gangrene, infection, trauma, neoplastic disease, or congenital deformity. Irrespective of the diagnosis, the following questions should be addressed before undertaking either an attempt at limb salvage, or performing an amputation:

1. Will limb salvage outperform amputation and prosthetic limb fitting? If all transpires as one could reasonably predict, will the functional independence of the patient following limb salvage/reconstruction be greater, or less than, amputation and prosthetic limb fitting. This will vary greatly with age, vocational ability, medical health, lifestyle, education, and social status.
2. What is a realistic expectation of functional capacities at the completion of treatment? A realistic appreciation of functional end results should be made with respect to both limb salvage and amputation. Consultation with physical medicine and rehabilitation, social work, and physical therapy can assist in determining reasonable outcome expectations.
3. What is the time and effort commitment required for both the treatment team and the patient? Both the physician and patient must have a reasonable understanding of the duration of the rehabilitation process, the inherent risks involved with revascularization, and the effort required for both.
4. What is the expected financial cost to the patient and resource consumption of the healthcare system? In the current medical-economic climate, one must realistically address these issues from both the patient and healthcare system perspective *(3,4)*.

Physical and Metabolic Considerations

Metabolic Cost of Amputation

The metabolic cost of walking is increased with proximal level amputations, being inversely proportional to the length of the residual limb and the number of joints preserved. With more proximal amputation, patients have a decreased self-selected, and maximum, walking speed. Oxygen consumption is increased. From an outcomes perspective, functional independence (functional independence measure score) is directly correlated with amputation levels. Distal level amputees achieve proportionally higher functional independence measure scores (Fig. 1) *(5–7)*.

Cognitive Considerations

It is suggested that many individuals with longstanding diabetes have cognitive and perceptual deficits *(8–11)*. There are certain specific cognitive capacities that are necessary for individuals to become successful prosthetic users: memory, attention, concentration, and organization. In order for patients with these deficiencies to become successful prosthetic users, they require either specific, successful education and training, or the physical presence of a caregiver that can provide substitute provision of these skills.

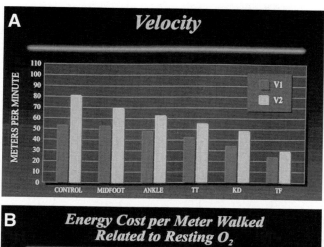

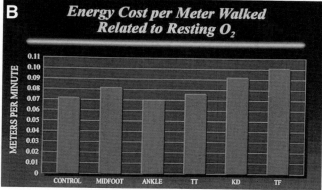

Fig. 1. (A) Walking velocity compared with surgical amputation level. V1 is self-selected walking speed. V2 is maximum walking speed. **(B)** Oxygen consumption per meter walked compared with surgical amputation level. Note that the metabolic cost of walking is increased with more proximal level amputation.

Load Transfer and Weight Bearing

Our feet act as uniquely adapted end organs of weight bearing. Following amputation, the residual limb must assume the tasks of load transfer, adapting to uneven terrain, and propulsion, utilizing tissues that are not biologically engineered for that purpose. The weight bearing surface of long bones is wider than the corresponding diaphysis. This increased surface area dissipates the force applied during weight bearing over a larger surface area, and the more accommodative articular cartilage and metaphyseal bone allow cushioning and shock absorption during weight bearing.

Direct load transfer, i.e., end bearing, which is achieved in disarticulation amputations at the knee and ankle joint levels, takes advantage of the normal weight bearing characteristics of the terminal bone of the residual limb. The overlying soft tissue envelope acts to cushion the bone, much as the heel pad and plantar tissues function in the foot.

Indirect load transfer, or total contact weight bearing, is necessary in diaphyseal transtibial and transfemoral amputation levels, in which the surface area and stiffness of the terminal residual limb require unloading. The weight-bearing load must be applied to the entire surface area, with the soft tissue envelope acting as a cushion *(12)* (Fig. 2).

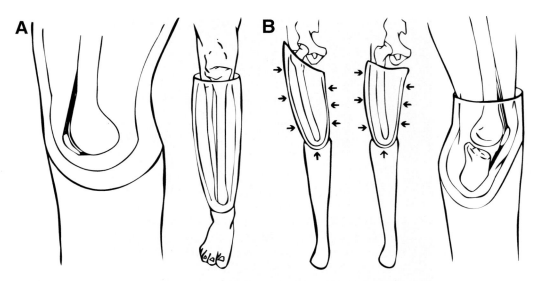

Fig. 2. (A) Direct load transfer (endbearing) is accomplished in knee disarticulation and Syme's ankle disarticulation amputation levels. **(B)** Indirect load transfer (total contact) is accomplished in transtibial and transfemoral amputation levels.

Soft Tissue Envelope

The soft tissue envelope acts as the interface between the bone of the residual limb and the prosthetic socket. It functions both to cushion the underlying bone, and dissipate the pressures and forces applied during weight bearing. Ideally, it should be made up of a mobile, nonadherent muscle mass, and full thickness skin. If the soft tissue envelope is adherent to bone, the shear forces will produce skin blistering, ulceration, and tissue breakdown. It should be durable enough to tolerate the direct pressures and pistoning within the prosthetic socket.

Healing Parameters

Vascular Perfusion

Amputation wounds generally heal by collateral flow, so arteriography is rarely a useful diagnostic tool to predict wound healing. Doppler ultrasound has been a utilized to assess blood flow in the extremity before amputation. An ankle–brachial index of 45 in the patient with diabetes has been considered adequate for healing as long as the systolic pressure at the ankle was 70 mmHg or higher. These values are falsely elevated, and nonpredictive, in at least 15% of patients with peripheral vascular disease, because of the noncompressibility and noncompliance, of calcified peripheral arteries *(13)*. This has prompted many to use transcutaneous oximetry as a measure of the oxygen-delivering capacity of the cardiovascular system to the area in question *(4,14)*. It actually records the oxygen delivering capacity of the vascular system to the skin at the proposed level of surgery. Values of 30 mmHg or higher have a 90% healing rate. Values between 20 and 29 mmHg have a 70% healing rate and values less than 20 are associated with failure rates greater than 50%. Edema and cellulitis may falsely lower the oxygen values and make this exam invalid *(4,14)*. Peripheral Vascular consultation should be obtained for patients who do not have adequate inflow on these exams. When transcutaneous oxygen measurement is not locally available, the

Vascular laboratory can measure toe pressures as an indicator of arterial inflow to the foot. This is owing to the observation that arteries of the hallux do not seem to be calcified, as do the vessels of the leg *(15–18)*. The accepted threshold toe pressure is 30 mmHg.

Nutrition and Immunocompetence

Preoperative review of nutritional status is obtained by measuring the serum albumin and the total lymphocyte count (TLC). The serum albumin should be at least 3.0 gm/dL and the TLC should be greater than 1500. The TLC is calculated by multiplying the white blood cell count by the percent of lymphocytes in the differential. When these values are suboptimal, nutritional consultation is helpful before definitive amputation. If possible, surgery in patients with malnutrition or immunodeficiency should be delayed until these issues can adequately be addressed. When infection or gangrene dictates urgent surgery, surgical debridement of infection, or open amputation at the most distal viable level, followed by open wound care, can be accomplished until wound healing potential can be optimized *(19–21)*. At times, such as with severe renal disease, the nutritional values will remain suboptimal and distal salvage attempts may still be pursued, but at known higher risk for failure.

Glucose control is also important as high glucose levels will deactivate macrophages and lymphocytes and may impair wound healing. High glucose levels have also been associated with other postoperative infections including those of the urinary tract and respiratory system. Ideal management involves maintenance of glucose levels below 200 mg/dL *(22)*. However, caution must be taken in managing the perioperative patient's glucose with calorie reduction, as this process may lead to significant protein depletion and subsequent wound failure. A minimum of 1800 calories daily should be provided to avoid a negative nitrogen balance that could accompany depletion of protein stores.

The combined wound healing parameters of vascular inflow and nutritional status have been studied and shown to significantly affect healing rates for pedal amputations. Attempting to optimize nutrition and perfusion preoperatively, when medically possible, will limit the risk of wound complications and failure.

Perioperative Considerations

Pedal amputations may be performed under local or regional anesthesia. The effectiveness of local anesthetics may be impaired by the presence of infection and may need to be administered proximal to any cellulitis. When amputating above the ankle, spinal or general anesthesia will be necessary. Spinal anesthesia is contraindicated in the patient with sepsis demonstrated by fever over 100°F.

Culture specific antibiotic therapy should be continued perioperatively. If the focus of infection is completely removed with amputation, then the antibiotics may be discontinued 24 hours after surgery. If, however, infection remains a concern, then antibiotics are continued for a soft tissue course of 10–14 days, or 6–8 weeks for bone infection.

Tourniquets may be needed to control bleeding at surgery. The surgeon must ensure that the tourniquet is not placed over a vascular anastomosis site or distal to an area of infection. The patient with severe vascular compromise will not require a tourniquet.

Preoperative Summary

Preoperative planning for distal limb salvage procedures should include the measurement of serum albumin, TLC and tissue perfusion. With satisfactory values in all three categories, healing rates as high as 90% may be attainable. However, at least 10% of even ideal cases may fail. With impaired nutrition or perfusion the risk of failure becomes even greater. The patient should be informed of these risks. Efforts should be made to use this information to plan procedures at levels that will limit the patient's exposure to multiple revision attempts. A single surgical session for a transtibial amputation may be preferable to multiple futile attempts at distal salvage in severely compromised or borderline cases.

RAY AMPUTATIONS

Indications

Single toe amputation or ray resection may be performed for irreversible necrosis of a toe without medial or lateral extension. Deep infection of an ulcer to bone is also an appropriate indication for toe amputation. If uncontrollable infection extends to the metatarsal-phalangeal joint, or metatarsal head, ray resection is appropriate. This procedure is also useful for infection or necrosis of the toe, requiring more proximal resection to obtain viable wound margins.

Ray resection is an excellent method of decompressing deep fascial infection limited to one compartment of the plantar structures of the foot, be that medial, lateral or central. In such cases the wound is always left open to allow continued drainage, and may be followed by a more proximal, definitive procedure when the acute infection is stable, if healing parameters are acceptable, for a distal limb salvage procedure *(23)*.

Procedure

Ray resections are performed at our institution as a wedge excision of the involved toe and metatarsal. Longitudinal incisions are made parallel to the involved ray, and converge on the dorsal and plantar surfaces of the foot. If ulceration is present, as frequently occurs plantar to the metatarsal head, the ulcer is resected along with the wedge of soft tissue that includes the affected toe. The initial incisions are carried to bone, and the toe is disarticulated at the metatarsal-phalangeal joint. The periosteum of the metatarsal is reflected as far proximally as necessary down the shaft of the bone in order to assure that the resection is performed at a level of viable, noninfected bone. The bone is usually cut at the proximal diaphysis, or diaphyseal-metaphyseal junction. It is rarely necessary to do the extensive dissection required to disarticulate the metatarsal cuneiform joint.

Once the bone is removed from the wound, the foot is compressed from proximal to distal to assure that there is no remaining ascending purulent drainage. If the flexor or extensor compartments reveal pus on compression, then they are opened and irrigated to clean out any remaining apparent infection. If the ray resection was performed for metatarsal or plantar space infection, it is usually left open to facilitate drainage, and allow for healing by second intention. This usually occurs in 6 weeks with patients who exhibit acceptable healing parameter, and avoid full weight bearing on the operated foot (Fig. 3).

Postoperative Care

The only ray resection that should be closed primarily is that performed for infection localized to the toe, with clearly viable wound edges, and no suggestion of proximal infection. In this case a gauze dressing is applied and the patient is maintained in a post-operative shoe until healed. A cane or walker is utilized for protected weight bearing.

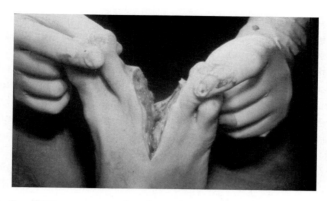

Fig. 3. Patient after third ray amputation for a diabetic ulcer and osteomyelitis. Note that the plantar ulcer was also excised.

In cases in which the wound is left open, culture directed antibiotics should be administered for soft tissue or bone infection depending on the extent of the infection. Infectious disease service consultation is advisable. The wound itself should be treated according to the surgeon's preferred protocol. If a significant space is present this should be packed with saline soaked gauze or alginate dressings. Packing should be sufficient to absorb excess drainage, but not aggressive enough to interfere with wound contraction. The amount of packing should decrease each week as the wound contracts and granulates. The foot should be protected from full weight bearing during this time with crutches, a walker, or wheelchair with a leg lift as necessary.

Once healing has been achieved the patient should have a prescription for protective foot gear. If there is evidence of pressure keratosis developing adjacent to the ray resection site, the patient should be seen in clinic as necessary to pare the callus in order to prevent transfer ulceration. Such visits may be necessary every 1, 2, or 3 months.

Complications

Persisting infection is rare if the wound was adequately debrided at the time of the ray resection. However, if residual infection is suspected, follow-up surgical debridement should be done. Wound failure may be owing to inadequate healing parameters, such as impaired blood flow, or abnormal serum albumin. Such metabolic wound failures may require more proximal amputation to obtain healing.

The most common late complication of ray resection is transfer lesion and reulceration. If pressure keratosis cannot be managed with debridement and prescription shoes, then resection of the remaining metatarsal heads, or more proximal amputation may become necessary *(24)*.

TRANSMETATARSAL AND LIS FRANC AMPUTATION

Indications

The indications for amputation in a diabetic foot include irreversible necrosis of a significant portion of bone or tendon, uncontrollable infection, or intractable pain. If ulceration is present for a prolonged period of time, not responsive to nonsurgical treatment, and is causing significant disability, amputation of the ulcerated part may be a necessary step to rehabilitation. If the amputation is to be at the level of the toes, foot, or ankle, attention should be directed at well-established vascular and metabolic parameters to assure a reasonable chance for healing success.

McKittrick advocated the transmetatarsal amputation in 1949 *(25)* for infection or gangrene of the toes in patients with diabetes in 1949. Wagner subsequently recommended its use in patients with diabetic foot complications in 1977 *(26),* advocating preoperative vascular review. He advised that Doppler studies demonstrating an ankle–brachial artery index greater than 0.45 could predict healing of the procedure with 90% accuracy. The authors' group reviewed 64 transmetatarsal and Lis Franc amputations in 1986 *(27).* These amputations were performed for gangrene of the forefoot, or forefoot ulcers resistant to nonsurgical attempts at healing. Their results indicated that patients with Doppler ankle-brachial artery index above 0.5, combined with serum albumin levels greater the 3 gm/dL and TLCs greater than 1500/cm^3 healed at a rate of 92%. Those patients lacking one or more of these three indicators healed at a rate of 38%.

Amputation of a single toe or metatarsal may be successfully performed for patients with a localized ulceration if preoperative healing indices are satisfactory. However, there can be significant transfer ulceration following such procedures leading to later complications, even if early healing is achieved *(23).*

This experience suggests that transmetatarsal amputation may be a more definitive procedure for the management of forefoot ulceration. Transmetatarsal amputation may be considered for patients with more than one ulceration or site of necrosis of the forefoot. Likewise this procedure may be considered in cases with significant nonhealing ulceration and other foot deformity that is likely to lead to subsequent ulcer. However, transmetatarsal amputation, in itself, does not assure that no further ulceration of the foot is likely.

In our long-term review of midfoot amputations, including transmetatarsal and Lis Franc procedures, 9 out of 64 feet sustained new ulcerations within the first year after healing the primary procedure *(28).* The source of these ulcerations included hypertrophic new bone formation, and subsequent varus or equinus deformity. These dynamic deformities were more likely in Lis Franc amputations, in which muscle imbalance was likely to occur because of the loss of the attachments of the peroneals and extensors (Figs. 4 and 5).

Plantar ulceration under the metatarsals may deter the surgeon from a transmetatarsal amputation, favoring a more proximal, yet more poorly functional, procedure because of the inability to preserve a long plantar flap for closure of the procedure. However, Sanders has demonstrated that a V-shaped excision of the ulceration, with the apex proximal, and the base at the junction of the dorsal and plantar flaps, allows conversion of the wound from a simple transverse incision to a T-shaped closure *(29).* This produces a longer, ulcer free, flap that can be closed over a transmetatarsal procedure, rather than requiring a more proximal Lis Franc operation to eliminate the plantar ulcer.

The specific indications for transmetatarsal amputation remain similar to McKittrick's, ulcer or gangrene of the toes. Thanks to Sanders plantar flap modification (Fig. 6), metatarsal head ulceration is also an appropriate indication for this procedure, when not responding to nonsurgical treatment. Ulceration or infection of a single toe may be

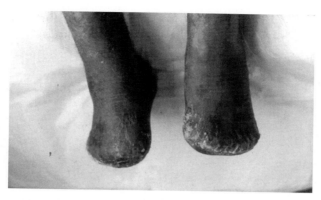

Fig. 4. Bilateral transmetatarsal amputation. The wounds are well healed in 6 weeks.

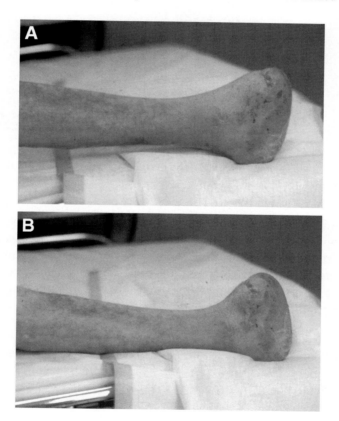

Fig. 5. (A) After Lis Franc amputation, equinus may develop and lead to reulceration at the distal stump. **(B)** Percutaneous tendoachilles lengthening was performed on this patient to improve ankle dorsiflexion and reduce the risk of ulcer.

treated with an isolated ray resection, understanding a risk of transfer ulceration. If that risk is increased by obvious ulcerative deformity in other parts of the foot, then transmetatarsal or the slightly more proximal Lis Franc amputation becomes more appropriate. All of these procedures are most likely to heal when albumin, lymphocyte count,

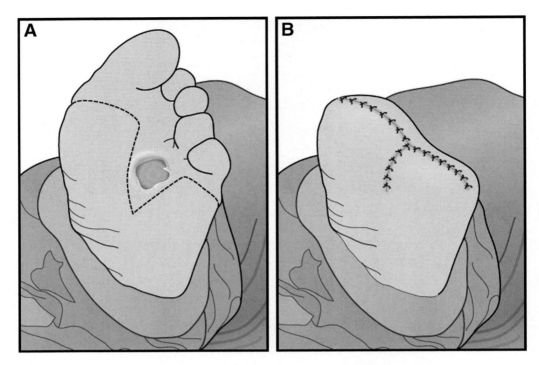

Fig. 6. (A) The Sander's technique for plantar flap revision with transmetatarsal amputation in the presence of a distal plantar ulcer. **(B)** The margins of the ulcer site are then approximated with closure as shown.

and arterial inflow meet recognized minimal standards described above. Before definitive midfoot amputation acute infection should be stabilized by incision and drainage, debridement or ray resection. Residual infected tissue present at the time of the definitive procedure can be expected to compromise success, and should be eliminated in a staged procedure, if necessary. If these criteria cannot be met, then higher amputation may be more appropriate.

Technique

This procedure can be performed with monitored anesthesia care, and spinal or ankle block. General anesthesia is rarely necessary. Appropriate medical clearance should be obtained regarding glycemic management and cardiovascular risks.

The transmetatarsal and Lis Franc amputations differ in technique mainly at the point of detachment of the forefoot from the hindfoot. The transmetatarsal procedure is osteotomized through the metatarsal bases, leaving the insertion of tibialis anterior, peroneus longus, and peroneus brevis in tact. The metatarsal osteotomy should be performed through the proximal metaphysis, in order to avoid long plantar metatarsal shafts and irregular parabola that might later result in plantar stump ulceration. The Lis Franc amputation requires disarticulation at the metatarsal cuneiform and cuboid joints, resulting in loss of the tendon insertions mentioned previously. The writer has made occasional attempts to preserve the base of the fifth metatarsal and peroneus brevis insertion, but this is not always practical.

The procedure begins with a dorsal incision across the metatarsal bases, from the medial to the lateral side of the foot, deferring the plantar incision for the time being. If no tourniquet is used, staging the incision like this avoids dealing with bleeding from both the top and bottom of the foot at the same time. The incision is carried to bone through the dorsal tendons and neurovascular structures. Significant vessels, such as dorsalis pedis, are identified and ligated. The periosteum of the metatarsal bases is incised and reflected using an elevator to expose either the site of the intended osteotomy, or the metatarsal tarsal articulation.

If a transmetatarsal amputation is to be performed, the osteotomies are now initiated. Using a power saw the first metatarsal is cut, directing the plane slightly medially and plantarly. The second, third, and fourth metatarsals are cut, taking care to produce a smooth parabola, leaving no stump particularly longer than the adjacent bone. The fifth metatarsal is cut last, directing the plane slightly lateral and plantar. At this point the plantar incision is made, initiated at a 90° or less angle to the dorsal incision, carried distally to the sulcus, around the metatarsal heads, and then posteriorly along the lateral side of the foot to the fifth metatarsal base. The incision should be carried to bone as much as possible. If plantar metatarsal head ulceration is present, it should be excised using a V-shaped wedge, directing the apex distally, and the base proximally at the level of the distal transverse incision. When this is closed, it results in a T-shaped flap (Fig. 3).

The metatarsals may now be lifted from the plantar flap from proximal to distal, dissecting along the metatarsal shafts in order to preserve as much of the soft tissue structures in the plantar flap as possible. The remaining distal attachments of the metatarsal heads are cut, and the forefoot is removed. Significant vascular structures should be ligated. The entire wound should be thoroughly irrigated. Remaining fibrous, ligamentous, and exposed tendinous structures should be cleanly cut from flap. Minimal debulking of remaining intrinsic muscle structures may be performed if necessary to obtain approximation. However, as much of the viable tissue of the plantar flap as possible should be preserved.

The technique is similar for a Lis Franc amputation, except that the metatarsal cuneiform and cuboid articulations are detached instead of the metatarsal osteotomy. The first cuneiform is invariably long, and needs to be ronguered or cut proximally to a smooth parabola with the remaining metatarsals. This cut should be directed slightly medially and plantarly. Articular cartilage from the remaining tarsals is ronguered to bleeding cancellous bone. Since adapting Sanders' plantar flap technique, the writer performs very few Lis Franc procedures because of the obvious functional disadvantage of varus and equinus associated with this procedure. If a Lis Franc is the only option, tibialis anterior is released from the medial side of the first cuneiform, and a percutaneous tendo-Achilles lengthening is performed.

Before closure, the wound should be thoroughly irrigated. If a tourniquet was used it should be released, and significant hemorrhaging vessels ligated. Because the procedure leaves relatively little dead space, drains are rarely necessary. The wound is closed in two to three layers, starting with sutures place in the middle of the planar flap musculature, and approximated to the intermetatarsal or intertarsal ligamentous structures. Then subcutaneous sutures passed from the distal deeper layers of the flap to the dorsal retinaculum. Finally the skin is closed with mattress or simple interrupted sutures of 3-0 nylon as needed to obtain a satisfactory incision line.

Postoperative Care

Mild compression, and protection of flap from tension are the writer's objectives in immediate postoperative wound care. In order to accomplish this, a soft gauze roll dressing is applied from the foot to the ankle. Moderated compression is applied, with minimal force directed from plantar to dorsal in order to protect the plantar flap from undue stress on the incision line. Then, two to three layers of cast padding are applied from the foot to the tibial tuberosity, maintaining the foot an ankle in neutral position, neither dorsiflexed or plantar flexed. Finally, several layers of 5 × 30 inch plaster of Paris splints are applied posteriorly from the tip of the stump to the calf, proximal to the knee. The splints are wrapped with another two layers of cast padding, and an ace wrap secures the entire dressing. This resembles a Jones dressing, protecting the wound from any contusions, and from any dorsal or plantar tension.

This dressing is left in place for approx 48 hours before the wound is inspected. A similar dressing is maintained for 2–4 weeks until the incision line is clearly stable. During this time the patient is instructed in the use of crutches, a walker, or wheel chair with leg elevation. Little or not weight bearing on the operated foot is allowed until the wound is clearly stable, and free of risk of major dehiscence. Occasional superficial dehiscence may occur, especially in high-risk patients. This is treated like any other grade 1 ulcer with cleansing, debridement, and topical wound care measures until healed. Major postoperative dehiscence, infection, or necrosis of the plantar flap will likely require revision surgery.

Complications

Wagner has stated that distal amputations can be expected to heal up to 90% of the time in patients with diabetes who exhibit adequate circulation as determined by Doppler examination demonstrating ankle–brachial artery index of 0.45 or better *(26)*. The authors' group confirmed that healing could be achieved in more than 90% of patients with diabetes undergoing midfoot amputation if ankle–brachial artery index is over 0.5, serum albumin is greater than 3.0 gm/dL, and TLC in more than 1500/cm^3 *(27)*. However, we have also noted that up to 42% of midfoot amputations may suffer some form of complication, even though the majority ultimately heal their surgical wounds *(28)*. The complications include early wound dehiscence, and late reulceration, which can be treated successfully to result in limb salvage in most cases. Patients most likely to suffer wound dehiscence include those with marginal vascular indices, low serum albumin. This is especially true in renal failure patients. These prognostic indicators should be taken into consideration in preoperative planning and discussed with the patient. Those at high risk for failure may be better served by a higher amputation more likely to heal with one operation.

Biomechanical abnormality resulting from muscle imbalance can result in dynamic varus, producing lateral foot ulceration. This is particularly true in Lis Franc amputations because of the varus pull of an unopposed tibialis anterior. Tibialis anterior tendon transfer in some cases can successfully treat this. Armstrong and associates *(30)* noted that bone regrowth after partial metatarsal amputation resulted in a significantly increased risk of reulceration. This regrowth was likely to occur in metaphyseal procedures, in males, when manual bone cutting equipment was utilized. In our experience, these reulcerations can be treated with aggressive exostectomy of the underlying bone and standard subsequent wound care.

Long-Term Follow-Up Needs

Patients with a history of ulceration remain at high risk for reulceration, even after the foot has been returned to grade 0 by a surgical procedure. The patient who has undergone any form of partial foot amputation should be placed in a high-risk foot clinic for regular follow-up visits. Both short- and long-term complications have been recognized. Even though the benefits of distal limb salvage are well accepted, biomechanical review and management visits must be included in after care for the amputation to be successful *(31)*. Early on, the wound should be protected with a posterior splint or cast and limited weight bearing. Rehabilitation should include crutch or walker training, if feasible. If the patient cannot use gait assistive devices, a wheel chair with leg lift, and instruction in wheel chair mobility and transfer techniques should be provided. These protective measures should be continued until wound is clearly healed.

Later, protective foot care, or even a plastizote-lined ankle foot orthosis may need to be prescribed for adequate protection. Although many patients may function well with an oxford shoe and anterior filler, others may need more elaborate orthotic management. Custom-made short shoes, rocker bottom shoes with a steel shank and anterior filler, or conventional shoes with an ankle foot orthosis have all been advocated. Each patient should be observed carefully as the return to full ambulation to determine the need for orthotic management. Computer assisted pressure mapping may be helpful in determining the success of any device in off-loading residual pressure points. If keratotic lesions should develop, these should be considered preulcerative and debrided regularly before ulceration can occur *(32,33)*.

Transmetatarsal and Lis Franc amputation have the benefit of improved function and patient acceptance over higher amputation for individuals suffering from serious forefoot infection, ulceration, or gangrene. However, these operations must be recognized as high-risk procedures. Nevertheless, with appropriate preoperative planning, meticulous surgical technique, protective postoperative care, and long-term follow-up, midfoot amputations can be successful limb salvage techniques for most patients undergoing these procedures.

CHOPART AMPUTATION

Indications

Francoise Chopart described disarticulation through the midtarsal joint while working at the Charitable Hospital in Paris in the 1800s *(31)*. The operation has been thought to have limited applications because the residual partial foot is susceptible to progressive equinovarus deformity. The Chopart amputation is gaining new favor because the length of the limb is retained and the potential complications of the procedure are frequently successfully addressed. Combining ankle fusion with hindfoot amputation allows apropulsive ambulation with a modified high-topped shoe *(35–38)*.

Amputation levels are usually chosen on the basis of tissue viability and residual limb function. A Chopart level amputation may be considered when the longer transmetatarsal or Lis Franc amputation level is not an option because of the extent of forefoot tissue destruction. Half of all patients undergoing an initial nontraumatic amputation will likely require an amputation of the contralateral limb *(39)*. There is a higher metabolic requirement for ambulation in those patients who undergo more proximal amputations. Therefore the decision on amputation level should attempt to maximize the patients mobility and independence by preserving length whenever possible, thus making the Chopart amputation useful in cases in which more distal foot procedures are not feasible.

An open Chopart amputation is useful to provide resection of grossly infected forefoot structures, as a stage-I procedure, anticipating a higher definitive procedure, such as a Boyd or Syme's amputation. The open Chopart amputation procedure disarticulates the foot at the level of the calcaneocuboid and talonavicular joints, leaving the articular surfaces intact. The proximal spread of infection may be less likely with the cancellous spaces unopened *(40)*. During the open Chopart procedure, care must be taken to visualize and resect all necrotic and/or nonviable tissue. Compression of the limb proximal to the open amputation site is done manually to identify purulent drainage from the compartments of the leg. If purulence is expressed with compression then the affected compartment must be incised and irrigated to provide adequate drainage. Once the acute infection is resolved and the healing parameter indices are reviewed, the open Chopart is may be revised to a definitive level. If the surgeon anticipates that the acute infection may be stabilized, and heal at the Chopart level is likely to occur, then care must be taken during the open Chopart procedure to retain sufficient skin and subcutaneous tissue to account for shrinkage and provide coverage of the stump.

The prerequisite for a definitive Chopart amputation is that the plantar heel pad and ankle/subtalar joint articulations are not compromised *(41)*. A closed or definitive Chopart amputation is considered if the forefoot infection extends proximal to the metatarsal bases and neither a transmetatarsal nor a Lis Franc amputation can be salvaged. Reyzelman et al. *(42)* suggest that a Chopart amputation is more advantageous than a short transmetatarsal or a Lis Franc amputation because it does not disrupt the transverse arch of the foot. The disruption of the transverse arch creates an overpowering of the tibialis anterior, tibialis posterior, and gastrocnemius muscle to the peroneus brevis muscle. The muscle imbalance created in the short transmetatarsal or Lis Franc amputation may lead to a varus rotation of the residual foot. A frontal plane rotation of the weight-bearing surface of a Chopart amputation is less likely to occur, unless the calcaneus or ankle is structurally in varus *(43)*. The Chopart amputation does, however, lead to an equinus deformity because of the unopposed pull of the Achilles tendon. An Achilles lengthening and/or performing a tibialis anterior transfer at the time of the definitive closure may address this.

Technique

The dorsal incision begins from the tuberosity of the navicular extending dorsolateral to the midcuboid level. The medial and lateral incisions are carried distally to the midshaft level of the first and fifth metatarsal and continued transversely at this level along the plantar aspect of the foot. These incisions form a fishmouth with dorsal and plantar flaps. The incisions are deepened to expose the talonavicular and calcaneocuboid joints. The tibialis anterior should be identified and preserved for later transfer to the talar neck. The remaining soft tissue structures are incised to complete the disarticulation of the forefoot from the rearfoot. The articular cartilage of the talus and calcaneus should be resected creating a flush surface when the definitive procedure is being performed. The tibialis anterior tendon may be attached to the talar neck at this time with either a

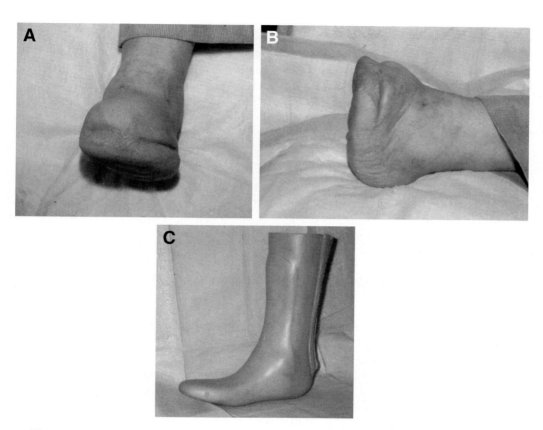

Fig. 7. (A) and **(B)** show a Chopart level amputation that was primarily closed. A percutaneous Achilles tenotomy was also performed to reduce the high risk of equinus deformity. **(C)** A variety of chopart prostheses have been advocated. This prosthesis has a posterior closure.

drill hole or suture. If a tourniquet has been utilized, it is deflated and hemostasis is achieved. The skin edges are then reapproximated and secured with the suture or staples. A drain is necessary only if there is significant loose soft tissue, or if excessive bleeding is anticipated, to prevent hematoma formation. The Achilles tendon is lengthened by either double or triple hemisection technique or by tenotomy after the wound is closed to limit later equinus deformity (Fig. 7A,B). A sterile compressive dressing and a posterior splint are applied to the lower extremity.

Postoperative Care

The patient is maintained nonweight bearing in a posterior splint or below knee cast until the wound is healed for up to 6 weeks if necessary. The Chopart amputee without equinus is capable of ambulating in an extra depth shoe with a forefoot filler but functions best with a polypropylene solid AFO prosthesis with foam filler *(40)*. The prosthesis helps to eliminate or minimize the pistoning motion of the distal amputation in a normal shoe. If the Chopart amputee has an equinus then they should be fitted for clamshell prosthesis (Fig. 7C) *(44)*.

Complications

The usual potential complications of infection or wound failure may occur with this procedure, as with any distal amputation. These are more likely if the procedure is preformed on patients who do not meet the generally accepted vascular and nutritional parameters described for transmetatarsal amputation. Care must be taken to fashion the flaps to provide adequate coverage for the residual stump without closing under excessive tension, as this may lead to wound dehiscence. Equinus deformity can still occur in time even if Achilles lengthening is performed. The development of a plantar ulceration in an equinus positioned stump is a common occurrence and may lead to revision surgery. As always, close postoperative follow-up and early intervention may minimize these problems.

In spite of these shortcomings the Chopart amputation remains useful as an early incision and drainage procedure to stabilize acute infection. It is also useful as a definitive procedure in selected cases because of its advantage of limb length and tissue preservation.

TRANSMALLEOLAR AMPUTATION: THE SYME'S PROCEDURE

Indications

Hindfoot amputation, to be successful, must produce a reliable result with a long-lasting and functional residual limb. Chopart's amputation at the Talo-navicular and calcaneal-cuboid joints creates significant muscle imbalance frequently resulting in ankle equinus and ulceration. The Boyd amputation has also been advocated *(45)*. This procedure involves fusion of a portion of the calcaneus to the distal tibia. The advantage is that the heel pad remains well anchored to the calcaneus. An additional problem becomes evident in attaining union of the tibia to calcaneus. There may also be difficulty in prosthetic fitting. The residual limb remains long and there is inadequate space to place a dynamic response prosthetic foot without raising the height of the contralateral limb to compensate for this addition. It is unknown whether this height difference results in gait problems for the patient with diabetes.

The Syme's amputation is performed through the malleoli and results in with physiological weight bearing throughout the residual limb. The fat pad takes load directly and transfers this directly to the distal tibia *(46)*. With the use of dynamic response feet this amputation level results in decreased energy expenditure with ambulation compared with higher procedures or midfoot amputation *(47–50)*. Contraindications for this procedure include local infection or gangrene at the level of the amputation, and inadequate nutritional and vascular parameters to sustain distal healing. Healing may be achieved using this procedure with serum albumin levels as low as 2.5 g/dL *(46)*. Heel ulceration has been considered as a contraindication to a Syme's procedure in the past. However, a recent report suggested that an anterior flap may be useful in patients with a nonviable heel pad *(49)*. A long-term review of this procedure modification in a significant series of patients has not yet been performed.

Procedure

The incision is placed anteriorly across the ankle mortise and then in a stirrup fashion across the anterior heel at the level of the malleoli. The incision is deepened at the anterior ankle and the ankle capsule is incised transversely. The ankle ligaments are

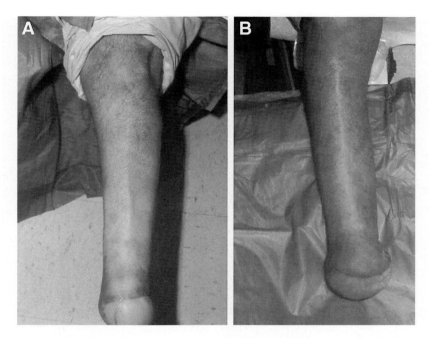

Fig. 8. (**A**) A well performed Syme's amputation with tapered stump and heel pad. (**B**) A more bulbous residual limb with medial and lateral flairs is a typical appearance. If these lateral prominences become problematic, wedge excision of these tissues may become necessary.

released sharply and the talus is displaced anteriorly in the mortise. A bone hook is placed into the talus and used to anteriorly distract the talus so that soft tissues may be freed from the talus and the calcaneus. Care is exercised at the posterior calcaneus to prevent buttonholing of the skin while releasing the soft tissues. Once free, the residual foot is removed from the wound and the wound is thoroughly irrigated. The residual tendons are gently distracted 0.5–1 cm and sectioned. If needed the anterior ankle vessels may be ligated with appropriate suture. Anterior and posterior margins of the distal tibia may require debridement to diminish excessive spurring. Two drill holes may be placed in posterior tibia and/or the anterior tibia. A heavy absorbable suture (0) may be utilized through the drill holes to anchor the plantar fascia to the distal tibia. The anterior aspect of the residual plantar fascia is sewn into the anterior ankle capsule and the subcutaneous tissues and skin are closed in layers. A medium hemovac drain is placed before closure. A posterior splint or a short leg cast is placed. The drain is removed 24–48 hours after surgery.

Postoperative Care

The patient may begin assisted/partial weight bearing at 3 to 5 days and is maintained in a short leg cast for 3 to 6 weeks. The patient is then advanced to a fiberglass cast temporary prosthesis with a rubber bumper distally. Once the patients' limb has matured and there is minimal residual edema, the patient is fitted for a Canadian Syme's prosthesis with a dynamic response foot (Figs. 8 and 9). Full activity is resumed. The need for physical therapy gait training is unusual.

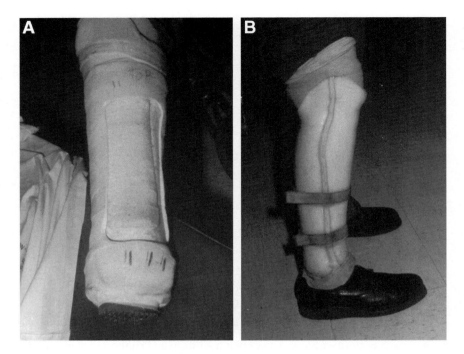

Fig. 9. (A) A fiberglass cast with a distal rubber bumper and a medial window is used as a temporary prosthesis to allow early ambulation for the Syme's amputation patients. **(B)** A thermoplastic variation of a temporary prosthesis with a prosthetic foot attached. In a patient with very limited ambulation, this may also serve as permanent prosthesis.

Complications

Healing rates for this level vary from 70% to 80%. Early complications with the wound may occur in up to 50% of the patients. Most of these problems may be treated with local wound care, total contact casting and culture specific antibiotic therapy. Other problems include heel pad migration and new bone formation. Heel pad migration has become less frequent with anchoring of the fascia. Should new bone formation become significant or cause ulceration, exostectomy may become necessary *(46)*.

TRANSTIBIAL OR BELOW KNEE AMPUTATION

Indications

Individuals with transtibial amputation provide the largest population of patients that are capable of achieving meaningful rehabilitation and functional independence following lower extremity amputation. The most predictable method of obtaining a durable residual limb is with a posterior myofasciocutaneous flap *(3)*. This level takes advantage of the plastic surgical tissue transfer technique of a composite tissue flap without dissection between layers, thus minimizing the risk for devascularization of the overlying skin.

Procedure

The optimal length of the tibial bone cut is the junction between the proximal and middle quarters of the tibia. A simple rule of thumb is 5 inches (12 to 15 cm) distal to the knee joint. The length of the posterior flap should be the length of the diameter of the limb at

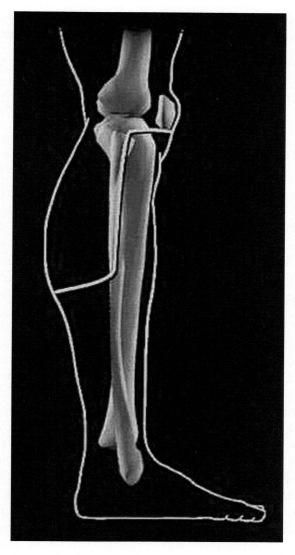

Fig. 10. Posterior myofasciocutaneous flap used in transtibial amputation level.

the level of the amputation, plus 1 cm. The longitudinal component of the flap should be between one-third and one-half of the width of the limb, depending on the size of the patient. Thinner patients require more bulk to create a functional residual limb (Fig. 10).

The muscle of the flap should be beveled to obtain good soft tissue padding without being too bulky (Fig. 5). The tibia is transected with a power saw, taking careful attention to beveling the anterior surface. The fibula is cut just proximal to the tibia, in order to provide an optimal bony surface for load transfer. The posterior gastrocnemius muscle fascia should be sutured to the anterior-distal residual tibia via drill holes or to the enveloping periosteum of the tibia. The lateral aspect of the flap is secured to the transected anterior compartment fascia. Securing the gastrocnemius muscle flap to the tibia serves two purposes: (1) it creates a cushioned soft tissue interface to alleviate the shear forces of weight bearing in prosthesis, and (2) control of the residual tibia positions the tibia in optimal alignment for effective load transfer to the prosthesis *(51)*. A suction drain is generally used under the flap, and the skin is reapproximated without tension.

Postoperative Care

Postoperatively, a rigid plaster dressing is applied *(52)*. Weight bearing with prosthesis is initiated at 5–21 days, based on the experience and resources of the rehabilitation team (Fig. 11).

KNEE DISARTICULATION

Indications

Knee disarticulation is generally performed in patients with the biological capacity to heal a surgical wound at the transtibial level, but they are not projected to walk with a prosthesis *(53,54)*. In selected patients, it provides an excellent direct load transfer residual limb for weight bearing in a prosthesis. In limited household walkers, or in feeble amputees with limited ambulatory capacity, this level takes advantage of the intrinsically stable polycentric four-bar linkage prosthetic knee joint. The enhanced inherent stability of this prosthetic system decreases the risk for falls in this limited ambulatory population.

Procedure

The currently recommended technique takes advantages of the accepted transtibial posterior myofasciocutaneous flap *(55)*. The skin incision is made transversely midway between the level of the inferior pole of the patella and the tibial tubercle, at the approximate level of the knee joint. The length of the posterior flap is equal to a diameter plus 1 cm (as with transtibial). The width of the flap again varies with the size of the patient, ranging between the posterior and middle thirds of the circumference of the leg (Fig. 12). The patellar ligament is detached from the tibia, and the capsule of the knee joint is incised circumferentially. The cruciate ligaments are detached from the tibia. A full-thickness posterior myofasciocutaneous flap is created along the posterior surface of the tibia. The soleus muscle is generally removed, unless it is needed to provide bulk. The gastrocnemius muscle is transected at the level of the posterior skin incision, with no creation of a tissue plane between the muscle and skin layers. The patellar ligament is then sutured to the distal stumps of the cruciate ligaments with nonabsorbable suture. The posterior gastrocnemius fascia is then sutured to the patellar ligament and retained knee joint retinaculum. The skin is reapproximated, and a rigid postoperative plaster rigid dressing.

Postoperative Care

Early weight bearing with a preparatory prosthesis or pylon can be initiated when the tissues of the residual limb appear secure. A locked knee or polycentric four-bar linkage prosthetic knee joint can be used, depending on the walking stability of the patient.

TRANSFEMORAL, OR ABOVE KNEE AMPUTATION

Indications

Gottschalk has clearly shown that the method of surgical construction of the transfemoral residual limb is the determining factor in positioning the femur for optimal

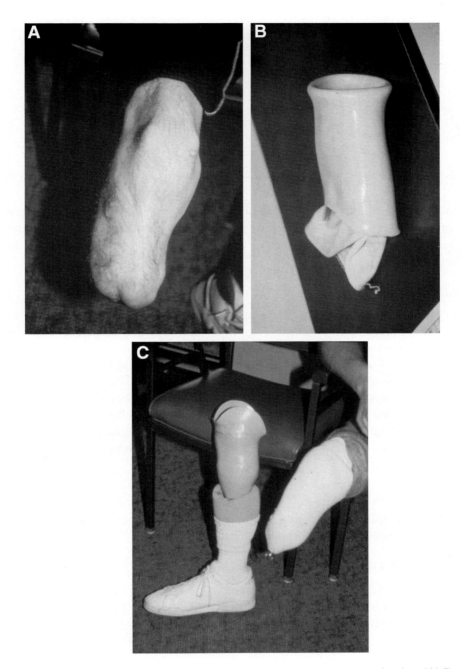

Fig. 11. This is the most common transtibial prosthetic socket system used today. (**A**) Residual limb of transtibial amputee. (**B**) Silicone suspension sleeve. The silicone sleeve snugly fits the residual limb, much like a condom. The bolt at the bottom locks into the (**C**) prosthesis.

load transfer *(56)*. Standard transfemoral amputation with a fish-mouth incision disengages the action of the adductor musculature. By disengaging the adductor muscles, the femur assumes an abducted, nonfunctional position. This relative functional

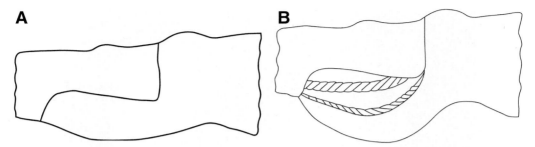

Fig. 12. (A) and **(B)** Posterior myofasciocutaneous flap used in knee disarticulation amputation.

shortening of the abductors produces an apparently weak abductor gait pattern. By using an adductor-based myocutaneous flap, the adductor muscles can be secured to the residual femur, allowing the femur to be appropriately prepositioned within the prosthetic socket *(57)*.

Procedure

Using the "rule-of-thumb," the bone cut is 5 inches above the knee joint. The soft tissue envelope is made up of a medial-based myofasciocutaneous flap (Fig. 13). The flap, including adductor magnus insertion, is dissected off of the femur. After securing hemostasis and cutting the bone, the adductor muscles are secured to the lateral cortex of the femur via drill holes, under normal resting muscle tension. The anterior and posterior muscle flaps are also secured to the residual femur via drill holes. Careful attention is taken to secure the muscles to the residual femur with the hip positioned at neutral flexion-extension, so that to avoid an iatrogenic hip flexion contracture, so often produced by repairing the soft tissues with the residual limb being propped on bolsters during wound closure.

Postoperative Care

An elastic compression dressing is applied, and weight bearing with a preparatory prosthesis is initiated when the wound appears secure.

HIP DISARTICULATION

Few hip disarticulation amputees become functional prosthetic users. Whether sitting in a chair, or "sitting" in a prosthetic socket, the weight-bearing platform can be enhanced by retaining the femoral head within the socket.

Rehabilitation

Amputation surgery should be considered as reconstructive surgery following removal of a nonfunctional organ of locomotion. As such, the concept of rehabilitation should begin before surgery. It cannot be sufficiently stressed that optimal functional outcomes can generally be achieved when the treatment team establishes reasonable goals. If functional walking is not reasonable, possibly independent wheelchair transfer for ambulation is most appropriate. The treatment team should have a reasonable expectation of goals outcomes at the end of treatment, before initiating

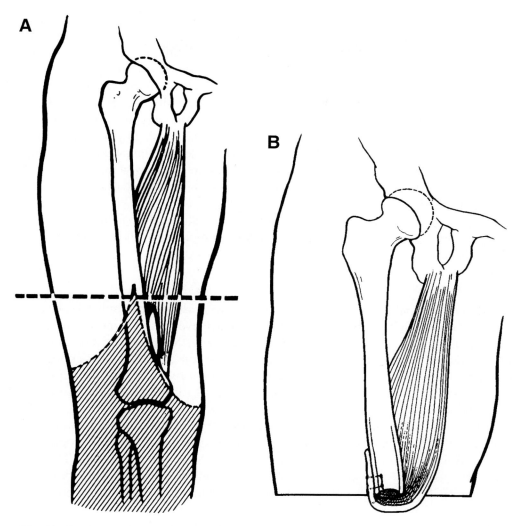

Fig. 13. (A) Skin incision for adductor myofasciocutaneous transfemoral amputation technique. **(B)** Schematic of muscle attachment.

treatment. When one measures results from an ambulatory perspective or from a measure of achieving activities of daily living, amputees are less functional or independent with more proximal level amputees. Unilateral ankle disarticulation amputees walk and functional at a level very comparable with their age and disease-matched counterparts. Although 87% of transtibial amputees will be functional walkers at 2 years, 36% would have died *(58)*. Ambulatory knee disarticulation amputees fare somewhat less well from both ambulatory and independence perspectives. Very few diabetic, dysvascular transfemoral amputees, or bilateral amputees, will become functional walkers.

Residual limb care in the early postoperative period can enhance, or detract, from good surgical technique. Specific wound care is related to the circumstances of the surgery. The use of rigid postoperative plaster dressings in transtibial or knee disarticulation amputations controls swelling, decreases postoperative pain, and protects the limb from trauma. The rigid plaster dressing is changed at 5- to 7-day intervals, with early postoperative prosthetic limb fitting and weight bearing being initiated between 5 and 21 days following surgery. Immediate postoperative prosthetic fitting should be reserved for patients with very stable, secure residual limbs. Generally, the residual limb of the transfemoral amputee is managed with a suspended compression dressing. Weight bearing with a prefabricated, or custom, prosthetic socket and training pylon can be initiated when the wound appears secure. With more proximal level amputation, these multiple system involved individuals are more likely to require walking aids, with almost all dysvascular diabetic amputees requiring the use of a walker or crutches for their limited range of walking.

When the treatment team develops reasonable, realistic goals, patients are capable of achieving the highest level of functional walking compatible with their multiple organ system disease.

CONCLUSION

Partial foot amputations are frequently used to successfully accomplish limb salvage. If below knee or higher amputation is required to achieve healing, many patients return to community ambulation, still utilizing and stressing the remaining limb. Once any form of amputation has occurred the patient must be considered at high risk for further amputation *(29)*. The principles of managing any high-risk foot must be applied, and regular review and management services are essential for preserving the salvaged and contralateral limb.

Patient education, shoe review with appropriate prescription or recommendation, and regular professional foot exams are the mainstay of any preventive program *(32)*. Regular follow-up must be initiated after healing has been accomplished. The patient should be instructed in regular self-foot exams, and the effects of sensory neuropathy. Potentially ulcerative pressure points should be identified and accommodated with orthotics and, or, shoes as needed. Recurring pressure keratosis should be acknowledged as a potential ulceration, and debrided as necessary to prevent the callus from becoming hemorrhagic or ulcerative. This may require intervals as little as every 4 weeks *(33)*.

It has been the authors' experience that no surgical procedure is effective, in itself, in preventing subsequent foot ulcers. The patient with any form of lower extremity amputation must be considered at high risk for further ulceration. Careful clinical follow-up, orthotic care, and debridement of chronic focal pressure keratosis are far more effective in preventing ulceration or further amputation than any operation.

REFERENCES

1. Adler AI, Boyko EJ, Ahroni JH, Smith DG. Lower extremity amputation in diabetes. The independent effects of peripheral vascular disease, sensory neuropathy and foot ulcers. *Diabetes Care* 1999;22(7):1029–1035.
2. Burgess EM, Romano RL, Zettl JH. *The Management of Lower Extremity Amputations*, US Government Printing Office, Washington, DC, 1969.

3. Pinzur MS, Bowker JH, Smith DG, Gottschalk FA. Amputation surgery in peripheral vascular disease, in *Instructional Course Lectures, The American Academy of Orthopaedic Surgeons.* C.V. Mosby, St. Louis, 1999, Vol. 48, pp. 687–692.

4. Pinzur MS, Sage R, Stuck R, Ketner L, Osterman H. Transcutaneous oxygen as a predictor of wound healing in amputations of the foot and ankle. *Foot Ankle* 1992;13:271–272.

5. Pinzur MS, Gold J, Schwartz D, Gross N. Energy demands for walking in dysvascular amputees as related to the level of amputation. *Orthopaedics* 1992;15:1033–1037.

6. Waters RL, Perry J, Antonelli D, et al. Energy cost of walking of amputees: the influence of level of amputation. *J Bone Joint Surg* 1976;58A:42–46.

7. Waters RL. The energy expenditure of amputee gait, in *Atlas of Limb Prosthetics*, (Bowker J, Michael J, eds.), Mosby Year Book, St. Louis, 1992, pp. 381–387.

8. Worral G, Moulton N, Briffett E. Effect of type II diabetes mellitus on cognitive function. *J Fam Pract* 1993;36:639–643.

9. Kruger S, Guthrie D. Foot care knowledge retention and self-care practices. *Diabetes Educ* 1992;18:487–490.

10. Thompson FJ, Masson EA. Can elderly diabetic patients cooperate with routine foot care? *Age Aging* 1992;21:333–337.

11. Pinzur MS, Graham G, Osterman H. Psychological testing in amputation rehabilitation. *Clin Orthop* 1988;229:236–240.

12. Pinzur MS. New concepts in lower-limb amputation and prosthetic management, in *Instructional Course Lectures, The American Academy of Orthopaedic Surgeons.* C.V. Mosby, St. Louis, 1990, Vol. 39, pp. 361–366.

13. Emanuele MA, Buchanan BJ, Abraira C. Elevated leg systolic pressures and arterial calcification in diabetic occlusive vascular disease. *Diabetes Care* 1981;4:289–292.

14. Wyss CR, Harrington RM, Burgess EM, Matsen FA. Transcutaneous oxygen tension as a predictor of success after an amputation. *J. Bone Joint Surg* 1988;70A:203–207.

15. Pahlsson HI, Wahlberg E, Olofsson P, Swedenborg J. The toe pole test for evaluation of arterial insufficiency in diabetic patients. *Eur J Endovasc Surg* 1999;18:133–137.

16. Carter SA, Tate RB. The value of toe pulse waves in determination of risks for limb amputation and death in patients with peripheral arterial disease and skin ulcers or gangrene. *J Vasc Surg* 2001;33:708–714.

17. Ubbink DT, Tulevski II, de Graaff JC, Legemate DA, Jacobs JHM. Optimisation of the noninvasive assessment of critical limb ischaemia requiring invasive treatment. *Eur J Endovasc Surg* 2000;19:131–137.

18. Misuri A, Lucertini G, Nanni A, et al. Predictive value of trancutaneous oximetry for selection of the amputation level. *J Cardiovasc Surg* 2000;41(1):83–87.

19. Dickhaut SC, Delee JC, Page CP. Nutrition status: importance in predicting wound healing after amputation. *J Bone Joint Surg Am* 1984;64:71–75.

20. Haydock DA, Hill GL. Improved wound healing response in surgical patients receiving intravenous nutrition. *Br J Surg* 1987;74:320–323.

21. Jensen JE, Jensen TG, Smith TK, et al. Nutrition in orthopaedic surgery. *J Bone Joint Surg Am* 1982;64:1263–1272.

22. Mowat AG, Baum J. Chemotaxis of polymorphonuclear leukocytes from patients with diabetes mellitus. *N Engl J Med* 1971;248:621–627.

23. Gianfortune P, Pulla RJ, Sage R. Ray resection in the insensitive or dysvascular foot: a critical review. *J Foot Surg* 1985;24:103–107.

24. Pinzur MS, Sage R, Schwaegler P. Ray resection in the dysvascular foot. *Clin Orth Related Res* 1984;191:232–234.

25. McKittrick LS, McKittrick JB, Risley TS. Transmetatarsal amputation for infection or gangrene in patients with diabetes mellitus. *Ann Surg* 1949;130:826–831.

26. Wagner FW. Amputations of the foot and ankle. *Clin Ortho* 1977;122:62–69.

27. Pinzur M, Kaminsky M, Sage R, Cronin R, Osterman H. Amputations at the middle level of the foot. *JBJS* 1986;68-A:1061.
28. Sage R, Pinzur MS, Cronin R, Preuss HF, Osterman H. Complications following midfoot amputation in neuropathic and dysvascular feet. *JAPMA* 1989;79:277.
29. Sanders LJ. Transmetatarsal and midfoot amputations. *Clin Podiatr Med Surg* 1997;14: 741–762.
30. Armstrong DG, Hadi S, Nguyen HC, Harkless LB. Factors associated with bone regrowth following diabetes-related partial amputation of the foot. *JBJS* 1999;81:1561–1565.
31. Mueller MJ, Sinacore DR. Rehabilitation factors following transmetatarsal amputation. *Phys Ther* 1994;74:1027–1033.
32. Mayfield JA, Reiber GE, Sanders LJ, Janisse D, Pogach L. Preventive foot care in people with diabetes. *Diabetes Care* 1998;21:2161–2177.
33 Sage RA, Webster JK, Fisher SG. Out patient care and morbidity reduction in diabetic foot ulcers associated with chronic pressure callus. *JAPMA* 2001;91:275–291.
34. Christie J, Clowes CB, Lamb DW. Amputation through the middle part of the foot. *J Bone Joint Surg Br* 1980;24:473–474.
35. McDonald A. Choparts amputation. *J Bone Joint Surg Br* 1955;37:468–470.
36. Lieberman JR, Jacobs RL, Goldstock L, et al. Chopart amputation with percutaneous heel cord lengthening. *Clin Orthop* 1993;296:86–91.
37. Chang BB, Bock DE, Jacob RL, et al. Increased limb salvage by the use of unconventional foot amputations. *J Vasc Surg* 1994;19:341–349.
38. Bingham J. The surgery of partial foot amputation in *Prosthetics and Orthotic Practice* (Murdoch G, ed.) Edward Arnold, London, 1970; p. 141.
39. Roach JJ, Deutscsh A, McFarlane DS. Resurrection of the amputations of lisfranc and chopart for diabetic gangrene. *Arch Surg* 1987;122:931–934.
40. Wagner FW. The dysvascular foot: a system for diagnosis and treatment. *Foot Ankle* 1981;2: 64–122.
41. Early JS. Transmetatarsal and midfoot amputations. *Clin Orth Related Res* 1999;361: 85–90.
42. Reyzelman AM, Suhad H, Armstrong DG. Limb salvage with Chopart's amputation and tendon balancing. *JAPMA* 1999;89:100–103.
43. Cohen-Sobel E. Advances in foot prosthetics, in *Advances in Podiatric Medicine and Surgery* (Kominsky SJ, ed.), Mosby Year Book, St. Louis, 1995, pp. 261–273.
44. Cohen-Sobel E, Cuselli M, Rizzuto J. Prosthetic management of a Chopart amputation variant. *JAPMA* 1994;84:505–510.
45. Grady JF, Winters CL. The Boyd amputation as a treatment for osteomyelitis of the foot. *JAPMA* 2000;90(5):234–239.
46. Pinzur MA, Stuck RM, Sage R, Hunt N, Rabinovich Z. Syme ankle disarticulation in patients with diabetes. *J Bone Joint Surg* 2004;85-A:1667–1672.
47. Pinzur M, Morrison C, Sage R, et al. Syme's two-stage amputation in insulin requiring diabetics with gangrene of the forefoot. *Foot Ankle* 1991;11:394–396.
48. Pinzur M. Restoration of walking ability with Syme's ankle disarticulation. *Clin Orth Related Res* 1999;361:71–75.
49. Robinson KP. Disarticulation at the ankle using an anterior flap: a preliminary report. *J Bone Joint Surg Br* 1999;81(4):617–620.
50. Waters RL, Perry J, Antonelli D, et al. Energy cost of walking of amputees: the influence of level of amputation. *J Bone Joint Surg Am* 1976;58:42.
51. Pinzur MS, Reddy N, Charuk G, Osterman H, Vrbos L. Control of the residual tibia in trans-tibial amputation. *Foot Ankle Int* 1996;17:538–540.
52. Pinzur MS. Current concepts: amputation surgery in peripheral vascular disease, in *Instructional Course Lectures, The American Academy of Orthopaedic Surgeons.* C.V. Mosby, St. Louis, 1997, Vol. 46, pp. 501–509.

53. Pinzur MS, Smith DG, Daluga DG, Osterman H. Selection of patients for through-the-knee amputation. *J Bone Joint Surg* 1988;70A:746–750.
54. Pinzur MS. Knee disarticulation: surgical procedures, in *Atlas of Limb Prosthetics*, (Bowker JH, Michael JW, eds.), Mosby Year Book, St. Louis, 1992, pp. 479–486.
55. Pinzur MS, Bowker JH. Knee disarticulation. *Clin Orthop* 1999;361:23–28.
56. Gottschalk F, Kourosh S, Stills M. Does socket configuration influence the position of the femur in above-knee amputation? *J Prosthet Orthot* 1989;2:94–102.
57. Gottschalk F. Transfemoral amputation, in *Atlas of Limb Prosthetics*, (Bowker JH, Michael JW, eds.), Mosby Year Book, St. Louis, 1992, pp. 501–507.
58. Pinzur MS, Gottschalk F, Smith D, et al. Functional outcome of below-knee amputation in peripheral vascular insufficiency. *Clin Orthop* 1993;286:247–249.

19

Soft Tissue Reconstructive Options
for the Ulcerated or Gangrenous Diabetic Foot

Christopher E. Attinger, MD

INTRODUCTION

Diabetic foot and ankle wounds usually occur because of acute or repetitive trauma in an insensate and biomechanically unstable foot. The body is unable to heal the wound owing to persistent trauma, biomechanical abnormality, infection, inadequate blood flow, ineffective immune system, or poor nutrition and the acute wound converts into a chronic wound. The goal is to transform the chronic wound into an acute healing wound with healthy granulation tissue, neoepithelialization, and wrinkled skin edges. The steps to achieve a healthy healing wound include establishing a correct diagnosis, ensuring a good local blood supply, debriding the wound to a clean base, correcting the biomechanical abnormality, and nurturing the wound until it shows signs of healing. The subsequent reconstruction can then usually be accomplished by simple techniques 90% of the time and complex flap reconstruction in 10% of cases. It may involve partial foot amputation to develop a sufficient tissue envelope to close the wound or to stabilize the foot biomechanically.

DEFINITION

Chronic wounds or ulcers are wounds arrested in the inflammatory phase of wound healing. Their surface is chronically infected and contains an overabundance of proteases that overwhelm local growth factors preventing them from being effective. Collagenases prevent an adequate collagen framework from being laid down. Elastases destroy local growth factors that guide the rebuilding process. Bacteria and their surrounding biofilm inhibit efforts to sterilize the wound and continue to contribute to the protease-rich wound environment.

In patients with diabetes, healing is seriously affected by poorly controlled blood glucose levels. Glucose levels above 300 inhibit the white blood cells from effectively destroying invading bacteria and directing the wound healing effort. High glucose levels glycosylate the red blood cell wall stiffening it. The end result is an increase in blood viscosity. Taking red blood cell deforming drugs (e.g., Trental®, Arentis Pharmaceuticals, Bridgewater, Connecticut or Pletal® Otaka American Pharmaceuticals, Bethesda, Margland can help restore red blood cell flexibility and decrease blood viscosity. High glucose levels also contribute to the stiffening of joints and tendons by glycosylating collagen and thereby

From: *The Diabetic Foot, Second Edition*
Edited by: A. Veves, J. M. Giurini, and F. W. LoGerfo © Humana Press Inc., Totowa, NJ

decreasing its flexibility. The most obvious manifestation of this occurs in the achilles tendon resulting in loss of foot dorsiflexion. This then places excessive pressure on the skeletal arch of the foot as well as the plantar forefoot during gait and contributes to Charcot collapse and forefoot ulceration.

More than 60% of diabetic ulcers have insufficient blood flow owing to peripheral vascular disease. The atherosclerotic disease is usually manifest below the popliteal artery and involves one or more of the three lower leg arteries: the anterior tibial artery, the posterior tibial artery, and/or the peroneal artery. Correction depends on the vascular surgeon's ability to correct the defect using endovascular techniques as well as traditional distal bypasses.

Given the complexity of issues involved in a chronic diabetic wound, resolution mandates a team effort. The team should include a diabetologist to bring the sugars under control, an infectious disease specialist to optimize antibiotic therapy, a foot and ankle surgeon to address the existing biomechanical abnormalities, a vascular surgeon to improve local blood flow, a wound specialist to convert the chronic wound in a healthy healing wound, and a plastic surgeon to close wounds that require flap reconstruction. Frequently, one of the treating physicians possess two or more of the necessary skill sets to treat diabetic wounds; i.e., the vascular surgeon, orthopedic surgeon, plastic surgeon, diabetologist, or infectious disease specialist can also be an expert in wound healing techniques.

ESTABLISHING A DIAGNOSIS

History

A thorough patient history is taken from the patient, family and friends, EMT, and/or referring doctor to help determine the wound's etiology. The origin (usually traumatic) and age of the wound are determined. The trauma is usually related to biomechanical abnormalities causing excessive local pressure during gait, changes in shoe wear, penetrating trauma, or excessive heat (hot water foot baths). The patient's tetanus immunization status is obtained and the patient is inoculated if revaccination is indicated. It is important to ask what previous topical therapy was applied to the wound because certain topical agents can contribute to the wound's chronicity *(1)* (e.g., caustic agents such as hydrogen peroxide, 10% iodine, Dakin's solution, and so on).

A careful medical history is obtained emphasizing possible manifestations of atherosclerotic disease to the heart, nervous system, kidneys, eyes, and lower extremity. For patients on dialysis, the onset and type of dialysis is documented. The venous aspect of circulation is likewise evaluated by noting abnormalities in blood coagulation, liver disease, heart failure, previous venous thrombi, and pulmonary emboli. The extent of the neuropathy present is then explored, loss of sensation, muscle weakness, loss of ability to sweat, and so on. The patient's ability to monitor and treat his/her blood sugars is carefully examined. Finally, the nutritional status is assessed: the recent weight gain or loss, the quality of the diet. Their smoking status is documented and a complete list of medications and drug allergies is obtained.

A social history is then obtained to determine the level of activity, the level of home help available, and the type of work they are involved in. This can help to assess the patient's ability to comply with the treatment regimen because these wounds can involve up to 6 months of inactivity (i.e., Ilizarov treatment of a Charcot collapse). The patient's lack of compliance is the single biggest reason for postoperative wound complications (>20%).

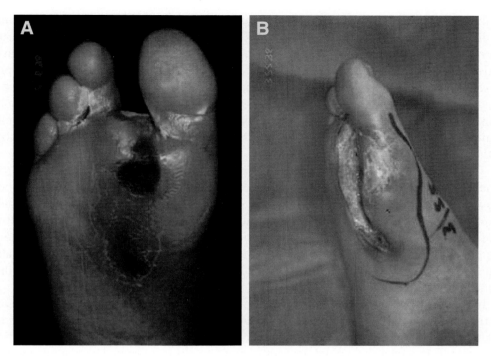

Fig. 1. If a foot presents with cellulitis (**A**), the border of the erythema is delineated and dated with indelible ink. If there is necrosis or ulceration, the wound should be debrided. After debridement, deep cultures of the wound are obtained and broad spectrum antibiotics are started. The delineated borders of the initial erythema are then assessed. If, after 4–6 hours, the cellulitis has extended beyond the inked boundary, either the antibiotics are inadequate and/or the wound has been inadequately debrided. In this case, the redness has receded and therefore the initial therapy is appropriate (**B**).

Physical Exam

The wound is then assessed carefully by measuring its size and depth. The area is obtained by multiplying the length of longest axis and by the width of the widest axis perpendicular to it. Depth measured and the exposed layers of tissue are documented, epidermis, dermis, subdermal fat, fascia, muscle tendon, joint capsule, joint, and/or bone. A metallic probe is used to assist in the evaluation of the depth of the wound. If the probe touches bone, there is an 85% chance that osteomyelitis *(2)* is present. If tendon is involved, the infection is very likely to have tracked proximally or distally. One should check for bogginess proximally and distally along the potentially involved tendon sheaths. If the suspicion is strong that a distal infection has spread proximally, the proximal areas in which the tendon sheaths are readily accessible should be aspirated (i.e., extensor retinaculum, tarsal tunnel, and so on). The wound is then photographed.

If cellulitis is present, the border of the erythema is delineated with indelible ink. After deep cultures of the wound are obtained and broad spectrum antibiotics are started, the spread or retreat of the erythema can be continuously assessed. If, after 4–6 hours, the cellulitis has extended beyond the inked boundary, either the antibiotics are inadequate and/or the wound has been inadequately debrided (Fig. 1). It is important not to confuse cellulitis with dependent rubor seen in patients with chronic ischemia or chronic wound. If the erythema disappears when the affected leg is elevated above the level of the heart, then the erythema is due to dependent rubor. With dependent rubor, inflammation is usually absent and the skin should have visible wrinkling. If the erythema persists despite elevation, the wound has surrounding cellulitis and needs antibiotic treatment ± debridement. Dependent rubor can also be often seen at a fresh operative site and should not be confused with postoperative cellulitis. Again, rapid resolution of the erythema with elevation and presence of wrinkled skin at the incision edge indicate dependent rubor rather than cellulitis.

The blood flow to the area is then evaluated by palpation and/or hand-held Doppler *(3)*. The presence of palpable anterior and posterior tibial pulses suggests adequate blood flow. If one of the pulses is absent, then the pulses should be evaluated with a Doppler. A triphasic Doppler signal indicates normal blood flow, biphasic adequate blood flow, and monophasic warrants further investigation. If the quality of flow is questionable, a formal noninvasive arterial Doppler evaluation has to be performed. If the flow is inadequate, the patient should then be referred to a vascular surgeon who specializes in distal revascularizations.

In the face of undetermined or inadequate blood flow, debridement should be delayed until blood flow status has been assessed and corrected. However, immediate debridement is called for regardless of the vascular status when wet gangrene, ascending cellulitis from a necrotic wound, or necrotizing fasciitis is present. The wound can then be kept clean with dressing changes until revascularization. If the wound manifests progressive gangrene, maggots can be applied to locally debride necrotic tissue as the patient awaits revascularization *(4,5)*. After successful bypass surgery, it then takes 4–10 days to maximize surrounding tissue oxygen level *(6)*. Definitive debridement and aggressive wound care should follow as soon as possible thereafter.

Sensation must also be assessed. Lack of protective sensation can be established when the patient is unable to feel 10 g of pressure (5.07 Semms-Weinstein monofilament). This prevents patients from sensing damage owing to excessive local pressure (prolonged decubitus position, tight shoes, clothes or dressings, biomechanical abnormalities, or the presence of foreign bodies).

The biomechanical abnormality caused by motor dysfunction, skeletal abnormalities and/or a tight achilles tendon cause high focal plantar pressures during gait and the local tissue at those sites eventually breaks down under the repetitive stress of normal ambulation (on average, a person takes 10,000 steps a day) when the patient in insensate. The motor neuropathy is most often seen in the intrinsic muscles of the foot with resultant hammer toe formation. Skeletal abnormalities can include a prominent metatarsal head, Charcot collapse, and so on. These are best evaluated by weight-bearing X-ray views. Because the elasticity of the Achilles tendon is affected by diabetes, it should also be carefully evaluated *(7)*. The patient's ability to dorsiflex the supinated foot tests the elasticity of the achilles tendon (Fig. 2). If the patient can dorsiflex the foot more than 15° with the knee straight and bent, then the tendon has sufficient plasticity. If the foot can only be dorsiflexed when the knee is bent, then the Gastrocnemius portion of the Achilles tendon is tight. If the foot cannot dorsiflex when the knee is straight or bent, then both the Gastrocnemius and Soleus portions of the Achilles tendon are tight. Open or percutaneous release of the Achilles tendon *(8)*

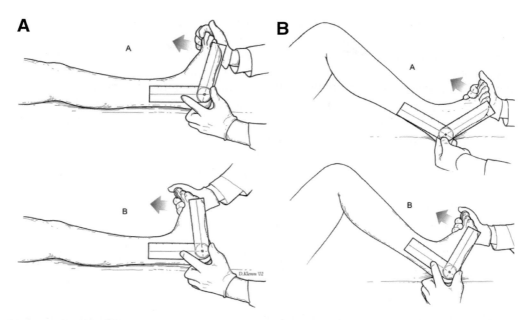

Fig. 2. The patient's ability to dorsiflex the supinated foot tests the elasticity of the Achilles tendon. If the patient can dorsiflex the foot more than 150 with the leg straight (**A**) and bent (**B**), then the tendon has sufficient plasticity. If the foot can only be dorsiflexed when the knee is bent, then the Gastrocnemius portion of the achilles tendon is tight.

decreases forefoot pressure in the equino-varus foot during gait sufficiently to allow for the rapid healing of plantar forefoot ulcers. The release results in a permanent decrease in pushoff forces which have show decreasing ulcer recurrence rate by 50% at 25 months out from surgery *(9,10)*. Unless correction of the underlying biomechanical abnormality is part of the entire treatment plan, debriding and good wound care may prove futile.

Testing

Blood work should be obtained. The immediate blood glucose level and chronic glucose level (hemoglobin A1C) should be assessed. Hemoglobin A1C over 6% indicate poor control of blood glucose levels (7% = average plasma glucose level of 170 mg/dl, 8% = 205, 9% = 240, 10% = 275, and 11% = 310). High blood sugar in the face of a low hemoglobin A1C can indicate acute infection. The white blood cell count and differentiation is also very helpful in monitoring systemic infection. The numbers, however, can look deceptively normal in renal failure diabetic patients. A sedimentation rate can be helpful as a tracking tool during treatment of an infection. The kidney function should be evaluated especially because many of these patients may require an angiogram.

An X-ray is critical to evaluate the underlying bone architecture. It may not pick up acute osteomyelitis because it can take up to 3 weeks for osteomyelitis to appear on X-ray. An MRI or nuclear scan is usually superfluous if the surgeon plans to evaluate the affected bone during the debridement. However, these studies can be useful when the extent of osteomyelitis in the suspected bone is unclear or when there is suspicion that other bones may be involved.

Noninvasive arterial studies are useful adjuncts to help assess the quality of blood flow to the foot. Ankle–brachial indices are inaccurate in patients with diabetes because their arterial walls calcify, preventing the cuff from compressing the vessel. Because the digital arteries are less likely to calcify, toe pressures higher than 50 mmHg indicate adequate flow. Pulse volume recordings that contain at least 15 small boxes in height indicate adequate arterial flow volumes. Tissue oxygen levels can be very useful if the laboratory tests them reliably. Levels lower than 20 mmHg indicate poor healing potential, level between 20 and 40 mmHg indicates possible healing and levels higher than 40 mmHg indicate good healing potential. Because no one test is totally accurate, the combination of all the above tests help provide the clinician with a more complete picture of the actual blood flow.

DEBRIDEMENT

The Role of Debridement in Wound Healing

Debriding a wound is defined as removing necrotic tissue, foreign material, and infecting bacteria from wound. Necrotic tissue, foreign material, and bacteria impede the body's attempt to heal by producing or stimulating the production of proteases, collagenases, and elastases that overwhelm the local wound healing process *(11)*. In this process, the building blocks (chemotactants, growth factors, growth receptors, mitogens, and so on) necessary for normal wound healing are destroyed. This hostile environment is one in which bacteria can proliferate and further inhibit wound healing. Bacteria produce their own wound inhibiting enzymes as well and consume many of the scarce local resources (oxygen, nutrition, and building blocks) that are necessary for wound healing. They also protect themselves from destruction by secreting a protective biofilm *(12)*. Steed reviewed the data of platelet-derived growth factor's effect on the healing of chronic diabetic wounds *(13)* and made the seminal observation that wounds healed more successfully when the wound debridement was performed weekly rather than more sporadically. The scheduled removal of wound healing inhibitors (such as proteases, collagenases, and elastases) allowed the wound to progress beyond the inflammatory phase and into the proliferative phase.

Debriding a wound adequately consists of removing all nonviable tissue until healthy viable tissue is reached. The body naturally autodebrides any necrotic tissue but this is a slow and frequently unpredictable process especially in the setting of a chronic wound. It is usually faster and safer to debride a wound surgically, with maggots, and/or with topical agents. Debridement should be performed after the diagnosis has been established and the steps to improving the local environment are underway. In the setting of an ischemic limb, debridement should usually be delayed until the leg has been revascularized so that potentially viable tissue is not prematurely removed or exposed to desiccation. However, immediate debridement should always be performed in the setting of wet gangrene or necrotizing fasciitis regardless of the vascular status of the leg.

When debriding, use atraumatic surgical techniques to avoid damaging the healthy tissue left behind. Such tissue should be protected as it is the source of growth factors, nutrients, and building blocks required for subsequent healing. To leave a maximal amount of viable tissue behind, avoid traumatizing techniques such as crushing the skin edges with forceps or clamps, burning tissue with electrocautery, or tying off large clumps of tissue with sutures *(14)*.

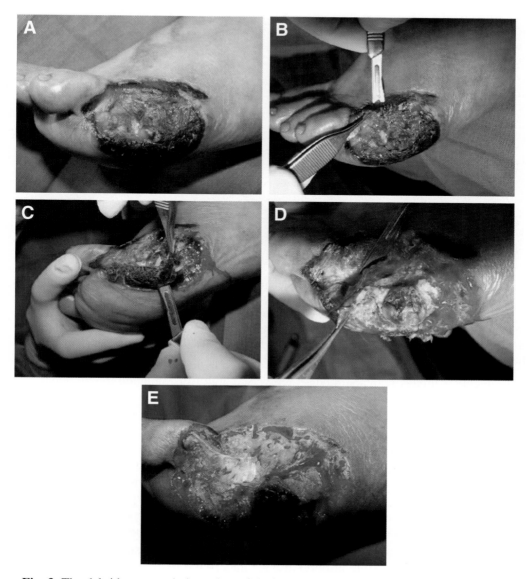

Fig. 3. The debridement technique that minimizes the risk of taking normal tissue is to take thin slices after thin slices of necrotic tissue until only normal tissue remains. Grasp the tissue to be removed with the pickup and use no. 10 or no. 20 blade to sliceoff thin layer after thin layer. Change surgical blades frequently, as they dull quickly.

The principal debriding technique consists of removing the grossly contaminated or ischemic tissue en masse. Surgical tools include a scalpel blade, mayo scissors, curettes, and rongeurs as well as power tools including a sagital saw and a power burr. However, when debridement approaches viable tissue, the technique is to take thin slices of tissue after thin slices of tissue until only normal tissue remains (Fig. 3). Grasp the tissue to be removed with the pickup and use a no. 10 or a no. 20 blade to slice off tissue, thin layer by thin layer, until healthy tissue appears. Change surgical blades frequently, as they

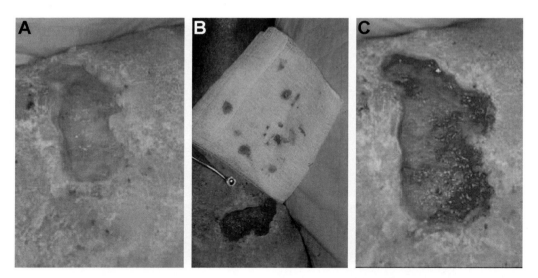

Fig. 4. Curettes with sharp edges are very helpful for removing the proteinaceous coagulum **(A)** that accumulates on top of both fresh and chronic granulation tissue. A curette is the ideal tool to remove coagulum **(B)**. Because the coagulum contains a high concentration of metalloproteases, its removal allows the growth factors that are naturally produced by the wound base **(C)**, that are topically applied (Regranex) or that are produced by bioengineered skin (Apligraf, Dermagraft) to be effective.

dull quickly. Curettes with sharp edges are very helpful for removing the proteinaceous coagulum that accumulates on top of both fresh and chronic granulation tissue (Fig. 4). Rongeurs are useful for removing hard-to-reach soft tissue and for debriding bone. An air-driven or electrical sagittal saw can serially saw off the bone until normal cortex and marrow appears. Cutting burrs and rasps permit fine debridement of bone surface until the telltale punctate bleeding at the freshened bone surface appears.

Newly available is a hydro-surgical debrider (VersaJet©, Smith & Nephew, Hull, United Kingdom) that use a high power water jet (up to 15,000 psi) to debride tissue (Fig. 5). The Venturi effect caused by this high pressure water jet stream sucks the underlying tissue into the stream of water and separates it from the underlying tissue. The debrider works rapidly to take thin slice after thin slice of tissue with minimal surrounding tissue trauma. More importantly, the underlying tissue is relatively unharmed by the jet stream and as such can proceed unimpeded as the source for new wound healing. The chief advantage of the VersaJet is that it allows for a very accurate control of the depth of cut and hence minimizes the risk of accidentally removing viable tissue. It is also very useful in preparing smooth recipient wound beds for skin grafts.

The basic tools of debridement used in an office include pickups, knife, scissors, and a curette. Surgical tools, not disposable suture removal kits, are recommended because the latter are usually dull, and they crush and damage the normal tissue left behind. Here again it is critical not to harm the underlying tissue as it will serve as the source for future wound healing. As such, one has to use gentle wound handling techniques such as sharp dissection instead of cautery resection, skin hooks to retract the tissue, pinpoint use of the cautery to minimize the amount of charred tissue left behind, and so on *(14)*.

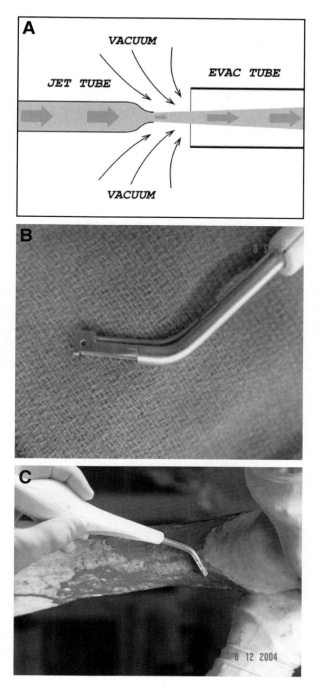

Fig. 5. The hydro-surgical debrider (VersaJet©, Smith & Nephew, Hull, United Kingdom) uses a high power water jet (up to 15,000 psi) to debride tissue. The Venturi effect caused by this high pressure water jet stream sucks the underlying tissue into the stream of water and separates it from the underlying tissue (**A**). The debrider (**B**) works rapidly to take thin slice after thin slice of tissue with minimal surrounding tissue trauma (**C**).

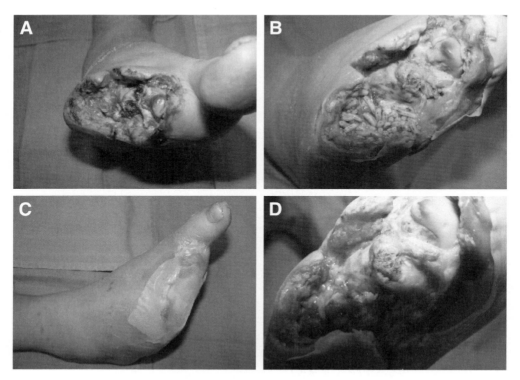

Fig. 6. The use of biosurgery with maggots is an extremely effective alternative to debriding a wound when the patient cannot tolerate surgery, debriding dressing, or topical agents. Maggots are the larvae of the Phoenicia sericata (green blow fly) and are irradiated so that they cannot metamorphose into the pupae phase. Thirty maggots consume 1 g tissue/day, consuming only necrotic tissue and bacteria and leaving any viable tissue intact. This partial necrotic forefoot (**A**) has maggots placed on it to prepare the wound for closure (**B**). the wound is sealed with a semipermeable membrane so that the maggots cannot escape (**C**). After 2 days of treatment, the wound's edge are clean and have begun to granulate (**D**).

The standard debriding dressing, i.e., wet-to-dry, can also be effective. The moist gauze is allowed to dry on the wound and then is ripped off the wound bed. Although this effectively removes dead tissue, it also removes viable tissue, can lead to wound desiccation, and is very painful in the sensate patient. Topical enzymatic debriding agents are effective, but they work slowly and can be painful. (If painful, the concentration can be decreased by diluting it with a wound gel.)

Debridement should be performed as often as necessary until the wound is deemed clean and ready for reconstruction. The wound is watched closely and redebrided as long as there is devitalized tissue. The use of biosurgery with maggots is an extremely effective alternative to debriding a wound when the patient cannot tolerate surgery, debriding dressing, or topical agents (Fig. 6) *(4,5)*. Maggots are the larvae of the *Phoenicia sericata* (green blow fly) and are irradiated so that they cannot metamorphose into the pupae phase. Thirty maggots consume 1 g tissue per day, consuming only necrotic tissue and bacteria and leaving any viable tissue intact. Maggots are painless and are very effective against antibiotic-resistant organisms. Maggots are the only agents that destroy all antibiotic-resistant bacteria including *MRSA* or *VRE*. They are applied on the wound and covered with a semipermeable dressing. They are changed for every 2 days. However, to use them, one must first obtain the cooperation of both the patient and hospital staff.

In between debridements, topical antibiotics can help reduce the bacterial load, silver sheeting (Acticoat©, Smith & Nephew, Hull, United Kingdom) or silver sulfadiazine works well for all wounds. Mupirocin (Glaxo-Smith-Kline, San Antonio, TX) is useful for MRSA, one-fourth strength acetic acid, gentamycin ointment for pseudomonas infections, bacitracin for minimally infected wounds. It is important to remember that patients can develop an allergy to these ointments and they should be discontinued when these develop. Topical steroids can help treat the allergic skin reaction that may ensue around the ulcer. Alternatively, the vacuum-assisted closure device (VAC©, Kinetics Concept, Inc., San Antonio, Texas) can be applied postdebridement to help reduce the bacterial flora. The negative pressure applied to the wound reduces the bacterial load over a 5-day period *(15)*.

What to Debride

Debriding Skin

Remove nonviable skin as soon as possible. If the border between live and dead tissue is clearly demarcated, excise the skin along that border. If the border is not obvious, start at the center of the wound and remove concentric circles of skin until bleeding tissue is reached. When excising skin, look for bleeding at the normal skin edge. Clotted venules at the skin edge indicate that the local microcirculation has been completely interrupted and that further excision is necessary (Fig. 7). Only when there is normal arterial and venous bleeding at the edge of the wound can one be satisfied that the cutaneous debridement has been adequate.

Debriding Subcutaneous Tissue

Subcutaneous tissue consists of fat, vessels, and nerves. Because of the decreased concentration of blood vessels in the subcutaneous fat, bleeding at the tissue's edge is not always a reliable indicator. Healthy fat has a shiny yellow color and is soft and resilient. Dead fat has a gray pallor to it, which is hard, and is not pliable. Debride fat until soft, yellow, and normal-looking fat appears. After debridement, fat must be kept in a moist environment to prevent desiccation. Again, the presence of clotted veins within the fat represents an interruption in the local blood flow and the fat should be debrided to clean bleeding fat.

To minimize damage to the surrounding tissue, coagulate the small blood vessels using bipolar cautery. Ligate the vessels if they are larger than 2–3 mm using metal Ligaclips which is the least-reactive foreign body material. For vessels larger than 3 mm, a suture ligature should be used. To minimize the risk of infection, only a monofilament suture should be used, preferably nonabsorbable.

Debriding Fascia, Tendon, and Muscle

Healthy fascia has a hard, white, and glistening appearance. When dead, it looks dull, soft, and stringy and is in the process of liquefying. Debride all necrotic fascia until solid, normal-looking bleeding fascia, or healthy underlying fascia appears. The viable fascia must be kept moist during the postdebridement period to avoid desiccation.

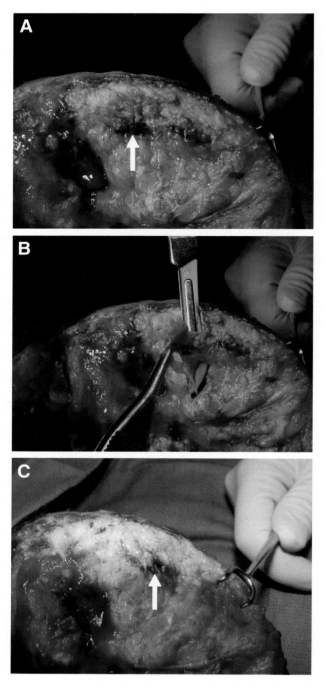

Fig. 7. When excising skin, look for bleeding at the normal skin edge. Clotted venules at the skin edge (**A**) indicate that the local microcirculation has been completely interrupted and that further excision is necessary. Thin slice after thin slice of the tissue containing clotted veins (**B**) should be removed until normal tissue appears (**C**). Note that in the final picture there is still a small localized area of clotted tissue that needs to be removed.

Infected necrotic tendon looks dull, soft, and partially liquefied. To ensure that any hidden necrotic tendon is also removed, make a proximal and distal incision along the path of the exposed tendon (Fig. 8). When the extensor tendons on the dorsum of the foot become exposed, it is hard to preserve them unless they are quickly covered with healthy tissue. If the tendons remain in place as the wound healing progresses, they usually become infected and will impede further healing until they are removed. With the larger achilles or anterior tibial tendon, debride only the portion that is necrotic or infected. Leave the hard, and shiny tendon underneath intact. The remaining tendon must be kept moist and clean, as it will granulate in. The tendon can then be skin grafted. Granulation formulation can be accelerated either with the VAC (first cover the tendon with a Vaseline mesh gauze), with a dermal template, cultured skin substitutes, or with the combined use of topical growth factor and hyperbaric oxygen.

Examine the underlying muscle. Healthy muscle has a bright red, shiny, and resilient appearance, and it contracts when grasped with forceps or touched with cautery. In neuropathic patients, the muscle may have a pale, possibly yellowish, color and may appear nonviable. It will have some tone, however, and will bleed when cut. Frankly dead muscle will be swollen, dull, and grainy when palpated, and it falls apart when pinched. If the muscle's viability is questionable, err on the side of caution and remove only what is not bleeding and appears dead. Subsequently, serially debride the wound until only viable muscle remains.

Debriding Bone

The key to debriding bone is to remove only what is dead and infected and leave hard bleeding bone behind. Be careful not to shatter proximal viable bone. In this regard, power tools are safer to use than rongeurs or chisels. In the larger bones, use a cutting burr to remove thin layer by thin layer of bone until punctate bleeding (paprika sign) appears. Copious irrigation is necessary to ensure that the heat generated by the burr does not damage the healthy bone. The best way to debride the osteomyelitic smaller long bones (phalanx, metacarpals, or metatarsals) is to cut slices of bone serially until normal bleeding bone appears (Fig. 9).

Obtain cultures of the bone remaining after debridement as well as of the debrided osteomyelitic bone. Debridement is finished once the infected bone has been removed and only bleeding, healthy bone remains. If the wound is closed after all infected bone has been removed, just 1 week of appropriate antibiotics is necessary postoperatively *(16)*. Only when there is a question that the bone left behind (e.g., calcaneus or tibia) may still harbor osteomyelitis is a longer course of antibiotics required.

Vacuum-Assisted Closure Device (VAC)

Once the wound is *clean* and *adequately vascularized*, then it can be covered with a VAC dressing. The VAC applies subatmospheric pressure to a wound via a closed suction mechanism *(15,17)*. This speeds up the formation of granulation, sterilizes the wound, and reduces tissue edema. The mechanisms by which this occurs are poorly understood. However, it is felt that the removal of inhibitory wound healing factors, decrease in edema, increased blood flow as well as the alteration of the cellular cytoskeleton plays a role in sterilizing the wound and stimulating the rapid formation of new tissue.

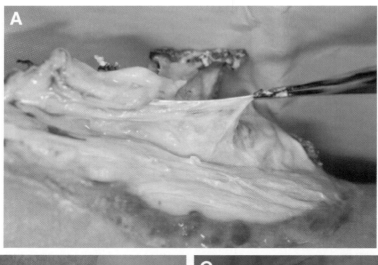

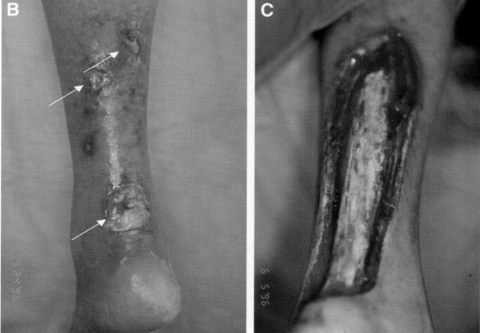

Fig. 8. Infected necrotic tendon looks dull, soft, and partially liquefied (**A**). It should be debrided to clean hard normal-looking tendon. For smaller tendons it usually means loss of that tendon. However, for the necrotic Achilles or anterior tibial tendon, much of the tendon can usually be spared. Note that in picture (**B**), the lesion originated at the distal tendon and spread proximally to the mid calf (**B**). To ensure that all necrotic tendon is removed, it is therefore important to explore proximal and distal to the exposed tendon to make sure all necrotic tendon has been removed (**C**).

The VAC system consists of a polyurethane ether foam sponge with pores sizes ranging from 400 to 600 µm which is placed directly on the wound surface. A non-collapsible evacuation tube with a fenestrated distal end surrounded by an adhesive

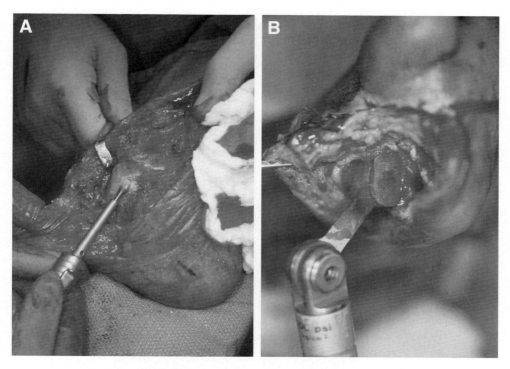

Fig. 9. In the larger bones, use a cutting burr to remove thin layer by thin layer of bone until punctate bleeding (paprika sign) appears **(A,B)**. Copious irrigation is necessary to ensure that the heat generated by the burr does not damage the healthy bone. The best way to debride the osteomyelitic smaller long bones (phalanx, metacarpals, or metatarsals) is to cut slices of bone serially until normal bleeding bone appears **(C,D)**.

dressing is placed on the outer surface of the sponge. The fenestrations at the end of the tube establish communication between the lumen of the tube and the foam sponge. A scissor or scalpel blade is used to tailor the shape of the sponge to the contours of the wound. The wound, with sponge and evacuation tube in place, is then covered with an impermeable adhesive drape that extends 3–5 cm over the adjacent normal skin (Fig. 10). A small hole is made in the impermeable sheet over the sponge. If that site is not on a potential weight-bearing portion of the foot, then the distal end of the suction tubing is placed over the site. If the sponge is over a potential weight-bearing portion of the foot (i.e., heel) a sponge bridge is attached to the site so that the drainage port is now on a nonweight-bearing portion of the foot. The proximal end of the evacuation tube is then connected via a drainage canister to an adjustable vacuum pump (Fig. 11). The pump creates suction that allows subatmospheric pressure to be applied to the entire wound surface. The open-cell nature of the foam enables equal distribution of the applied suction to the entire surface of the wound. The drainage canister collects any fluid that is expressed from the wound. The subatmospheric pressure can be applied in a constant or intermittent mode with pressures up to 125 mmHg. The intermittent mode has been found to stimulate the formation of granulation tissue more rapidly and maintain increased blood flow for longer periods of time.

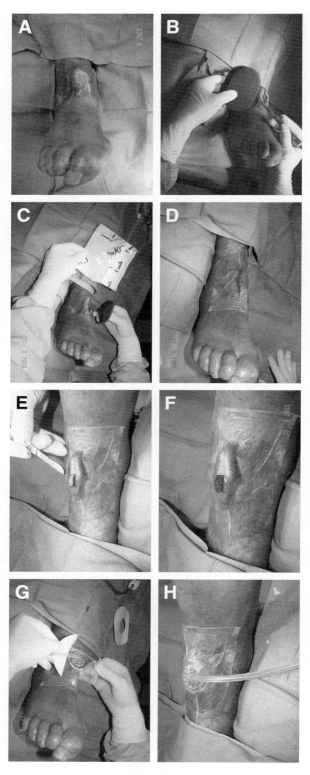

Fig. 10.

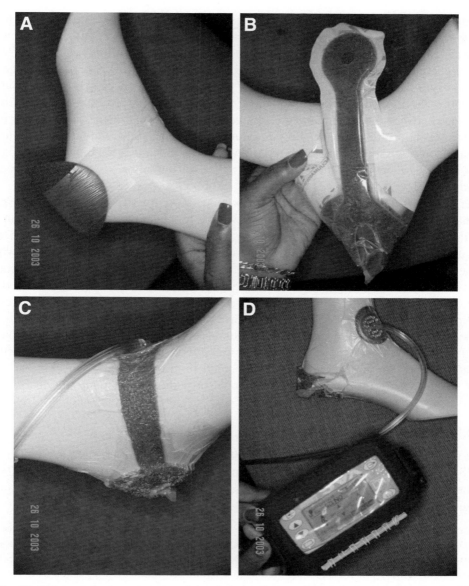

Fig. 11. If the sponge is over a potential weight-bearing portion of the foot such as the heel **(A)** a sponge bridge **(B)** is attached to the site so that the drainage port is now on a nonweight-bearing portion of the foot **(C,D)**. The distal end of the catheter is hooked up to the portable suction device.

Fig. 10. *(See Opposite Page)* **(A–I)** The VAC **(C)** system consists of a polyurethane ether foam sponge with pores sizes ranging from 400 to 600 m which is placed directly on the wound surface **(A)**. A scissor or scalpel blade is used to tailor the shape of the sponge to the contours of the wound **(B)**. The wound, with sponge, is then covered with an impermeable adhesive drape that extends 3–5 cm over the adjacent normal skin **(C,D)**. A small hole is made in the impermeable sheet over the sponge **(F,G)**. The distal end of the evacuation tube is placed over the fenestration **(H,I)**. The proximal end of the suction tubing is then connected via a drainage canister to an adjustable vacuum pump. The pump creates subatmospheric pressure that is then applied to the entire wound surface.

If the VAC is being placed over sensitive structures such as a neurovascular bundle or a tendon, then one should place vaseline mesh (Adaptec©, Johnson & Johnson Gateway, LLC, Piscataway, NJ) or silicone mesh (Mepitel©, Mölnlycke Health Care, Göteborg, Sweden) between the wound and sponge to minimize potential damage to the underlying structure. With long-term VAC use, the wound can develop an odor. This can be addressed in one of two ways: one can either interpose a layer of silver (Acticoat) between the wound and the sponge or one can stop the VAC for a day or two and use an acetic acid and gauze dressing during that time. If the wound is ischemic or still has necrotic tissue in it, the use of the VAC is counter-indicated. In the former case, it can cause further necrosis of the wound edges. In the latter case, an infection can develop.

The VAC has changed the way chronic wounds are currently being treated *(18)*. It stimulates conversion of a debrided chronic wound to a healing acute wound. It can be used in almost any kind of wound, providing the wound is clean and well vascularized. The quality of the granulation tissue is more vascular than that normally produced without the VAC *(19)*. Small wounds can heal by secondary intention more rapidly with the VAC. If more involved reconstruction is planned, the surgeon is no longer rushed to cover the wound *(20)* with a microsurgical free flap and can electively plan the reconstruction. In addition, the reconstructive plans are usually simplified because the VAC shrinks the size of the wound so that most wounds can be closed with a combination of local flaps and skin grafts. The VAC has limited effectiveness if the surgeon expects it to heal a wound over an exposed fracture or joint. In those cases, the safer option is to cover the exposed joint or fracture with a local or pedicled flap while the rest of the wound is skin grafted.

WHEN IS THE WOUND READY TO CLOSE?

The wound is ready to close when all the abnormal parameters surrounding the wound have been corrected and when all signs of inflammation have disappeared (Fig. 12). It can then be allowed to heal by secondary intention, closed by delayed primary closure, skin grafted or covered with a flap.

1. Erythema: the wound itself should have no surrounding erythema. Cellulitis should not be confused with dependent rubor owing to ischemia or recent local surgery. If there is surrounding erythema that goes away immediately with elevation, then the wound has dependent rubor. Otherwise, if it persists, then inflammation still exists. If the wound initially had massive cellulitis, there usually is a sloughing of the superficial epithelium in which the cellulitis had previously been.
2. Induration: the wound edges should have minimal if any induration. Wrinkled skin lines at the wound's edge are one of the most reliable signs that inflammation has largely resolved. Induration may be absent in patients who lack normal immunological response (i.e., renal failure, steroid dependence).
3. Pain: pain should have subsided in a wound with resolving inflammation. Decreasing pain, however, is a less reliable indicator than resolving erythema or induration.
4. Fresh granulation within the wound: this shows that there is sufficient blood supply and a hospitable environment for the wound to go through the final stages of wound healing.
5. Neoepithelialization at wounds edge: the presence of new epithelium at the wounds edge reflects a healthy wound that is on its way to healing by secondary intention.

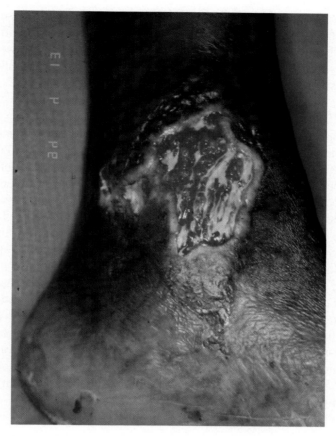

Fig. 12. The wound is ready to close when all signs of inflammation have disappeared: erythema, induration, and swelling. There should be wrinkled skin lines at the edge of the wound and neoepithelialization occurring at the border of the wound. The wound can then be allowed to heal by secondary intention, closed by delayed primary closure, skin grafted, or covered with a flap.

6. Wound surface sterility: if quantitative counts are available, then a count of less than 10^5 bacteria per gram of tissue signifies that the wound is ready to successfully be skin grafted *(21)*. Alternatively, if an allograft or xenograft placed on the wound takes, then the wound bed is sterile enough for a skin graft to take.

CLOSURE TECHNIQUES

Closure techniques include allowing the wound to heal by secondary intention or by closing it with: (1) delayed primary closure, (2) skin graft, (3) local flap, (4) pedicled flap, and (5) free flap. If surgical closure is chosen, there should be two setups of instruments in the operating room. The first set of instruments is used to debride the wound. Culturing those instruments postdebridement yield a quantitative culture of up to 10^3 bacteria. Reusing those same instruments during the closure would needlessly recontaminate the freshly debrided wound and increase the risk for postoperative infection. The debrided wound should be cleansed using pulsed lavage and then redraped. If a VersaJet is used to debride the wound, then one can dispense with two sets of instruments and the pulsed lavage. In either case, the wound should be redraped, surgeon should change gloves and a new set of uncontaminated instruments should be used. These steps ensure that the wound is as clean as possible before closure thereby decreasing the risk of subsequent infection and tissue necrosis.

Promoting Healing by Secondary Intention

A healthy granulating wound normally decreases in surface area by at least 10–15% per week *(22)*. The biomechanical abnormality that caused the wound should be addressed. If the wound is on the plantar forefoot and the etiology is an equino-varus deformity from a tight Achilles tendon and/or a hammer toe, the tendon should be lengthened, and/or the hammer toe corrected. The plantar foot should then be unweighted. If the wound is located near a joint surface (i.e., ankle), the involved joint should be immobilized by a splint or external fixator to prevent shear forces from disrupting the ongoing repair. A moist dressing on the wound allows for more rapid epithelialization of the wound *(23)*. If the wound fails to respond to the above conservative measures, healing adjuncts should be implemented.

When dealing with wound healing adjuncts, it is important to keep their cost in mind. Xenograft costs approx \$50 per role of 400 cm^2, growth factor \$400–\$500/15 g, and cultured skin derivatives \$1000/40 cm^2 of tissue. Application of the VAC is approx \$125 per day, whereas hyperbaric oxygen costs in excess of \$500 per day. In order to accurately estimate the total cost of a given option, one also has to factor in the cost of visiting nurses, hospital stay and operative costs. Whenever clinically applicable, one should first start with the least expensive and move up the ladder when a given treatment fails to bring about the desired results.

Adjuncts to Help the Wound Heal

Several adjuncts can help a wound heal by secondary intention if it fails to respond to conservative therapy:

1. Platelet-derived growth factor: This gel has been shown effective in diabetic wounds when they are well vascularized, clean, and regularly debrided *(24)*. Removing the proteinaceous coagulum from the wound surface before applying the growth factor is important because the coagulum contains metalloproteases that will digest the applied growth factor before the latter can affect the wound. Patients are given scrub brushes or soft toothbrushes and are instructed to scrub the wound surface every time before applying the growth factor. Alternatively, if pain is an issue in treating the wound surface aggressively, a topical debriding agent can be used in between each application of the growth factor. The use of a protease modulating matrix (Promogran©, Johnson & Johnson Gateway, LLC, Piscataway, NJ) *(25,26)* on top of the applied growth factor is thought to increase the effectiveness of the growth factor by neutralizing wound healing inhibitors such as metalloproteinase and elastase *(27)*.
2. Temporary coverage: Xenograft (pigskin) *(28)* or allograft (cadaver skin) *(29)* provides an excellent temporary dressing over clean healthy wounds. They are an excellent, inexpensive temporary dressing that provides a collagen-based scaffolding for new tissue to grow into. If the temporary graft initially "takes," it turns pink indicating that the underlying bed is sterile and well enough vascularized for a split-thickness skin graft to successfully take. In healthy patients, rejection starts at approx 7–9 days. In the immune compromised patient, it can take up to 1 month before the temporary skin graft is rejected.

3. Cultured skin substitutes: Although these are not skin graft substitutes *per se*, they are bioengineered skin equivalents that provide a moist living surface producing an entire array of local growth factors to the underlying wound bed. They are made by allowing live human fibroblasts to migrate into and populate the collagen scaffolding. This scaffolding can then be covered with a layer of epidermis grown separately. These products come in two commercial forms: combined dermal-epidermal graft (Apligraf©, Organogenesis Inc. Canton, MA) or a dermal graft (Dermagraft©, Smith & Nephew, Hull, United Kingdom). They have been shown to be effective in healing both venous stasis ulcers *(30,31)* and diabetic ulcers *(32,33)*. A classification system based on the graft's appearance after it has been applied has to be designed to help the clinician judge its potential effectiveness *(34)*. However, if the biomechanical problem that led to the initial ulceration are not also addressed, the graft will not be very effective in healing the wound.

For the cultured skin substitute to be effective, the wound base should be well vascularized and free of necrotic or infected tissue. The skin substitute should be applied and treated like a skin graft (*see* pp. 415–417). Meshing Apligraf before application is thought to stimulate the production of growth factors. To ensure optimal results, there should be minimal motion present at the wound site. A compressive four ply dressing or Jones dressing is effective in doing this. An alternative is applying a VAC to help better fixate the graft, keep the wound bed sterile, and further stimulate the formation of granulation tissue *(35)*. If there is a yellowish necrotic appearance to the wound base, the cultured skin is probably no longer effective and should be replaced after the base has been debrided *(34)*. Otherwise, the skin substitute can be reapplied every 6 weeks if necessary.

4. Hyperbaric oxygen: Hyperbaric oxygen supplies the body with oxygen at two to three times normal atmospheric pressures. Hyperbaric oxygen saturates existing hemoglobin and dissolves sufficient free oxygen in the blood plasma to increase the concentration of oxygen at the wounds edge. The increase of oxygen at the wound's edge significantly increases the oxygen gradient between the edge and the hypoxic center of the wound bed. The higher the gradient, the stronger the body's wound healing response *(36,37)* and more rapid the promotion of angiogenesis, collagen synthesis, and neoepithelialization. In addition, hyperbaric oxygen potentiates the white blood cells ability to destroy bacteria *(38)*.

Hyperbaric oxygen is most effective if there is adequate vascular inflow. Before undergoing hyperbaric oxygen treatment, candidates should undergo an oxygen challenge test to see whether there is a rise in the local tissue oxygen pressure after exposing the lungs to increased oxygen content. Breathing in 100% oxygen should lead to at least a 10 mmHg. rise in tissue oxygen levels around the wound site. Diving in a chamber at two atmospheres should increase the tissue oxygen level to above 300 mmHg. Otherwise, the hyperbaric oxygen treatments unlikely to be effective.

One should monitor the wound closely for changes to make sure that the treatment is positively affecting the wound. Combining platelet-derived growth factor with hyperbaric oxygen treatments is more effective together than either treatment alone (Fig. 13) *(39)*. Therefore, if the clinical decision is to begin hyperbaric oxygen therapy to stimulate wound healing, growth factor should probably be applied to the wound at the same time to maximize the benefits of hyperbaric oxygen. Hyperbaric oxygen has been shown to increase limb salvage in patients with diabetes in a double-blind randomized study *(40)*.

Closing a Wound by Delayed Primary Closure

The wound edges have to be freshly debrided and the wound should be closed without tension. Wounds can be safely closed by approximating to the point of blanching at the suture track and then waiting until the edges turn pink again. If this does not occur, the

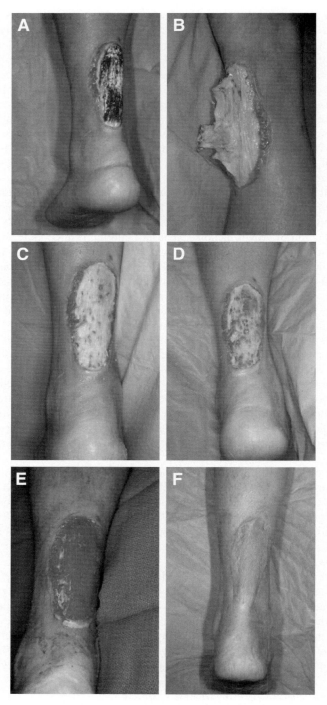

Fig. 13. This elderly patient with diabetes presented with gangrene of the Achilles tendon (**A**). The wound was debrided by removing the loose filmy and necrotic portions of the tendon (**B**). The wound was then treated with the combination of hyperbaric oxygen and topical growth factor. Granulation appeared at week 1 (**C**), increased at week 2 (**D**), and covered the entire week by week 3 (**E**). The wound was then skin grafted and the patient survived an additional 2 years without problems.

sutures have to be relaxed. Because the leg, ankle, and foot consist of a circumferential soft tissue envelope around a boney pillar, it is easy to apply excessive circumferential pressure when a wound is closed too tightly. It is therefore important to check distal arterial pulses pre- and postclosure to avoid compromising distal blood flow. Because one is dealing with a previously infected wound, deep sutures should be avoided and the wound should be closed with as few monofilament (least reactive) sutures as possible. This minimizes the amount of foreign material within the wound that can potentiate subsequent infection *(41)*. Closing with vertical mattress sutures creates good tissue eversion along the wound's edge without requiring deeper sutures. Interrupted suture closure gives the surgeon more option when addressing a seroma or hematoma. Removal of one or two of the overlying sutures rather than opening the entire closure is usually sufficient to adequately drain the underlying seroma or hematoma (Fig. 14).

Often the skin edges are too far apart to close primarily (i.e., postfasciotomy and postfracture). Gradual reapproximation of the skin edges is possible by serial operations every 2–3 days in which the skin edges are approximated up to the point of blanching with horizontal mattress sutures. A VAC can be placed over the remaining soft tissue gap to help decrease the edema and make the surrounding tissue more mobile. Alternatively, skin staples can be placed at the wound edges and a vessel loop is threaded through them much like tying up shoe laces *(42)*. The band is tightened daily until the edges touch and then the wound can be allowed to heal by secondary intention or formally closed using vertical mattress sutures. Alternatively, spring loaded approximating devices (Proxiderm©, Progressive Surgical Products, Westbury, NY) can be applied to both wound edges *(43)*. Proxiderm is the soft tissue equivalent of the Ilizarov although a significant amount of ingenuity is required when applying the postoperative dressing to prevent the devices from being displaced. If done carefully, the skin will sufficiently relax over time so that the wound edges can then be primarily closed.

One should remember that any wound need not be closed provided that the critical structures such as the neurovascular bundle, bone, tendon or joint are covered. The remaining wound gap can heal by secondary intention. This can be accelerated with the use of the VAC. Alternatively, the granulating bed can later be skin grafted.

Skin Graft

This is the simplest of all coverage techniques with the only prerequisite is wound with a bed of healthy granulation tissue. The superficial layer of granulation tissue is removed to ensure that there is minimal bacterial contamination within the interstices of the granulation buds. The use of the VersaJet in this setting is ideal because one can precisely adjust the depth of debridement and rapidly establish a smooth and level recipient bed. The wound is then redraped and clean instruments are used.

Preferable donor sites include the *ipsi*-lateral thigh, leg, or instep. The size of the defect is measured to determine the amount of skin graft needed. The area needed is then drawn on the donor site. The appropriate width skin graft guide (1, 2, 3, or 4 inches) should be used to harvest the appropriate size skin graft. The thickness of the harvest is set at 15 per 1000 inches which is an effective compromise between adequate take rate and skin graft contraction *(44)*. If the skin at the donor site is flabby or hard to stabilize, the area should be tumesced by injecting sufficient normal saline into the donor site until the entire site is firm. This then provides a stable platform from which to successfully

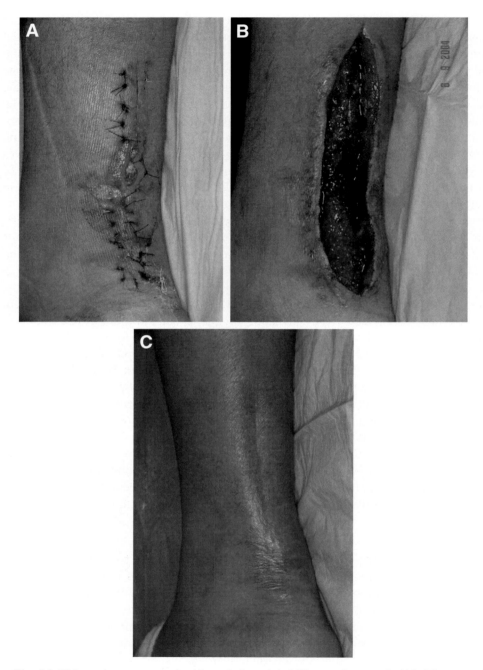

Fig. 14. This patient presented with an infected Achilles tendon repair (**A**). The wound was opened, the tendon debrided and the infected Ethibond suture removed. A VAC was placed on the wound until the cultures were back and the tissue edges are soft (**B**). The wound was then debrided and closed in the operating room. It healed without complications (**C**).

harvest the skin graft. The skin graft harvester is turned on and then brought down to the donor site with uniform pressure being applied on the head of the harvester. When the designated graft has been harvested, the machine is lifted off the donor site. The

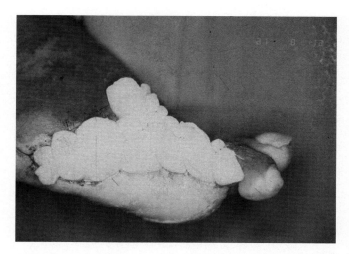

Fig. 15. To prevent shearing forces from disrupting the graft, a bolster can be tied over the graft. Bolster stitches are placed around the graft by going through the edge of the skin graft and wound bed, tying the suture, and leaving one end long enough to then tie over the bolster. Vaseline gauze is then placed on the graft and wet unwrung cotton balls are placed on top of the gauze. The long ties are then tightly tied over the cotton balls which wrings out excess fluid as the cotton balls conform to the underlying recipient bed. The result is application of uniform pressure over the entire skin graft. The bolster dressing is removed 7–10 days later.

harvested skin graft can then be meshed (1/1) to allow for a natural egress of the inevitable build up of underlying fluid or blood. Alternatively the graft can be pierced with a no. 11 blade several times to allow for egress of excess fluid. Seroma or hematoma underneath a skin graft is the most frequent cause of skin graft failure.

The skin graft is then placed on the donor site. If meshed, spreading of the mesh is avoided to ensure a more rapid complete take. Otherwise, the raw areas between the meshed skin have to then epithelialize, which increases both scarring and the time to full healing. Spraying the donor site with topical thrombin just before placing the skin graft helps control bleeding at the recipient site *(45)*. Some centers are using fibrin glue instead because it also fixes the graft to the underlying bed. Otherwise, the graft can be secured to the recipient site using skin clips or absorbable monofilament suture. To prevent shearing forces from disrupting the graft, a bolster can be tied over the graft. For a bolster dressing, bolster monofilament ties are placed through the edge of the graft and wound. The suture is tied and one end is left long so that it can then serve as the bolster tie. Vaseline gauze is then placed on the graft and wet unwrung cotton balls are placed on top of the gauze. The bolster stitches are then tightly tied over the cotton balls which wrings out excess fluid as the cotton balls are forced to conform to the underlying recipient bed. The result is application of uniform pressure over the entire skin graft. The bolster dressing is removed 7–10 days later (Fig. 15).

The VAC is an alternative method of covering fresh skin grafts and provides successful skin graft take rates of as high as 95% *(17,46)*. The VAC facilitates maximal contact between the skin graft and the bed, helps stabilizes the skin graft on the bed to counteract shear forces, and removes any excess fluid that could disrupt the contact between the graft and the underlying bed (Fig. 16). It has been shown to be more effective that bolster

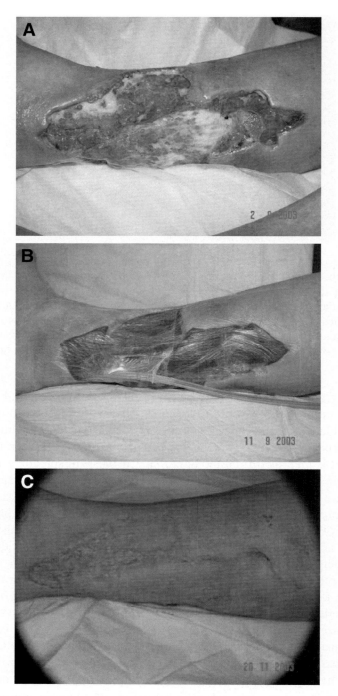

Fig. 16. The VAC facilitates maximal contact between the skin graft and the bed (**A**), helps stabilizes the skin graft on the bed to counteract shear forces while removing any excess fluid. The fresh skin graft is first covered with a nonadherent dressing (silicone or vaseline mesh). A sheet of silver ions can then interposed between the mesh and VAC sponge to ensure better bacterial control. The VAC sponge is then placed on top (**B**) and continuous pressure is applied for 3–5 days postoperatively. The graft is then allowed to fully heal with a simple semiocclusive dressing such as vaseline gauze (**C**).

dressing in ensuring high initial skin graft takes *(47)*. The fresh skin graft is first covered with a nonadherent dressing (silicone or vaseline mesh). A sheet of silver ions can then interposed between the mesh and VAC sponge to ensure better bacterial control. The VAC sponge is then placed on top and continuous pressure is applied for 3–5 days postoperatively.

When considering skin grafting over bone, tendon or joint, creating a neodermis improves the chances of skin graft flexibility and durability. Integra® artificial dermis (Integra LifeSciences Holding Company, Plainsboro, NJ) is composed of an overlying removable silicone film (to prevent desiccation) with an underlying dermal matrix of cross-linked bovine collagen and chondroitin sulfate *(48,49)*. The dermal layer functions as a dermal template to facilitate the migration of the patient's own fibroblasts, macrophages, lymphocytes, and endothelial cells as well as new vessels. The sheet of Integra is meshed, cut to fit the wound and affixed to the site with staples or suture. Over the ensuing week(s), a new cell populated dermis is formed. The revascularization process is accelerated three- to fourfold by placing a VAC over Integra *(50)*. Then, the silicone layer can be removed so that a thin skin autologous skin graft (8/1000 inches to 10/1000 inches) can be placed on it (Fig. 17).

For lower leg wounds, an Unna boot dressing over a skin graft allows the patient to ambulate immediately postoperatively. If the graft is in an area in which joint motion could disrupt the graft off of its bed (i.e., ankle or distal forefoot) then immobilization with a posterior splint, cast or external fixator and nonweight bearing for two or more week is critical for the graft to take successfully. For heel wounds, the Ilizarov frame is very useful because it not only immobilizes the ankle but it also suspends the foot in mid air so that the patient cannot disrupt the graft (Fig. 18). If the graft is on the plantar aspect of the foot, there should be no weight bearing until the skin graft has matured (usually 6 weeks). For wounds on the weight-bearing portions of the foot (heel, lateral midfoot, under the metatarsal heads), plantar glabrous skin grafts are the ideal source of autographs because they permit the regeneration of the normal glabrous plantar surface *(51)*. These should be harvested from the nonweight-bearing portion of the plantar foot, the instep. The instep is infiltrated with normal saline to create a smooth but firm harvesting surface. The graft is harvested at a thickness of 30/1000 inches. The instep should be covered with a thin autograft (8 to 10/1000 inches) from the thigh so the donor site can heal without problem. The glabrous skin graft is then inset over the recipient site and sewn in with a 5–0 monofilament suture. Because of its thickness, the graft takes longer to heal and weight bearing should not be allowed until the graft has completely healed. The graft may take up to 6–8 weeks to heal but should hold up better than a normal skin graft to the normal wear and tear that occurs with ambulation.

Local Flaps

Local flaps are flaps with unidentified blood supply adjacent to a given defect that are either rotated on a pivot point or advanced forward to cover the defect. They come in various shapes (square, rectangular, rhomboid, semicircular, or bilobed) *(52)*. They usually consist of skin and the underlying fat or skin, fat, and the underlying fascia. They, however, can also include the muscle. It is important to carefully preplan the flap by first accurately determining the size of the defect after debridement. The flap should be designed in the area in which the tissue is the most mobile. Using a template when

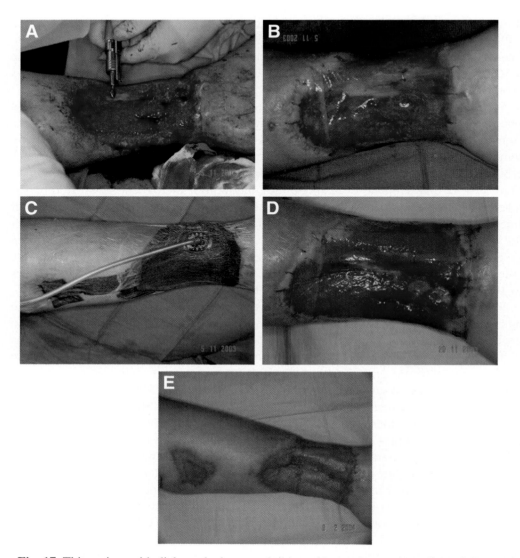

Fig. 17. This patient with diabetes had exposed tibia and large almost circumferential wound just above the ankle **(A)**. The sheet of Integra is meshed, cut to fit the wound and affixed to the site with staples or suture **(B)**. A VAC is placed over the Integra to speed up the vascularization of the dermal template **(C)**. Once that has occurred **(D)**, the silicone layer can be removed so that a thin skin autologous skin graft (8/1000 inches to 10/1000 inches) can be placed on it. The skin graft is covered with silicone mesh and a VAC for 3–5 days and then a normal dressing is place on the graft as it continues to heal **(E)**.

designing the flap and holding its base at the pivot point as it is being swung into the defect is the best way of estimating the adequateness of the design.

The ratio of length to width is critical for the survival of the tip of the flap *(53)*. Because the blood flow to the skin in the foot and ankle is not as developed as in the face, the length to width ratio should not exceed a 1:1 or 1:1.5 ratio. The viability of such a flap is increased when one can Doppler out a cutaneous perforator at the base of

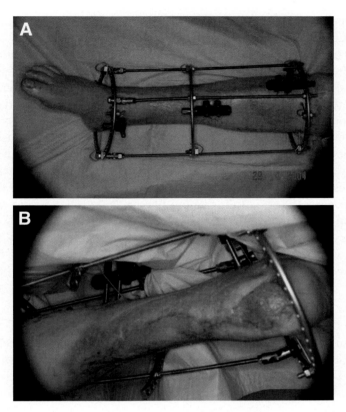

Fig. 18. For heel ulcers, the Ilizarov frame is very useful because it suspends the foot in mid air so that the patient cannot disrupt the graft during the healing process. The Ilizarov can also stabilize the ankle in neutral position to avoid the development of equino-varus deformity.

the planned flap. To ensure adequate tension free coverage, a slightly larger pattern should be used than what would anatomically be necessary. When moving the flap to cover the defect, it is important that the flap fill the defect without tension to avoid compromising the blood flow to its distal end. A force *(54)* of 25 mmHg. causes enough venous congestion for flap necrosis unless the tension is released within 4 hours. Seeing the distal flap pale as it is being sewn in is cause for concern. If a 4-0 or larger nylon stitch breaks as the flap is being sewn in, that also is cause for concern. If the flap cannot remain pink when inset, it should be rotated back into its bed and delayed for 4–7 days while it develops more robust blood supply. During that time, the VAC can be placed on the open wound to ensure that no edema develops.

Atraumatic technique *(14)* is a necessary prerequisite when dissecting the flap (bipolar cautery, sharp dissection rather than cautery dissection, grasping flap with skin hooks rather than pickups, and so on) and when insetting the flap (half buried horizontal mattress or simple vertical mattress stitch with nonreactive suture). This minimizes the risk of damaging the tissue edges that can become ischemic and/or become a site of entry for infection. In order to help takeoff tension of the distal end of the flap, the stitches are biased to bring the flap toward the distal edge of the defect. This minimizes tension at the most vulnerable distal of the flap: its distal end.

Local flaps are very useful in coverage of foot and ankle wounds because they only need to be of sufficient size to cover the exposed tendon, bone, or joint. The rest of the wound can then be covered with a simple skin graft. This combination of limited local flap and skin graft frequently obviates the need of larger pedicled or free flaps. If correctly designed, a local flap can also improve the surgical exposure of the underlying tissue if corrective surgery has to be performed *(55)*. The harvesting of an appropriately designed flap often improves the exposure of joints, bone or tendons sufficiently to avoid making an extra incision. In addition, local flaps are a very useful mode of reconstruction when trying to close a wound through an Ilizarov type fixator. This is because the frame often makes it impossible to perform the extensive dissection required for pedicled flaps or to provide the necessary space to perform the microsurgical anastomosis for free flaps.

In order to increase the size of the random flap beyond the 1:1.5 ratio without risking necrosis, the flap should to be delayed for 4–10 days *(56)*. The simplest way to this is to incise both sides of the flap and undermine it. The incisions are then closed. This interrupts vertical blood flow from the underlying muscle or artery to the center of the flap and forces the blood to flow from the base of the flap toward the tip and vice versa. When the flap has been sufficiently delayed, the tip is incised and the flap is elevated and rotated into position.

Flaps That Rotate Around a Pivot Point

These random flaps rotate around a single pivot point and therefore need to be planned carefully to avoid excessive tension along the radius of the arc of rotation. The rotation flap is designed when a pie-shaped triangular defect is created to remove a lesion or preexistent defect. The base of the triangle lies along the hypothetical circumference of a semicircular flap that can then be rotated into the defect. The most useful application of this type flap is on the plantar aspect of the foot in which the flap is elevated off the plantar fascia and rotated in position. It can also be used over the plantar forefoot (Fig. 19), at both malleoli and on the dorsum of the foot *(57,58)*. If vascular anatomical considerations dictate, the flap can also include underlying fascia and or muscle.

Transposition flaps are rectangular flaps that can be rotated up to 90°. The end of the flap has to be longer than the distance between the pivot point and the edge of the defect so that when the flap is rotated, it can fit in without tension. Preplanning the rotation with gauze or paper is the key to avoiding excessive tension on the distal end of the flap at inset. The donor site can usually be closed primarily. Otherwise, it may require skin grafting. The dog ear that results from rotating the flap should not be addressed at the initial surgery. The dog ear will usually flatten down. However, if it is still a problem once the flap has healed, the dog ear can be safely removed. This is the most frequently used flap to cover the malleoli or exposed tibial-talar fusion around an Ilizarov frame (Fig. 20).

Advancement Flaps

Advancement flaps are moved directly forward to fill a defect without rotation or lateral movement. A rectangle of skin is dissected out and should include, at a minimum, skin and subcutaneous tissue. The flap is advanced into the defect. This may create a folding of the tissue at both ends of its base (burrow's triangles) which can be removed so that the skin can be sutured together without causing any irregularities in the contour. It is also important that the tension on the flap is adjusted so that there is no blanched area when it is in its new position.

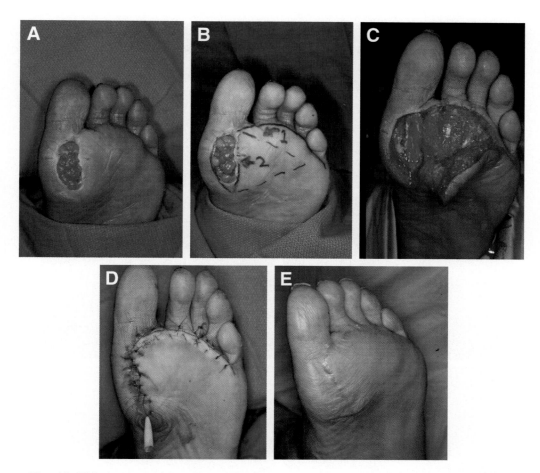

Fig. 19. This is a morbidly obese diabetic patient with an ulcer under the first MTP **(A)**. Potential flaps for closure included a rotation flap and a V to Y advancement flap **(B)**. The wound was debrided and a rotation flap was chosen as the mode of reconstruction. The flap was elevated with great care to preserve the neurovascular bundles to the toes **(C)**. The flap is sewn into position with biased stitches to prevent tension on the distal end of the flap **(D)**. The flap went on to heal despite poor compliance in keeping weight off the foot during the healing phase **(E)**.

A V–Y flap is a "V" shaped flap that, when advanced, forms a "Y" (Fig. 21). The V–Y flap depends on direct underlying perforators to stay alive. For that reason, no undermining whatsoever can be done when dissecting out this flap. It is important to realize that the maximum advancement is limited to 1–2 cm. Therefore, if the defect is larger, double opposing V–Y flaps can be used to close defects of up to 3–4 cm wide. The flap is especially useful for defects on the sole of the foot *(59)*. On the plantar foot, the incisions are carried *through* the plantar fascia without undermining to allow for *maximum* mobility and viability of the flap. The flap should be designed as large as possible to ensure the inclusion of as many perforators as possible.

Pedicled Flaps

Pedicled flaps have identifiable blood vessels feeding the flap. They can contain various tissue combinations including cutaneous, fasciocutaneous, muscle, musculocuta-

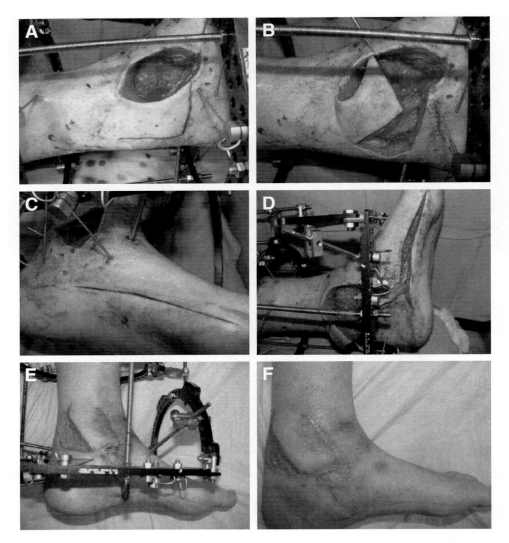

Fig. 20. This patient with diabetes developed an infected Charcot ankle joint. The infected joint was resected and the remaining foot and ankle were stabilized using an Ilizarov frame (**A**). The defect was debrided and the upper half of the exposed joint was covered with a local flap (**B**) while the distal portion of the defect was covered with an abductor hallucis muscle flap (**C,D**). The wound went on to heal without incident (**E,F**).

neous, osteocutaneous, osteo-musculocutaneous type flaps, and so on. These flaps work well if they were not involved in the initial trauma, infection, or radiation field. Otherwise, the flaps are stiff, difficult to dissect out and difficult to transfer. In addition, the flap has to be soft and pliable because the vascular pedicle is usually intolerant of any twisting or turning that occurs when the flap is swung into its new position.

These flaps are often more difficult to dissect and have a higher complication rate than performing a free flap that can run as high as 30–40% *(60)*. Harvesting a pedicled flap often places a donor site deficit on the foot and ankle that has to be skin grafted. However, pedicled flaps allow the surgeon to perform a rapid operation with a short hospital stay that yields excellent long lasting results. The anatomy and techniques of dissection are discussed in flap

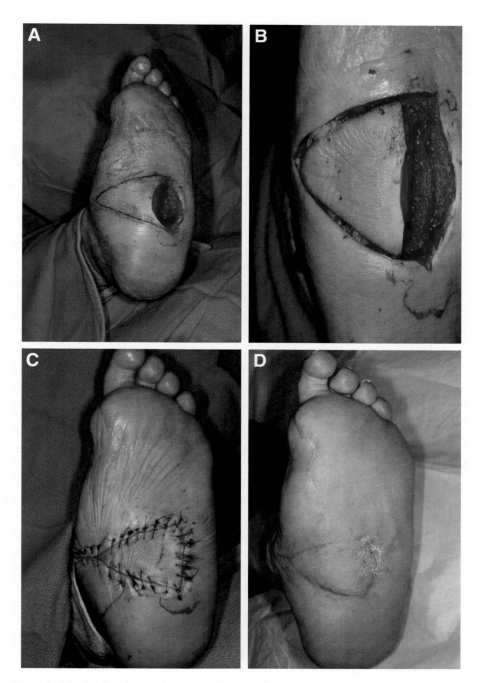

Fig. 21. A V–Y flap is a "V" shaped flap (**A,B**) that, when advanced, forms a "Y" (**C**). The V–Y flap depends on direct underlying perforators to stay alive. For that reason, no undermining whatsoever can be done when dissecting out this flap. On the plantar aspect of the foot, the maximum advancement is limited to 1–2 cm.

anatomy books *(61,62)*. It is important to practice these flap on cadaver legs as the dissections are often tedious and can be difficult. The distal reach of the flap often provides insufficient tissue so that it is very important to understand the size limitations of each flap.

Lower Leg and Ankle Flaps: Muscle

The lower leg muscles are poor candidates for pedicled flaps because most of them have segmental minor pedicles as their blood supply and therefore only a small portion of the muscle can safely be transferred. The distal portion of some of these muscles can be used to cover small defects around the ankle medially, anteriorly, laterally *(63)*. For small and proximal defect, the muscle flap can usually be separated from its distal tendon to minimize the loss of function.

The extensor hallucis longus (EHL) m. (anterior tibial artery) can cover small defects that are as distal as 2 cm above the medial malleolus. The extensor digitorum longus (EDL) m. and peroneus tertius m. (anterior tibial artery) are used for small defects as distal as 2.1 cm above the medial malleolus. The peroneus brevis m. (peroneal artery) can be used for small defects as distal as 4 cm above the medial malleolus. The flexor digitorum longus m. (posterior tibial artery) can be used for small defects as distal as 6 cm above the medial malleolus. The soleus muscle (popliteal, peroneal and posterior tibial artery) is the only type 2 muscle in the distal lower leg in which the minor distal pedicles can be safely detached and the muscle with its intact proximal major pedicles can be rotated to cover large (10 × 8 cm) anterior lower leg defects as distal as 6.6 cm above the medial malleolus. It can be harvested as a hemisoleus for small defects *(64)* and as an entire soleus for larger defects. All the just described muscles usually have to be skin grafted for complete coverage. In addition the ankle has to be immobilized to avoid dehiscence and ensure adequate skin graft take. The use of external frames can be very useful with the former and the use of the vacuum-assisted closure device for the latter.

If a larger flap or wider angle of rotation is needed, one of the three major lower leg arteries with the relevant minor perforators has to be taken with the muscle flap. The sacrifice of a major artery should only be considered if all three arteries are open and there is excellent retrograde flow. These flaps are usually harvested distally and therefore the accompanying artery depends on retrograde flow. Because these flaps are larger, the tendon is also taken with the muscle. It is therefore important to tenodese the distal portion of the severed tendon to the tendon of a similar muscle so that the function is not lost. For example, if the distal EHL muscle is harvested, the EHL tendon distal to the harvest should be tenodesed to the EDL so that the hallux maintains its position during gait (Fig. 22). Because the loss of the anterior tibial tendon is so debilitating, the distal muscle should not be harvested unless the ankle has been or is being fused.

Lower Leg and Ankle Flaps: Fasciocutanous Flaps

Fasciocutaneous flaps are useful for reconstruction around the foot and ankle although the donor site usually has to be skin grafted *(65)*. The retrograde peroneal flap (retrograde peroneal artery) *(66)* is useful for ankle, heel, and proximal dorsal foot defects. Its blood flow is retrograde and depends on an intact distal peroneal arterial–arterial anastomosis with either or both the anterior tibial artery and/or posterior tibial artery. The dissection is tedious and it does sacrifice one of the three major arteries of the leg. A similar retrograde anterior tibial artery flap *(67)* fasciocutaneous flap (retrograde anterior tibial artery) has been described for coverage in young patients with traumatic wounds over the same areas. Because the anterior compartment is the only compartment of the leg whose muscle depends solely on the anterior tibial artery, only

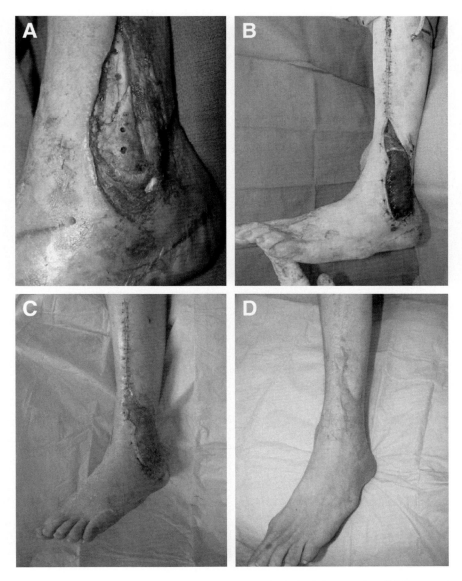

Fig. 22. The EHL muscle is harvested with the distal third of the anterior tibial artery to cover the lateral distal exposed fibula **(A,B)**. The muscle is skin grafted **(C)**. The EHL tendon distal to the harvest is tenodesed to the EDL so that the hallux maintains its position during gait **(D)**.

the lower half of the artery can be safely harvested as a vascular leash. The retrograde sural nerve flap *(68)* (retrograde sural artery) is a versatile neurofasciocutaneous flap that is useful for ankle and heel defects (Fig. 23). The sural artery travels with the sural nerve and receives retrograde flow from a peroneal perforator 5 cm above the lateral malleolus. The artery first courses above the fascia and then goes deep to the fascia at mid calf although the accompanying lesser saphenous vein remains above the fascia. The venous congestion often seen with this flap can be minimized if the pedicle is harvested with 3 cm of tissue on either side of the pedicle and with the overlying skin

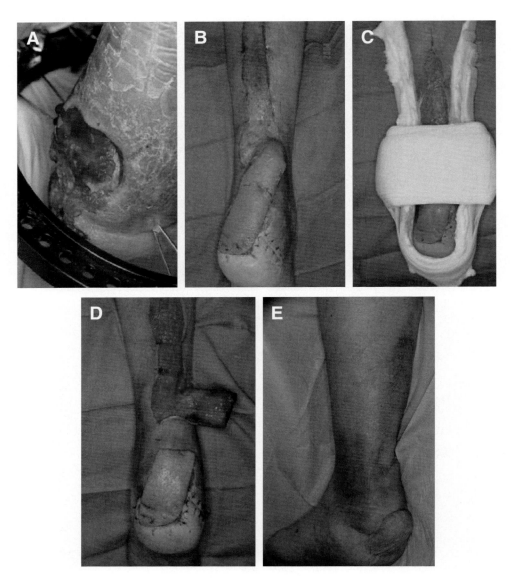

Fig. 23. The retrograde sural nerve flap is a versatile neurofasciocutaneous flap that is useful for ankle and heel defects. The patient has a heel ulcer with osteomyelitis of the calcaneus **(A)**. A sural artery flap is dissected out and inset over the defect **(B)**. A cast is designed to off weight the heel **(C)**. Alternatively an Ilizarov can be applied to off weight the heel during healing. After 2 weeks, the pedicle is cut and the defect is skin grafted **(D)**. The flap goes on to heal **(D)**.

intact *(69)*. Problems with the venous congestion can be avoided if the flap is delayed 4–10 days earlier by tying off the proximal lesser saphenous vein and sural artery. The inset of the flap is critical to avoid kinking of the pedicle. Ingenious splinting often has to be designed to keep pressure off of the pedicle while the flap heals (the use of the Ilizarov external frame can be very useful in this regard). The major donor deficit of the flap is the loss of sensibility along the lateral aspect of the foot and a skin grafted depression at the posterior calf donor site that may pose a problem if the

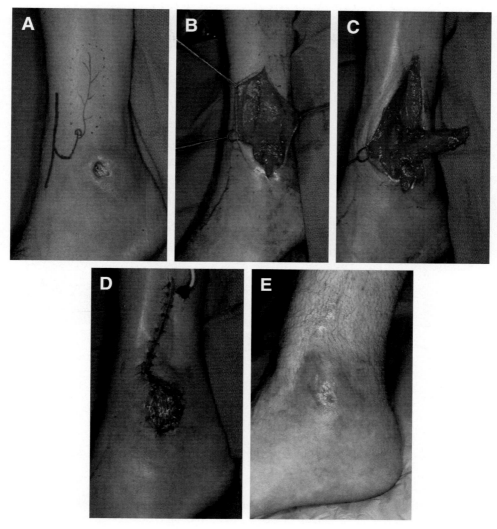

Fig. 24. The supramalleolar flap based on the superior cutaneous branch of the anterior perforating branch of the peroneal artery can be used for lateral malleolar (**A**) as well as for dorsal foot defects. When harvested as fasciocutaneous flap (**B,C**), it is then skin grafted (**D**). Because of the new blood supply, the ulcer heals without problems (**E**).

patient later has to undergo a below the knee amputation. The supramalleolar flap (superior cutaneous branch of the anterior perforating branch of the peroneal artery) can be used for lateral malleolar and heel defects as well as for dorsal foot defects (Fig. 24) *(70)*. It can be either harvested with the overlying skin or as a fascial layer that can then be skin grafted. When harvested as a fascial layer only, the donor site can be closed primarily. Small fasciocutaneous flaps based on individual perforators can also be designed over the row of perforators originating from the posterior tibial artery medially and the peroneal artery laterally *(71)*. Although the reach and size of the flap is limited, it can be expanded by applying the delay principle. These local flaps have proven to be extremely useful in the closure of soft tissue defects around the ankle in patients in an

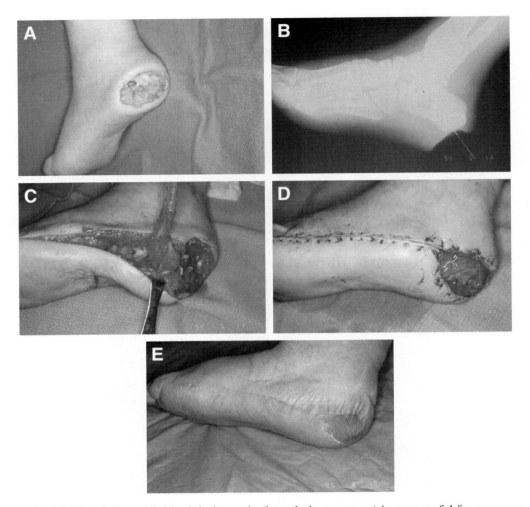

Fig. 25. The abductor digiti minimi muscle (lateral plantar artery) is very useful for coverage of small mid and posterior lateral defects of the sole of the foot and lateral calcaneal osteomyelitis. The dominant pedicle lies very close to its origin and provides sufficient blood supply so that the minor more distal pedicles can be safely ligated.

Ilizarov frame because accessibility to the normal flaps or recipient vessels is always a problem (*see* Fig. 20).

Foot Flaps: Muscle Flaps

The muscle flaps in the foot have a type 2 vascular pattern with a proximal dominant pedicle and several distal minor pedicles are useful to cover relatively small local defects *(72,73)*. The abductor digiti minimi muscle (lateral plantar artery) is very useful for coverage of small mid and posterior lateral defects of the sole of the foot and lateral distal ankle (Fig. 25). Its dominant pedicle is just distal and medial to its origin off of the calcaneus and it has a thin distal muscular bulk *(74)*. The abductor hallucis brevis muscle (medial plantar artery) is larger and can be used to cover medial defects of the mid and hindfoot as well as

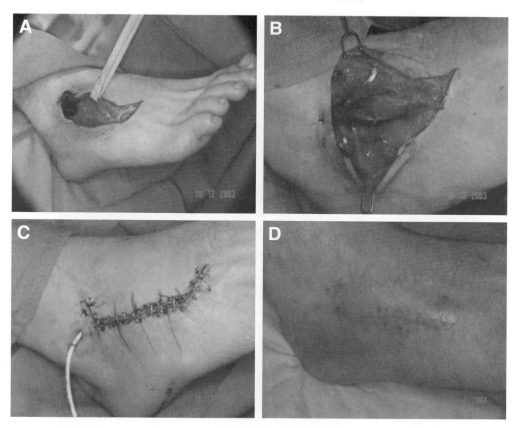

Fig. 26. The extensor digitorum brevis m. (lateral tarsal artery) has disappointingly little bulk but can be used for local defects over the sinus tarsi or lateral calcaneus. The muscle can either be rotated in a limited fashion on its dominant pedicle, the lateral tarsal artery, or in a wider arc if harvested with the distal anterior tibial artery (antegrade flow) or the proximal dorsalis pedis artery (retrograde flow).

the medial distal ankle (*see* Fig. 20). Its dominant pedicle is at the takeoff of the medial plantar artery and its relatively thin distal muscular bulk can be difficult to dissect off the flexor hallucis brevis muscle. The extensor digitorum brevis m. (lateral tarsal artery) has disappointingly little bulk but can be used for local defects over the sinus tarsi or lateral calcaneus (75). The muscle can either be rotated in a limited fashion (Fig. 26) on its dominant pedicle, the lateral tarsal artery, or in a wider arc if harvested with the entire dorsalis pedis artery. The flexor digitorum brevis m. (type 2, lateral plantar artery) can be used to cover plantar heel defects (76). Because the muscle bulk is small, it works best if it is used to fill a defect that can be covered with plantar tissue (Fig. 27).

Foot Flaps: Fasciocutaneous Flaps

The most versatile fasciocutaneous flap of the foot is the medial plantar flap that is the ideal tissue for the coverage of plantar defects (77–79). It can also reach medial ankle defects. It can be harvested to a size as large as 6 × 10 cm, has sensibility, and has a wide arc of rotation if it is taken with the proximal part of the medial plantar artery. It can be harvested on the superficial medial plantar artery (cutaneous branch of the

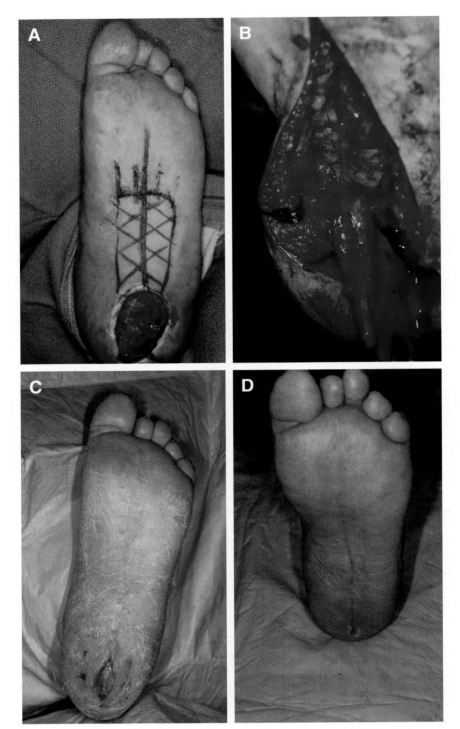

Fig. 27. The flexor digitorum brevis m. (type 2, lateral plantar artery) can be used to cover plantar heel defects. Because the muscle bulk is small, it works best if it is used to fill a defect that can be covered with plantar tissue. Skin grafting the muscle often leads to breakdown because of the lack of bulky soft tissue. This diabetic patient had developed a plantar ulcer from calcaneal gait after a percutaneous release of her Archilles tendon. The Achilles tendon was shortened by 2 cm and the defect **(A)** was filled with the flexor digitorum brevis muscle **(B)**. The plantar fascia was closed over it. The wound initially dehisced **(C)** but went on to heal brevis minimal postoperative compliance **(D)**.

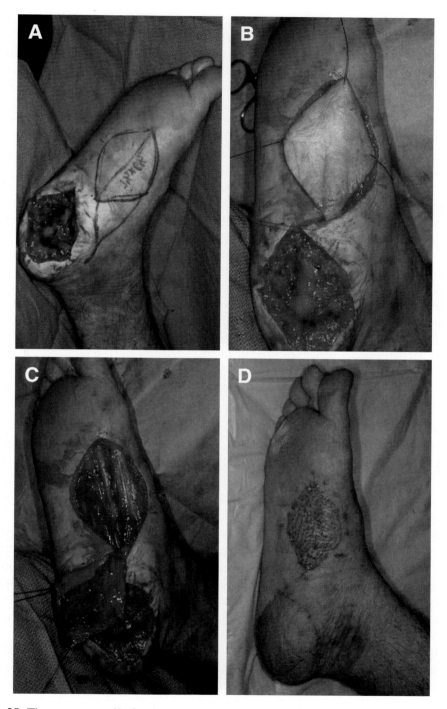

Fig. 28. The most versatile fasciocutaneous flap of the foot is the medial plantar flap that is the ideal tissue for the coverage of plantar defects. It can be harvested on the superficial medial plantar artery (cutaneous branch of the medial plantar artery) or on the deep medial plantar artery (deep branch of the medial plantar artery). The flap below is based on the deep medial plantar artery.

medial plantar artery) or on the deep medial plantar artery (deep branch of the medial plantar artery) (Fig. 28). It is preferable to harvest the flap with the superficial branch if the artery can be dopplered because it will minimally disrupt the existing foot vascular blood supply. However, if it is to be harvested with retrograde flow, the flap should be harvested with the deep branch of the medial plantar artery. The lateral calcaneal flap (calcaneal branch of the peroneal artery) is useful for posterior calcaneal and distal Achilles defects (Fig. 29) *(80)*. Its length can be increased by harvesting it as an "L" shape posterior to and below the lateral malleolus *(81)*. It is harvested with the lesser saphenous vein and sural nerve. Because the calcaneal branch of the peroneal artery lies directly on top of periosteum, there is a great danger of damaging or cutting it during harvest. The dorsalis pedis flap (dorsalis pedis and its continuation, the first dorsal metatarsal artery) can be either proximally or distally based for coverage of ankle and dorsal foot defects *(82)*. A flap wider than 4 cm usually requires skin grafting on top of extensor tendon paratenon which leaves the dorsum of the foot with less than ideal coverage. The loss of the dorsalis pedis can pose problems unless the collateral circulation is intact. Because the donor site is vulnerable both from a vascular and tissue breakdown perspective, this flap is now rarely used. The filet of toe flap (digital artery) is useful for small forefoot web space ulcers and distal forefoot problems although the reach of the flap is always less than expected *(83)*. The technique involves removal of the nail bed, phalangeal bones, extensor tendons, flexor tendons, and volar plates while leaving the two digital arteries intact. A variation of this is the very elegant Toe Island flap in which a part of the toe pulp is raised directly over the *ipsi*-lateral digital neurovascular bundle *(84,85)*. The flap is then elevated with its long vascular leash to cover a distal defect. The leash is buried under the intervening tissue.

Complications Associated With Pedicled Flaps

Once the flap has been successfully raised, it can still fail because of tension at the insetting (refer to introductory section on local flaps), inadequate evaluation the blood flow, twisting of the pedicle, hematoma, and/or infection. Failure to appropriately evaluate the direction of arterial flow, whether it be antegrade or retrograde, can lead to flap loss. The direction of flow is easily determined with a Doppler. Occluding the artery proximally and distal to the location in which the artery is being dopplered allows the surgeon to determine whether the flow is antegrade or retrograde or both. Partial or complete occlusion of the vascular pedicle occurs when the artery and vein feeding the flap are twisted as the flap is placed into the recipient site. This occurs if the vascular pedicle is skeletonized and the flap is rotated at a sharp angle or if the base of the flap is indurated and inflexible (chronic scar tissue and radiation). Proper flap design and donor site selection should prevent this from occurring.

Hematoma creates pressure on the flap which can limit venous return and eventually can lead to flap necrosis. The presence of free blood in the deep space is also a cause for concern because the red blood cells themselves release superoxide radicals *(86)* that can contribute to flap necrosis. Hematoma can be prevented by meticulous hemostasis, topical agents and closed suction drainage. Postoperatively, it is important to visualize the flap and an occlusive transparent dressing facilitates this. If there is any suspicion of existing hematoma, then the wound should be explored and the hematoma evacuated. If the flap was closed with interrupted sutures, removal of one or two stitches allows for evacuation

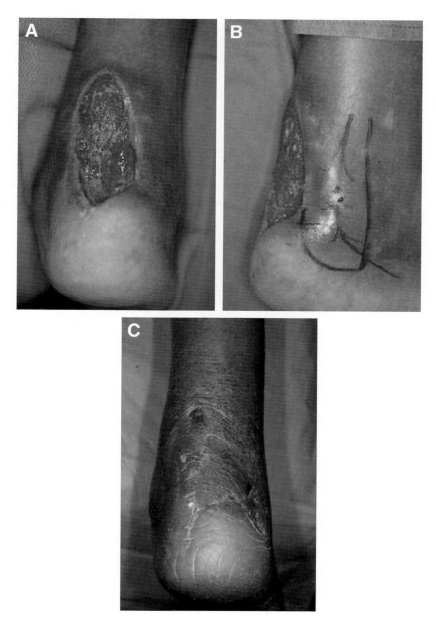

Fig. 29. The lateral calcaneal flap (calcaneal branch of the peroneal artery) is useful for posterior calcaneal and distal Achilles defects. It is harvested with the lesser saphenous vein and sural nerve. Because the calcaneal branch of the peroneal artery lies directly on top of periosteum, there is a great danger of damaging or cutting it during harvest.

of the hematoma without risking the disruption of the whole repair. It is important to flush the space with normal saline to get rid of any remaining hemolyzed blood. If the hematoma cannot be removed in this way, the patient should be returned to the OR for formal evacuation. Applying a bandage that does not allow for normal postoperative soft tissue swelling can also impede blood flow.

Infection can damage or destroy a flap by increasing the metabolic demand of the flap so that it outstrips existing blood supply. Infection damages capillary bed, which short-circuits vascular flow and leads to arterial occlusion. It is therefore important not to plan a reconstruction before all signs of infection are gone. This means that the skin edges are soft with no surrounding induration or erythema, that the pain has diminished and that there are signs of healing (granulation and neoepithelialization). This may require serial debridements that may take up to 1 month before the wound is ready.

Microsurgical Free Flap

The microsurgical free flap is the most complex reconstruction that paradoxically enjoys the highest success rate (>95%) *(87)*. Although it is beyond the scope of this chapter to cover the technical aspects of microsurgery, I would refer the reader to many excellent texts *(88–93)* that cover the field. However, it is important to mention some of the key points for using this type of reconstruction successfully. A distal flap is harvested from the body with its vascular pedicle that is then attached to the local recipient vessels using microsurgical techniques. The key is to have accessible and open recipient artery and vein(s) to which the flap vessels can be anastomosed. The recipient artery should not be sacrificed by performing an end-to-end anastomosis; instead an end to side should always be performed. Two vein anastomoses should always be performed whenever possible to ensure adequate outflow. The flap is then carefully tailored to the defect and inset. The better the fit, the less likely the need for later revision of a bulky flap. This obviously is very important because the reconstructed foot will have to fit inside a shoe *(94)*.

The key to choosing the appropriate flap is the distance between the recipient vessel and the existing defect. That distance can be decreased by harvesting a larger flap and removing normal tissue between the defect and the recipient vessel. The longest pedicles are the Serratus muscle and the radial forearm flap. Muscle flaps with a skin graft work the best to cover osteomyelitis and defects on the sole of the foot *(95)*. Good donor muscles include the gracilis muscle from the ipsi-lateral leg, the rectus abdominus muscle, the serratus muscle, and the latissimus dorsi muscle. The latter should be avoided whenever possible as sacrifice of the latissimus dorsi m. may affect the patient's ability to crutch walk and will definitely hinder the patient's ability to propel himself/herself in a wheelchair. Muscles can be aggressively trimmed to better fit a given defect as long as the main vascular pedicle remains intact (Fig. 30).

Fasciocutaneous and cutaneous flaps work better on the nonweight-bearing portions of the foot (i.e., dorsum of the foot and ankle). Flaps that are frequently used include the radial forearm flap, the lateral arm flap, the lateral thigh flap, and the para-scapular flap (Fig. 31). The key in choosing the appropriate flap is to match the depth of the defect with the relative thickness of the harvested flap. This can be difficult in obese patients. Trimmed muscle with skin graft or fascial flaps with skin graft may be more appropriate.

RECONSTRUCTIVE OPTIONS BY LOCATION OF DEFECT

Forefoot Coverage

Toe ulcer or gangrene is best treated with a limited amputation that uses all remaining viable tissue so that the amputated toe is as long as possible when closed.

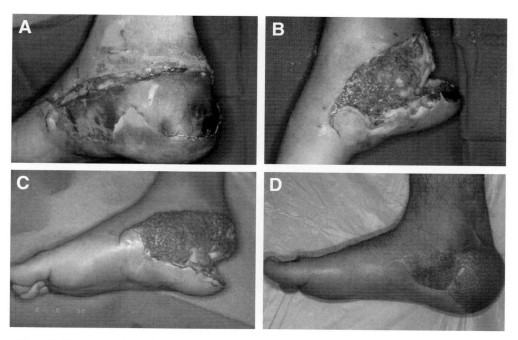

Fig. 30. This diabetic patient had an avulsion injury over the right heel (**A**). The wound was serially debrided (**B**) until a healthy base wound healing base was achieved (**C**). A serratus muscle flap with skin graft was used to over the heel. This is the appearance of the foot 5 years later (**D**).

The surgeon should attempt to at least preserve a sufficient portion of the proximal phalanx to act as a spacer preventing the adjacent toes from drifting into the empty space. If the hallux is involved, attempts should be made to preserve as much length as possible because of its critical role in ambulation *(96)*. A toe island flap from the second toe is an excellent way to fill a defect on the hallux without having to resort to shortening it.

Ulcers under the metatarsal head(s) occur because biomechanical abnormalities place excessive or extended pressure on the plantar forefoot during the gait cycle. Although hammer toes are contributing factors and should be corrected, the principle cause of the abnormal biomechanical forces is usually a tight Achilles tendon that prevents ankle dorsiflexion beyond the neutral position. A percutaneous release of the achilles tendon is performed if both portions of the achilles tendon are tight while a gastrocnemius recession is performed if only the gastrocnemius portion of the achilles tendon is tight. With the release of the achilles tendon, forefoot pressures drops dramatically and the ulcer(s), if it does not involve bone, should heal by secondary intention in less than 6 weeks *(97,98)*. This decrease in pushoff strength persists and prevents recurrent ulceration by more than 50% over the next 25 months *(9,10)*.

The complications associated with the gastrocnemius recession are far less than those associated with the percutaneous achilles tendon release. The primary complication of a gastrocnemius recession is a hematoma from tears in the underlying soleus muscle. On the other hand, an overaggressive percutaneous release of the Achilles tendon leads to calcaneal gait and eventual plantar heel ulcers (13–14%) that are extremely difficult to heal (*see* Fig. 27). Healing may require retightening the Achilles tendon or ankle fusion in addition to treating the ulcer.

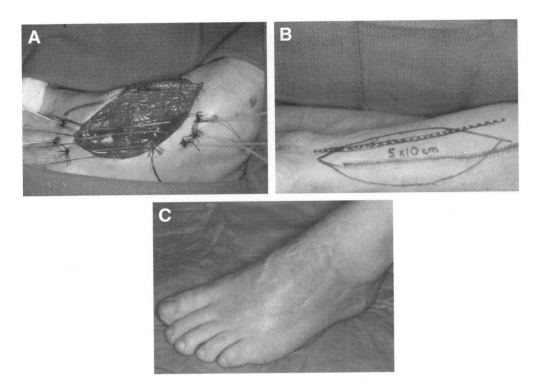

Fig. 31. This defect occurred after resection of a sarcoma. The radial forearm flap was harvested with tendon and nerve. The reconstruction included tenodesing the proximal and distal toe extensors with a vascularized palmaris tendon. Sensory innervation was obtained by anastamosing the lateral antecubital nerve to the superficial peroneal nerve.

For patients with normal ankle dorsiflexion who have a stage 1–3 plantar ulcer under metatarsal head owing to a plantarly prominent metatarsal head, the affected metatarsal head can be elevated with preplanned osteotomies and internal fixation. The metatarsal head is thus shifted 2–3 mm superiorly. Upward movement with its attendant pressure relief is usually sufficient for the underlying ulcer to heal by secondary intention. There should not be any transfer lesions to the other metatarsal heads because the anatomic metatarsal head parabola will be preserved. However, if the metatarsal head has osteomyelitis, it should be shaved or resected. The ulcer should heal by secondary intention if all weight is kept off the forefoot as it heals. The small deep forefoot ulcers without an obvious bony prominence can also be closed with a local flap: a filleted toe flap, a toe island flap, a bilobed flap, a rotation flap, a Limberg flap, or a V–Y flap. For larger ulcers in which the metatarsal head has been resected, consideration should be given to ray amputation. Resecting the more independent first or fifth metatarsal causes less biomechanical disruption than the second, third, or fourth metatarsal because the middle metatarsals operate as a cohesive central unit.

All efforts should be made to preserve as much of the metatarsals as possible if more than one is exposed because they are so important to normal ambulation. Local tissue is often insufficient to do this in the forefoot and therefore a microsurgical free flap should be considered. If ulcers are present under several metatarsal heads or if a transfer lesion from one of the resected metatarsal head to a neighboring metatarsal has occurred, consideration should be given to doing a panmetatarsal head resection. This is performed with two or three dorsal incisions and great care is taken to preserve the proportional lengths of each metatarsal so that the normal distal metatarsal parabola is preserved. Removing the metatarsal heads while leaving the flexors and extensors to the toes intact helps prevent the inevitable equino-varus deformity that accompanies loss of the distal extensors.

If more than two toes and the accompanying metatarsals heads have to be resected, then a transmetatarsal amputation *(99)* should be performed. The normal parabola with the second metatarsal being the longest is preserved. All bone cuts should be made so that the plantar aspect of the cut is shorter than the dorsal one. If the extensor and flexor tendons of the fourth and fifth toe are intact, they should be tenodesed with the ankle in the neutral position. This helps prevent the subsequent equino-varus deformity from the loss of extensor forces that usually leads to breakdown under the distal fifth metatarsal head. If the achilles tendon is tight, it should be lengthened *(100)*. As much plantar tissue as possible should be preserved so that the anterior portion of the amputation consists of healthy plantar tissue. When there are existing medial or lateral defects, the remaining plantar flap should be appropriately rotated to cover the entire plantar forefoot. Dog ears should be resected so that the distal end is as normally tapered as possible and easy to fit into a shoe with a simple orthotics and filler.

The most proximal forefoot amputation is the Lisfranc amputation in which all the metatarsals are removed *(101)*. The direction of the blood flow along the dorsalis pedis and lateral plantar arteries should be evaluated. If both have antegrade flow, then the connection between the two can be sacrificed. However, if only one of the two vessels is providing blood flow to the entire foot, the connection has to be preserved. To prevent an equino-varus deformity, one can either address the anterior tibialis tendon or the Achilles tendon. The anterior tibial tendon can be split so that the lateral half is inserted into the cuboid bone. Alternatively, the Achilles tendon has to be lengthened. The Lisfranc amputation can be closed with volar or dorsal flaps if there is sufficient tissue. If there is not adequate tissue for coverage, a free muscle flap with skin graft should be used. Postoperatively, the patient's foot should be placed in slight dorsiflexion until the wound has healed.

Midfoot Coverage

Defects on the medial aspect of the sole are nonweight bearing and are best treated with a skin graft. Ulcers on the medial and lateral plantar midfoot are usually owing to Charcot collapse of the midfoot plantar arch. If the underlying shattered bone has healed and is stable (Eichenholtz stage 3), then the excess bone can be shaved via a medial or lateral approach although the ulcer can either be allowed to heal by secondary intention or can be covered with a glabrous skin graft or a local flap. For small defects, useful local flap includes the V–Y flap, the rotation flap, the bilobed flap, the rhomboid flap, or the transposition flap. If a muscle flap is needed, a pedicled abductor hallucis flap medially or an abductor digiti minimi flap laterally works well. For slightly larger defects, large V–Y flaps, random large medially based rotation flaps or pedicled medial plantar fasciocutaneous flap can be successful. Larger defects should be filled with free muscle flaps covered by skin grafts. Great care should be taken to inset the flap at the same height as the surrounding tissue. If the midfoot bones are unstable (Eichenholz stage 1 or 2), then they can be excised with a wedge excision. The bones on either side of the resection are then fused to recreate the normal arch of the foot and held in place with an Ilizarov frame. The shortening of the skeletal midfoot usually leaves enough loose soft tissue to close the wound primarily or with a local flap.

Hindfoot Coverage

Plantar heel defects or ulcers are among the most difficult of all wounds to heal. If they are the result of the patient being in a prolonged decubitus position, they are also usually a reflection of severe vascular disease. A partial calcanectomy may be required to develop enough of a local soft tissue envelope to cover the resulting defect. Although patients can ambulate with a partially resected calcaneus, they will need orthotics and molded shoes. If there is an underlying collapsed bone or bone spur causing a hindfoot defect, the bone should be shaved down. These ulcers are usually closed with double V–Y flaps or larger medially based rotation flaps. Plantar heel defects can also be closed with pedicled flaps that include the medial plantar fasciocutaneous flap or the flexor digiti minimi muscle flap. Posterior heel defects are better closed with extended lateral calcaneal fasciocutaneous flap or the retrograde sural artery fasciocutaneous flap. If the defect is large, then a muscle free flap with skin graft should be used. The flap should be carefully tailored so there is no excess tissue and it blends in well with the rest of the heel. Medial or lateral calcaneal defects usually occur after fracture and attempted repair. If this results in osteomyelitis of the calcaneus, the infected bone should be debrided and antibiotic beads should be placed. The defect can usually be covered with the abductor hallucis muscle flap medially or the abductor digiti minimi flap laterally. The exposed muscle is then skin grafted. After 6 weeks or more, the beads can be replaced with bone graft. Consideration should be given to applying an Ilizarov frame during the healing phase for heel defect because it protects the soft tissue repair from pressure by suspending the heel and immobilizes the ankle so that sheer forces cannot disrupt the repair.

The two hindfoot amputations are the Chopart and Symes amputations. The Chopart amputation leaves an intact talus and calcaneus while removing the mid and forefoot bones of the foot. To avoid going into equino-varus deformity, a minimum of two centimeters of the achilles has to be resected so that the connection between the two parts of the achilles tendon have no chance of healing together. When the amputation has healed, a calcaneal-tibial rod can be used to further stabilize the ankle. The Symes amputation should be considered if there is insufficient tissue to primarily close a Chopart amputation and the talus and calcaneus are involved with osteomyelitis. The tibia and fibula are cut just above the ankle mortise and the deboned heel pad swung anteriorly. The heel pad has to be anchored to the anterior portion of the distal tibia to prevent posterior migration. The amputation can be difficult to shape because large dog ears occur when the heel pad is brought up anteriorly. These dog ears contain part of the blood supply to the heel so they cannot be easily removed. They can be carefully trimmed at the initial operation or 4–6 weeks later to allow for alternative blood flow patterns to be established. The ultimate goal

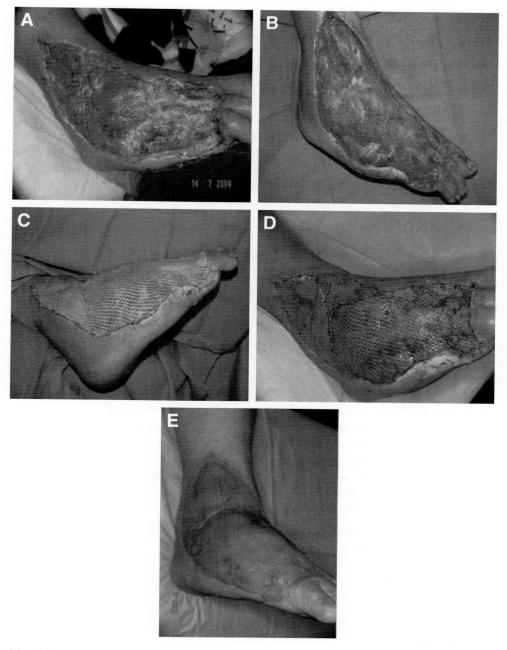

Fig. 32. This patient developed necrotizing fasciitis with α-hemolytic streptococcus that destroyed the entire dorsum of the foot (**A**). After multiple debridements, the wound was covered with Integra and a VAC. The Integra (**B**) was then covered with a skin graft (**C**) and the wound went on to heal without incident (**D,E**).

is a thin, tailored stump that can fit well into a patellar weight-bearing prosthesis. A poorly designed Symes amputation is a prosthetist's nightmare and can lead to repeated breakdown of the stump.

Dorsum of the Foot

The defects on the dorsum of the foot are often treated with simple skin grafts. If the tissue covering the extensor tendons is thin or nonexistent, a dermal regeneration template (Integra) should be applied. When the dermis is vascularized, a thin skin autograft is then applied (Fig. 32). Local flaps that can be used for small defects include rotation, bilobed, rhomboid or transposition flaps. Possible pedicled flaps include the extensor digitorum brevis muscle flap, the dorsalis pedis flap, the supramalleolar flap, and the sural artery flap. The EDB muscle's reach can be increased by cutting the dorsalis pedis artery above or below the lateral tarsal artery, depending on where the defect is and whether there is adequate antegrade and retrograde flow. The reach of the supramalleolar flap can be increased by cutting the anterior perforating branch of the peroneal artery before it anastomoses with the lateral malleolar artery. For defects at the sinus tarsus the EDB flap works well. The most appropriate microsurgical free flap is a thin fasciocutaneous flap to minimize bulk. The radial forearm flap is an excellent choice because it is sensate and provides a vascularized tendon (palmaris tendon) to reconstruct lost extensor function. Thin muscle flaps with skin grafts or fascial flaps are effective options as well.

Ankle Defects

Soft tissue around the ankle is sparse and has minimal flexibility. If there is sufficient granulation tissue, a skin graft will work well. To encourage the formation of a healthy wound bed, the VAC ± Integra can be used (*see* Fig. 32). The achilles tendon, if allowed sufficient time to form a granulating bed, will tolerate a skin graft that will hold up well over time. Local flaps do not need to cover the entire defect because only the critical area of the wound such as exposed tendon, bone or joints needs to be covered whereas the rest of the wound can be skin grafted. Useful local flaps include rotation, bilobed, or transposition flaps. Local flaps can easily be individually designed off posterior tibial and peroneal arterial perforators. Pedicled flaps include the supramalleolar flap, the dorsalis pedis flap, the retrograde sural artery flap, the medial plantar flap, abductor hallucis muscle flap, the abductor digiti minimi muscle flap and the extensor digitorum brevis muscle flap. Free flaps can either be fasciocutaneous or muscle with skin graft but they should be kept thin. In order to ensure good healing, the ankle should be temporarily immobilized with an external fixator.

SUMMARY

Treating diabetic foot ulcers and gangrene can only be done effectively by using a team approach which at the minimum includes a wound care team, a vascular surgeon, a plastic surgeon, an infectious disease specialist, an endocrinologist, and a prosthetist. The wound needs to be accurately assessed, debrided, and cultured. The vascular and medical status has to be optimized. The repair is then dictated by how much of the foot remains postdebridement and how the foot can be closed in the most biomechanically stable construct possible. This may involve skeletal manipulation, tendon lengthening, and or partial foot amputations. Soft tissue reconstruction can be as simple as allowing the wound to heal by secondary intention or as complex as covering it with a microsurgical free flaps. Wound healing adjuncts such as growth factor, cultured skin, and hyperbaric are be helpful in preparing the wound bed for closure. More than 90% of the wound can be closed utilizing simple methods from healing by secondary intention to skin grafting. Utilizing this approach should decrease the primary and secondary major amputation rate to below 5%.

REFERENCES

1. Rodeheaver GT. Wound cleansing, wound irrigation, wound disinfection, in *Chronic Wound Care* (Krasner D, Kane D. eds.), 2nd ed. Health Management Publication, Inc., Wayne PA, 1997, pp. 97–108.
2. Grayson ML, Gibbons GW, Balogh K, et al. Probing to bone in infected pedal ulcers: a clinical sign of osteomyelitis in diabetic patients. *JAMA* 1995;273:721–723.
3. Attinger CE, Cooper P, Blume P, Bulan EJ. The safest surgical incisions and amputations using the angiosome concept and doppler on arterial–arterial connections of the foot and ankle. *Foot Ankle Clin N Am* 2001;6:745–801.
4. Wolff H, Hansson C. Larval therapy—an effective method of ulcer debridement, *Clin Exp Dermatol* 2003;28:134.
5. Sherman RA, Sherman J, Gilead L, et al. Maggot therapy in outpatients. *Arch Phys Med Rehabil* 2001;81:1226–1229.
6. Rhodes GR, King TA. Delayed skin oxygenation following distal tibial revascularization. Implications for wound healing in late amputations. *Am Surg* 1986;52:519–525.
7. Grant WP, Sullivan R, Sonenshine DE. Electron microscope investigation of the effects of diabetes mellitus on the Achilles tendon. *J Foot Ankle Surg* 1997;36:1.
8. Armstrong DG, Stacpoole-Shea, Nguyen H. Lengthening of the Achilles tendon in diabetic patients who are at high risk for ulceration of the foot. *Adv Ortho Surg* 1999;23:71.
9. Mueller MJ, Sinacore DR, Hastings MK, et al. Effect of Achilles tendon lengthening on neuropathic plantar ulcers, a randomized clinical trial. *J Bone Joint Surg Am* 2003; 85a:1436.
10. Maluf KS, Mueller MJ, Hastings MK, et al. Tendon Achilles lengthening for the treatment neuropathic ulcers causes a temporary reduction in forefoot pressure associated with changes in plantar flexor power rather than ankle motion during gait. *J Biomech* 2004;37:897.
11. Falanga V. Growth factors and chronic wounds: the need to understand the microenvironment. *J Dermatol* 1992;19:667.
12. Edwards R, Harding KG. Bacteria and wound healing. *Curr Opin Inf Dis* 2004;17:91.
13. Steed DL, Donohoe D, Webster MW, et al. Effect of extensive debridement and treatment on the healing of diabetic foot ulcers. *J Am Coll Surg* 1996;183:61–64.
14. Edgerton MT. *The Art of Surgical Technique*, Williams and Wilkins, Baltimore, 1988.
15. Morykwas MJ, Argenta LC, et al. Vacuum assisted closure: a new method for wound control and treatment: animal studies and basic foundation. *Ann Plast Surg* 1997;38:553–562.
16. Lipsky BA, Berendt AR, Deery HG, et al. Diagnosis and treatment of diabetic foot infections. *Clin Inf Dis* 2004;39:885.
17. Argenta LC, Morykwas MJ. Vacuum-assisted closure: a new method for wound control and treatment: clinical experience. *Ann Plast Surg* 1997;38:563–576.
18. DeFranzo AJ, Argenta LC, Marks MW, et al. The use of vacuum-assisted closure therapy for the treatment of lower extremity wounds with exposed bone. *Plast Reconstr Surg* 2004;113:1339.
19. Joseph E, Hamori CA, BergmanS, et al. A prospective randomized trial of vacuum assisted closure versus standard therapy of chronic non-healing wounds. *Wounds* 2000;12:60.
20. Byrd HS, Spicer TE, Cierny G III. Management of open tibial fractures. *Plast Reconstr Surg* 1985;76:719.
21. Krizek TJ, Robson MC. The evolution of quantitative bacteriology in wound management. *Am J Surg* 1975;130:579.
22. Sheehan P, Jones P, Caselli A, et al. Percent change in wound area of diabetic foot ulcers over a 4 week period is a robust indicator of complete healing in a 12 week prospective trial. *Diabetes Care* 2003;26:1879.

23. Haimowitz JE, Margolis DJ. Moist wound healing, in *Chronic Wound Care* (Krasner D, Kane D, eds.), 2nd ed. Health Management Publication, Inc., Wayne PA, 1997, pp. 49–56.

24. Steed DL. The diabetic study group: clinical evaluation of recombinant human platelet derived growth factor for treatment of lower extremity diabetic ulcers. *J Vasc Surg* 1995;21:71–81.

25. Cullen B, Smith R, McCulloch, et al. Mechanism of action of Promogran, a protease modulating matrix for the treatment of diabetic foot ulcers. *Diabetes Care* 2002;25:1892.

26. Veves A, Sheehan P, Pham HT. A randomized controlled trial of Promogran (a collagen/oxidized regenerated cellulose dressing) vs standard treatment in the management of diabetic foot ulcers. *Arch Surg* 2002;137:822.

27. Morbach S, Hoffmeier H, Ochs HR. An in-use observational study of the treatment of diabetic foot ulcers with Promogram & Regranex gel, Poster, 17th Clinical Symposium On Advances In Skin & Wound Care & in the 13th European Tissue Repair Society Meeting.

28. Bromberg BE, Song IC, Mohn MP. The use of pigskin as a temporary biological dressing. *Plast Reconstr Surg* 1965;36:80.

29. Bondoc CC, Butke JF. Clinical experience with viable frozen human skin and frozen skin bank. *Ann Surg* 1971;174:371.

30. Omar AA, Mavor AI, Jones AM, et al. Treatment of venous leg ulcers with Dermagraft. *Eur J Vasc Endovasc Surg* 2004;6:666.

31. Falanga V, Sabolinski M. A bilayered skin construct (APLIGRAF) accelerates complete closure of hard to heal venous stasis ulcers. *Wound Repair Regen* 1999;7:201.

32. Veves A, Falanga V, Armstrong DG. Graftskin, a human skin equivalent, is effective in the management of non-infected neuropathic diabetic foot ulcers. *Diabetes Care* 2001;24:290–295.

33. Marston WA, Hanft J, Norwood P, et al. The efficacy and safety of Dermagraft in improving the healing of chronic diabetic foot ulcers: results of a prospective randomized study. *Diabetes Care* 2003;26:1701.

34. Saap LJ, Donohue K, Falanga V. Clinical classification of bioengineered skin use and it correlation with healing of diabetic and venous ulcers. *Dermatol Surg* 2004;30:1095–1100.

35. Espensen EH, Nixon BP, Lavery LA, et al. Use of subatmospheric (VAC) therapy to improve bioengineered tissue grafting in diabetic foot wounds. *J Am Podiatr Med Assoc* 2002;92:396.

36. Hunt TK, Pai MP. The effect of varying ambient oxygen tensions on wound metabolism and collagen synthesis. *Surg Gyn Obstet* 1972;135:561.

37. Pai MP, Hunt TK. Effect of varying oxygen tension on healing in open wounds. *Surg Gyn Obstet* 1972;135:756–757.

38. Hohn DC, Mackay RD, Halliday B, et al. The effect of oxygen tension on the microbiocidal function of leukocytes in wounds and in vitro. *Surg Forum* 1976;27:18–20.

39. Bonomo SR, Davidson JD, Tyrone JW, et al. Enhancement of wound healing by hyperbaric oxygen and transforming growth factor beta3 in a new chronic wound model in aged rabbits. *Arch Surg* 2000;135:1148.

40. Faglia E, Favales F, Aldeghi A, et al. Adjunctive systemic hyperbaric oxygen therapy in treatment of severe prevalently ischemic diabetic foot ulcer; a randomized study. *Diabetes Care* 1996;19:1338–1343.

41. Connolly WB, Hunt TK, Zederfeldt B, et al. Clinical comparison of wound closed by suture and adhesive tape. *Am J Surg* 1969;117:318.

42. Janzing HM, Broos PL. Dermotraction: an effective technique for the closure of fasciotomy wounds: a preliminary report of 15 patients. *J Orthop Trauma* 2001;15:438.

43. Gorecki PJ, Cottam D, Ger R, et al. Lower extremity compartment syndrome following a laparoscopic Roux-en-Y gastric bypass. *Obes Surg* 2002;2:289.

44. Rudolph R, Ballantyne DL. Skin grafts, in *Plastic Surgery* (McCarthy JG, ed.),Vol. 1, WB Saunders, Philadelphia, PA, 1990, pp. 221–274.

45. Currie LJ, Sharpe JR, Martin R. The use of fibrin glue in skin grafts and tissue engineered skin replacement: a review. *Plast Reconstr Surg* 2001;108:1713.

46. Blackburn JH, Boemi L, Hall WW, et al. Negative Pressure dressings as a bolster for skin grafts. *Ann Plast Surg* 1998;40:453.

47. Scherer LA, Shiver S, Chang M, et al. The vacuum assisted closure device: a method of securing skin grafts and improving skin graft survival. *Arch Surg* 137:930.

48. Moiemen NS, Staiano JJ, Ojeh NO, et al. Reconstructive surgery with a dermal regeneration template: clinical and histological study. *Plast Reconstr Surg* 2001;108:93.

49. Frame JD, Still J, Lakhel-LeCoadau A, et al. Use of dermal regeneration template in contracture release procedures: a multicenter evaluation. *Plast Reconstr Surg* 2004;113:1330.

50. Molnar JA, Defranzo AJ, Hadaegh A, et al. Acceleration of Integra incorporation in complex tissue defects with subatmospheric pressure. *Plast Reconstr Surg* 2004;113:1339.

51. Banis JC. Glabrous skin graft for plantar defects. *Foot Ankle Clin* 2001;6:827.

52. Paragas LK, Attinger C, Blume PA. Local flaps. *Clin Podiatr Med Surg* 2000;17:267.

53. Hallock GG. Distal lower leg local random fasciocutaneous flaps. *Plast Reconstr Surg* 1990;86:304.

54. Sundell B. Studies in the circulation of pedicle skin flaps. *Ann Chir Gynaecol Fenn* 1963;133(Suppl 53):1.

55. Blume PA, Paragas LK, Sumpio BE, Attinger CE. Single stage surgical treatment for non infected diabetic foot ulcers. *Plast Reconstr Surg* 2002;109:601.

56. Taylor GI, Corlett RJ, Caddy CM, Zelt RG. An anatomic review of the delay phenomenon: II. Clinical applications. *Plast Reconstr Surg* 1992;89(3):408–416.

57. Hidalgo DA, Shaw WW. Anatomic basis of plantar flap design. *Plast Reconstr Surg* 1986;78:627.

58. Shaw WW, Hidalgo DA. Anatomic basis of plantar flap design: clinical applications. *Plast Reconstr Surg* 1986;78:637.

59. Colen LB, Repogle SL, Mathes SJ. The V-Y plantar flap for reconstruction of the forefoot. *Plast Reconstr Surg* 1988;81:220.

60. Attinger CE, Ducic I, Cooper P, Zelen CM. The role of intrinsic muscle flaps of the foot for bone coverage in foot and ankle defects in diabetic and non diabetic patients. *Plast Reconstr Surg* 2002;110:1047.

61. Masqualet AC, Gilbert A. An atlas of flaps, in *Limb Reconstruction*, J.B. Lippincott Co., Philadelphia, 1995.

62. Mathes SJ, Nahai F. *Reconstructive Surgery: Principles, Anatomy & Technique*, Churchill Livingston Inc., New York, NY, 1997.

63. Hughes LA, Mahoney JL. Anatomic basis of local muscle flaps in the distal third of the leg. *Plast Reconstr Surg* 1993;92:1144.

64. Tobin GR. Hemisoleus and reversed hemi-soleus flaps. *Plast Reconstr Surg* 1987;79:407.

65. Cormack GC, Lamberty BGH: *The Arterial Anatomy of Skin Flaps*, 2nd ed., Churchill Livingston, London, 1994.

66. Yoshimura M, Imiura S, Shimamura K, et al. Peroneal flap for reconstruction of the extremity: preliminary report. *Plast Reconstr Surg* 1984;74:420.

67. Dong JS, Peng YP, Zhang YY, et al. Reverse anterior tibial artery flap for reconstruction of foot donor site. *Plast Reconstr Surg* 2003;112:1604.

68. Hasegawa M, Torii S, Katoh H, et al. The distally based sural artery flap. *Plast Reconstr Surg* 1994;93:1012.

69. Baumeister SP, Spierer R, Erdman D, et al. A realistic complication analysis of 70 sural artery flaps in a multimorbid patient group. *Plast Reconstr Surg* 2003;112:129.

70. Masqualet AC, Beveridge J, Romana C. The lateral supramalleolar flap. *Plast Reconstr Surg* 1988;81:74.

71. Hallock GG. Distal lower leg local random fasciocutaneous flaps. *Plast Reconstr Surg* 1990;86:304.

72. Ger R. The management of chronic ulcers of the dorsum of the foot by muscle transposition and free skin grafting. *Br J Plast Surg* 1976;29:199.

73. Attinger CE, Ducic I, Cooper P, Zelen CM. The role of intrinsic muscle flaps of the foot for bone coverage in foot and ankle defects in diabetic and non diabetic patients. *Plast Reconstructr Surg* 2002;110:1047.

74. Attinger CE, Cooper P. Soft tissue reconstruction for calcaneal fractures or osteomyelitis. *Foot Ankle Clin N Am* 2001;32:135.

75. Leitner DW, Gordon L, Buncke HJ. The extensor digitorum brevis as a muscle island flap. *Plast Reconstr Surg* 1985;767:777.

76. Hartrampf CR Jr, Scheflan M, Bostwick J III. The flexor digitorum brevis muscle island pedicle flap, a new dimension in heel reconstruction. *Plast Reconstr Surg* 1980; 66:264.

77. Morrison WA, Crabb D McC, O'Brien B McC et al. The instep of the foot as a fasciocutaneous island flap and as a free flap for heel defects. *Plast Reconstr Surg* 1972;72: 56–63.

78. Harrison DH, Morgan BDG. The instep island flap to resurface plantar defects. *Br J Plast Surg* 1981;34:315–318.

79. Masqualet AC, Romana MC. The medial pedis flap, a new fasciocutaneous flap. *Plast Reconstr Surg* 1990;85:765.

80. Grabb WC, Argenta LC. The lateral calcaneal artery skin flap. *Plast Reconstr Surg* 1981;68:723–730.

81. Yan A, Park S, Icao T, Nakamura N. Reconstruction of a skin defect of the posterior heel by a lateral calcaneal flap. *Plast Reconstr Surg* 1985;75:642–646.

82. McCraw JB, Furlow LT Jr. The dorsalis pedis arterialized flap: a clinical study. *Plast Reconstr Surg* 1975;55:177–185.

83. Emmet AJJ. The filleted toe flap. *Br J Plast Surg* 1976;29:19.

84. Snyder GB, Edgerton MT. The principle of island neurovascular flap in the management of ulcerated anaesthetic weight-bearing areas of the lower extremity. *Plast Reconstr Surg* 1965;36:518.

85. Kaplan I. Neurovascular island flap in the treatment of trophic ulceration of the heel. *Br J Plast Surg* 1976;29:19.

86. Manson P, Anthenelli RM, Im MJ, et al. The role of oxygen free radicals in ischemic tissue injury in island skin flaps. *Ann Surg* 1983;198:87.

87. Khouri RK, Cooley BC, Kunselman AR, et al. A prospective study of microvascular free-flap surgery and outcome. *Plast Reconstr Surg* 2000;105:2279.

88. Buncke HJ. *Microsurgery: transplantation–Replantation*, Lea & Fiebiger, Philadelphia, 1991.

89. O'Brien BM, Morrison WA. *Reconstructive Microsurgery*, *Churchill Livingstone*, New York, NY, 1987.

90. Shaw Ww, Hildalgo DA. *Microsurgery in Trauma*, Futura Publishing Company, Mount Kisco, New York, 1987.

91. Strauch B, Han-Liang Y. *Atlas of Microvascular Surgery: Anatomy and Operative Procedures*, Thieme, New York, 1993.

92. Mathes SJ, Nahai F. *Reconstructive Surgery: Principles, Anatomy, & Technique*, Churchill Livingston, New York, 1997.

93. Serafin D. *Atlas of Microsurgical Composite Tissue Transplantation*, W.B Saunders, Philadelphia, 1996.

94. Goldberg JA, Adkins P, Tsai T. Microvascular reconstruction of the foot: weight bearing patterns, gait analysis, and long term follow up. *Plast Reconstr Surg* 1992;92:904.

95. May JW, Rohrich RJ. Foot reconstruction using free microvascular muscle flaps with skin grafts. *Clin Plast Surg* 1986;13:681.

96. Mann RA, Poppen NK, O'Konski M. Amputation of the great toe: a clinical and biomechanical study. *Clin Ortho Relat Res* 1988;226:192.
97. Armstrong DG, Stacpoole-Shea S, Nguyen H, Harkless LB. Lengthening of the Achilles tendon in diabetic patients who are at high risk for ulceration of the foot. *J Bone Joint Surg* 1999;81-A:535–538.
98. Lin SS, Lee TH, Wapner KL. Plantar forefoot ulceration with equinus deformity of the ankle in diabetic patients: the effect of tendo-Achilles lengthening and total contact casting. *Orthop* 1996;19:465–475.
99. Chrzan JS, Giurini JM, Hurchik JM. A biomechanical model for the transmetatarsal amputation. *JAPMA* 1993;83:82.
100. Barry DC, Sabacinski KA, Habershaw GM, et al. Tendo achillis procedures for chronic ulcerations in diabetic patients with transmetatarsal amputations. *JAPMA* 1993;83:97.
101. Bowker JH. Partial foot amputations and disarticulations. *Foot Ankle* 1997;2:153.

20

Role of Growth Factors in the Treatment of Diabetic Foot Ulceration

David L. Steed, MD

PRINCIPLES OF WOUND HEALING AND GROWTH FACTOR THERAPY

Wound healing is the process of tissue repair and the tissue response to injury. It is a complex biological process involving chemotaxis, cellular reproduction, matrix protein production and deposition, neovascularization, and scar remodeling (1). Growth factors are polypeptides that control the growth, differentiation, and metabolism of cells, and regulate the process of tissue repair (2,3). The role of growth factors in wound healing and specifically in diabetic ulcer healing is the subject of this chapter.

The three phases of wound healing—inflammation, fibroplasia, and maturation—are each controlled by growth factors that are present in only small amounts, yet powerful in their influence on wound repair. There is great interest in manipulating the cellular environment of the wound with proteins, growth factors, and gene therapy.

The first phase of wound healing is the inflammatory response, initiated immediately after the injury (4). Vasoconstriction limits hemorrhage to the site of wounding. As blood vessels are damaged and blood leaks from within the lumen, platelets come into contact with collagen in the wall of the vessel beneath the endothelium. Platelets are activated by the collagen and initiate coagulation. Serotonin and thromboxane are released and enhance vasoconstriction locally, keeping the healing factors within the wound. Simultaneously, vasodilatation occurs, allowing new factors to be brought into the wound. Vasodilatation is mediated by histamine, released by the platelets, mast cells, and basophils. There is also an increase in vascular permeability allowing blood borne factors to enter this area. Arachidonic acid is produced and serves as an intermediate for production of prostaglandins and leukotrienes. These proteins are intense vasodilators which increase vascular permeability, along with histamine, bradykinin, and complement. Thromboxane also increases platelet aggregation and local vasoconstriction.

Platelets control hemorrhage by initiating clotting through the coagulation system. The intrinsic system is activated by Hageman factor, known as factor XII, as it comes into contact with collagen. In the presence of kininogen, a precursor of bradykinin and prekallikrein, factor XII activates factor XI, then factor IX, and then factor VIII. Thromboplastin triggers a response in the extrinsic system. Thromboplastin is formed as phospholipids and glycoproteins are released by blood coming into contact with the injured tissues. Factor VII is activated in the presence of calcium. Both the intrinsic and

From: *The Diabetic Foot, Second Edition*
Edited by: A. Veves, J. M. Giurini, and F. W. LoGerfo © Humana Press Inc., Totowa, NJ

extrinsic systems activate the final common pathway, producing fibrin and leading to fibrin polymerization. To balance the coagulation cascade, the fibrinolytic system is activated. This system monitors clotting to prevent coagulation from extending beyond the wound. It is activated by the same factors that initiate coagulation and thus regulates the process.

The complement cascade is activated by platelets and neutral proteases. This system produces potent proteins known as anaphylotoxins, which cause mast cells to degranulate and release histamine. Substances released by the inflammatory process are chemoattractants for neutrophils. These cause margination of white blood cells and then migration of these white blood cells into the wound. The neutrophils are phagocytes for bacteria. Wounds can heal without white blood cells, but the risk of infection is increased. Neutrophils produce free oxygen radicals and lysosomal enzymes for host defense. The neutrophils are later removed from the wound by tissue macrophages.

Monocytes enter the wound space and become tissue macrophages. They take over control of the wound environment by the third day. Wounds cannot heal without the macrophage. These cells regulate the production of growth factors including platelet-derived growth factor (PDGF), tumor necrosis factor (TNF), and transforming growth factor (TGF)-β; thus they control protein production, matrix formation, and remodeling. Extracellular matrix (ECM) is a group of proteins in a polysaccharide gel made up of glycosaminoglycans and proteoglycans produced by the fibroblast. These proteins are structural such as collagen and elastin, or are involved in controlling cell adhesion such as fibronectin and laminin *(5)*. Thrombospondin and von Willebrand factor are other adhesion molecules. Fibronectin is also a chemoattractant for circulating monocytes and stimulates its differentiation into tissue macrophages.

The second phase of wound healing is fibroplasia and begins with macrophages and fibroblasts increasing in number in the wound, whereas white blood cells decrease as fewer enter the wound. The inflammatory response ends as the mediators of inflammation are no longer produced, and those already present are inactivated or removed by diffusion or by macrophages. Fibroplasia begins around the fifth day following injury and may continue for 2 weeks. This begins the process of matrix formation, especially collagen synthesis. Angiogenesis is the process of rebuilding the blood supply to the wound *(6)*. Fibroblasts are attracted to the wound and replicate in response to fibronectin, PDGF, fibroblast growth factor (FGF), TGF-β, and C5a, a product of the complement system. Fibroblasts produce proteoglycans and structural proteins. The cellular matrix is made up of hyaluronate and fibronectin which allow for cellular migration through chemotactic factors formed in the wound. Fibronectin binds proteins and fibroblasts in the matrix and provides a pathway along which fibroblasts can move. Fibronectin also plays a role in epithelialization and angiogenesis.

Collagen is the most common protein in the mammalian world and is produced by the fibroblast. It is a family of at least 12 proteins, rich in glycine and proline, and bound in a tight triple helix. Cross-linking between the three strands of collagen provides for a very stable molecule, resistant to breakdown. Macrophages control the release of collagen from fibroblasts through growth factors such as PDGF, epidermal growth factor (EGF), FGF, and TGF-β. Collagen is remodeled for several years in a healing wound. Elastin is the other major structural protein and contains proline and lysine. It is present as random coils, allowing both stretch and recoil. It is present in much smaller amounts than collagen.

Angiogenesis occurs by the budding of existing capillaries after stimulation by FGF. Endothelial cells proliferate and migrate through the healing wound, allowing connections between the capillaries to form a vascular network in the wound space. This capillary network provides an avenue of access for new healing factors into the wound and ends when the wound has an adequate blood supply. Hypoxia triggers angiogenesis; thus it appears as if this process if controlled by oxygen tension *(7,8)*.

Epithelialization occurs as cells migrate from the edge of the wound over a collagen-fibronectin surface. This process results in mature skin covering the wound. Scar contracture then occurs as the wound matures.

The final phase of wound repair is maturation or scar remodeling. Wound remodeling involves a number of proteins including hyaluronidase, collagenase, and elastase. Hyaluronate in the matrix is replaced by dermatan sulfate and chondroitin sulfate. These proteins reduce cell migration and allow cell differentiation. Plasmin, which is formed from plasminogen, degrades fibrin. Urokinase, produced by leukocytes, fibroblasts, endothelial cells, and keratinocytes, activates collagenase and elastase. Collagenase, which allows collagen remodeling, is secreted by macrophages, fibroblasts, epithelial cells, and white blood cells. It is able to break the collagen triple helix to allow remodeling. The scar becomes less hyperemic and less red in appearance as blood supply is reduced. The scar remodels and wound strength increases for up to 2 years following injury, yet the total collagen content of the wound does not change.

GROWTH FACTORS

Growth factors are polypeptides that initiate the growth and proliferation of cells and stimulate protein production *(2,3)*. They are named for their tissue of origin, their biological action, or the cell on which they exert their influence. Growth factors may have paracrine or autocrine function whereby they affect not only adjacent cells but also have a self-regulating effect. Some are transported plasma bound to large carrier proteins and thus serve an endocrine function. They are produced by a variety of cells including platelets, macrophages, epithelial cells, fibroblasts, and endothelial cells. Growth factors are chemoattractants for neutrophils, macrophages, fibroblasts, and endothelial cells. Growth factors bind to specific receptors on the cell surface to stimulate cell growth. Although present in only minute amounts, they exert a powerful influence on wound repair.

The growth factors involved in wound healing include PDGF, TGF-β, EGF, FGF, and insulin-like growth factor (IGF; Table 1). The platelet that is critical to the initiation of the wound-healing process is rich in growth factors. Growth factors initially released in the wound space by platelets are subsequently degraded by proteases. Other cells that have been drawn into the wound space such as inflammatory cells, fibroblasts, and epithelial cells are also involved in growth factor production. Macrophages also release factors such as TNF. Keratinocytes are stimulated by EGF, IGF-1, TGF-α, and interleukin (IL)-1. Wound remodeling occurs under the control of collagenase, produced in response to EGF, TNF, IL-1, and PDGF. Thus, all of wound healing is under the direct or indirect control of growth factors. It is reasonable then to speculate that exogenous growth factors applied to the wound may influence healing.

Table 1
Growth Factors, Their Sources and Actions

Growth factor	Cell of origin	Action
PDGF	Platelets	Chemoattractant and mitogen for fibroblasts, smooth muscle cells, macrophages, inflammatory cells.
TGF-α	Endothelium Fibroblasts Macrophages Keratinocytes Hepatocytes Eosinophiles	Mitogens for keratinocytes and fibroblasts. Angiogenesis factor.
TGF-β	Platelets Macrophage Fibroblasts Keratinocytes Lymphocytes	Chemoattractant for neutrophils, macrophages, fibroblasts. Stimulates collagen synthesis, granulation tissue formation, reepithelialization.
VEGF	Endothelial cells	Potent mitogen for endothelial cells
EGF	Platelet Kidney Salivary gland Lacrimal gland	Promotes epidermal regeneration. Increases fibroblasts in a wound.
FGF	Fibroblasts Endothelial cells Smooth muscle cells Chrondrocytes	Mitogen for endothelial cells. Angiogenesis factor.
KGF	Fibroblasts	Stimulates keratinocytes.
IGF	Liver Lung Heart Lung Pancreas Brain Muscle	Stimulate synthesis of glycogen and transport of glucose and amino acids across cell membranes. Increase collagen synthesis by the fibroblast.

PLATELET-DERIVED GROWTH FACTOR

PDGF has been studied more widely than any other growth factor and is approved for clinical use. PDGF has a molecular weight of 24,000 Daltons. It is a potent chemoattractant and mitogen for fibroblasts, smooth muscle cells, and inflammatory cells. PDGF is produced by platelets, macrophages, vascular endothelium, and fibroblasts *(9)*. It is made up of two chains, an A and a B chain, held together by disulfide bonds in three dimeric forms, AA, AB, and BB. There is a 60% amino acid homology between the two chains. Human platelets contain all three forms of PDGF in a ratio of about 12% AA, 65% AB, and 23% BB. The B chain is quite similar to the transforming gene of the simian sarcoma virus, an acute transforming retrovirus. The human proto-oncogene C-*sis* is similar the viral oncogene V-*cis* and encodes for the B chain of PDGF.

There are two PDGF receptors, α- and β-receptor. The α receptor recognizes both the A and B chains of PDGF and thus can bind to the AA form, the AB form, and the BB form. The β receptor recognizes only the B chain, and thus binds only to the BB form and weakly to the AB form. Most cells have many times more β-receptors than α-receptors. Cells with PDGF receptors include fibroblasts, vascular smooth muscle cells, and some microvascular endothelial cells. PDGF acts with TGF-β and EGF to stimulate mesenchymal cells. Although PDGF is produced by endothelial cells of the vascular system, the endothelial cells do not respond to PDGF. Rather, they work in a paracrine manner to stimulate adjacent smooth muscle cells. Smooth muscle cells also act in an autocrine fashion and produce PDGF.

PDGF is stabile to extremes of heat, a wide range of pH, and degradation by proteases. The principle cells involved in the early stages of wound healing all synthesize and secrete PDGF. Platelets, among the first cells to enter the wound, are the largest source of PDGF in the human body. Circulating monocytes are attracted to the wound and become tissue macrophages. These cells also produce PDGF. PDGF stimulates the production of fibronectin and hyaluronic acid, proteins which are important components of provisional matrix. Collagenase, a protein important in wound remodeling, is also produced in response to PDGF. There are no reported cases of a human deficient in PDGF suggesting that PDGF is critical to the survival of the individual.

PDGF has been manufactured by recombinant DNA technology. In animal models, it has been shown to improve the breaking strength of incisional wounds when applied topically as a single dose. It also accelerated acute wound healing. By 3 months, however, there was no difference in wound healing as compared with untreated wounds suggesting that although PDGF accelerated wound healing, the wound healing was quite similar to normal healing. Wounds treated with PDGF had a marked increase in inflammatory cells entering the wound, including neutrophils, monocytes, and fibroblasts. As a result of this cellular response, granulation tissue production was also increased. Despite the fact that PDGF does not directly affect keratinocytes, wounds in animals were shown to have an increased rate of epithelialization. This is probably owing to the influence from macrophages and fibroblasts attracted into the wound space by PDGF. Wounds treated topically with PDGF have an increase in neovascularization, although PDGF does not directly stimulate endothelial cells. Thus, it appears as if PDGF accelerates wound healing by accelerating the normal sequences of healing. The healed wounds appear to be normal in all aspects.

PDGF has been studied extensively in clinical trials. The effectiveness of recombinant human PDGF-BB in healing was first studied in decubitus ulcers *(10,11)*. Patients were treated with PDGF topically and followed for 28 days. There was a greater amount of wound closure in patients treated with the highest dose of PDGF. The lower doses had little effect. In another trial, patients with decubitus ulcers were treated with 100 or 300 µg/mL or placebo again for 1 month. The ulcer volume was significantly reduced in the PDGF-treated patients. No significant toxicity related to PDGF was noted. Complete wound closure was not an end point in either study and thus the question regarding whether PDGF could accomplish complete wound healing in humans was not answered.

A randomized prospective double blind trial of recombinant PDGF-BB was performed in patients with diabetic neurotrophic foot ulcers *(12)*. Patients were treated with PDGF at a dose of 2.2 µg/cm^2 of wound in vehicle, carboxymethylcellulose, or vehicle alone for 20 weeks or until complete wound closure occurred. Patients had wounds of at least 8-week duration, were considered to be free of infection, and had an adequate blood supply as demonstrated by a transcutaneous oxygen tension (TcPO$_2$) of at least 30 mmHg. All wounds were debrided by completely excising the wound prior to entry into the study and as needed during the trial. In these patients with chronic nonhealing wounds, 48% healed following treatment with PDGF, whereas only 25% healed with vehicle alone ($p < 0.01$). The median reduction in wound area was 98.8% for PDGF-treated patients but only 82.1% for those treated with vehicle. There were no significant differences in the incidence or severity of adverse events in either group. This was the first clinical trial to suggest that a growth factor, PDGF, could be applied topically and be effective and safe in accelerating the healing of chronic wounds in humans.

In another trial using recombinant human PDGF in the treatment of similar patients with diabetic foot ulcers, those patients treated with PDGF-BB had an increase in the incidence of complete wound closure of 43% as compared with placebo ($p = 0.007$). PDGF also decreased the time to achieve complete wound closure by 32% ($p = 0.013$) when compared with the placebo.

In reviewing patients treated with PDGF or vehicle alone, it was noted that those patients receiving the best wound care healed better whether PDGF or vehicle was applied. Debridement proved to be critically important. The benefits from PDGF will be minimized if the wounds are not treated properly. The vehicle, carboxymethylcellulose, was tested to determine if it was inert in wound healing. It did provide a moist environment for wound healing but did not improve healing significantly. PDGF is approved for use in the United States and is sold as Regranex.

TRANSFORMING GROWTH FACTOR

The growth factor studied most extensively after PDGF is TGF-β. Transforming growth factors are made up of two polypeptide chains, α and β. TGF-α has a 30% amino acid homology with EGF. It is named because of its ability to reversibly stimulate the growth of cells. Cancer cells do this also. TGF-α is produced by many different cells including macrophages, keratinocytes, hepatocytes, and eosinophiles *(13)*. TGF-α and EGF are mitogens for keratinocytes and fibroblasts, but TGF-α is a more potent angiogenesis factor. Both TGF-α and EGF bind to the EGF receptor but their specific actions may be different partly owing to differences in their binding. As yet there have been no clinical trials of wound healing with TGF-α.

TGF-β has no amino acid homology with TGF-α or any other group of growth factors. TGF-β is a group of proteins which can reversibly inhibit growth of cells especially those of ectodermal origin. TGF-β is structurally similar to bone morphogenic protein.

TGF-β is produced by a variety of cells including platelets, macrophages, fibroblasts, keratinocytes, and lymphocytes. TGF-β is a chemoattractant for neutrophils, macrophages, and fibroblasts and stimulates collagen synthesis, granulation tissue formation, and reepithelialization *(14,15)*. Nearly all cells have receptors for TGF-β and have the potential to respond to it. TGF-β can stimulate or inhibit the growth or differentiation of many different cells. It appears as if TGF-β is the most widely acting group of growth factors.

There have been three forms of TGF-β isolated, TGF-β_1, TGF-β_2, and TGF-β_3. The actions of the three different forms of TGF-β are very similar. TGF-βs have a molecular weight of about 25,000. They reversibly stimulate growth of fibroblasts and thus received their name. TGF-βs are potent stimulators of chemotaxis in inflammatory cells and trigger cells to produce ECM. Thus, the TGF-β is important in wound healing. TGF-β may be associated with scarring. Increased TFG-β has been found in fibroblasts of human hypertrophic burn scar and in keloids *(16–19)*. TGF-β was tested in diabetic wounds in three different doses in a collagen sponge *(20)*. There was also a standard care arm in the trial. There was a significant improvement in the healing of diabetic ulcers treated with each of the three doses of TGF-β compared with collagen sponge. In this study, the patients treated with standard care healed better than those patients treated with TGF-β. The role of TGF-β in treating patients with chronic wounds remains undetermined.

VASCULAR ENDOTHELIAL GROWTH FACTOR

Vascular endothelial growth factor (VEGF) is quite similar to PDGF. It has a molecular weight of 45,000 Daltons. It has a 24% amino acid homology to the B chain of PDGF. VEGF, however, binds different receptors than PDGF and has different actions. Although it is a potent mitogen for endothelial cells, it is not a mitogen for fibroblasts or vascular smooth muscle cells as is PDGF. VEGF is angiogenic and may play a role in wound healing by way of this property. VEGF antibodies reduce angiogenesis and granulation tissue formation *(21)*. There has been interest in using VEGF to stimulate the development of collateral arteries in patients with vascular disease, but as yet there is no proof that it will be of benefit clinically in wound healing.

EPIDERMAL GROWTH FACTOR

EGF is a small molecule similar to TGF-α. EGF is produced by the platelet and found in high quantities in the early phase of wound healing. The active form has a molecular weight of 6200 Daltons. EGF is produced by the kidney, salivary glands, and lacrimal glands, and thus is found in high concentrations in urine, saliva, and tears. EGF promotes epidermal regeneration in pigs and corneal epithelialization in rabbits. It also increases the tensile strength of wounds in animals. EGF increases wound healing by stimulating the production of proteins such as fibronectin. Although EGF does not stimulate collagen production, it increases the number of fibroblasts in the wound. These cells produce collagen and improve the wound strength. EGF shares a receptor with TGF-α.

EGF has been studied in a randomized trial of healing of skin graft donor sites *(22)*. Donor sites treated with silver sulfadiazine containing EGF had an accelerated rate of epidermal regeneration as compared with patients treated with silver sulfadiazine alone. EGF reduced the healing time by 1.5 days. These results did not have clinical significance;

however, this was the first trial to demonstrate a benefit from treatment with a single growth factor in human wounds. In another trial, EGF was used in an open label study with a crossover design in patients with chronic wounds *(23)*. Patients with chronic wounds were treated with silver sulfadiazine. In those who did not heal, silver sulfadiazine containing EGF was then used. Improvement was noted in many of these patients. The results of these studies suggest that EGF may be of benefit in wound healing, although as yet, there is not enough data to confirm this.

FIBROBLAST GROWTH FACTOR

FGF is a group of heparin bound growth factors. There are two forms: acidic FGF (aFGF) and basic FGF (bFGF). Both molecules have molecular weights of 15,000. There is a 50% amino acid homology among the two molecules. They are commonly bound to heparin or to heparan sulfate, which protects them from enzymatic degradation. FGF can be produced by fibroblasts, endothelial cells, smooth muscle cells, and chondrocytes. In addition to endothelial cells, FGFs can stimulate fibroblasts, keratinocytes, chondrocytes, and myoblasts. There are at least four different FGF receptors identified thus far. They appear to have a similar function. Both aFGF and bFGF are found in the ECM in the bound form. Matrix degradation proteins then acts to release aFGF or bFGF. Acidic FGF is similar to endothelial cell growth factor, whereas bFGF is similar to endothelial cell growth factor II. Both aFGF and bFGF are similar to keratinocyte growth factor (KGF). These proteins are mitogens for cells of mesodermal and neuroectodermal origin. FGFs are potent mitogens for endothelial cells and function as angiogenesis factors by stimulating growth of new blood vessels through proliferation of capillary endothelial cells. To date, there are no clinical trials which have proven FGF to be of benefit in clinical wound healing.

KERATINOCYTE GROWTH FACTOR

KGF is closely related to the FGFs. It is a protein with a molecular weight of 2800 and has a significant amino acid homology with the FGFs. Although KGF is found only in fibroblasts, it stimulates keratinocytes, not fibroblasts. It may share a receptor with FGF. KGF-2 was used in a randomized prospective blinded trial of patients with venous stasis ulcers *(24)*. There appeared to be a benefit from treatment with KGF-2. The role of KGF-2 in wound healing is still, however, unclear.

INSULIN-LIKE GROWTH FACTOR

IGFs, or somatomedins, are proteins that have a 50% amino acid homology with proinsulin and have insulin-like activity *(25)*. There are two forms of this growth factor, IGF-1 and IGF-2. IGF-1 and IGF-2 are anabolic hormones that can stimulate the synthesis of glycogen and glycosaminoglycans. They can also increase the transport of glucose and amino acids across cell membranes. They increase collagen synthesis by fibroblasts. At this time, there are no clinical trials reported using IGFs. Both are secreted as large precursor molecules that are then cleaved to an active form. IGF-1 is identical to Somatomedin-C, whereas IGF-2 is similar to somatomedin. These growth factors are found in the liver, heart, lung, pancreas, brain, and muscle. IGF-2 is also synthesized by many different tissues but is particularly prominent during fetal development and plays a significant role in fetal growth. IGF-1 and IGF-2 have separate receptors. The actions of pituitary growth hormone may be mediated through IGF-1. IGF-1 then causes cell division. IGF-1 is produced predominantly in the liver. It is found in high concentrations in platelets and is released into the wound when clotting occurs. Levels of IGF-1 and IGF-2 depend on many different factors, such as age, gender, nutritional status, and hormone level. Growth hormone is a regulator of IGF-1 and IGF-2 as are prolactin, thyroid hormone, and sex hormones. Elevated levels of somatomedins are found in patients with acromegaly.

PLATELET RELEASATES

In the first 2 days following injury, growth factors are produced and released by platelets. Thereafter, growth factor production is taken over by macrophages. Within the α-granules of the human platelet are multiple growth factors that are released when platelets are activated and degranulate. These include PDGF, TGF-β, FGF, EGF, platelet factor 4, platelet-derived angiogenesis factor, and β-thromboglobulin. A purified platelet releasate can be prepared by stimulating platelets to release the contents of their α-granules by using thrombin. Use of a platelet releasate in wound healing has theoretical advantages. The growth factors that are released are identical to and in the same proportion as those factors normally brought into the wound by the platelet. Preparation of a platelet releasate is simple and inexpensive because the platelets can be harvested from peripheral blood. Platelets readily release the contents of their α-granules when stimulated with thrombin. Growth factors are preserved in banked blood. Thus, large quantities of growth factors can be retrieved from the platelets of pooled human blood. There may, however, be disadvantages to using a platelet releasate. Not all growth factors promote wound healing. There is a signal for wound healing to stop. A platelet releasate might concentrate factors that heal the wound as well as those which signal the wound healing process to end. There is also the possibility of transmission of an infectious agent if the platelet releasate applied to the wound is from another individual. This risk could be reduced if the releasate were harvested from a single donor or from the patient himself.

There has been considerable experience with the use of platelet releasates in wound healing. A preliminary report described the use of an autologous platelet releasate in six patients with chronic lower extremity ulcers from connective tissue diseases. A homologous platelet releasate was used to treat 11 patients with leg ulcers from diabetes and 8 patients with leg ulcers secondary to chronic venous insufficiency *(26)*. No benefit was observed from using the platelet releasate; however, this study pointed out the importance of topical growth factor application only in the context of good wound care and in a narrowly defined group of patients. Growth factors cannot be expected to have a positive influence on wound healing unless they are applied in a comprehensive wound care program. The underlying etiology of these wounds such as venous hypertension, diabetic neuropathy, or ischemia must be addressed. In another trial, 49 patients with chronic wounds were treated with an autologous platelet releasate *(27)*. There appeared to be a correlation with complete wound healing and initial wound size. This was the first clinical trial to suggest a benefit from a platelet releasate applied topically.

A randomized trial of platelet releasate vs a platelet buffer was conducted in patients with ulcers secondary to diabetes, peripheral vascular disease, venous insufficiency, or vasculitis *(28)*. This study suggested a benefit from the treatment of leg ulcers in these 32 patients from a topically applied growth factor preparation. The growth factor preparation was added to microcrystalline collagen, a potent stimulator of platelets. The exact contribution from the collagen to the healing of these wounds was not defined.

Two other trials suggested a benefit from a platelet releasate. In one trial, patients were treated for 3 months with silver sulfadiazine *(29)*. Only 3 of the 23 lower extremity wounds healed; however, when the platelet releasate was then applied, the remaining ulcers healed. Another study of 70 patients suggested a similar benefit from a platelet releasate *(30)*. Despite evidence that platelet releasates are of benefit, another trial observed very different result. In a randomized prospective double-blind placebo controlled trial, topical platelet releasate was applied to the leg ulcers of 26 patients. The ulcers were secondary to diabetes, peripheral vascular disease, or chronic venous insufficiency *(31)*. Wounds treated with the platelet releasate increased in size that is worsened, whereas wounds in the control group improved. This study suggested that a platelet releasate might be detrimental to wound healing.

Thirteen patients with diabetic neurotrophic ulcers were enrolled in a randomized trial of a platelet releasate vs saline placebo *(32)*. A benefit was seen in those treated with the platelet releasate. By 20 weeks of therapy, five of seven patients healed using the platelet releasate, whereas only two of six patients healed using the saline placebo. By 24 weeks of treatment, three additional patients in the control group healed, suggesting that the platelet releasate stimulated more rapid healing but did not result in a greater proportion of healed wounds.

Although there is some evidence to suggest that they may be of benefit from a platelet releasate applied topically to lower extremity wounds, the inconsistency of the results as well as the concern about transmission of infectious agents in using a homologous preparation leaves their role in human wound healing undefined.

Living skin equivalents (LSEs) are approved for use in humans. These LSEs are tissue grafts made from keratinocytes and dermal fibroblasts harvested from neonatal foreskin using tissue-engineering biotechnology *(33)*. A graft cultured on a synthetic scaffold can be cryopreserved to prolong the viability of the cells and their metabolic activity *(34)*. When placed on a wound, an LSE serves as a drug-delivery system providing matrix proteins and growth factors including PDGF, TGF-β, VEGF, and KGF to the wound *(35)*. LSEs have no professional antigen-presenting cells, such as endothelial cells, leukocytes, Langerhans cells, or dermal dendritic cells; thus, they do not activate T cells and cause rejection. Fibroblasts and kerotinocytes do not express HLA class II antigens and thus do not activate unprimed allogenic T cells. The cells of the LSE are preprogrammed to die and are replaced by the patient's own cells in the healed wound. They stimulate epithelial cells to grow across the wound from the margin. LSEs have been shown to be of benefit in healing diabetic ulcers in certain cases *(36)*.

In summary, growth factors exert a powerful influence over wound healing, controlling the growth, differentiation, and metabolism of cells. There are only a few reports in which growth factors applied topically can exert a positive influence on wound repair;

however, there is no doubt that they control wound healing. It is likely that their actions will be defined and we will thus be able to control the wound environment to achieve a complete and durable wound healing.

REFERENCES

1. Edington HE. Wound healing, in *Basic Science Review for Surgeons* (Simmons RL, Steed DL, eds.), WB Saunders, Philadelphia, 1992, pp. 41–55.
2. McGrath MH. Peptide growth factors and wound healing. *Clin Plast Surg* 1990;17:421–432.
3. Rothe MJ, Falanga V. Growth factors and wound healing. *Clin Dermatol* 1992;9:553–559.
4. Steed DL. Mediators of inflammation, in *Basic Science Review for Surgeons* (Simmons RL, Steed DL, eds.), WB Saunders, Philadelphia, 1992, pp. 12–29.
5. Grinnel F. Fibronectin and wound healing. *Am J Dermatopathol* 1982;4:185–192.
6. Folkman T, Lansburn M. Angiogenic factors. *Science* 1987;235:442–447.
7. Knighton DR, Hunt TK, Schewenstuhl A. Oxygen tension regulates the expression of angiogenesis factor by macrophages. *Science* 1983;221:1283–1290.
8. Knighton DR, Silver IA, Hunt TK. Regulation of wound healing angiogenesis: effect of oxygen gradients and inspired oxygen concentration. *Surgery* 1981;90:262–269.
9. Lynch SE, Nixon JC. Role of platelet-derived growth factor in wound healing: synergistic effects with growth factors. *Proc Natl Acad Sci USA* 1987;84:7696–7697.
10. Robson M, Phillips L. Platelet-derived growth factor BB for the treatment of chronic pressure ulcers. *Lancet* 1992;339:23–25.
11. Mustoe T, Cutler N. A phase II study to evaluate recombinant platelet-derived growth factor-BB in the treatment of stage 3 and 4 pressure ulcers. *Arch Surg* 1994;129:212–219.
12. Steed DL, Diabetic Ulcer Study Group: clinical evaluation of recombinant human platelet-derived growth factor for the treatment of lower extremity diabetic ulcers. *J Vasc Surg* 1995;21:71–81.
13. Sporn MB, Robert AB. Transforming growth factor. *JAMA* 1989;262:938–941.
14. Assoian R, Komoriya A, Meyers C, Miller D, Sporn M. Transforming growth factor-beta in human platelets. Identification of a major storage site, purification, and characterization. *J Biol Chem* 1983;258:7155–7160.
15. O'Kane S, Ferguson M. Transforming growth factor beta and wound healing. *Int J Biochem Cell Biol* 1997;29:63–78.
16. Ghahary A, Shen Y, Scott PG, Gong Y, Tredget E. Enhanced expression of mRNA for transforming growth factor-beta, type I and type III procollagen in human post-burn hypertrophic scar tissues. *J Lab Clin Med* 1993;122:465–473.
17. Schmid P, Itin P, Cherry G, Bi C, Cox D. Enhanced expression of transforming growth factor-beta type I and type II receptors in wound granulation tissue and hypertrophic scar. *Am J Pathol* 1998;152:485–493.
18. Wang R, Ghahary A, Shen Q, Scott P, Roy K, Tredget E. Hypertrophic scar tissues and fibroblasts produce more transforming growth factor-beta 1 mRNA and protein than normal skin and cells. *Wound Repair Regen* 2000;8:128–137.
19. Lee T, Chin G, Kim W, Chau D, Gittes G, Longaker M. Expression of transforming growth factor beta 1, 2, and 3 proteins in keloids. *Ann Plast Surg* 1999;43:179–184.
20. McPherson J, Pratt B, Steed D, Robson M. Healing of diabetic foot ulcers using transforming growth factor—beta in collagen sponge. Abstracts of the meeting of the European Tissue Repair Society, 1999.
21. Howdieshell T, Callaway D, Webb W, et al. Antibody neutralization of vascular endothelial growth factor inhibits wound granulation tissue formation. *J Surg Res* 2001;96:173–182.
22. Brown GL, Curtsinger L, Nanney LB. Enhancement of wound healing by topical treatment with epidermal growth factor. *N Engl J Med* 1989;321:76–80.

23. Brown GL, Curtsinger L. Stimulation of healing of chronic wounds by epidermal growth factor. *Plast Recontr Surg* 1991;88:189–194.
24. Robson M, Steed D, Jensen J. Keratinocyte growth factor 2 in the treatment of venous leg ulcers. Abstracts of the World Congress of Wound Healing, 2000.
25. Spencer EM, Skover G, Hunt TK. Somatomedins: do they play a pivotal role in wound healing? in *Growth Factors and Other Aspects of Wound Healing: Biological and Clinical Implications* (Barbul A, Pines E, Caldwell M, eds.), Alan R Liss, New York, 1988.
26. Steed DL, Goslen B, Hambley R, et al. Clinical trials with purified platelet releasate, in *Clinical and Experimental Approaches to Dermal and Epidermal Repair: Normal and Chronic Wounds* (Barbul A, ed.), Alan R Liss, New York, 1990, pp. 103–113.
27. Knighton DR, Ciresi KF. Classifications and treatment of chronic nonhealing wounds. *Ann Surg* 1986;104:322–330.
28. Knighton DR, Ciresi K. Stimulation of repair in chronic, nonhealing, cutaneous ulcers using platelet-derived wound healing formula. *Surg Gynecol Obstet* 1990;170:56–60.
29. Atri SC, Misra J. Use of homologous platelet factors in achieving total healing of recalcitrant skin ulcers. *Surgery* 1990;108:508–512.
30. Holloway GA, Steed DL, DeMarco MJ, et al. A randomized controlled dose response trial of activated platelet supernatant topical CT-102 (APST) in chronic nonhealing wounds in patients with diabetes mellitus. *Wounds* 1993;5:198–206.
31. Krupski WC, Reilly LM. A prospective randomized trial of autologous platelet-derived wound healing factors for treatment of chronic nonhealing wounds: a preliminary report. *J Vasc Surg* 1991;14:526–532.
32. Steed DL, Goslen JB, Holloway GA. CT-102 activated platelet supernatant, topical versus placebo: a randomized prospective double blind trial in healing of chronic diabetic foot ulcers. *Diabetes Care* 1992;15:1598–1604.
33. Rennekampff H, Kiessig V, Hansbrough J. Current concepts in the development of cultured skin replacements. *J Surg Res* 1996;62:288–295.
34. Hansbrough J, Franco E. Skin replacements. *Clin Plast Surg* 1998;25:407–423.
35. Yannas I. Studies on the biological activity of the dermal regeneration template. *Wound Repair Regen* 1998;6:518–524.
36. Pollak R, Edington H, Jensen J. A human dermal replacement for the treatment of diabetic foot ulcers. *Wounds* 1997;9:175–183.

21

Living Skin Equivalents for the Diabetic Foot Ulcer

Thanh Dinh, DPM and Aristidis Veves, MD, DSc

INTRODUCTION

Foot ulceration remains the leading diabetic complication requiring hospitalization *(1)*. Treatment of the diabetic foot ulcer is often a complex process that involves a multidisciplinary approach. Despite best efforts, failure to heal a diabetic foot ulcer can lead to amputation *(2)*. As the incidence of diabetes in the general population is expected to rise, the prevalence of ulcerations and amputations will follow. The resulting cost to society can be measured in direct costs attributed to treatment, as well as indirect costs in lost productivity. The total cost of diabetic foot ulcerations in the United States has been estimated to approach $4 billion annually, as extrapolated from the costs of ulcer care and amputations *(3)*. However the costs are measured, diabetic foot ulcerations represent a major public health challenge of growing proportions.

TREATMENT

Over the last decade, significant strides have been made in the treatment of diabetic foot ulcerations. Prevention remains the best means of averting the potentially devastating results of diabetic foot ulcerations. It has been estimated that up to 80% of diabetic foot ulcers are preventable with routine clinical examination of the "at-risk" foot *(4)*. In the event that a foot ulceration develops, a multi-disciplinary team approach to treatment has been demonstrated to be the most beneficial and cost-effective method, in addition to preventing amputation *(5)*.

Treatment of diabetic foot ulcerations varies greatly depending on the severity of the ulceration as well as the presence of ischemia. However, the cornerstones of treatment for full-thickness ulcers should consist of: adequate debridement, offloading of pressure, treatment of infection, and local wound care. Despite good wound care incorporating all of the above treatment principles, one study demonstrated only 24% of ulcers healed after 12 weeks and only 31% of ulcers healed after 20 weeks *(6)*.

Evidence of poor wound healing despite strict adherence to wound care guidelines has led to further investigation into the pathophysiology of the diabetic foot ulcer. The observed "faulty wound healing" has been attributed to a disruption in the normal healing process *(7)*. This disruption results in cessation or stalling of wound healing, with a resultant hostile chronic wound environment.

From: *The Diabetic Foot, Second Edition*
Edited by: A. Veves, J. M. Giurini, and F. W. LoGerfo © Humana Press Inc., Totowa, NJ

IMPAIRED WOUND HEALING

The normal wound healing process involves the timely expression of numerous growth factors that promote cellular migration and proliferation, production of new connective tissue matrix and collagen deposition *(8)*. All three of these physiological processes are altered in the diabetic state and contribute to the poor healing observed in diabetic foot ulcers. The importance of growth factors and their function in normal wound healing is discussed elsewhere in this book. However, in discussion of advanced wound care products, it is important to recognize the unique biochemical characteristics of the chronic diabetic foot ulcer in order to understand how living skin equivalents influence wound healing.

Normal wound healing transitions through three overlapping phases: inflammation, proliferation, and maturation. Instead of progressing in an orderly and timely fashion, it is now clear that diabetic ulcers are "stuck" in the inflammation phase of the wound healing process. During this delay there is a cessation of epidermal growth and migration over the wound surface *(9)*. A common characteristic of all chronic wounds is the elevation of the levels of matrix metalloproteinases (MMPs) that results in increased proteolytic activity and inactivation of the growth factors that involved in the wound healing process *(10)*. Additionally, these chronic wounds have been found to exhibit deficiencies in growth factors and cytokines along with elevated levels of inhibitory proteases. As a result, impaired wound healing is manifested in aberrant protein synthesis, cellular activity, and growth factor secretion.

At present, the term chronic wound simply refers to a wound that has been disrupted during the normal, controlled inflammatory phase or the cellular proliferative phase. However, a number of studies have attempted to describe the chronic wound based on the length of time present and failure to demonstrate significant improvement within that time interval. In a Consensus Development Conference, the American Diabetes Association defined a chronic wound as one that failed to "continuously progress towards healing." Furthermore, wounds that remained unhealed after 4 weeks was a source of concern, and were associated with worse outcomes, including amputation *(11)*. Regardless of the definition, what remains clear is the fact that the chronic wound fails to heal in a timely fashion and this can be attributed to an altered biochemical wound environment.

Treatment of the chronic wound initially focused on bolus doses of exogenous growth factors. Topically applied recombinant human platelet-derived growth factor (rhPDGF)-BB (becaplermin) in conjunction with good wound care, significantly increased the incidence of complete wound closure and significantly reduced the time to complete closure of chronic diabetic neuropathic ulcers *(12)*. As a result of the promising findings, the development of a replacement tissue to overcome the deficiencies found in chronic wounds was undertaken.

SKIN GRAFTING

Skin is an important organ, covering the entire body and providing the first line of defense against many offending organisms. When skin integrity is lost, infection, illness, major disability, and even death can occur. Therefore, coverage of large skin defects is essential for protection against disease and disability. The birth of skin grafting can be traced back to 1869, when a Swiss surgeon named Reverdin reported on the hastening of the healing of granulating wounds by what he called "epidermic" grafts *(13)*. These "epidermic" grafts were allografts of superficial skin excised in small (approx 2 × 3 mm) pinches. Since its inception, the technique of skin grafting has been perfected to allow for coverage of skin defects in various scenarios such as burns, traumatic injuries with skin loss, epidermolysis bullosa, and chronic wounds.

Although skin grafting provides a valuable and immediate means of soft tissue coverage in most wounds, there are significant disadvantages to its use in the diabetic foot ulcer. The most obvious advantage to skin grafting is the immediate provision of skin coverage. In addition to immediate coverage, skin grafting also appears to stimulate wound healing with revascularization of the skin graft to the host bed. However, in the patient with diabetes, the skin from the donor site may also exhibit faulty wound healing characteristics that could potentially result in secondary wound complications at the donor site. Therefore investigation into suitable skin substitutes with skin-like characteristics was undertaken for use in instances where a donor site was unavailable, or undesirable.

Since the 1970s, scientists have been able to grow human skin cells in vitro *(14)*. With the advent of cultured epithelial autografts, the problem of allograft rejections was eliminated, as was the problem of skin donor availability *(15)*. However, cultured epithelial autografts could spontaneously blister and also took time to produce, typically a couple of weeks *(16)*. And so the search for an optimal wound dressing with more immediate availability continued.

In 1987, the term "tissue engineering" was coined at a National Science Foundation meeting *(17)*. This term described the application of engineering to the development of biological substitutes to restore, maintain, or improve function. The goal at this time was to create a readily available tissue replacement with the biological and pharmacological properties of human skin *(18)*. Advances in tissue engineering over the last decade has lead to the development of living skin equivalents (LSE) that have shown effectiveness in diabetic foot ulcers compared to standard care and has been used as adjunctive therapy for the difficult to heal wounds. LSEs have also demonstrated effectiveness in other wounds such as burns, venous ulcers, decubitus ulcers, and epidermolysis bullosa.

LIVING SKIN EQUIVALENTS

Cadaveric Allograft

Cadaveric allograft skin has been used to provide temporary coverage for full-thickness burns by most burn centers in the United States *(19)*. Cadaver skin closes and protects the wound, and therefore can be lifesaving in instances of large skin defects such as burns. The cadaver skin is often removed at a later date, leaving a well-vascularized wound base that makes subsequent skin grafting more readily to take. Unfortunately, the demand for cadaver skin is high and is often not available for immediate use. It can also pose problems with graft rejection and transmission of disease because many transmittable diseases cannot be screened effectively and some diseases may not have been expressed at the time the skin is harvested *(20,21)*. Cadaver allograft skin can be treated chemically to decrease fears of transmittable diseases, however, this results in an inert acellular dermal matrix *(22)*. Cryopreservation affords longer storage and immediate availability, but also make the allograft more susceptible to sloughing off the wound bed.

Epidermal Replacements

The technology for epidermal replacement was developed in the 1970s *(23)*. Epithelial cells were procured from a full-thickness skin biopsy, thus allowing the use of a patient's own keratinocytes to promote wound closure. Serial cultivation resulted in expansion of the epithelial cells into broad sheets, which were recultured until confluent thin layers of undifferentiated cells were obtained. These sheets were then attached to a petroleum gauze carrier for easier handling.

There were high hopes that use of epidermal replacements would be beneficial in the treatment of burn patients. As a result, these cultured autologous grafts were used in a wide range of burn centers *(24,25)*. However, engraftment rates were suboptimal and, when successful, the epithelium was fragile and showed a lack of durability *(26)*.

At present, there exists only one cultured epidermal autograft produced and manufactured in the United States (Epicel, Genzyme Tissue Repair Corporation, Cambridge, MA). Because the grafts are grown from a patient's own skin cells, they are not rejected by the patient's immune system. However, this technique is expensive, requires a biopsy and takes 2–3 weeks to culture sufficient epithelium for grafting. Furthermore, Epicel sheets are thin and fragile and must be handled with extreme care during and after application. Studies have found that healed epithelium can be very fragile and the skin prone to contraction and breakdown *(26)*. Many of the imperfections associated with epithelial wound closure may be attributable to the absence of a dermal element because the epidermis is fragile without a dermal bed. The dermal element plays an important role in wound healing, affecting epithelial migration, differentiation, attachment, and growth. Therefore, efforts to develop dermal analogs were undertaken.

Dermal Replacements

Initial developments of dermal replacements consisted of a composite graft with a collagen-based dermal analog of bovine collagen and an outer temporary epidermal substitute layer of silicone (Integra, Integra Life Sciences Corporation, Plainsboro, NJ) *(27)*. The dermal replacement layer of Integra consists of a porous matrix of fibers of bovine type 1 collagen that is crosslinked with chondroitin-6-sulfate, and glycosaminoglycan (GAG) extracted from shark cartilage. The porous matrix is designed to serve as a template for infiltration of the patient's fibroblasts, macrophages, lymphocytes, and capillaries. The outer silicone layer of Integra serves as a temporary epidermis and allows for water flux, protection from microbial invasion, and prevention of burn wound desiccation. Although Integra has been successfully used on burns, it is not currently indicated for use in diabetic foot ulcers or other chronic wounds. It is also important to note that implantation is a two-stage procedure. After application of the Integra, the neodermis requires approx 3 weeks for vascularization to the wound bed. Following this, the temporary silicone layer is removed and a second operative procedure is required for application of an autograft. As a result, the process can be both lengthy and costly.

DERMAGRAFT

Dermal replacements underwent further evolution with the introduction of a living dermal equivalent that contained allogenic neonatal fibroblasts impregnated on a bioabsorbable polyglactin mesh (Dermagraft, Advanced Tissue Sciences Inc, La Jolla, CA).

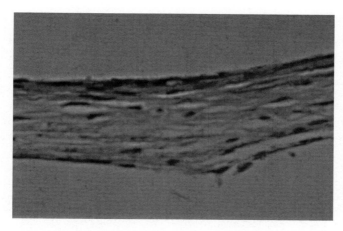

Fig. 1. The cross section of Dermagraft showing collagen fibers in parallel bundles.

There are three major production steps in the manufacturing of Dermagraft. First, fibroblasts from human neonatal foreskin are screened, enzymatically treated, and either banked or placed into a tissue culture. Next, allogenic dermal fibroblasts are seeded onto a bioabsorbable polyglactin mesh. Finally, the cells proliferate and produce dermal collagen, growth factors, GAGs, and fibronectin during a 2- to 3-week period.

The final structure is similar to the metabolically active papillary dermis of neonatal skin. Demagraft contains growth factors and matrix proteins instrumental to wound healing such as: platelet-derived growth factor (PDGF)-A, insulin-like growth factor (IGF), mitogen for keratinocytes (KGF), heparin binding epidermal growth factor (HBEGF), transforming growth factors (TGF-α, TGF-β_1, TGF-β_3), vascular endothelial growth factor (VEGF), and secreted protein acidic and rich in cysteine (SPARC). The matrix proteins and growth factors remain active after implantation onto the wound bed *(27,28)*. No exogenous human or animal collagen, GAG, or growth factors are added. Dermagraft has been shown to stimulate angiogenesis possibly by upregulating cellular adhesion molecules in response to growth factor stimulation *(28)*. Preclinical studies in animals indicated that Dermagraft incorporates itself quickly into the wound and vascularized well. Preclinical data also indicated that Dermagraft might limit wound contraction and scarring.

Dermagraft is designed to replace the dermal layer of the skin and to provide stimulus to improve wound healing. The histological cross-section shows human collagen fibers arranged in parallel bundles (Fig. 1). Dermagraft is supplied as a 2-inch by 3-inch graft in a sealed plastic bag (Fig. 2) on dry ice. Dermagraft must be stored at –70°C. Dermagraft must be rapidly thawed and warmed before application on to the wound. The top of the package is cut and the tissue is rinsed with sterile saline. The package is translucent so the wound can be traced and Dermagraft is cut to the wound size. It is then can be removed form the package and applied to the wound. Secondary dressing is used to keep the implant in place and keep the wound moist. Dermagraft acts on wound by cell colonization and provision of growth factors and cytokines. Because of cryopreservation, the cells can lose some viability and therapeutic effect *(29)*.

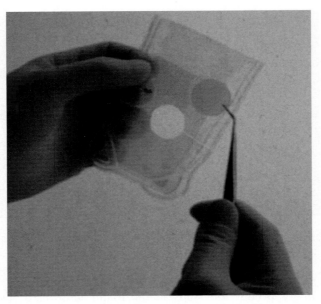

Fig. 2. Dermagraft is supplied in a translucent bag. It can be used to trace the ulcer then cut the specimen to fit the ulcer.

EFFICACY OF DERMAGRAFT IN DIABETIC FOOT ULCERS

A pilot study was performed to assess the efficacy of Dermagraft diabetic foot ulcers for the duration of 12 weeks *(30)*. Fifty patients were enrolled and divided into four treatment groups. Group A patients received one piece of Dermagraft weekly for a total of eight pieces and eight applications plus control treatment. Group B patients received two pieces of Dermagraft every 2 weeks for a total of eight pieces and four applications plus control treatment. Group C patients received one piece of Dermagraft every 2 weeks for a total of four pieces and four applications plus control treatment. Group D patients received conventional treatment only. Patients in all groups had very similar demographic characteristics. After 12 weeks, group A patients achieved more wound healing than other groups. Wound closure in the group A patients (50%) after 12 weeks was significantly better than the control group (8%, $p = 0.03$). There were no reported adverse events in this study.

As a result of the encouraging pilot study, a large, prospective, randomized control study was conducted to investigate the effectiveness of Dermagraft on diabetic foot ulcers *(31)*. A total of 281 patients were enrolled at 20 centers. Patients were randomized to receive either Dermagraft weekly for a total of eight applications or only conventional wound care. One-hundred and twenty-six patients were enrolled in the standard wound care group, with 31.7% healing rate by the end of week 12. One-hundred and nine patients received Dermagraft treatment, resulting in a 38.5% healing rate by the end of week 12. The healing rates between the two groups were found to be a statistically nonsignificant result ($p = 0.14$).

Further analysis revealed that a specific range of metabolic activity of Dermagraft was associated with higher complete healing rate by week 12 *(32)*. Seventy-six patients received metabolically active products at least at the first application, and 48.7% of these achieved wound healing by week 12 ($p = 0.008$). Sixty-one patients received

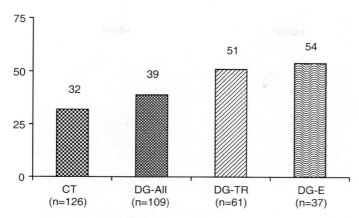

Fig. 3. Results of Dermagraft study. A 32% of the control (CT) achieved wound healing compared to 39% of patients who received Dermagraft (DG-All) treatment ($p = 0.14$). Patients who received metabolically active products at the first two applications and the majority of the following application (DG-TR) achieved 51% healing rate by week 12 ($p = 0.006$). Patients who received metabolically active products at all time (DG-E) achieved 54% healing rate ($p = 0.007$).

metabolically active products at the first two applications and as well as many of the subsequent applications, and 50.8% of these patient had complete wound closure by week 12 ($p = 0.006$). Thirty-seven patients received the correct metabolically active products at all applications, and they achieved the highest healing rate of 54.1% by week 12 ($p = 0.0067$) (Fig. 3). A supplemental study using Dermagraft within the therapeutic range reported healing rates of diabetic foot ulcers above 50% at 12 weeks *(33)*.

A subsequent study involving more centers and larger patient population was concluded recently. In a randomized, controlled, multicenter study at 35 centers throughout the United States, 314 patients were randomized to either the Dermagraft treatment group or control (conventional therapy) *(34)*. Except for the application of Dermagraft (applied weekly for up to 7 weeks), treatment of study ulcers was identical for patients in both groups. All patients received pressure-reducing footwear and were allowed to be ambulatory during the study.

The results demonstrated that patients with chronic diabetic foot ulcers of more than 6 weeks duration experienced a significant clinical benefit when treated with Dermagraft vs patients treated with conventional therapy alone. With regard to complete wound closure by week 12, 30% of Dermagraft patients healed compared with 18.3% of control patients ($p = 0.023$). The overall incidence of adverse events was similar for both the Dermagraft and control groups, but the Dermagraft group experienced significantly fewer ulcer-related adverse events.

COMPOSITE REPLACEMENTS

Composite replacements are allogenic, bilayered skin equivalents consisting of a well-differentiated human epidermis and a dermal layer of bovine collagen containing human fibroblasts. A composite cultured skin (CSS, Ortec International Inc, New York, NY) was developed that consists of neonatal keratinocytes and fibroblasts cultured in distinct bovine type 1 collagen layer. This has limited use and studied for patients with burns and epidermolysis bullosa *(35)*.

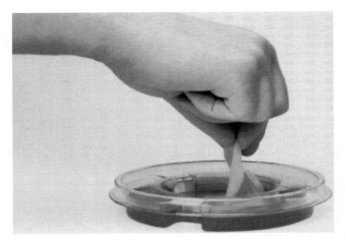

Fig. 4. Apligraf is manufactured in a culture medium disk approx 3 inch in diameter. It looks and feels like human skin. In can be lifted off the disk and transferred to the wound.

APLIGRAF

Apligraf is a composite graft is made up of a cultured living dermis and sequentially cultured epidermis, derived from neonatal foreskin (Graftskin, Organogenesis Inc., Canton, MA). Apligraf is a bilayered skin construct, consists of four components: extracellular matrix, viable allogenic dermal fibroblasts, epidermal keratinocytes, and a stratum corneum. The extracellular matrix of Apligraf consists of type-1 bovine collagen (acid-extracted from bovine tendon and subsequently purified) organized into fibrils and fibroblast-produced proteins. This matrix promotes the ingrowth of cells, provides the scaffold for the three-dimensional structure of Apligraf, and provides mechanical stability and flexibility to the finished product.

The dermal fibroblasts produce growth factors to stimulate wound healing, contribute to the formation of new dermal tissue, and provide factors that help to maintain the overlying epidermis. The epidermal keratinocytes form the epidermis. They produce growth factors to stimulate wound healing and achieve biological wound closure. The stratum corneum provides a natural barrier to mechanical damage, infection, and wound desiccation. The dermal fibroblasts and keratinocytes are separated from normally discarded infant human foreskin. Apligraf is processed under aseptic conditions and thus requires similar handling. Blood samples of the maternal parent of the foreskin donor is tested and compared to normal ranges. Test for many infectious agents are performed and include anti-HIV virus antibody, HIV antigen, Hepatitis, Rapid Plasma Reagin, Glutamic pyruvic transaminase, Epstein–Barr, and Herpes simplex. The cells are also tested for many infectious agents and also for their lack of tumorigenic potential.

Apligraf is supplied as a circular sheet approx 3 inch in diameter (44 cm^2) in a plastic container with a gel-cultured medium (Fig. 4). Apligraf looks and feels like human skin. Histological sections showed that Apligraf only lacks blood vessels, sweat glands, and hair follicles when compared to human skin (Fig. 5). Apligraf contains all cytokines present in human skin (Table 1). The specimen is in a sealed plastic bag that can be kept at room temperature for up to 5 d. Once the bag is opened, the product must be applied

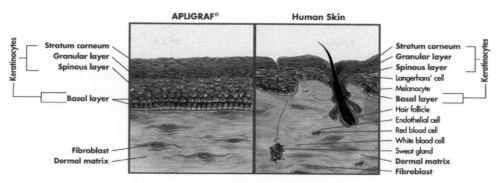

Fig. 5. Histology comparison between Apligraf and human skin. They are very similar. Apligraf lack Langerhans' cell and melanocyte at the epidermis level. In the dermis level, Apligraf does not contain any hair follicle, sweat gland, endothelial cell, or any blood cells.

Table 1
Cytokine Expression in Apligraf and Human Skin

	Human keratinocytes	Human dermal fibroblasts	Apligraf	Human skin
FGF-1	+	+	+	+
FGF-2	−	+	+	+
FGF-7	−	+	+	+
ECGF	−	+	+	+
IGF-1	−	−	+	+
IGF-2	−	+	+	+
PDGF-AB	+	+	+	+
TGF-α	+	−	+	+
IL-1α	+	−	+	+
IL-6	−	+	+	+
IL-8	−	−	+	+
IL-11	−	+	+	+
TGF-β1	−	+	+	+
TGF-β3	−	+	+	+
VEGF	+	−	+	+

Apligraf contains all the cytokines of those present in human skin.

within 30 minutes. The color of the gel medium will change to indicate when the product is no longer usable. The epidermal layer is closest to the lid of the plastic container, and has a matted or dull finish. The dermal layer rests on the insert membrane closest to the gel medium, and has a glossy appearance.

Apligraf can be trimmed to size and applied to the ulcer with the dermal layer in contact with the wound bed. The wound bed should be debrided extensively to be free of necrotic tissue. Apligraf can overlap the wound edge onto normal surrounding tissues without causing any harm. Apligraf can be "mesh" to cover larger wound. Apligraf does not need to be sutured in but it can be done to ensure the implant does not shift of the

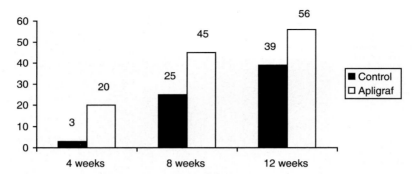

Fig. 6. Results of Multicenter Apligraf study. The difference between the control and Apligraf treatment is apparent early in the study. At week 4, 3% of patients who received control treatment had wound healing compared to 20% of patients who received Apligraf once a week for the first 4 weeks. At week 8, 25% of control patients achieved wound healing compared to 45% of the Apligraf treated patients. By 12 weeks, 39% of the control patients achieved complete wound healing compared to 56% of the patients who received Apligraf treatment ($p = 0.0026$).

target wound. Secondary dressings are used to keep the implant in place and to maintain a moist wound environment.

EFFICACY OF APLIGRAF IN DIABETIC FOOT ULCERS

A multicenter, prospective, randomized control clinical trial was conducted to study the efficacy of Apligraf in the treatment of chronic diabetic foot ulcers *(35)*. Two-hundred and eight patients enrolled in 24 centers across the country. The efficacy of the treatment was studied for 12 weeks, followed by another 3 months of safety follow-up. Ninety-six patients were randomized to control group. This group received saline moistened gauze treatment in addition to good wound care and offloading techniques. One-hundred and twelve patients were randomized to the treatment group. These patients received Apligraf once a week for the first 4 weeks with a maximum of five applications. After week number four, patients in the treatment groups received similar dressing regiments as the control group.

Apligraf quickly showed the difference in treatment (Fig. 6). After 4 weeks, 20% of patients who received Apligraf achieved wound healing compared to 3% in the control group. After 8 weeks, 45% of patients who received Apligraf treatment healed their ulcers compared to 25% of the control group. By the end of week 12, 56% (63/112) of Apligraf-treated patients had complete wound closure compared to 39% (36/96) of the control ($p = 0.0026$). Among the patients who had complete wound closure, the median time to 100% wound closure for Apligraf group was 65 days compared to 90 days for the control group. The recurrence rate was similar in both treatment groups. By 6 months after initiation of therapy, 8% (5/63) of the Apligraf-treated patients had recurrent ulcer compared to 17% (6/36) of the control group.

Because Apligraf could heal more ulcers in a shorter time, safety data also revealed that patients treated with Apligraf had a lower incidence of osteomyelitis and lower frequency of amputation. The incidence of adverse events was similar in the two treatment groups during the study.

CLINICAL APPLICATION

The exact mechanism of action of living skin equivalents is still under much discussion and research. It is believed that LSEs act as a "smart matrix" by inducing the expression of growth factors and cytokines that contribute to wound healing *(36)*. This concept is substantiated by the observation that wounds treated with LSEs exhibit wound healing from the edges of the wound bed.

It is postulated that the donor allogenic cells from LSEs are responsible for the delivery of growth factors and cytokines integral to wound healing. What remains unclear is how long these donor allogenic cells remain active in the wound site. Using polymerase chain reaction analysis, Phillips et al. detected allogenic donor cell DNA after the initial month of grafting *(37)*. However, the allogenic DNA did not appear to persist after 2 months of grafting.

Some LSEs may become vascularized with time and lead to graft integration analogous to autologous skin grafting. Using laser Doppler imaging, Newton et al. assessed blood flow in seven diabetic foot ulcers treated with eight applications of Dermagraft on a weekly basis *(38)*. It was found that blood flow increased by an average of 72% at the base of five out of seven diabetic foot ulcers. This angiogenesis may be responsible for the effectiveness of LSEs in the treatment of diabetic foot ulcers.

Rejection of the LSE or development of immune sensitization does not appear to be a problem. It is thought that this may be because of the fact that neonatal fibroblasts lack the HLA-DR surface antigens, which are responsible for generating allograft rejection *(39)*.

As in many studies, patients with severe medical conditions such as end-stage renal failure on dialysis are often excluded. Some of the authors' patients with diabetes who had end-stage renal disease on hemodialysis were able to achieve complete wound healing on their chronic ulcers using Apligraf in addition to normal good wound care and offloading technique.

COST EFFECTIVENESS AND QUALITY OF LIFE

A major criticism of LSEs is the significant cost associated with their use. This has been a difficult issue to study because of the variation in healthcare cost from one region to another.

However, recent investigation has found that treatment with Apligraf is more cost effective because of its greater effectiveness offsetting the added cost of the product *(40)*. The investigators concluded that the cost effectiveness benefit was realized at the 5-month mark and treatment with Apligraf resulted in a 12% reduction in costs over the first year of treatment compared to standard wound care. Using modeling techniques over a 52-week period, Dermagraft treated diabetic foot ulcers was also felt to be more cost effective than standard wound care based on its ability to heal more wounds over that time period.

A similar conclusion was reached with the use of Apligraf for venous stasis ulcerations. Schonfeld et al. *(41)* estimated that ulcers treated with Apligraf cost $20,041 annually, compared to $27,493 for those treated with compression therapy and wound care. Furthermore, they found that treatment with Apligraf led to 3 months more in the healed state.

Obviously, faster wound healing can lead to reduction in treatment costs. What is more difficult to measure, however, is the health-related quality of life. Mathias et al. attempted to evaluate whether the use of Apligraf contributed to improved quality of life in patients. Based on a telephone questionnaire, 79% of respondents felt that their health was "much better" following treatment with Apligraf *(42)*. The respondents also reported that the greatest improvement was reported in pain symptoms.

REFERENCES

1. Gibbons G, Eliopolos G. Infection of the diabetic foot, in *Management of Diabetic Foot Problems* (Kozak G, Hoar CJ, Rowbotham J, Wheelock F, Gibbons G, Campbell eds.), Saunders, Philadelphia, 1984, pp 97–102.
2. Reiber GE, Boyko EJ, Smith DG. Lower extremity foot ulcers and amputations in diabetes, in *National Diabetes Data Group ed. Diabetes in America,* 2nd ed. National Institutes of Health, Washington, 1995, pp 409–428.
3. Bakker K, Rauwerda JA, Schaper NC. *Diabetes Metab Res Rev* 2000;16(Suppl 1): S1.
4. Helm PA, Walker SC, Pulliam GF. Recurrence of neuropathic ulcerations following healing in a total contact cast. *Arch Phys Med Rehabil* 1991;72:967–970.
5. Apelqvist J, Larson J. What is the most effective way to reduce the incidence of amputation in the diabetic foot? *Diabetes Metab Res Rev* 2000;16(Suppl 1):S75–83.
6. Margolis DJ, Kantor J, Berlin JA. Healing of diabetic neuropathic foot ulcers receiving standard treatment: a meta-analysis. *Diabetes Care* 1999; 22(5):692–695.
7. Loots MA, Lamme EN, Zeegelaar J, Mekkes JR, Bos JD, Middelkoop E. Differences in Cellular infiltrate and extracellular matrix of chronic diabetic and venous ulcers versus acute wounds. *J Invest Dermatol* 1998;111:850–857.
8. Witte MB, Barbul A. General principles of wound healing. *Surg Clin North Am* 1997;77: 509–528.
9. Jude EB, Boulton AJ, Ferguson MW, Appleton I. The role of nitric oxide synthase isoforms and arginase in the pathogenesis of diabetic foot ulcers: possible modulatory effects by transforming growth factor beta 1. *Diabetologia* 1999;42:748–757.
10. Loots MA, Lamme EN, Zeegelaar J, Mekkes JR, Bos JD, Middelkoop E. Differences in Cellular infiltrate and extracellular matrix of chronic diabetic and venous ulcers versus acute wounds. *J Invest Dermatol* 1998;111:850–857.
11. American Diabetes Association, Inc. Consensus Development Conference on Diabetic Foot Wound Care, 7–8 April 1999, Boston, MA. *Diabetes Care* 1999;22:1354–1360.
12. Wieman TJ, Smiell JM, Su Y. Efficacy and safety of a topical gel formulation of recombinant human platelet-derived growth factor-BB (becaplermin) in patients with chronic neuropathic diabetic ulcers. A phase III randomized placebo-controlled double-blind study. *Diabetes Care* 1998;21(5):822–827.
13. Reverdin JL. Greffe epidermique. *Bull Soc Imperiale Chir Paris* 1869; 493.
14. Rheinwald JG, Green H. Serial cultivation of strains of human epidermal keratinocytes: the formation of keratinizing colonies from single cells. *Cell* 1975;6:331–343.
15. O'Connor NE, Mulliken JB, Banks-Schlegel S, et al. Grafting of burns with cultured epithelium prepared from autologous epidermal cells. *Lancet* 1981;1:75–78.
16. Phillips TJ. Cultured skin grafts: past, present and future. *Arch Dermatol* 1988;124: 1035–1038.
17. Eaglstein WH, Falanga V. Tissue engineering for skin: an update. *J Am Acad Dermatol* 1998;39(6):1007–1010.
18. Kirsner RS, Falanga V, Eaglstein WH. Biology of skin grafts: grafts as pharmacologic agents. *Arch Dermatol* 1993;129:481–483.
19. Greenleaf G, Hansbrough JF. Current trends in the use of allograft skin for burn patients and reflections on the future of skin banking in the United States. *J Burn Care Rehabil* 1995;15:428.

20. Greenleaf G, Cooper ML, Hansbrough JF. Microbial contamination in allografted wound beds in patients with burns. *J Burn Care Rehabil* 1991;12:442.
21. Kealey GP. Disease transmission by means of allografts. *J Burn Care Rehabil* 1997;18:10–11.
22. Kolenik SA III, Lefell DJ. The use of cryopreserved human skin allografts in wound healing following Mohs surgery. *Dermatol Surg* 1995;21:615–620.
23. Rheinwald JG, Green H. Serial cultivation of strains of human epidermal keratinocytes: the formation of keratinizing colonies from single cells. *Cell* 1975;6:331–343.
24. Phillips TJ, Gilchrest BA. Clinical applications of cultured epithelium. *Epithelial Cell Biol* 1992;1:39–46.
25. Limova M, Mauro T. Treatment of leg ulcers with cultured epithelial autografts: treatment protocol and five year experience. *Wounds* 1995;7:170–180.
26. Sheridan RL, Tompkins RG. Cultured autologous epithelium in patients with burns of ninety percent or more of the body surface. *J Trauma* 1995;38:48–50.
27. Burke JF, Yannas IV, Quinby WC, et al. Successful use of physiologically acceptable artificial skin in the treatment of extensive burn injury. *Ann Surg* 1981;194:413–428.
28. Jiang WG, Harding KG. Enhancement of wound tissue expansion and angiogenesis by matrix-embedded fibroblasts (Dermagraft), a role of hepatocyte growth factor/scatter factor. *Int J Mol Med* 1998;2:203–210.
29. Mansbridge J, Liu K, Patch R, Symons K, Pinney E. Three-dimensional fibroblast culture implant for the treatment of diabetic foot ulcers: metabolic activity and therapeutic range. *Tissue Eng* 1998;4(4):403–411.
30. Gentzkow GD, Iwasaki SD, Hershon KS, et al. Use of Dermagraft, a cultured human dermis, to treat diabetic foot ulcers. *Diabetes Care* 1996;19(4):350–354.
31. Pollak RA, Edington H, Jensen JL, Kroeker RO, Gentzkow GD and the Dermagraft Diabetic Ulcer Study Group. A human dermal replacement for the treatment of diabetic foot ulcers. *Wounds* 1997;9:175–178.
32. Naughton G, Mansbridge J, Gentzkow G. A metabolically active human dermal replacement for the treatment of diabetic foot ulcers. *Artif Organs* 1997;21(11):1203–1210.
33. Bowering CK. The use of Dermagraft in the treatment of diabetic foot ulcers. *Today's Ther Trends* 1998;16:87–96.
34. Marston MA, Hanft J, Norwood P, Pollack R. The efficacy and safety of Dermagraft in improving the healing of chronic diabetic foot ulcers: results of a prospective randomized trial. *Diabetes Care* 2003;26(6):1701–1705.
35. Veves A, Falanga V, Armstrong DG, Sabolinski ML. Graftskin, a human skin equivalent, is effective in the management of noninfected neuropathic diabetic foot ulcers. *Diabetes Care.* 2001;24:290–295.
36. Sabolinski ML, Alvarez O, Auletta M, et al. Cultured skin as a "smart material" for healing wounds: experience in venous ulcers. *Biomaterials* 1996;17:311–320.
37. Phillips TJ, Manzoor J, Rojas A, et al. The longevity of a bilayered skin substitute after application to venous ulcers. *Arch Dermatol* 2002;138(8):1079–1081.
38. Newton DJ, Khan F, Belch JJF, Mitchell MR, Leese GP. Blood flow changes in diabetic foot ulcers treated with dermal replacement therapy. *J Foot Ankle Surg* 2002;41:233–237.
39. Falanga V, Margolis D, Alverez O, et al. Healing of venous ulcer and lack of clinical rejection with an allogenic cultured human skin equivalent. *Arch Dermatol* 1998;134:293–300.
40. Redekop WK, McDonnell J, Verboom P, Lovas K, Kalo Z. The cost effectiveness of Apligraf treatment of diabetic foot ulcers. *Pharmacoeconomics* 2003;21(16):1171–1183.
41. Schonfeld WH, Villa KF, Fastenau JM, Mazonson PD, Falanga V. An economic assessment of Apligraf (Graftskin) for the treatment of hard-to-heal venous leg ulcers. *Wound Repair Regen* 2000;8(4):251–257.
42. Mathias SD, Prebil LA, Boyko WL, Fastenau J. Health-related quality of life in venous leg ulcer patients successfully treated with Apligraf: a pilot study. *Adv Skin Wound Care* 2000; 13(2):76–78.

22

Lower Extremity Arterial Reconstruction in Patients With Diabetes Mellitus

Principles of Treatment

Kakra Hughes, MD, David Campbell, MD and Frank B. Pomposelli Jr., MD

INTRODUCTION

Foot problems remain the most common reason for hospitalization for patients with diabetes mellitus *(1,2)*. Approximately 20% of the 12–15 million patients with diabetes in the United States can expect to be hospitalized for a foot problem at least once during their lifetime, and account for an annual health care cost for this problem alone in excess of one billion dollars *(3)*. The primary pathological mechanisms of neuropathy and ischemia set the stage for pressure necrosis, ulceration, and multimicrobial infection, which if improperly treated ultimately leads to gangrene and amputation *(4)*. Understanding how the factors of neuropathy, ischemia, and infection are impacting on an individual patient with a foot complication and simultaneously effecting proper treatment for all factors present is essential to foot salvage. Although this chapter focuses on the treatment of ischemia owing to arterial insufficiency, it is important to remember that ischemia is accompanied by infection in approx 50% of patients in our experience *(5)*, and that most, if not all, patients will have peripheral neuropathy present as well. Although focusing on correction of ischemia, often by operative reconstruction or percutaneous intervention, the vascular surgeon cannot ignore these other factors if foot salvage is ultimately to be successful.

VASCULAR DISEASE IN PATIENTS WITH DIABETES

A detailed discussion of vascular disease in patients with diabetes can be found elsewhere in this book. The most important principle in treating foot ischemia in patients with diabetes is recognizing that the cause of their presenting symptoms is macrovascular occlusion of the leg arteries resulting from atherosclerosis. In the past, many clinicians incorrectly assumed that gangrene, nonhealing ulcers and poor healing of minor amputations, or other foot procedures were because of microvascular occlusion of the arterioles—so-called "small vessel disease" *(6)*. This concept, although erroneous and subsequently refuted in several studies *(7–11)*, persists to this day. In the minds of many clinicians and their patients this concept has resulted in a pessimistic attitude toward treatment of ischemia that all too often leads to an unnecessary limb amputation without an attempt at arterial revascularization. This attitude and approach is antiquated,

From: *The Diabetic Foot, Second Edition*
Edited by: A. Veves, J. M. Giurini, and F. W. LoGerfo © Humana Press Inc., Totowa, NJ

inappropriate, and must be discouraged in the strongest of terms. In the authors' opinion, rejection of the small vessel theory alone could well decrease the 40-fold increased risk of major limb amputation a person with diabetes faces during his or her lifetime as compared with a person who does not have diabetes.

ATHEROSCLEROSIS IN DIABETES

Although histologically similar to disease in persons without diabetes, atherosclerosis in the patient with diabetes has certain clinically relevant differences. Previous studies have confirmed that diabetes mellitus is a strong independent risk factor for atherosclerotic coronary *(12,13)*, cerebrovascular *(14)*, and peripheral vascular disease *(14)*. Patients with diabetes face a higher likelihood of cardiovascular mortality. In addition, generalized atherosclerosis is more prevalent and progresses more rapidly in patients with diabetes. In those patients presenting with ischemic symptoms of the lower extremity, gangrene, and tissue loss are more likely to be present compared with persons without diabetes. Diabetic patients with coronary atherosclerosis are more likely to have so-called "silent ischemia"—absence of typical anginal symptoms or pain with myocardial infarction, particularly in those patients with significant polyneuropathy *(15)*.

These findings suggest that arterial reconstruction in these patients carries a higher risk of adverse outcome, particularly myocardial infarction and/or death. In fact, both Lee *(16)* and Eagle *(17)* have listed diabetes mellitus as an independent risk factor for adverse cardiac outcomes in patients undergoing major surgery. Our personal experience however, in well over 3000 patients undergoing lower extremity arterial reconstruction in the last decade, refutes this position. In a recent study of nearly 800 lower extremity bypass procedures performed in patients with diabetes followed for a minimum of 5 years after surgery, the in-hospital mortality rate was 1% and the long-term graft patency, limb salvage, and patient survival rates were comparable or better than patients without diabetes treated in the same time period *(18)*. More recently, we have reviewed the results of more than 6500 patients (62% with diabetes) undergoing major *(19)* vascular operations—carotid, aortic, or lower extremity arterial reconstruction—and have found that diabetes alone did not confer a higher mortality or cardiac morbidity rate. In our opinion, careful perioperative management, including an aggressive approach toward invasive cardiac monitoring in the early postoperative period has been responsible for the low-cardiac morbidity and mortality rate in these high-risk patients.

From the vascular surgeon's perspective, the most important difference in lower extremity atherosclerosis in patients with diabetes is the location of atherosclerotic occlusive lesions in the artery supplying the leg and the foot *(8,10)*. In patients without diabetes, atherosclerosis most commonly involves the infrarenal aorta, iliac arteries, and superficial femoral artery with relative sparing of the more distal arteries. In patients with diabetes however, the most significant occlusive lesion occurs in the crural arteries distal to the knee—the anterior tibial artery, peroneal artery or posterior tibial artery—but with sparing of the arteries of the foot (Figs. 1 and 2). This pattern of occlusive disease, known as "tibial artery disease," requires a different approach to vascular reconstruction and presents special challenges for the surgeon (discussed later). Moreover, patients with diabetes who smoke may have a combination of both patterns of disease, making successful revascularization more complex.

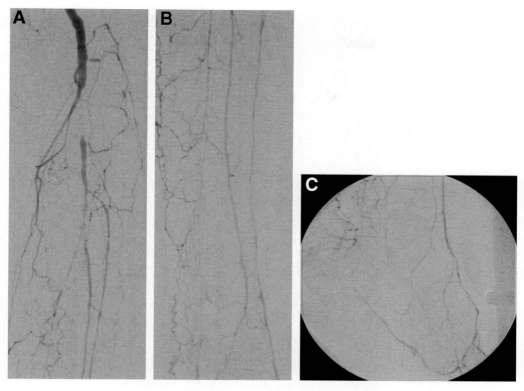

Fig. 1. Intra-arterial digital subtraction arteriogram of the left lower leg and foot of a patient presenting with an ischemic foot lesion; more proximal vessels are not shown because they were all widely patent. **(A)** Knee view: the distal popliteal artery is occluded, and the proximal posterior tibial, anterior tibial, and peroneal arteries are either occluded or severely narrowed. **(B)** Calf view: the peroneal and anterior tibial arteries are patent but severely narrowed. The peroneal artery occludes at the ankle. The posterior tibial artery is occluded and never seen. **(C)** Lateral foot view: the dorsalis pedis artery is widely patent, with runoff into patent tarsal branches, which fill a plantar artery through the pedal arch.

PATIENT SELECTION

Many patients with diabetes will have evidence of peripheral vascular disease manifested by absence of palpable leg or foot pulses with either minimal or no symptoms. In these patients, their disease is well compensated and no treatment is necessary other than education about vascular disease including signs and symptoms and reduction of associated risk factors, particularly cessation of smoking. Regular follow-up examinations, usually at a 6- to 12-month interval, are reasonable. Many clinicians will obtain baseline noninvasive arterial testing at this point, although this is not mandatory. Many such patients have associated coronary and carotid atherosclerosis, which may also be asymptomatic. Routine screening for disease in these territories in the absence of signs or symptoms, based solely on evidence of lower extremity atherosclerosis, may be appropriate in individual patients but probably not cost effective, as a routine, in all such patients.

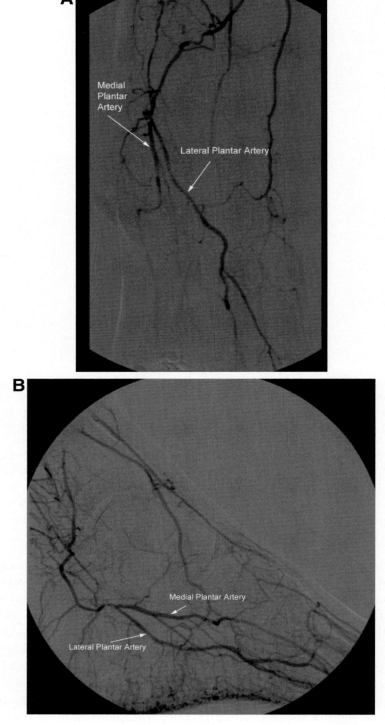

Fig. 2. Preoperative antero–posterior (**A**) and lateral (**B**) arteriogram of the foot of a patient undergoing a plantar artery bypass.

In patients presenting with typical symptoms mandating treatment, several factors must be taken into consideration. Certain patients may not be appropriate for arterial reconstruction such as those with dementia and/or other organic brain syndromes who are nonambulatory or bedridden and have little likelihood of successful rehabilitation. Similarly, patients with severe flexion contractures of the knee or hip are poor candidates. Patients with terminal cancer with very short life expectancy or similar lethal comorbidities do poorly with vascular reconstruction and are also probably better served by primary amputations. Patients with an unsalvageable foot owing to extensive necrotizing infection, even when ischemic, likewise require primary amputation. However, in other patients presenting with infection complicating ischemia, proper control of spreading infection must be accomplished before arterial reconstruction. Broad-spectrum intravenous antibiotics to cover Gram-positive, Gram-negative, and anaerobic organisms should be started immediately after cultures are taken, because most infections in patients with diabetes are multimicrobial *(1,19)*. Once culture data is available antibiotics can then be appropriately adjusted. In addition, those patients with abscess formation, septic arthritis, necrotizing fasciitis, and so on, should undergo prompt incision, drainage and debridement including partial open toe, ray, or forefoot amputation *(20)* as indicated (Fig. 3).

In our series of pedal bypasses, secondary infection was present at the time of presentation in more than 50% of patients *(21)*. Infection places an increased metabolic demand on already ischemic tissues and may accelerate and exacerbate tissue necrosis. Because many patients with diabetes have a blunted neurogenic inflammatory response, typical inflammatory signs of infection may be absent or diminished. It is, therefore, imperative that all ulcers be carefully probed and inspected and superficial eschars unroofed to look for potential deep space abscesses, which are not readily apparent from visual inspection of the foot. The need to control spreading infection may delay vascular reconstruction for several days, but waiting longer than necessary in order to sterilize wounds is inappropriate and may result in further necrosis and tissue loss. Signs of resolving spreading infection include reduction of fever, resolution of cellulitis, and lymphangitis, particularly in areas of potential surgical incisions and return of glycemic control, which is probably the most sensitive indicator of improvement. During this period which rarely extends beyond 4 or 5 days, contrast arteriography and other presurgical evaluations such as testing for coronary disease when necessary can be performed so that vascular reconstruction may be undertaken without additional delay.

There are occasional patients in whom infection cannot be totally eradicated before bypass. Patients with severe ischemia may have inadequate blood flow to distal sites to deliver adequate tissue penetration of antibiotics until arterial blood flow has been adequately restored. It is important in these patients to continue antibiotics coverage for several days following arterial reconstructive surgery. Occasionally, patients may seem to have worsening of their infection after revascularization because of the enhanced inflammatory response that is possible once arterial blood flow has been restored.

It is important to realize that age alone is not a contraindication to arterial reconstruction. We have successfully performed these procedures in selected patients over the age of 90. When selecting patients for arterial reconstruction the functional and physiological status of the patient is far more important than chronological age. In fact, a limb salvaging arterial reconstruction may mean the difference for an elderly patient between continued independent living and the need for permanent custodial nursing home care. We recently

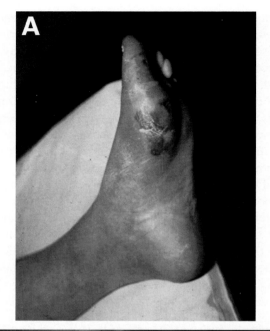

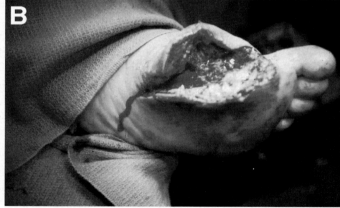

Fig. 3. Photographs of the right foot of a patient with diabetes who presented with a rapidly spreading infection as a result of a plantar ulcer over the first metatarsal. **(A)** Marked swelling and erythema of the medial forefoot is evident. There was palpable crepitus and malodorous drainage owing to involvement of the bone, joint, and flexor tendon with gas-forming bacteria. **(B)** Control of this infection required an emergent open first ray amputation. Cultures grew multiple organisms including *Staphylococcus aureus*, *Proteus,* and anaerobes.

evaluated our results with arterial reconstruction in a cohort of patients who were 80 years of age or older at the time of arterial reconstruction, evaluating both the rate of success of initial procedure and two important quality of life outcomes—the ability to ambulate and whether or not the patients returned to their own residences following surgery. At 1 year following surgery, the vast majority (>80%) was still ambulatory and residing in their homes either alone or with relatives *(22).*

Patients with limb ischemia who present with signs and symptoms of coronary disease such as worsening angina, recent congestive heart failure, or recent myocardial infarction need to have stabilization of their cardiac disease before arterial reconstruction. Occasionally angioplasty or even coronary artery bypass grafting may be required before lower extremity surgery, although in our experience this has been unusual. Virtually all diabetic patients with lower extremity ischemia have occult coronary disease *(23)*. Consequently, screening tests such as dipyridamole–thallium imaging are almost always abnormal to some degree. Attempting to quantify the degree of abnormality with such testing has occasionally proved useful in stratifying those patients at excessive risk for perioperative cardiac morbidity or mortality, however, most such patients with severely abnormal scans usually have obvious clinical signs or symptoms as well *(24)*. As a result, we rely mostly on the patient's clinical presentation and electrocardiogram in determining when further evaluation is needed and use imaging studies selectively in those patients with unclear or atypical symptoms. In asymptomatic patients who are reasonably active with no acute changes on an electrocardiogram, no further studies are generally undertaken. We recently conducted a retrospective review of asymptomatic patients with diabetes at our institution undergoing elective infrainguinal arterial reconstruction and noted that preoperative cardiac evaluation did not improve or predict postoperative morbidity and mortality *(25)*. It has also been shown in a prospective randomized study that coronary artery revascularization before elective vascular surgery does not significantly alter the long-term outcome *(26)*. We have found that frequent use of invasive perioperative cardiac monitoring, including pulmonary arterial catheters along with anesthesia management by personnel accustomed to treating patients with ischemic heart disease, and managing patients in a specialized, subacute, monitored unit with cardiac monitoring capabilities, in the early postoperative period, has significantly reduced perioperative cardiac morbidity and mortality in our patients. It is also of interest that in a relatively recent prospective randomized trial, the type of anesthesia given (i.e., spinal, epidural, or general endotracheal) did not affect the incidence of perioperative cardiac complications *(27)* or graft thrombosis *(28)*.

Patients presenting with renal failure present special challenges. When acute renal insufficiency occurs, most commonly following contrast arteriography, surgery is delayed until renal function stabilizes or returns to normal. Most such patients will demonstrate a transient rise in serum creatinine without other symptoms. It is rare that such patients will become anuric or require hemodialysis. Withholding contrast arteriography in patients with diabetes and compromised renal function is, therefore, generally inappropriate and unnecessary. If there are significant concerns about renal function, however, magnetic resonance angiography can often provide adequate images to plan arterial reconstruction *(29)*.

The appropriate treatment of ischemic peripheral vascular disease in patients with endstage renal disease has yet to be clearly elucidated. Many such patients have severe, advanced atherosclerosis with target arteries that are often heavily calcified. Gangrene and tissue loss are frequently present and the healing response in such patients is poor, even with restoration of arterial blood flow. Moreover, some such patients will require amputation even with patent arterial bypass grafts. Many studies in the past have recommended caution when proceeding with lower extremity operative revascularization in this patient group on the basis of poor patient survival and limb salvage rates (ranging from 38% to 62% at 2 years) *(30–32)*. Others have, more recently, advocated arterial reconstruction citing improving morbidity and mortality results *(33,34)*. We recently reported our experience with 177 lower extremity arterial bypasses in patients with endstage renal disease *(35)* of whom 92% had diabetes. Primary patency and limb salvage rates at 1 year were 84% and 80%, respectively. In-hospital mortality rate was 3% and 30-day mortality was 5%. Patient survival, however, sharply declined with 60% survival at 1 year, 18% at 3 years and only 5% at 5 years. Increasing age and number of years on dialysis were identified as negative predictors of limb salvage and survival. It appears then that whereas the technical outcome of infrainguinal bypass grafting in patients with endstage renal disease is satisfactory, the abysmal survival rate may call into question the overall benefit of arterial reconstruction in this patient population. Furthermore, whereas our study did not allow us to predict which patients would benefit from operative reconstruction, it appears as though certain factors such as heel gangrene may be important, on the basis of our observation that 52% of such patients needed amputation in spite of patent grafts. Careful patient selection, therefore, is of utmost importance.

EVALUATION AND DIAGNOSTIC STUDIES

Patients requiring surgical intervention for lower extremity arterial insufficiency usually present with severely disabling intermittent claudication or signs and symptoms of limb threatening ischemia. Intermittent claudication is pain, cramping, or a sensation of severe fatigue in the muscles of the leg, which occurs with walking and is promptly relieved by rest. Many patients adjust their lifestyles to minimize or eliminate any significant walking. The location of discomfort can give hints to the location of the disease. Patients with aortoiliac atherosclerosis will often complain of buttock and thigh pain, whereas patients with femoral disease will typically have calf discomfort, although patients with aortoiliac occlusive disease can have calf claudication as their only presenting symptom. Patients with tibial arterial occlusive disease will also have calf claudication and may also complain of foot discomfort or numbness with walking. Nocturnal muscle cramping, which is a common complaint among patients with diabetes, is not a typical symptom of vascular disease, even though it may involve the calf muscles, and should not be mistaken for intermittent claudication.

Most patients with intermittent claudication do not require operative or endovascular intervention. Studies on the natural history of claudication have demonstrated that progression to limb threatening ischemia is uncommon *(36,37)*. Many patients respond to conservative treatment measures such as cessation of tobacco use, correction of risk factors for atherosclerosis, weight reduction when necessary and an exercise program involving walking *(38)*. Additionally, two medications have traditionally been utilized: pentoxifilline, 400 mg orally three times daily or cilostazol, 100 mg orally twice daily, which have been demonstrated to improve walking distance in patients with claudication because of atherosclerosis *(39–41)*. Both drugs are generally well tolerated but need to be taken for several weeks before improvement in walking distance can be appreciated. In the authors' experience, pentoxifilline has been disappointing in relieving claudication symptoms. Cilostazol has been more effective, but has more side effects and is contraindicated in patients with a history of congestive heart failure. In most cases, we start with exercise and risk factor reduction alone as a first step and add a medication later if necessary. Surgical intervention for claudication is reserved for those patients who are severely disabled with a very limited functional capacity, unable to work owing to their symptoms, or who have not responded to more conservative treatment. In the authors' experience, patient noncompliance is the most common reason for failure of conservative treatment measures.

Recent emerging reports have shown a significantly beneficial effect of 3-hydroxy-3-methylglutaryl-coenzyme A inhibitors (HMG-CoA reductase inhibitors, or statins) in the management of vascular disease. A broad range of atheroprotective properties of these cholesterol-lowering agents have been demonstrated beyond their effect on lipid metabolism. Statins have been shown to prevent new or worsening symptoms of claudication, to improve walking distance, walking velocity, and overall ambulatory performance *(42–45)*. Recently published studies from our institution and others have suggested an associated decrease in perioperative cardiac complications *(46,47)* and mortality *(48)* in vascular surgical patients. Furthermore, statin use has been linked to improved patency of autogenous infrainguinal bypass grafts *(49)* as well as a reduction in the incidence of graft failure following coronary artery bypass *(50)*. Other studies have shown that statins are associated with a reduction in cardiovascular events in patients with coronary artery disease *(51–54)*. In the light of all of these beneficial effects, it is the authors' opinion that routine use of statins in vascular surgical patients should be strongly encouraged.

Most patients with diabetes referred for vascular intervention have limb threatening ischemic problems which, if not promptly treated, are likely to ultimately result in amputation. The most common presenting problem is a nonhealing ulcer with or without associated gangrene and infection. Many patients will initially develop an ulcer as a result of neuropathy, which will then not heal in spite of proper treatment towing to associated arterial insufficiency, the so-called neuropathic ischemic ulcer. Some patients are referred after a minor surgical procedure in the foot fails to heal owing to ischemia. Patients with limb threatening ischemia can also present with ischemic rest pain with or without associated tissue loss. Ischemic rest pain typically occurs in the distal foot, particularly the toes. It is exacerbated by recumbency and relieved by dependency. Patients often give a history of noticing pain, numbness or paresthesias when retiring for bed, which is then relieved by placing their foot in a dependent position. Often times, it may not be recognized that placing the foot in a dependent position is the cause of relief and relief may be associated with other maneuvers such as walking and stamping the involved foot on the floor or getting up and taking an oral analgesic medication. It is important, but occasionally difficult, to differentiate rest pain from painful diabetic neuropathy, which may also be subjectively worse at night (Table 1). Neuropathic patients may also present with no rest pain in spite of overt severe foot ischemia because of the complete loss of sensation. Nocturnal muscle cramps are a common complaint but not because of arterial insufficiency.

The noninvasive vascular laboratory *(55,56)* is particularly useful in those patients with diabetes presenting with pain in the foot and absent pulses in which the etiology is unclear and may be resulting from either ischemia or painful diabetic neuropathy.

Table 1
Distinguishing Features of Ischemic Rest Pain and Painful Neuropathy

Rest pain	Neuropathy
Usually unilateral	Often bilateral
Consistently present	Waxes and wanes
Relieved by dependency of foot	Not relieved by dependency
Always associated with absent pulses	Pulses may be present and normal

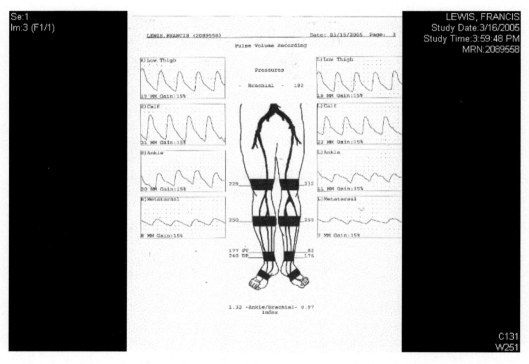

Fig. 4. A pulse volume recording obtained from a diabetic patient with a nonhealing left foot ulcer and absent distal pulses. The thigh waveforms depicted are normal with the forefoot tracings indicative of severe ischemia.

Patients with severe ischemia will usually have ankle brachial indices of less than 0.4. In patients with diabetes however, care must be taken in interpreting ankle pressures because many patients will have unexpectedly elevated ankle pressures owing to calcification of the arterial wall making vessels difficult to compress with a blood pressure cuff *(57)*. In fact, approx 10% of patients will have incompressible vessels making ankle pressures incalculable. Pulse volume recordings are useful in these patients because they are unaffected by calcification of vessels. Severely abnormal waveforms at the ankle or forefoot suggest severe ischemia (Fig. 4). Some centers have found toe pressures *(57)* and transcutaneous oxygen measurements *(58,59)* to also be useful in these patients, although we do not routinely use these two modalities in our practice.

Noninvasive arterial testing with exercise *(55,57)* is also useful in patients with claudication presenting with palpable distal pulses. Baseline studies are taken and then repeated with exercise, usually walking on a treadmill at a slight elevation until symptoms are reproduced. A subsequent reduction in arterial pressures or worsening of pulse volume waveforms suggests proximal stenotic lesions. Those patients with development of claudication who do not have an associated change in their noninvasive testing suggest another cause for claudication such as spinal stenosis (so-called pseudoclaudication). Following surgery, noninvasive testing can be used to quantify the degree of improvement in distal circulation. Arterial reconstructions with vein grafts are susceptible to the development of neointimal hyperplasia, which can lead to stricture and stenosis in vein grafts and ultimately graft thrombosis. Ultrasound evaluation of vein grafts with color flow duplex scanning is useful in detecting vein graft stenoses resulting from intimal hyperplasia *(60)*. When detected, significant stenoses can often be repaired by vein patch angioplasty, interposition grafts or balloon angioplasty, before graft thrombosis *(44,61,62)*.

Noninvasive testing however adds little to the evaluation of patients presenting with obvious signs of foot ischemia and absent foot pulses. For most patients a careful history and physical examination will detect significant arterial insufficiency. The most important feature of the physical examination is the status of the foot pulses. If the posterior tibial and dorsalis pedis artery pulses are nonpalpable in patients presenting with typical signs and symptoms of ischemia, no further noninvasive testing is necessary and contrast arteriography should be performed straight away.

The ultimate goal of lower extremity reconstruction is to restore perfusion pressure in the distal circulation by bypassing all major occlusions and if possible reestablish a palpable foot pulse. The outflow target artery (the point of the distal anastomosis) should be relatively free of occlusive disease and demonstrate unimpeded arterial flow into the arteries of the foot. In general, the most proximal artery distal to the occlusion meeting these two criteria is chosen. In order to make these determinations, the vascular surgeon needs a high quality, comprehensive, contrast arteriogram of the entire lower extremity circulation extending from the infrarenal aorta to the base of the toes. It is crucial to visualize the entire tibial and foot circulation because the former is the most common location of the most significant occlusive lesions and the latter is an important potential site for placement of the distal anastomosis of the bypass graft. Iliac artery atherosclerosis accompanies lower extremity atherosclerosis in approx 10–20% of patients with diabetes. When encountered and significant, balloon angioplasty of iliac lesions usually accompanied by stent placement, is almost always possible and will improve arterial inflow for bypass. This can usually be performed at the same time as the diagnostic arteriogram. For many years, our preference has been to exclusively use intra-arterial digital subtraction arteriography *(63)* to evaluate the lower extremity arterial circulation. With currently available equipment it is possible to obtain a complete survey from the infrarenal aorta to the base of the toes with approx 100 cc of contrast or half of the amount required for conventional arteriography. Although conventional arteriography can provide excellent views of the lower extremity arterial anatomy, we have found cases in which it failed to demonstrate a suitable outflow vessel that was subsequently seen by the digital subtraction method.

As stated previously, arteriography should almost never be withheld because of fear of exacerbating renal insufficiency. For patients with mild to moderate renal insufficiency (creatinine <2.5), hydration before angiography with normal saline—for about 12 hours—will usually prevent significant deterioration of renal function. At least one study has suggested that administration of a sodium bicarbonate solution (154 meq/L sodium bicarbonate solution given as a bolus of 3 cc/kg per hour for 1 hour before the procedure followed by an infusion of 1 cc/kg per hour for 6 hours after the procedure) is more effective than hydration with sodium chloride for prevention of contrast-induced nephropathy (64). Other studies have reported a reduction in the incidence of contrast nephropathy with the use of *N*-acetylcysteine (typically given as a dose of 600 mg orally twice daily the day before and the day of the procedure) (65,66). Whereas these strategies may, in fact, prevent a rise in serum creatinine, whether or not protection against a rise in serum creatinine confers any clinically significant benefit is a question yet to be answered. For patients with more marginal renal function, magnetic resonance arteriography can often provide adequate images of the distal circulation to plan the arterial reconstruction. Although some centers consider this technique as superior to contrast arteriography (29), we have found that intra-arterial digital subtraction arteriography continues to provide the best quality images and reserve magnetic resonance arteriography for those patients for whom the administration of contrast is potentially harmful or contraindicated.

VASCULAR RECONSTRUCTION

One of the most important developments in vascular surgery has been the demonstration that autogenous saphenous vein as opposed to prosthetic graft material gives the best short- and long-term results for distal bypass. In a large multicenter prospective randomized clinical trial, 6-year patency of saphenous vein grafts was more than four times that of prosthetic grafts (67).

For more than 50 years, the standard procedure performed for lower extremity arterial revascularization has been the reversed saphenous vein bypass (68). An inherent problem with reversing the vein, which is necessary to overcome the impediment of flow from valves, is a size discrepancy that results between the arteries and veins when they are connected. Vein grafts that have the diameter of less than 4 mm at the distal end can thrombose when connected directly to the much larger common femoral artery at the groin, owing to the size discrepancy. For many years, some vascular surgeons would routinely discard saphenous veins that were smaller than 4 mm at the distal end in order to prevent this cause of early graft thrombosis when performing an arterial bypass with reversed saphenous vein. Methods were developed to render the valves incompetent in order to allow the vein to be used nonreversed or "*in situ.*" However no procedure was widely accepted until the late 1970s when Leather and associates (69) described a new technique using a modified Mills valvulotome which cut the valves atraumatically and quickly. Vascular surgeons enthusiastically embraced the leather technique and began reporting improved results with the *in situ* bypass (70–72). This led some to conclude that the *in situ* bypass possesses some inherent biological superiority to the reversed saphenous vein graft (73). However evidence to support this concept is lacking (74). Moreover, when *in situ* bypasses are compared to more contemporary series of reversed saphenous vein bypasses no apparent superiority is evident *(75)*. In our own experience we have frequently used both procedures and have observed essentially identical results with either vein configuration *(76)*. The *in situ* technique, however, is an important advance in lower extremity reconstructive surgery and continues to be used widely by most vascular surgeons.

In the 1980s, Ascer and associates *(77)* reported the first series of bypass grafts with inflow (proximal anastomosis) taken from the popliteal artery. They showed equivalent results when compared with the traditional approach of taking inflow from the common femoral artery. These results have been confirmed by other groups *(78)* including our own *(79)* and has proven to be another important advance in arterial reconstruction in patients with diabetes. Because atherosclerotic occlusive disease often spares the superficial femoral artery in patients with diabetes, the popliteal artery can usually be readily used as a source of inflow for the distal vein graft. Doing so shortens the operative procedure and avoids potentially troublesome groin wound complications, which can accompany thigh and groin dissections. Short vein grafts also increase the likelihood that a vein bypass can be performed when the length of available conduit is limited. Theoretically, shorter vein grafts should also have higher flow rates and possibly better long-term patency. Our recent experience with extreme distal arterial reconstructions has shown that popliteal artery inflow is possible in about 60% of patients with diabetes undergoing vascular reconstruction in the lower extremity *(76)*.

When the saphenous vein is unavailable because of previous harvesting or vein stripping, alternative sources of conduit must be used. Although some surgeons will use a prosthetic graft in these circumstances, alternative vein grafts including contra lateral saphenous vein, arm vein, or lesser saphenous vein can be used. We have generally not harvested the contralateral saphenous vein in diabetic patients with absent distal pulses in the opposite extremity. Our experience has demonstrated that in patients with a missing ipsilateral saphenous vein, the likelihood of requiring another arterial reconstruction in the opposite extremity approaches 40% at 3 years following the first operation *(80)*. Moreover, in our tertiary care practice, many such patients do not have adequate available contralateral saphenous vein owing to its use for other vascular procedures or venous disease. When the ipsilateral saphenous vein is unavailable, our venous conduit of choice has been arm vein. Our recent results with arm vein grafts have been improved by examining the vein with the angioscope *(81)* to exclude segments with strictures or recanalization from trauma induced by previous venapuncture and thrombosis. Using the angioscope in this way to upgrade the quality of arm vein grafts has significantly improved our results with these grafts and further reduces the number of patients requiring the use of prosthetic conduit *(82)*. One potential disadvantage of arm vein grafts is their limited length although the use of popliteal artery inflow makes the use of shorter arm vein graft conduits possible in many patients. Moreover, the use of composite grafts made of various segments of arm vein including the cephalic–basilic vein loop graft *(83)* can provide enough conduit length to extend from the groin to the distal tibial and even foot vessels in many patients. Our results with arm vein grafts in more than 500 procedures have been reported *(84)*. Patency and limb salvage rates were 57.5% and 71.5%, respectively at 5 years. These results were inferior to those with *de novo* reconstructions done with saphenous vein, however significantly better than those reported with prosthetic conduits.

A review of arteriograms at our institution imaging the entire lower extremity circulation in patients evaluated for vascular surgery has demonstrated that in 10% of cases, a foot artery, usually the dorsalis pedis artery is the only suitable outflow vessel. In another 15% of patients the dorsalis pedis artery will appear to be a better quality outflow target vessel than other patent but diseased tibial vessels. As a result, we began performing bypasses to the dorsalis pedis artery in situations where no other bypass option existed and where we believed the patient was definitely facing amputation as the only alternative. Early results proved gratifying enough that we standardized our technique and indications to encompass all patients in which we thought the dorsalis pedis artery was the best bypass option even if more proximal outflow target arteries were present (64). Our results with bypass to the dorsalis pedis artery in more than 1000 patients have recently been reported (85) and demonstrated primary graft patency of 56.8% and limb salvage approaching 80% at 5 years (Fig. 5). Moreover, we have demonstrated that even in the presence of foot infection dorsalis pedis bypass can be safely performed as long as spreading sepsis is controlled before surgery (5). These results have compared favorably with other reports of pedal level arterial reconstruction (86–90) and are, comparable to results now routinely reported for popliteal and tibial artery reconstructions. Although pedal arterial bypass represents an "extreme" type of distal arterial reconstruction it is almost always possible, particularly when the vascular surgeon is flexible in terms of how the vein graft is prepared, and where the proximal anastomosis is placed.

We have also occasionally encountered instances in our practice when the only available outflow target for arterial reconstruction is a plantar (branch of the inframalleolar posterior tibial artery) or a tarsal (branch of the dorsalis pedis) artery in a patient who would otherwise undergo primary amputation. In these instances, we have performed bypasses to these very distal targets as an alternative to primary amputation. Our recently reported results of 98 bypass procedures to the plantar or tarsal arteries demonstrated a primary patency of 67% and a limb salvage rate of 75% at 1 year (91) (Fig. 5).

Distal arterial reconstruction presents special technical challenges for the vascular surgeon and requires meticulous attention to detail. The target arteries are usually small (1.0–2.0 mm in diameter) and often calcified owing to medial calcinosis. Because long-term success requires the use of venous conduit, harvesting an adequate venous conduit is essential and can often present problems, particularly when the ipsilateral saphenous vein is not available. In the early days of distal bypass surgery, many procedures were unsuccessful, resulting in amputation. Technical improvements in arteriography, surgical instruments, and sutures and techniques such as the *in situ* bypass have significantly improved the outcome of distal arterial bypass, and outstanding results are often reported in more contemporary series. These improvements have proved to be especially beneficial to patients with diabetes mellitus, because their occlusive disease almost always requires a bypass to this level. In particular, the development and application of bypasses to the dorsalis pedis artery has had a direct effect in our own experience on the likelihood of amputation in patients with diabetes presenting with limb-threatening ischemia. Since its inception, pedal bypass has resulted in a significant decline in all

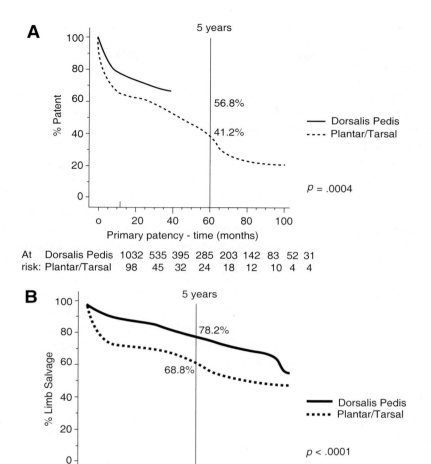

Fig. 5. Primary patency (**A**) and limb salvage (**B**) for patients undergoing bypasses to the dorsalis pedis artery and to the plantar/tarsal arteries.

amputations performed for ischemia *(70)*. Currently bypasses to the dorsalis pedis artery constitute about 30% of all lower extremity arterial reconstructions in our patients with diabetes.

It is important to remember, however, that foot artery bypass is not the only procedure applicable to patients with diabetes. In general, the goal of treatment is to restore maximal arterial flow to the foot because this provides the best chance for healing. The diagnostic preoperative arteriogram is the key piece of information necessary in planning an appropriate surgical procedure. If a bypass to the popliteal or tibial artery will restore maximal arterial flow and restoration of palpable foot pulses bypasses need not extend to the level of the foot. Since the quality of the venous conduit is the most important determinant in long-term success, using the shortest length of high-quality venous conduit necessary to achieve this goal is the basic rule. Each operation must be individualized based on the patient's available venous conduit and arterial anatomy as demonstrated on the preoperative arteriogram.

Successful arterial reconstruction with restoration of maximal arterial flow does not end a vascular surgeon's responsibility to the patient. Often, significant wounds and/or ulcerations may still be present on the foot. Devising an appropriate treatment plan to close the wounds and heal the foot is the ultimate treatment goal. Until the skin envelope is intact, the patient is still susceptible to infection despite excellent arterial circulation. The methods involved in healing open wounds and ulcerations in the diabetic foot after restoration of arterial flow are complex and extend beyond the purview of this chapter. A variety of treatment methods are used and are individualized according to the patient's clinical circumstances. Although many small ulcers may be left to heal by secondary intention, some may require toe or partial forefoot amputations especially when associated with gangrene and chronic osteomyelitis. For larger wounds, split thickness skin grafts are used when the area involved is not a weight-bearing surface. For patients with complex wounds of weight-bearing surfaces, particularly the heel, or when bone or tendons need to be covered, more sophisticated plastic surgical reconstructions involving local rotational flaps and even free tissue transfers have been occasionally employed in our practice. Proper application of these procedures requires the expertise of plastic surgeons in conjunction with foot and ankle orthopedic or podiatric surgeons to be successfully carried out.

CONCLUSION

This chapter has reviewed the principles of evaluation, diagnosis, and treatment of arterial disease in diabetic patients with lower extremity ischemia. Rejection of the small vessel hypothesis and understanding the location of atherosclerotic occlusive disease in the lower extremity of patients with diabetes is key to effecting proper treatment. Understanding the interplay of neuropathy and infection with ischemia and providing proper treatment for these problem as well as treating arterial insufficiency is essential to ultimate success. A thorough understanding of the pathophysiology of ischemia and a carefully planned approach, including the prompt control of infection when present, a high-quality digital subtraction arteriogram, and an appropriate distal arterial reconstruction to maximize foot perfusion should lead to rates of limb salvage in patients with diabetes which equal or exceed those achieved in nondiabetic patients with lower extremity ischemia.

REFERENCES

1. Gibbons GW, Eliopoulos GM. Infection of the diabetic foot In: *Management of Diabetic Foot Problems* (Kozak G, ed.), WB Saunders, Philadelphia, 1984.
2. Edmonds ME. The diabetic foot: pathophysiology and treatment. *Clin Endocrinol Metab* 1986;15:889–916.
3. Grunfeld C. Diabetic foot ulcers: etiology, treatment, and prevention. *Adv Intern Med* 1992;37:103–132.
4. Levin M. The diabetic foot: pathophysiology, evaluation and treatment, in *The Diabetic Foot* (Levin M, ed.), Mosby Year Book, St Louis, 1987.

5. Tannenbaum GA, Pomposelli FB Jr, Marcaccio EJ, et al. Safety of vein bypass grafting to the dorsal pedal artery in diabetic patients with foot infections. *J Vasc Surg* 1992;15:982–988 (Discussion 989–990).

6. Goldenberg SG, Alex M, Joshi RA. Nonatheromatous peripheral vascular disease of the lower extremity in diabetes mellitus. *Diabetes* 1959;8:261–273.

7. Barner HB, Kaiser GC, Willman VL. Blood flow in the diabetic leg. *Circulation* 1971; 43:391–394.

8. Conrad MC. Large and small artery occlusion in diabetics and nondiabetics with severe vascular disease. *Circulation* 1967;36:83–91.

9. Irwin ST, Gilmore J, McGrann S, Hood J, Allen JA. Blood flow in diabetics with foot lesions due to "small vessel disease." *Br J Surg* 1988;75:1201–1206.

10. LoGerfo FW, Coffman JD. Current concepts. Vascular and microvascular disease of the foot in diabetes. Implications for foot care. *N Engl J Med* 1984;311:1615–1619.

11. Strandness DE, Priest RE, Gibbons GE. Combined clinical and pathological study of diabetic and nondiabetic peripheral arterial disease. *Diabetes* 1964;13:366–372.

12. Kannel WB, McGee DL. Diabetes and cardiovascular disease. The Framingham study. *JAMA* 1979;241:2035–2038.

13. Smith JW, Marcus FI, Serokman R. Prognosis of patients with diabetes mellitus after acute myocardial infarction. *Am J Cardiol* 1984;54:718–721.

14. Petersen CM. Influence of diabetes on vascular disease and its complications, in *Vascular Surgery: A Comprehensive Review* (Moore WS, ed.), 6th ed., WB Saunders, Philadelphia, 2002.

15. Zarich S, Waxman S, Freeman RT, Mittleman M, Hegarty P, Nesto RW. Effect of autonomic nervous system dysfunction on the circadian pattern of myocardial ischemia in diabetes mellitus *J Am Coll Cardiol* 1994;24:956–962. (*see* comments)

16. Lee TH, Marcantonio ER, Mangione CM, et al. Derivation and prospective validation of a simple index for prediction of cardiac risk of major noncardiac surgery. *Circulation* 1999;100:1043–1049.

17. Eagle KA, Coley CM, Newell JB, et al. Combining clinical and thallium data optimizes preoperative assessment of cardiac risk before major vascular surgery. *Ann Intern Med* 1989;110:859–866.

18. Akbari CM, Pomposelli FB Jr, Gibbons GW, et al. Lower extremity revascularization in diabetes: late observations. *Arch Surg* 2000;135:452–456.

19. Hamdan AD, Saltzberg SS, Sheahan M, et al. Lack of association of diabetes with increased postoperative mortality and cardiac morbidity: results of 6565 major vascular operations. *Arch Surg* 2002;137:417–421.

20. Gibbons GW. The diabetic foot: amputations and drainage of infection. *J Vasc Surg* 1987;5:791–793.

21. Pomposelli FB Jr, Marcaccio EJ, Gibbons GW, et al. Dorsalis pedis arterial bypass: durable limb salvage for foot ischemia in patients with diabetes mellitus. *J Vasc Surg* 1995;21:375–384.

22. Pomposelli FB Jr, Arora S, Gibbons GW, et al. Lower extremity arterial reconstruction in the very elderly: successful outcome preserves not only the limb but also residential status and ambulatory function. *J Vasc Surg* 1998;28:215–225.

23. Nesto RW. Screening for asymptomatic coronary artery disease in diabetes *Diabetes Care* 1999;22:1393–1395 (editorial; comment).

24. Zarich SW, Cohen MC, Lane SE, et al. Routine perioperative dipyridamole 201Tl imaging in diabetic patients undergoing vascular surgery. *Diabetes Care* 1996;19:355–360.

25. Monahan TS, Shrikhande GV, Pomposelli FB, et al. Preoperative cardiac evaluation does not improve or predict perioperative or late survival in asymptomatic diabetic patients undergoing elective infrainguinal arterial reconstruction. *J Vasc Surg* 2005;41:38–45 (Discussion 45).

26. McFalls EO, Ward HB, Moritz TE, et al. Coronary-artery revascularization before elective major vascular surgery. *N Engl J Med* 2004;351:2795–2804.

27. Bode RH Jr, Lewis KP, Zarich SW, et al. Cardiac outcome after peripheral vascular surgery. Comparison of general and regional anesthesia. *Anesthesiology* 1996;84:3–13 (see comments).

28. Pierce ET, Pomposelli FB Jr, Stanley GD, et al. Anesthesia type does not influence early graft patency or limb salvage rates of lower extremity arterial bypass. *J Vasc Surg* 1997;25:226–232 (Discussion 232–233).

29. Carpenter JP, Baum RA, Holland GA, Barker CF. Peripheral vascular surgery with magnetic resonance angiography as the sole preoperative imaging modality. *J Vasc Surg* 1994;20:861–869 (Discussion 869–871).

30. Johnson BL, Glickman MH, Bandyk DF, Esses GE. Failure of foot salvage in patients with end-stage renal disease after surgical revascularization. *J Vasc Surg* 1995;22:280–285 (Discussion 285–286).

31. Leers SA, Reifsnyder T, Delmonte R, Caron M. Realistic expectations for pedal bypass grafts in patients with end-stage renal disease. *J Vasc Surg* 1998;28:976–980 (Discussion 981–983).

32. Harrington EB, Harrington ME, Schanzer H, Haimov M. End-stage renal disease—is infrainguinal limb revascularization justified? *J Vasc Surg* 1990;12:691–695 (Discussion 695–696).

33. Lantis JC 2nd, Conte MS, Belkin M, Whittemore AD, Mannick JA, Donaldson MC. Infrainguinal bypass grafting in patients with end-stage renal disease: improving outcomes? *J Vasc Surg* 2001;33:1171–1178.

34. Meyerson SL, Skelly CL, Curi MA, et al. Long-term results justify autogenous infrainguinal bypass grafting in patients with end-stage renal failure. *J Vasc Surg* 2001;34:27–33.

35. Ramdev P, Rayan SS, Sheahan M, et al. A decade experience with infrainguinal revascularization in a dialysis-dependent patient population. *J Vasc Surg* 2002;36:969–974.

36. Dormandy J, Heeck L, Vig S. The natural history of claudication: risk to life and limb. *Semin Vasc Surg* 1999;12:123–137.

37. McDermott MM, McCarthy W. Intermittent claudication. The natural history. *Surg Clin North Am* 1995;75:581–591.

38. Hertzer NR. The natural history of peripheral vascular disease. Implications for its management. *Circulation* 1991;83:I12–I19.

39. Dawson DL, Cutler BS, Hiatt WR, et al. A comparison of cilostazol and pentoxifylline for treating intermittent claudication. *Am J Med* 2000;109:523–530 (in Process Citation).

40. Dawson DL, Cutler BS, Meissner MH, Strandness DE Jr. Cilostazol has beneficial effects in treatment of intermittent claudication: results from a multicenter, randomized, prospective, double-blind trial. *Circulation* 1998;98:678–686.

41. Gillings DB. Pentoxifylline and intermittent claudication: review of clinical trials and cost-effectiveness analyses. *J Cardiovasc Pharmacol* 1995;25:S44–S50.

42. Pedersen TR, Kjekshus J, Pyorala K, et al. Effect of simvastatin on ischemic signs and symptoms in the Scandinavian simvastatin survival study (4S). *Am J Cardiol* 1998;81:333–335.

43. McDermott MM, Guralnik JM, Greenland P, et al. Statin use and leg functioning in patients with and without lower-extremity peripheral arterial disease. *Circulation* 2003;107:757–761.

44. Mondillo S, Ballo P, Barbati R, et al. Effects of simvastatin on walking performance and symptoms of intermittent claudication in hypercholesterolemic patients with peripheral vascular disease. *Am J Med* 2003;114:359–364.

45. Mohler ER 3rd, Hiatt WR, Creager MA. Cholesterol reduction with atorvastatin improves walking distance in patients with peripheral arterial disease. *Circulation* 2003;108:1481–1486.

46. O'Neil-Callahan K, Katsimaglis G, Tepper MR, et al. Statins decrease perioperative cardiac complications in patients undergoing noncardiac vascular surgery: the Statins for Risk Reduction in Surgery (StaRRS) study. *J Am Coll Cardiol* 2005;45:336–342.

47. Durazzo AE, Machado FS, Ikeoka DT, et al. Reduction in cardiovascular events after vascular surgery with atorvastatin: a randomized trial. *J Vasc Surg* 2004;39:967–975 (Discussion 975–976).

48. Poldermans D, Bax JJ, Kertai MD, et al. Statins are associated with a reduced incidence of perioperative mortality in patients undergoing major noncardiac vascular surgery. *Circulation* 2003;107:1848–1851.

49. Abbruzzese TA, Havens J, Belkin M, et al. Statin therapy is associated with improved patency of autogenous infrainguinal bypass grafts. *J Vasc Surg* 2004;39:1178–1185.

50. Christenson JT. Preoperative lipid control with simvastatin reduces the risk for graft failure already 1 year after myocardial revascularization. *Cardiovasc Surg* 2001;9:33–43.

51. Sacks FM, Pfeffer MA, Moye LA, et al. The effect of pravastatin on coronary events after myocardial infarction in patients with average cholesterol levels. Cholesterol and recurrent events trial investigators. *N Engl J Med* 1996;335:1001–1009.

52. Randomised trial of cholesterol lowering in 4444 patients with coronary heart disease: the Scandinavian Simvastatin Survival Study (4S). *Lancet* 1994;344:1383–1389.

53. Prevention of cardiovascular events and death with pravastatin in patients with coronary heart disease and a broad range of initial cholesterol levels. The Long-Term Intervention with Pravastatin in Ischaemic Disease (LIPID) Study Group. *N Engl J Med* 1998;339: 1349–1357.

54. Ridker PM, Rifai N, Clearfield M, et al. Measurement of C-reactive protein for the targeting of statin therapy in the primary prevention of acute coronary events. *N Engl J Med* 2001;344: 1959–1965.

55. Gahtan V. The noninvasive vascular laboratory. *Surg Clin North Am* 1998;78:507–518.

56. Raines J, Traad E. Noninvasive evaluation of peripheral vascular disease. *Med Clin North Am* 1980;64:283–304.

57. Weitz JI, Byrne J, Clagett GP, et al. Diagnosis and treatment of chronic arterial insufficiency of the lower extremities: a critical review *Circulation* 1996;94:3026–3049 (published erratum appears in *Circulation* 2000 29;102(9):1074).

58. White RA, Nolan L, Harley D, et al. Noninvasive evaluation of peripheral vascular disease using transcutaneous oxygen tension. *Am J Surg* 1982;144:68–75.

59. Hauser CJ, Klein SR, Mehringer CM, Appel P, Shoemaker WC. Superiority of transcutaneous oximetry in noninvasive vascular diagnosis in patients with diabetes. *Arch Surg* 1984;119: 690–694.

60. Bandyk DF, Seabrook GR, Moldenhauer P, et al. Hemodynamics of vein graft stenosis. *J Vasc Surg* 1988;8:688–695.

61. Carlson GA, Hoballah JJ, Sharp WJ, et al. Balloon angioplasty as a treatment of failing infrainguinal autologous vein bypass grafts. *J Vasc Surg* 2004;39:421–426.

62. Engelke C, Morgan RA, Belli AM. Cutting balloon percutaneous transluminal angioplasty for salvage of lower limb arterial bypass grafts: feasibility. *Radiology* 2002;223:106–114.

63. Blakeman BM, Littooy FN, Baker WH. Intra-arterial digital subtraction angiography as a method to study peripheral vascular disease. *J Vasc Surg* 1986;4:168–173.

64. Merten GJ, Burgess WP, Gray LV, et al. Prevention of contrast-induced nephropathy with sodium bicarbonate: a randomized controlled trial. *JAMA* 2004;291:2328–2334.

65. Birck R, Krzossok S, Markowetz F, Schnulle P, van der Woude FJ, Braun C. Acetylcysteine for prevention of contrast nephropathy: meta-analysis. *Lancet* 2003;362:598–603.

66. Ochoa A, Pellizzon G, Addala S, et al. Abbreviated dosing of *N*-acetylcysteine prevents contrast-induced nephropathy after elective and urgent coronary angiography and intervention. *J Interv Cardiol* 2004;17:159–165.

67. Veith FJ, Gupta SK, Ascer E, et al. Six-year prospective multicenter randomized comparison of autologous saphenous vein and expanded polytetrafluoroethylene grafts in infrainguinal arterial reconstructions. *J Vasc Surg* 1986;3:104–114.

68. Kunlin J. Le traitement de l'arterite obliterante par la greffe veinuse. *Arch Mal Coeur Vaiss* 1949;42:371.
69. Leather RP, Powers SR, Karmody AM. A reappraisal of the *in situ* saphenous vein arterial bypass: its use in limb salvage. *Surgery* 1979;86:453–461.
70. Buchbinder D, Rolins DL, Verta MJ, et al. Early experience with *in situ* saphenous vein bypass for distal arterial reconstruction. *Surgery* 1986;99:350–357.
71. Hurley JJ, Auer AI, Binnington HB, et al. Comparison of initial limb salvage in 98 consecutive patients with either reversed autogenous or *in situ* vein bypass graft procedures. *Am J Surg* 1985;150:777–781.
72. Strayhorn EC, Wohlgemuth S, Deuel M, Glickman MH, Hurwitz RL. Early experience utilizing the *in situ* saphenous vein technique in 54 patients. *J Cardiovasc Surg (Torino)* 1988;29:161–165.
73. Bush HL Jr, Corey CA, Nabseth DC. Distal *in situ* saphenous vein grafts for limb salvage. Increased operative blood flow and postoperative patency. *Am J Surg* 1983;145:542–548.
74. Cambria RP, Megerman J, Brewster DC, Warnock DF, Hasson J, Abbott WM. The evolution of morphologic and biomechanical changes in reversed and *in-situ* vein grafts. *Ann Surg* 1987;205:167–174.
75. Taylor LM Jr, Edwards JM, Porter JM. Present status of reversed vein bypass grafting: five-year results of a modern series. *J Vasc Surg* 1990;11:193–205 (Discussion 205–206).
76. Pomposelli FB Jr, Jepsen SJ, Gibbons GW, et al. A flexible approach to infrapopliteal vein grafts in patients with diabetes mellitus. *Arch Surg* 1991;126:724–727 (Discussion 727–729).
77. Ascer E, Veith FJ, Gupta SK, et al. Short vein grafts: a superior option for arterial reconstructions to poor or compromised outflow tracts? *J Vasc Surg* 1988;7:370–378.
78. Cantelmo NL, Snow JR, Menzoian JO, LoGerfo FW. Successful vein bypass in patients with an ischemic limb and a palpable popliteal pulse. *Arch Surg* 1986;121:217–220.
79. Stonebridge PA, Tsoukas AI, Pomposelli FB Jr, et al. Popliteal-to-distal bypass grafts for limb salvage in diabetics. *Eur J Vasc Surg* 1991;5:265–269.
80. Holzenbein TJ, Pomposelli FB Jr, Miller A, et al. Results of a policy with arm veins used as the first alternative to an unavailable ipsilateral greater saphenous vein for infrainguinal bypass. *J Vasc Surg* 1996;23:130–140.
81. Miller A, Campbell DR, Gibbons GW, et al. Routine intraoperative angioscopy in lower extremity revascularization. *Arch Surg* 1989;124:604–608.
82. Stonebridge PA, Miller A, Tsoukas A, et al. Angioscopy of arm vein infrainguinal bypass grafts. *Ann Vasc Surg* 1991;5:170–175.
83. Balshi JD, Cantelmo NL, Menzoian JO, LoGerfo FW. The use of arm veins for infrainguinal bypass in end-stage peripheral vascular disease. *Arch Surg* 1989;124:1078–1081.
84. Faries PL, Arora S, Pomposelli FB Jr, et al. The use of arm vein in lower-extremity revascularization: results of 520 procedures performed in eight years. *J Vasc Surg* 2000;31:50–59.
85. Pomposelli FB, Kansal N, Hamdan AD, et al. A decade of experience with dorsalis pedis artery bypass: analysis of outcome in more than 1000 cases. *J Vasc Surg* 2003;37:307–315.
86. Andros G, Harris RW, Salles-Cunha SX, Dulawa LB, Oblath RW, Apyan RL. Bypass grafts to the ankle and foot. *J Vasc Surg* 1988;7:785–794.
87. Darling RC 3rd, Chang BB, Shah DM, Leather RP. Choice of peroneal or dorsalis pedis artery bypass for limb salvage. *Semin Vasc Surg* 1997;10:17–22.
88. Levine AW, Davis RC, Gingery RO, Anderegg DD. *In situ* bypass to the dorsalis pedis and tibial arteries at the ankle. *Ann Vasc Surg* 1989;3:205–209.
89. Shanik DG, Auer AI, Hershey FB. Vein bypass to the dorsalis pedis artery for limb ischaemia. *Ir Med J* 1982;75:54–56.
90. Shieber W, Parks C. Dorsalis pedis artery in bypass grafting. *Am J Surg* 1974;128:752–755.
91. Hughes K, Domenig CM, Hamdan AD, et al. Bypass to plantar and tarsal arteries: an acceptable approach to limb salvage. *J Vasc Surg* 2004;40:1149–1157.

23
Angioplasty and Other Noninvasive Vascular Surgical Procedures

Sherry D. Scovell, MD

INTRODUCTION

The field of vascular surgery has undergone significant changes recently. Beginning with the development of less invasive techniques to manage general surgical pathology, such as laproscopic procedures, there has been a paradigm shift in the type of techniques that are available to treat patients. Historically, vascular surgery patients have been successfully treated with open surgical procedures in the majority of cases. Technology has allowed for the advent of change. In addition, the desire of patients to be treated with less invasive methods of management has pushed this technology as well as the clinical pattern of treatment.

Endovascular surgery is the management of vascular surgical disorders through less invasive methods of treatment. These methods of treatment have been around for many decades but have only recently been refined over the past few years. Currently, nearly every vascular disorder may be approached by either a classic open approach or a novel endovascular procedure. These distinctly diverse methods of treatment have their respective advantages and disadvantages and cannot be deemed equivalent. However, having two distinctly different methods of treatment available allows the vascular surgeon to fully evaluate the patient and decide which method would be best suited for treatment of that specific patient. The treatment may then be individualized to the particular patient, because now the vascular surgeon possesses the full armentarium of skills to treat patients with both open and endovascular surgery.

Patients with diabetes clearly have a predisposition to peripheral vascular disease, which is represented by cumulative damage to blood vessels. In the patient with diabetes, the pattern of lower extremity atherosclerosis has been found to involve the infrageniculate arteries with a relative sparing of the foot vessels (1). Just as this fact makes these patients particularly good candidates for distal bypass grafting, it also makes tibial intervention an attractive option. As patients with diabetes have atherosclerotic disease in the arteries to the lower extremities, they also manifest arterial occlusive disease in other vessels simultaneously, including the coronary circulation. This fact, coupled with the multiple medical comorbidities that often accompany diabetes, such as hypertension, hyperlipidemia, and renal vascular disease, makes less invasive alternatives especially attractive owing to the lower overall morbidity and mortality of the procedure as well as the quicker return to functional status.

From: *The Diabetic Foot, Second Edition*
Edited by: A. Veves, J. M. Giurini, and F. W. LoGerfo © Humana Press Inc., Totowa, NJ

This chapter will explore those less-invasive options that have recently been and currently are being refined to treat patients with severe peripheral vascular disease. In addition, the diabetic population has frequently been cited as a group, which may have worse outcomes than the nondiabetic population. We will examine what data is available exclusively in diabetic patients with respect to these interventional procedures.

HISTORY

The most basic interventional procedure is the angioplasty. By definition, angioplasty is the inflation of a balloon within an artery in the region of a plaque. This leads to fracture of that plaque allowing the expansion of the lumen. This concept was originally proposed by Dotter and Judkins in 1964 *(2)*. In general, angioplasty leads to reasonable patency rates but may also have complications. Arterial dissection is a frequent complication of angioplasty as might be expected following fracture of a plaque. If this dissection is flow limiting, it may lead to thrombosis of the vessel. In addition, lesions that are heavily calcified or eccentric may have residual stenosis after angioplasty. Additionally, some lesions may have significant recoil following angioplasty leading to a suboptimal result.

As a result of the above mentioned concerns, intravascular stents were developed to serve as a mechanical scaffolding that could be placed in the region of angioplasty to overcome these complications. A metallic stent is used to tack the intima and media down to the adventitia with the expectation of increasing overall patency rates.

Since then, there have been significant advances in technology with respect to balloons and catheters as well as stents. These advances combined with the low morbidity and mortality of percutaneous interventions had led to widespread acceptance of these procedures by physicians and patients alike.

PRESENTATION/INDICATIONS FOR ANGIOPLASTY

In general, patients with peripheral vascular disease present with claudication, rest pain, ulceration, or gangrene. Most patients with diabetes, however, present with limb-threatening ischemia, such as ulceration, gangrene, or rest pain instead of claudication because the classic pattern of arterial disease in patients with diabetes is in the distal vessels of the leg. These patients are often initially evaluated with noninvasive studies such as pulse volume recordings. However, the majority of patients ultimately require a method of defining the anatomy of the lower extremity arterial circulation and the associated stenoses or occlusions that are responsible for the above afflictions. This feat may be accomplished in a number of ways, including through the use of magnetic resonance angiography, duplex scanning, or arteriography. Contrast arteriography, however, remains the gold standard for this purpose.

ARTERIOGRAPHY

One of the essential steps in the evaluation of the patient with lower extremity peripheral vascular disease is the arteriogram. Through the cannulation of peripheral arteries, the injection of radio-opaque contrast agents into the arterial tree, and the capture of these images with digital subtraction techniques, a "road map" of the peripheral arterial circulation may be well defined *(3)*. In this manner, the vascular surgeon is able to

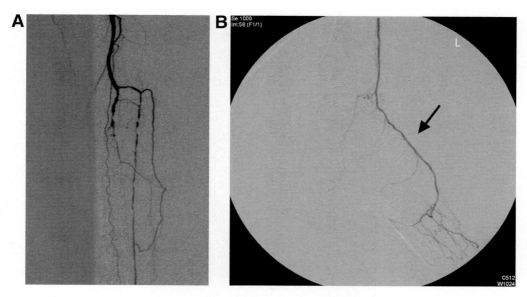

Fig. 1. (A,B) Tibial disease with sparing of the pedal vessels, which is typical in patients with diabetes.

specifically identify any and all critical regions of stenosis or occlusion along the arterial tree.

Proper angiographic technique is imperative in patients with diabetes. It is essential that the pedal vessels in the foot be adequately evaluated. This effort is especially critical in patients with diabetes as the tibial arteries are typically severely diseased with relative sparing of the foot vessels, such as the dorsalis pedis artery *(3)* (Fig. 1A,B). A common error of omission in patients with diabetes is to terminate the arteriogram once it is noted that the tibial vessels are occluded. There are, however, several technical maneuvers that can be performed in order to obtain adequate films of these distal foot vessels.

The angiographic catheter is typically inserted into the contralateral common femoral artery (CFA) and advanced into the distal aorta for abdominal aortic and subsequently pelvic views. However, before imaging the leg vessels, the distal external iliac artery (ipsilateral to the leg with the pathology) is cannulated selectively by positioning the catheter over the aortic bifurcation and placing the tip in the distal external iliac artery (Fig. 2). Images are then obtained from the level of the CFA to the dorsalis pedis artery in the foot. Magnified foot films are obtained in both lateral and anteroposterior projections thus allowing an accurate determination of the caliber and quality of the dorsalis pedis, posterior tibial, and plantar arteries. Additionally, these techniques allow the use of less-contrast agent as they are obtained selectively.

One of the distinct advantages of arteriography is that it is not only a diagnostic examination but allows for the physiological evaluation of stenotic lesions through the use of pressure gradient measurements across those lesions. Pressure measurements across the lesion in question is critical in evaluating whether the lesion is hemodynamically significant. This should be accomplished both with and without reactive hyperemia or with vasodilation. Nitroglycerine may be utilized at doses of 100 µg or 15–30 mg of

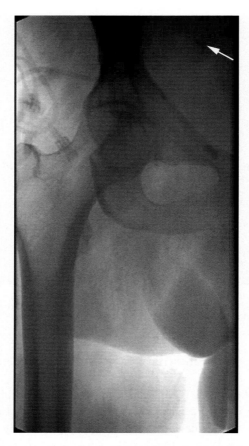

Fig. 2. The site of puncture is typically the femoral artery contralateral to the leg being evaluated. The catheter tip is then directed over the aortic bifurcation and placed in the distal external iliac artery of the leg to be studied.

papaverine may be substituted. A resting mean pressure gradient of greater that 5–7 mmHg and a post vasodilatation mean pressure gradient of greater than 10–15 mmHg in general define a hemodynamically significant lesion *(4)*. Pressure measurements should also be repeated following intervention to assure that the gradient has decreased or equalized and to evaluate technical success.

The arterial images created may then be utilized to determine whether the patient is best suited for endovascular or open surgical repair based on numerous factors such as lesion location and length as well as a host of others factors.

If an interventional procedure is deemed appropriate for the patient, it may be undertaken at the time of the initial arteriogram. Any significant arterial lesions uncovered may be treated through the use of angioplasty, stenting, and other novel techniques in the same setting as the diagnostic procedure.

These procedures, although essential, are invasive and not without complications. One complication that is slightly more common in patients with diabetes is that of acute renal failure. Adequate preprocedure hydration is essential to decrease the incidence of contrast-induced renal failure. This complication occurs less frequently owing to the introduction of nonionic contrast agents that are routinely utilized in diabetic populations *(5,6)*. In addition, for any patient with an elevated creatinine preprocedure, mucomyst or *N*-acetylcysteine is administered as well as a bicarbonate bolus which seems to be protective in patients with chronic renal insufficiency *(7)*. Other complications of interventional arterial procedures include bleeding, infection, pseudoaneurysm development, development of an arteriovenous fistula, and vessel thrombosis.

INTERVENTIONS

Typically, there are definite generalizations that may be followed as guidelines with respect to the interventional management of vascular disease. The results of interventional management are quite variable and dependent on multiple factors, including the length of the lesion and the location of the lesion in the arterial tree. In general, shorter lesions have more durable results when compared with longer lesions. As well, stenoses that are more proximal in the arterial tree, such as the common iliac artery, have more durable results than those located in distal vessels, such as tibial arteries. This is likely related to the fact that the more proximal vessels are larger in diameter and have higher flow rates. As would be expected, intervening on stenoses, in general, have longer lasting results when compared with occlusions. All of these factors need to be taken into consideration when determining if an endovascular procedure is appropriate for the patient.

As a result of the above generalizations, a classification system was developed in an attempt to characterize and further define outcomes. The Transatlantic Inter-Society Consensus (TASC) classification is a system that defines lesions based on the length, location, degree of calcification, and whether they are stenoses or occlusions *(8)*. This classification scheme is specific for each level of the arterial tree. When considering interventional management of stenoses or occlusions in the vascular tree, ultimately more proximal segments are classified and treated differently than those more distal in the arterial tree. For this reason, the TASC morphological classification system has been defined for each specific arterial segment. These defined regions are aortoiliac, femoropopliteal, and tibial.

Typically, TASC type-A lesions, or focal regions of stenosis, are best suited for endovascular management, whereas type-D lesions, which are occlusions, have the most durable results when treated with open surgical management. Although these generalizations are true, there are some type-D lesions that may warrant an attempt at endovascular management. The case in point would be a patient with multiple medical comorbidities who would not easily tolerate an extensive surgical procedure. An attempt at recanalization of the occluded arterial segment may be beneficial, especially in a patient with tissue loss, which may heal in a short time and not necessarily require long-term patency.

Another important consideration involves knowing the surgical options that are available to each individual patient. It is often prudent to preserve all viable surgical options available to the patient when performing an endovascular procedure. This is because longevity in interventional procedures cannot be expected or predicted at this point with any reasonable degree of certainty, and secondary surgical procedures may be required to prevent limb loss if the initial interventional procedure or procedures should fail.

BRIEF DESCRIPTION OF ANGIOPLASTY METHODS

As mentioned above, one major benefit of arteriography is that it may be both diagnostic and therapeutic. Most interventional procedures are undertaken at the time of the initial arteriogram. This allows the patient to undergo only one invasive procedure. Additionally, these interventions are typically performed under local anesthesia with monitored conscious sedation, which avoids the morbidity that may be associated with the fluctuations in blood pressure that can be seen with general anesthesia.

The small sheath that is used for arteriography is typically changed for a larger French sheath that will accommodate angioplasty balloons and stent delivery systems, which are typically higher profile than angiography catheters. The patient is systemically heparinized. Anticoagulation is necessary for the intervention as a short period of arterial occlusion is needed.

The appropriate diameter balloon and stent, depending on the location in the arterial tree, are chosen. Under fluoroscopy, the balloon is positioned around the region of stenosis and inflated. Typically, a repeat arteriogram of that region is preformed to evaluate the result of the angioplasty. If there is significant recoil, residual stenosis, or a flow-limiting dissection, placement of a stent is considered.

ASSESSMENT OF INTERVENTIONAL OUTCOMES

The success of an interventional procedure may be defined based on clinical, hemodynamic, and/or angiographic criteria. Clinical criteria refer to whether the initial indication for intervention has resolved. In the case of an ulcer, it may heal following an interventional procedure. If the artery restenoses after the ulcer has headed, there may not be any clinical consequences and thus, be defined as a clinical success. Typically, for patients with rest pain or life-limiting claudication, the symptoms recur if the area of the intervention restenoses. This would be a clinical failure.

Hemodynamic criteria refer to whether there is a pressure gradient across the region of previous intervention as measured at time of arteriography. Typically, before determining if a stenosis is significant, pressure measurements are taken in the artery proximal and subsequently distal to the lesion. These maneuvers may also be performed with the use of a vasodilator to mimic exercise or a hyperemic state. If there is a pressure gradient, the lesion is considered significant. Following intervention with either angioplasty or stent placement, repeat arterial pressures around the region of the lesion are again measured. A successful procedure is defined as no discernable residual pressure gradient. A failure would be defined as a continued pressure gradient across the region in question.

Finally, when arteriography uncovers an arterial lesion, the percent stenosis is typically calculated. To accomplish this task, the minimal luminal diameter of the stenotic segment is compared with the diameter of the normal adjacent artery. Once the intervention with angioplasty or stenting is undertaken, there should be less than 20% residual stenosis in the segment in question. Angiographic evidence for restenosis may be used to measure outcomes. The criterion for late angiographic success is typically defined as no evidence of recurrent stenosis greater than 50%. Failure is defined as progression to greater than or equal to 50% stenosis or the need for a repeat procedure on the initially treated segment of the artery. Typically, the percent restenosis is again determined by comparing the minimal luminal diameter of the stenotic region to the diameter of the adjacent normal artery.

AORTOILIAC LESIONS

The aorta and iliac arteries are well suited for interventional management. This fact is true because they are large diameter, high-flow vessels in the proximal arterial tree. They are easily accessed through the ipsilateral CFA. Aortoiliac artery lesions are classified

Table 1
Aortoiliac Lesions: TASC Classification

TASC type-A iliac lesions
   Single stenosis <3 cm of the CIA or EIA
TASC type-B iliac lesions
   Single stenosis 3–10 cm in length, not extending into the CFA
   Total of two stenoses <5 cm long in the CIA and/or EIA, not extending into the CFA
   Unilateral CIA occlusion
TASC type-C iliac lesions
   Bilateral 5–10 cm long stenosis of the CIA and/or EIA, not extending into the CFA
   Unilateral occlusion involving both the CIA and EIA
   Unilateral stenosis extending into the CFA
   Bilateral CIA occlusion
TASC type-D iliac lesions
   Diffuse, multiple unilateral stenoses involving the CIA, EIA, and CFA (usually >10 cm)
   Unilateral occlusion involving both the CIA and EIA
   Bilateral EIA occlusions
   Diffuse disease involving the aorta and both iliac arteries
   Iliac stenoses in a patient with an abdominal aortic aneurysm or other lesion requiring
      aortic or iliac surgery

by the extent of disease as well as their location in the proximal arterial tree. Above is the morphological stratification of iliac lesions *(9)* (Table 1).

In general, the iliac lesions that are classified as type-A lesions are best managed by endovascular management. Those classified as type-D lesions are typically best managed by open surgery. It would seem as if type-B lesions might be able to be successfully managed by endovascular means and type-C lesions best treated by open surgical methods, although the data in unclear at this point.

The TASC working group evaluated four studies regarding iliac artery interventions, which had carefully documented results and follow-up. In these series, the indication for intervention in the majority of patients was intermittent claudication in 77% *(9)*. Overall, the patency rates in patients treated for intermittent claudication were close to 80% at 1 year and 60% at 5 years. Interestingly, the patency rates for a successful recanalization of an occluded iliac artery were not significantly different from the patency rate for angioplasty of a stenotic region (Fig. 3A,B). Also, of note, interventions were less durable when performed on the external iliac artery when compared with the common iliac artery.

Arteriography in patients with diabetes often demonstrates multi-level disease. Therefore, iliac artery interventions may need to be coupled or staged with either distal open or percutaneous revascularization. As well results were better in patients with good runoff vessels and those being treated for less severe disease, such as those with intermittent claudication vs limb-threatening ischemia *(10)*.

In patients with diabetes, iliac artery lesions tend to be more eccentric and heavily calcified. These two factors/features may predict failure with angioplasty alone and primary stent placement in such cases may be warranted. In general, outcomes of iliac angioplasty and limb-salvage rates were similar in with and without diabetes with respect to long-term patency *(11)*.

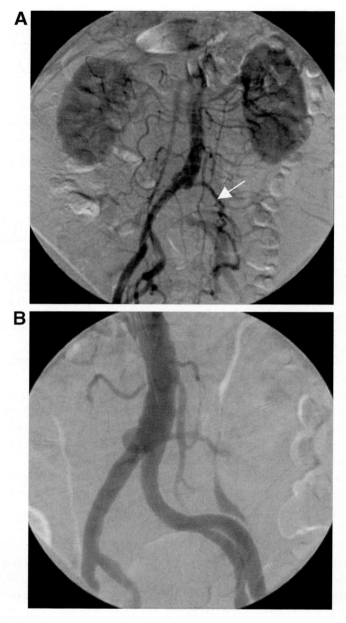

Fig. 3. (A,B) Iliac artery recanalization.

There are several contraindications to iliac artery angioplasty. In the past, diffuse disease in the iliac artery seemed to preclude endovascular management. This is not currently the case. Although external iliac angioplasty and stent placement, especially in women, tend to fare worse long term with respect to patency, this procedure is often undertaken, likely because of the ease of the procedure and the lower morbidity and mortality when compared with open surgery *(12)*. It is a contraindication to endovascularly treat an iliac stenosis that is in continuity with aneurysmal disease. This is because of the suggestion that manipulation of the balloon and stent in the region of the aneurysm

Table 2
Femoropopliteal Lesions: TASC Classification

TASC type-A femoropopliteal lesions
  Single stenosis up to 3 cm in length, not at the origin of the superficial femoral artery
  or the distal popliteal artery
TASC type-B femoropopliteal lesions
  Single stenoses or occlusions 3–5 cm long, not involving the distal popliteal artery
  Heavily calcified stenoses up to 3 cm in length
  Multiple lesions, each less than 3 cm (stenoses or occlusions)
TASC type-C femoropopliteal lesions
  Single stenosis or occlusion longer that 5 cm
  Multiple stenoses or occlusions, each 3–5 cm, with or without heavy calcification
TASC type-D femoropopliteal lesions
  Complete CFA or superficial femoral artery occlusions or complete popliteal and proximal
    trifurcation occlusions

may precipitate rupture of the adjacent aneurysm. These iliac stenoses may easily be treated in the operating room at the same time that the aneurysm is being repaired.

FEMORAL AND POPLITEAL ARTERIES

Intuitively, the results of intervention in the aortoiliac segment are more durable when compared with that of the femoropopliteal region. Rutherford and Durham constructed composite patency curves comparing these two regions. They discovered that intervention in the femoropopliteal region had an early failure rate that was twice as high as that in the aortoiliac region *(13)*. However, the longer-term failure rate seemed to be the same as with iliac angioplasty.

As in the aortoiliac arteries, there were found to be certain factors that seemed predictive of a favorable outcome in this region. The TASC working group defined a morphological classification system for stratification of femoropopliteal lesions as well *(9)* (Table 2). Of significance, patients with claudication as an indication as well as good distal runoff seemed to have a higher patency rate *(14)* (Fig. 4A,B). In addition, occlusions longer than 5 cm had a primary success rate of 12% compared with occlusions with lengths of less than 5 cm which had primary success rates of 32% *(15)*.

Additionally, patients without diabetes seemed to fare better with respect to patency in this region *(16–18)*. In a retrospective study, cumulative freedom from restenosis at 12 months was 77% in patients without diabetes and 22% in patients with diabetes *(19)*. For this reason, interventional management of the femoropopliteal segment in patients with diabetes should be utilized with caution and with lower patency expectations when compared with patients without diabetes.

TIBIAL ARTERIES

However, patients with diabetes typically manifest the majority of their disease in their infrageniculate arteries with relative sparing of the foot vessels. This is the reason that extreme distal arterial reconstruction is feasible in this patient population. It is also why tibial angioplasty will eventually play a large role in the care of these patients *(3)*.

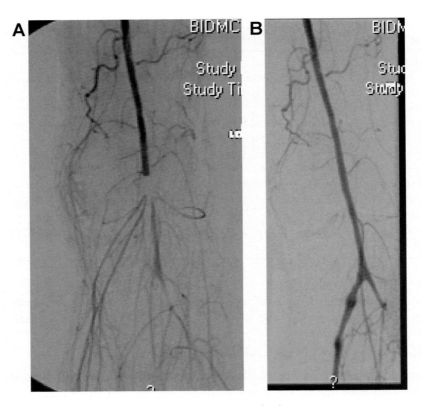

Fig. 4. (A,B) Popliteal angioplasty.

The role of angioplasty with respect to the tibial vessels has not been well defined as of yet. There have even been studies that suggest that angioplasty in the patient with diabetes should only be considered with respect to the proximal vessels, such as the iliac arteries. Recently, however, there has been a trend toward initially treating patients with interventional management, even in the diabetic population. The majority of published literature on angioplasty of the tibial arteries refers to short, focal stenoses *(20)*. However, there are some data to suggest that interventional management may be feasible in patients with longer segment stenoses or occlusions (Fig. 5A,B).

One of the largest studies till date on interventional management in patients with diabetes suggests that angioplasty, even in the tibial vessels, is not an unreasonable option *(21)*. In this study from Italy, 221 patients with diabetes underwent angiographic evaluation for ulceration. Of those, 219 patients were discovered to have significant evidence of arterial stenosis or occlusion and underwent angioplasty; 5.8% of patients had angioplasty in the femoral or popliteal regions; 42.4% had angioplasty of the infrapopliteal arteries, and 51.8% underwent angioplasty of vessels in both regions.

Worsening of the ulcer or the development of rest pain determined recurrence. In this case of suspected recurrence, the patient underwent ankle–brachial pressure measurements and TcPO$_2$ measurements followed by an arterial duplex examination of the region of previous angioplasty. The patients were also subjected to a repeat arteriogram. Clinical recurrence occurred in 7.3% (14 patients) of patients within an average time of 4.6 months (range 1–12 months). In 10 of these patients, a second angioplasty could be performed successfully thus permitting limb salvage.

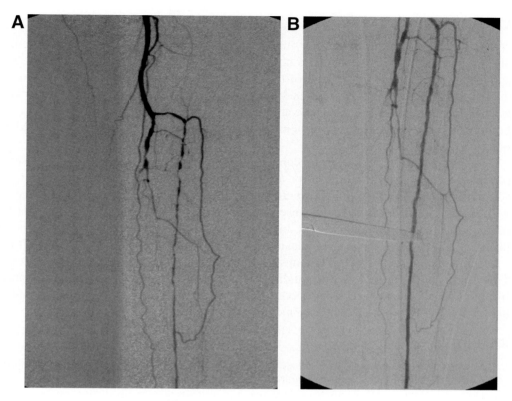

Fig. 5. (A,B) Tibial angioplasty.

The clinical recurrence rate in this series is quite low, especially in consideration of the length and location of the lesions treated. However, the lesions in this study were not uniform. These patients had a combination of focal lesions mixed with long segmental stenoses or occlusions as well as multiple lesions in the same vessel, which were often extremely calcified.

Much of the data in the literature today is similar to this study. The lesions are not typically uniform and as mentioned previously, the length of the lesion and whether it is a stenosis or an occlusion will play a significant role in the overall outcome of the intervention. In addition, long-term follow-up in these patients is lacking. However, it certainly remains an alternative for those diabetic patients with multiple medical comorbidities in which an operation is a less attractive option.

DIABETES AND ANGIOPLASTY

Diabetes mellitus was not associated with either early or late failure in iliac arteries with angioplasty and primary stenting *(22)*. With respect to angioplasty alone in this region, diabetes did seem to affect patient outcome *(23)*. With respect to the femoropopliteal segment, patients with diabetes do seem to exhibit lower long term patency rates when compared with patients without diabetes *(19)*. In the tibial vessels, there is not enough long-term data in the literature to comment about patency specifically in the diabetic population. However, this seems to be the region that will most affect outcome in the patient with diabetes, as the tibial vessels are typically diseased *(24)*.

CONCLUSIONS

These data and the emergence of interventional management of peripheral vascular disease in patients with diabetes has become a popular option, both with surgeons and patients alike. This fact is because of the high efficacy combined with the low risk of the procedure. Typically, these procedures are performed under local anesthesia with monitored conscious sedation. There are no incisions created by the procedure, and the prudent operator always preserves their surgical options if a bypass procedure should be required at a later time.

The high rate of restenosis or reocclusion is typically touted as the downfall of these procedures. However, the option for a repeat intervention or a surgical procedure is typically available in these cases. Angioplasty is particularly useful in diabetic patients with tissue loss or ulceration. In these patients, restenosis or reocclusion may not be detected if the vessel remains patent until the ulcer heals and subsequently occludes. In this manner, the restenosis or reocclusion is irrelevant as there is no longer tissue loss.

Overall, angioplasty with or without stenting is a viable option in patients with diabetes. This offers another alternative to patients with ulceration, rest pain, or less commonly, life-limiting claudication. It is a procedure that is less invasive and certainly becoming more popular with vascular surgeons and patients alike.

REFERENCES

1. LoGerfo FW, Gibbons GW, Pomposelli FB, et al. Trends in the care of the diabetic foot. Expanded role of arterial reconstruction. *Arch Surg* 1992;127:617–621.
2. Dotter CT, Judkins MP. Transluminal treatment of artherosclerotic obstruction: description of a new technique and a preliminary report of its application. *Circulation* 1964;30:654–670.
3. LoGerfo FW, Coffman JD. Current concepts. Vascular and microvascular disease of the foot in diabetics. Implications for foot care. *N Engl J Med* 1984;311:1615–1619.
4. Bonn J. Percutaneous vascular intervention: value of hemodynamic measurements. *Radiology* 1996;201:18–20.
5. Aspelin P, Aubry P, Fransson SG, Strasser R, Willenbrock R, Lundkvist J. Cost-effectiveness of iodixanol in patients at high risk of contrast-induced nephropathy. *Am Heart J* 2005;149: 298–303.
6. Lautin EM, Freeman NJ, Schoenfeld AH, et al. Radiocontrast-associated renal dysfunction: incidence and risk factors. *AJR Am J Roentgenol* 1991;157:66–68.
7. Blakeman BM, Littooy F, Baker WH. Intra-arterial digital subtraction angiography as a method to study peripheral vascular diseases. *J Vasc Surg* 1986;4:168–173.
8. Tepel M, van der Giet M, Schwarzfeld C, et al. Prevention of radiographic-contrast-agent-induced reductions in renal function by acetylcysteine. *N Engl J Med* 2000;343:210–212.
9. TASC. Management of peripheral arterial disease (PAD)/Transatlantic Inter-Society Consensus (TASC). *J Vasc Surg* 2000;31, Part 2.
10. Faries PL, Brophy D, LoGerfo FW, et al. Combined iliac angioplasty and infrainguinal revascularization surgery are effective in diabetic patients with multilevel arterial disease. *Ann Vasc Surg* 2001;15:67–72.
11. Spence LD, Hartnell GG, Reinking G, Gibbons G, Pomposelli F, Clouse ME. Diabetic versus nondiabetic limb-threatening ischemia: outcome of percutaneous iliac intervention. *AJR Am J Roentgenol* 1999;172:1335–1341.
12. Timaran CH, Prault TL, Stevens SL, Freeman MB, Goldman MH. Iliac artery stenting versus surgical reconstruction for TASC (Transatlantic Inter-Society Consensus) type B and type C iliac lesions. *J Vasc Surg* 2003;38:272–278.

13. Dormandy JA, Rutherford RB. Management of peripheral arterial disease (PAD). TASC Working Group. Transatlantic Inter-Society Consensus (TASC). *J Vasc Surg* 2000;31(Suppl): S1–S296.

14. Stanley B, Teague B, Raptis S, Taylor DJ, Berce M. Efficacy of balloon angioplasty of the superficial femoral artery and popliteal artery in the relief of leg ischemia. *J Vasc Surg* 1996;23:679–685.

15. Lofberg A, Karacagil S, Ljungman C, et al. Percutaneous transluminal angioplasty of the femoropopliteal arteries in limbs with chronic critical lower limb ischemia. *J Vasc Surg* 2001;34:114–121.

16. Rutherford RB, Durham J. Percutaneous balloon angioplasty for artheriosclerosis obliterans: long term results, in *Techniques in Vascular Surgery* (Yao JST, Pearce WH, eds.), Saunders, Philadelphia, PA, 1992, pp. 329–345.

17. Capek P, McLean GK, Berkowitz HD. Femoropopliteal angioplasty. Factors influencing long-term success. *Circulation* 1991;83:I-70–I-80.

18. Johnston KW. Femoral and popliteal arteries: reanalysis of results of balloon angioplasty. *Radiology* 1992;183:767–772.

19. Sabeti S, Mlekusch W, Amighi J, Minar E, Schillinger M. Primary patency of long-segment self-expanding nitinol stents in the femoropopliteal arteries. *J Endovasc Ther* 2005;12:6–12.

20. Matsi PJ, Manninen HI, Vanninen RL, et al. Femoropopliteal angioplasty in patients with claudication: primary and secondary patency in 140 limbs with 1–3-yr follow-up. *Radiology* 1994;191:727–733.

21. Ouriel K. Peripheral arterial disease. *Lancet* 2001;358:1257–1264.

22. Faglia E, Mantero M, Caminiti M, et al. Extensive use of peripheral angioplasty, particularly infrapopliteal, in the treatment of ischaemic diabetic foot ulcers: clinical results of a multi-centric study of 221 consecutive diabetic subjects. *J Intern Med* 2002;252:225–232.

23. Sullivan TM, Childs MB, Bacharach JM, Gray BH, Piedmonte MR. Percutaneous transluminal angioplasty and primary stenting of the iliac arteries in 288 patients. *J Vasc Surg* 1997;25: 829–839.

24. Johnston KW. Iliac arteries: reanalysis of results of balloon angioplasty. *Radiology* 1993; 186:207–212.

Psychosocial and Educational Implications of Diabetic Foot Complications

Katie Weinger, EdD, RN and Arlene Smaldone, DNSc, CPNP, CDE

INTRODUCTION

In recent years, clinicians have begun to recognize the impact that educational, psychosocial, and behavioral factors have on treatment success for leg and foot wounds. Furthermore, many now consider quality of life as an important outcome of treatment for those suffering from neuropathy, foot ulcerations, and amputations. However, although interest is increasing, behavioral aspects of the diabetic foot remain fledging science. Researchers are only now beginning to investigate the psychological response to diabetic foot ulceration and amputation and the behavioral and psychological factors that influence self-care. Although cross-sectional studies have explored these areas, little longitudinal data currently exists.

In this chapter, we review the current state of behavioral science pertaining to individuals with diabetic foot disease including barriers to prevention, precipitating factors, and therapeutic interventions. The first section describes some of the behavioral/psychological issues faced by individuals with diabetes during the course of their illness. We describe four phases of psychological responses and attempt to relate these phases to the prevention, diagnosis, or treatment of foot problems. Then, we discuss quality of life for those with peripheral neuropathy, lower extremity wounds, or amputations. Next, we discuss depression, its impact on self-care, signs and symptoms, and implications of treatment. Finally, we describe strategies and interventions that may be useful for clinicians either to incorporate into their clinical practice or as a referral for struggling patients.

PHASES OF PSYCHOLOGICAL RESPONSES AND EDUCATIONAL ASPECTS OF DIABETES

Individuals face significant events or crises at different points during the course of diabetes that challenge their usual ways of coping and dealing with stress (1–3). These events evoke heightened anxiety, feelings of helplessness, and temporary states of cognitive confusion. People facing crisis typically employ coping strategies they have used in the past that have varying levels of effectiveness (1). Some strategies such as denial or anger may actually interfere with health whereas other strategies using a more pragmatic approach serve to help incorporate information and skills into one's lifestyle (4). Those living with diabetes may face important stressors throughout the course of illness.

From: *The Diabetic Foot, Second Edition*
Edited by: A. Veves, J. M. Giurini, and F. W. LoGerfo © Humana Press Inc., Totowa, NJ

Four periods warrant special mention: onset of diabetes, health maintenance and prevention, early onset of complications, and the stage of illness in which complications dominate *(2,3)*. Each period has psychological and educational implications for the patient, family, and clinician regarding the prevention and treatment of foot problems.

Onset of Diabetes

The onset of diabetes is typically abrupt for those diagnosed with type 1 diabetes and for some diagnosed with type 2 diabetes. The patient and family, faced with the task of acquiring knowledge and "survival skills," must adapt quickly to a new and demanding regimen of insulin injections, blood glucose monitoring, nutrition, and other lifestyle adjustments. Both patients and families may experience a period of grief and mourning for loss of the healthy self and begin to adjust to the idea of living with a serious chronic illness. Prior experience with diabetes, such as having a family member or friend who has the disease, can color the response to the diagnosis. During times of crisis, individuals have difficulty both processing and retaining information *(1,5)*. Yet for most people with diabetes, diagnosis is the time when they receive diabetes education, and for many people, this education is the only formal education they receive during the course of their illness. Discussion of preventive measures such as foot care is often lost or simply not addressed when faced with the priorities of acquisition of "survival skills."

Onset of diabetes for those diagnosed with type 2 diabetes is typically more gradual and viewed as less cumbersome. Often, the perception of type 2 diabetes and treatment with oral medications for blood glucose control is considered a normal part of aging. Most individuals, if worried, are concerned about heart disease and hypertension, rather than their feet. Similarly, clinicians tend to stress more immediate concerns during their initial patient interactions. Prevention of foot complications is typically not addressed nor perceived as an immediate need by patients or clinicians.

Maintenance of Health and Prevention of Complications

During the maintenance phase, treatment, and education focus on prevention of complications, healthy lifestyle habits, and incorporating changes in lifestyle into family life. Individuals with diabetes develop diabetes "habits," self-care behaviors that can include key preventive practices such as foot care. People tend to remember and do those things that they perceive as most important, typically those instructions that clinicians particularly stressed *(6)*. Unfortunately, not all physicians and educators emphasize the importance of foot care. Many clinicians do not check feet at each visit *(7,8)*, but instead may focus on glycemic control in hopes that improved glycemia will prevent foot problems *(9)*. Evidence suggests that preventive foot care education can decrease the incidence of ulceration and need for amputation *(9–12)*. Unless special effort is made to teach by example during office visits, preventive foot care will be largely ignored. Clearly, both patients and clinicians need education about foot assessment *(13)* and preventive foot care *(12,14)*. Receiving education does not go hand-in-hand with the practice of self-care behaviors. Some patients may experience denial and resistance to treatment; these people typically have difficulty integrating preventive practices into their daily routines. Incorporating chronic illness into one's worldview takes time; health-care personnel play key roles in coaching and assisting the patient to achieve this effectively.

Early Onset of Complications

Complications of diabetes develop insidiously. Most patients go through a period of years before being affected by microvascular and macrovascular complications. Although the concept of complications should not be foreign to patients with diabetes, the onset and recognition of complications set a new disease trajectory affecting patients' relationships with family and providers and their self-image as a functioning, "healthy" person.

The prevalence of peripheral neuropathy is estimated to be 28.5% in patients with diabetes with most cases (62%) asymptomatic *(15)*. Patients who lack protective sensation are seven times more likely to develop a foot ulcer secondary to physical and/or thermal trauma *(16)*. Treatment of neuropathy or its sequelae, foot ulceration and/or amputation, accounts for about 27% of medical costs attributed to diabetes in the United States *(17)*. Neuropathy is often first identified on routine examination of the feet by either decreased reflexes or impaired localized sensation both of which have gone unnoticed by the patient. At this point, intervention remains directed at maintaining circulation and skin integrity through heightened attention to foot care. However, for many patients, hearing this "bad news" engenders high levels of stress and anxiety that serve to block the important communication occurring between provider and patient at this time *(1)*. Therefore, patients may be unable to effectively process what needs to be done to maintain their health. Furthermore, people often use the experiences of others to understand their own condition. Thus, patients may use the experiences of family and friends with diabetes to frame their assumptions about complications and may assume their own course will be fixed to a similar path. Often these assumptions are not communicated to their health provider. Yet these beliefs and assumptions about diabetic neuropathy and its management are fundamental to motivation and performance of preventive foot care behaviors *(18)*.

As neuropathy progresses, the patient is often faced with neuropathic foot pain which may be moderate-to-severe in intensity and difficult to control. Treatment is often not highly effective and patients must learn to live with discomfort that impacts their usual level of activity, ability to function, and sleep. Those with painful neuropathy may respond in one of two ways: maintenance of a high level of vigilance and a renewed interest in their health care practices that will facilitate preventive foot care or a more fatalistic response, "there's nothing I can do to control the course of events," which will inhibit motivation to perform preventive foot care behaviors *(18)*.

Evidence suggests that the risk of foot ulcers and their associated cost of care could be significantly reduced by appropriate screening and targeted preventive strategies geared toward good foot care *(10,12,19)*. However, to be successful, these strategies must use a patient-centered approach in order to understand how patients make sense of and emotionally respond to diabetes because these are intimately linked to employment of self-care behaviors *(20)*.

Complications Dominate

Foot ulceration affects 15–30% of patients with diabetes during their lifetime *(21,22)* and complications of nonhealing ulcers include infection, gangrene, and amputation of the affected limb. Foot ulcers are a causative factor in 85% of all nontraumatic lower limb amputations with resulting high morbidity and mortality *(23)*. Furthermore, those

Table 1
Psychosocial Consequences of Foot Ulcers or Amputations

Depression
Alterations in self-image as a disabled person vs a healthy functioning person
Alterations in body image
Disruptions in family relationships
Dependency/over dependency
Alterations in social relationships
Social isolation
Sleep disturbances
Disruption in sexuality or sexual functioning

who undergo amputation are at higher risk for loss of their remaining limb in the future
(24). Table 1 summarizes the psychosocial consequences of diabetic foot ulceration and
amputation.

Diagnosis of a foot ulcer sets a new level of intensity to the patient's treatment regimen. Consultation with a specialist may be required for wound management. Patients
will experience a double burden of illness—they still need to maintain or improve their
self-care behaviors for management of diabetes but now need to perform complex
wound care treatment regimens, establish relationships with new clinicians, and face
new implications for both long- and short-term outcome. The patient may be unable to
walk or drive a car, making him dependent on others for office visits, dressing changes,
obtaining treatment supplies, and routine activities of daily life. Sleep is disrupted by
pain and discomfort *(25,26)*. Treatment regimens are lengthy, complex, painful, and
often require hospitalization. In one study of diabetic patients with foot ulcers, 68%
reported negative psychological impact that comprised anxiety, depression, social isolation, and negative self-image *(27)*. These negative emotions resulting from ulcerations
may be because of the fear of amputation and frustration with the lengthy course of
treatment and its uncertainty regarding outcome *(25,28,29)*.

Adjustment to Amputation

Few studies have used longitudinal design to investigate the psychological response
to amputations. Thus, we currently rely on cross-sectional data to understand factors
that impact adjustment. Most of the studies that examine amputation include individuals
with traumatic and medical amputations and thus are not diabetes specific. However,
much of the information may apply to patients with diabetes. Phantom limb and stump
pain may affect adjustment to amputation *(30,31)*. Although phantom limb pain was
originally viewed as psychosomatic in origin, current views hold that it also may have
a physiological basis *(32,33)*. Phantom limb pain is common with one study
finding 69% of persons with amputations experiencing this problem *(34)*. Whether
psychological factors play any role in the origin of phantom limb pain is unclear.
However, the presence of phantom pain may impede adjustment to amputation *(31,35)*
as reports have found it associated with depression *(35–37)*, body image anxiety
(35,36,38), and stress *(30)*.

An individual with an amputation must cope with alterations in identity, with some
viewing themselves as disabled vs healthy *(30)*. People with amputations will probably

face the curiosity of society and the conscious or unconsciously labeling of "being different" *(30–32)*. These data suggest that helping individuals with a newly amputated limb prepare for societal response to their missing limb may be an important role for the health care team; patients need to know what to expect and anticipate how they feel and how they could respond.

QUALITY OF LIFE

People value feeling well and most individuals place high priority on either maintaining or improving the way they feel. Neuropathy and its sequelae of foot ulceration and amputation diminish one's perception of self and feeling of wellness as these patients cope with neuropathic pain, wound management and diminished mobility *(26)*. Treatment regimens for those faced with neuropathic pain are often complex and difficult for patients to understand, for example, carefully titrated dosing, different medication combinations, and alternate uses of medications such as antidepressants for pain. Despite this, pain is often difficult to control. Further, treatment of foot ulceration is often burdensome, imposes additional mobility restrictions, and is of long and uncertain duration. In one study of quality of life for those with foot ulceration *(39)* the mean duration of ulcer treatment was 43 weeks and others have reported that approx 70% of those receiving standard foot ulcer care will not heal after 20 weeks of treatment *(40)*. Although treatment duration is long, individuals with diabetic foot ulceration who seek timely care are more likely to heal today than a decade ago *(41)*. However promises of future improvement in health may not be a good motivator to follow complex treatment regimens when gains are associated with lifestyle restrictions of long duration and without guarantee of success *(42)*.

Many people with diabetes feel burdened to some degree by the rigorous demands of their disease. Quality of life is a multidimensional concept representing an individual's physical, emotional, and social well-being from his own unique perspective *(43)*. Health-related quality of life and disease-specific quality of life refer to the impact of health problems on one's everyday life: examples include the effect of disease and its treatment on a patient's functioning, health beliefs, and subjective feelings of well-being *(44)*. As such, health-related quality of life is subject to change over time and over the course of illness.

Quality of Life and Self-Care

Clinicians need to understand patients' quality of life in order to understand their motivation or lack of motivation for self-care including wound care. Rubin *(43)* noted that those affected by what he termed "diabetes overwhelmus" or poor quality of life often take a "to hell with it!" attitude toward their self-care, doing less than recommended to manage their diabetes resulting in diminished self-care. Thus, assessment of quality-of-life issues is important, because it may powerfully predict an individual's capacity to manage his disease and follow treatment recommendations.

Assessing Quality of Life

Currently no gold standard exists for the assessment of diabetes-specific quality of life and a variety of instruments have been developed and used by researchers to understand the influence of glycemic control, treatment regimens, and complications on the person affected by diabetes. Diabetes researchers have used both general health and disease-specific quality-of-life instruments in order to appreciate the challenges of diabetes from the patient perspective. Diabetes quality-of-life studies have focused primarily on describing the health state of individuals with varying levels of symptoms and complications.

The use of intensive insulin regimens prompted interest in diabetes specific quality of life and thus, in measuring diabetes patients' quality of life. The diabetes quality-of-life *(45)* measure was developed for use during the diabetes complications and control trial and subsequently adapted for youth *(46)*. Diabetes complications and control trial found that intensity of diabetes treatment regimen does not, in itself, impair quality of life for those treated with intensive insulin regimens *(47)*. The well-being questionnaire *(48)* is another diabetes-specific quality-of-life measure developed for use in a World Health Organization study evaluating new treatments for the management of diabetes.

The Problem Areas in Diabetes *(49,50)* (Fig. 1) is both a clinical tool and an outcomes measure to identify diabetes-related emotional distress. Twenty items cover a range of emotional issues common among those with both types 1 and 2 diabetes. High scores indicate greater emotional distress and a score of more than 40–50 merits referral to a mental health professional. The Problem Areas in Diabetes survey strongly correlates with both depression and self-care *(51)* and is responsive to change over time *(52)* thus making it useful in assessment of patients undergoing long-treatment regimens such as foot ulcer therapies. Identification of individual items of concern to the patient can serve as a point of conversation during the office visit.

General health-related quality-of-life measures (i.e., not focusing on a specific disease such as diabetes) also provide information on quality of life in patients with diabetes. The EuroQol quality-of-life tool (EQ-5D) has two components: a questionnaire that assesses mobility, self-care, usual activities, pain, anxiety, and depression and a visual analog scale that allows patients to indicate their quality on a scale of 0–100 *(39)*. Functional health status is another important aspect of quality of life; the Short Form 36 is a well-used measure in this area *(53)*. These measures, although not diabetes specific, allow comparison of quality-of-life issues for those with diabetes to both the general population and those with other chronic conditions.

The NeuroQoL *(54)* is a recently developed instrument designed to study the effect of neuropathy and foot ulceration on quality of life. Items for this measure were derived from interviews with patients directly affected by neuropathy and/or foot ulcers.

Thus, several tools are available for use by clinicians to assess quality of life and its impact on patients' self-care and motivation.

Effect of Diabetes and Neuropathic Complications on Quality of Life

Only a few studies have specifically examined the effect of foot ulcers and amputation on quality of life and these have primarily used generic rather than diabetes-specific instruments.

In general, quality of life is lower for those with diabetes compared with those unaffected by the disease *(55)*. Further, quality of life for patients with type 2 diabetes without complications and not on insulin was slightly higher compared to those with uncomplicated type 1 diabetes; scores for those with diabetes were similar to scores reported in other studies for adults with chronic obstructive pulmonary disease and osteoarthritis *(55)*. Similar findings have been reported by others *(56,57)*.

INSTRUCTIONS: Which of the following diabetes issues are currently a problem for you?
Circle the number that gives the best answer for you. Please provide an answer for each question.

	Not a problem	Minor problem	Moderate problem	Somewhat serious problem	Serious problem
1. Not having clear and concrete goals for your diabetes care?	0	1	2	3	4
2. Feeling discouraged with your diabetes treatment plan?	0	1	2	3	4
3. Feeling scared when you think about living with diabetes?	0	1	2	3	4
4. Uncomfortable social situations related to your diabetes care (e.g., people telling you what to eat)?	0	1	2	3	4
5. Feelings of deprivation regarding food and meals?	0	1	2	3	4
6. Feeling depressed when you think about living with diabetes?	0	1	2	3	4
7. Not knowing if your mood or feelings are related to your diabetes?	0	1	2	3	4
8. Feeling overwhelmed by your diabetes?	0	1	2	3	4
9. Worrying about low blood sugar reactions?	0	1	2	3	4
10. Feeling angry when you think about living with diabetes?	0	1	2	3	4
11. Feeling constantly concerned about food and eating?	0	1	2	3	4
12. Worrying about the future and the possibility of serious complications?	0	1	2	3	4
13. Feelings of guilt or anxiety when you get off track with your diabetes management?	0	1	2	3	4
14. Not "accepting" your diabetes?	0	1	2	3	4
15. Feeling unsatisfied with your diabetes physician?	0	1	2	3	4
16. Feeling that diabetes is taking up too much of your mental and physical energy every day?	0	1	2	3	4
17. Feeling alone with your diabetes?	0	1	2	3	4
18. Feeling that your friends and family are not supportive of your diabetes management efforts?	0	1	2	3	4
19. Coping with complications of diabetes?	0	1	2	3	4
20. Feeling "burned out" by the constant effort needed to manage diabetes?	0	1	2	3	4

Fig. 1. The Problem Areas in Diabetes questionnaire.

Complications of diabetes are the most important disease-specific determinant of quality of life for diabetes patients *(58)*. Quality of life is diminished not only for those affected by neuropathy and its sequelae but for their caregivers as well *(50,59)*. Coffee *(55)* reported progressively lower quality-of-life scores for those with symptomatic neuropathy and ulceration with the lowest scores reported for those with amputation indicating the increased health burdens presented by these complications. However, others suggest that those treated for foot ulceration may experience poorer quality of life than those with amputation because of the fear of ulcer recurrence, repeated episodes of infection, and potential life-long disability *(27,60)*.

Impact on Patient and Family

Qualitative studies using focus group *(25)* and in-depth interview *(26)* methodology offer insight into the experiences of those with foot ulceration and family members who participate in their care. Foot ulcers require the incorporation of a completely different lifestyle for both patients and their caregivers and have an equally negative impact on both the patient and caregiver. Reduced mobility and diminished sense of self restricts the patient's usual life regardless of age and has consequences on role function and sexuality. Although interest in sexual activity does not diminish *(61,62)*, many individuals with lower extremity amputations report problems such as loss of libido and erectile dysfunction *(62,63)*. Because of problems with autonomic neuropathy, sexual problems may be more prevalent among individuals with diabetes. Loss of employment is a problem for many affected by ulceration or amputation, particularly those in occupations which require a great deal of walking or standing and is associated with reduced self-esteem especially for younger patients.

Restrictions in mobility are particularly hard for diabetic patients with foot ulcers. Patients are generally concerned with becoming a burden on others in terms of their daily care, shopping, cooking, and transportation to frequent medical appointments *(25,26)*. Patients and their caregivers voice their perception of social isolation, patients because of the physical activity restrictions imposed by the ulcer and family members because of the time and intensity burden of caring for their ill family member *(25,26)*. One qualitative study reports *(25)* that despite their understanding that nonweight bearing would promote healing, nearly all patients could not comply either through necessity or frustration. The negative impact of foot ulceration on quality of life is pervasive for both patient and family and fraught with uncertainty about whether the ulcer will heal and, if so, whether it will recur in the future.

Implications for the Practitioner

Focusing attention on physical care of the feet without attention to the psychosocial features of health-related quality of life has important limiting effects on both patient care and strategies for intervention *(26)*. Greater understanding of quality of life specific to lower extremity ulcers by physicians is important to allow for improved patient-physician communication, adherence to treatment regimens and increase in patient satisfaction and quality of care. Further, assessment of the impact of diabetes on the patient is important to identification of patients who may have a more difficult time in either complying with the demands of more demanding self-care regimens, or may benefit from referral to a mental health professional for counseling. The Problem Areas in Diabetes scale is particularly useful in this area.

DEPRESSION AND DEPRESSIVE DISORDERS

Depression is a serious psychiatric disorder that interferes with interpersonal relationships, quality of life, and the ability to perform and function. Both amputation and diabetes are independently associated with depression, placing these individuals at

Table 2
Symptoms of Depression

Loss of pleasure or interest in activities	Pessimism
Tearfulness and crying spells	Significant weight or appetite loss when
Irritability[a]	not dieting; failure to gain age
Increased sense of worthlessness or guilt	appropriate weight[a]
Recurrent thoughts of suicide or death	Indecisiveness
Suicide threats or attempts	Social withdrawal or isolation
Loss of concentration[b]	Insomnia or hypersomnia[a]
Decrease in recent memory[b]	Psychomotor slowing[a]
Fatigue; loss of energy[b]	Psychomotor agitation

[a]Depressed mood and four other symptoms below for more than 2 weeks may indicate major depression.
[b]Symptoms that may also reflect poorly controlled diabetes and/or hypoglycemia.

extremely high risk of depression and its consequences *(64–66)*. Depression may accompany amputation in the general population with older people experiencing more depression within the first 2 years following amputation and younger individuals experiencing more depression over the longer term *(67)*.

Diabetes and Depression

The prevalence of depression for people with diabetes is about two to three times that of the general population *(65,66)*. Comorbid depression occurs in all age groups, and ethnic minorities experience depressive symptoms and depression at rates that equal those of adult Caucasians *(68–71)*. In addition, severity of depressive symptoms is associated with poor adherence to dietary recommendations and medication regimen, functional impairment and higher health care costs in primary care diabetes patients *(72)*. High levels of diabetes-related emotional distress are associated with poor adherence to self-care behavior recommendations *(51)*. Thus, dysthymia, subclinical depression, and diabetes-related emotional distress can impact the success of diabetes treatment, diabetes self-care, and one's ability to care for their wound or amputation. Unfortunately, depression in diabetes is both underrecognized and, when recognized, undertreated *(73–76)*.

To further complicate the picture, depression among people with diabetes is also associated with the presence of other serious complications: retinopathy, macrovascular complications of cardiovascular disease, neuropathy, nephropathy, hypertension, and sexual dysfunction *(68,77–80)*. Thus, individuals with depression and peripheral vascular disease may also be coping with other serious comorbidities.

Depression may present with cognitive, physical, affective, or attitudinal symptoms. Table 2 lists symptoms that typically mark depression, although most people present with only some of these symptoms. The physical and cognitive symptoms often overlap with poorly controlled diabetes, making the diagnosis more difficult. Several short assessment tools such as the Beck Depression Inventory *(81)*, the Hospital Anxiety and Depression Scale *(82)*, or the Brief Symptom Inventory *(83)* are useful for screening for depression. Asking simple questions such as "during the past month, have you been bothered by feeling down, depressed, or hopeless?" and "during the past month, have you been bothered by little interest or pleasure in doing things?" can be as successful as surveys when screening for depression *(84)*. If a person experiences depressed mood or loss of interest or pleasure in usual activities and at least four other depressive symptoms for a duration of at least 2 weeks, then depression must be considered *(85)*. Major depression must be considered when these symptoms are accompanied by deterioration in glycemic control or the inability to function in the home or at work.

Treatment of Depression

Depressive disorders are usually responsive to treatment with medications or psychotherapy. Both treatments are effective used alone or in combination *(77,86)*. Although the primary care provider typically initiates pharmacotherapy, knowledge of when to institute a mental health referral is important *(87)*. Those with suicidal ideation are at serious risk and need immediate referral to psychiatric care. As depression improves and symptoms begin to remit, patients are more energetic and therefore at greater risk of suicide. A mental health professional can also help (1) evaluate the success of current therapy, (2) institute combination therapy using counseling as well as medication, (3) individualize pharmacotherapy, and (4) evaluate the need for hospitalization.

STRATEGIES TO IMPROVE SELF-CARE BEHAVIORS

Several techniques are available to for use by clinicians to help patients improve their self-care behaviors. This section describes these techniques, some of which can be easily incorporated into an office visit or other patient encounter.

Reinforcing Information

Most people remember only a small portion of the information that they receive during medical appointments. Studies that compared the information retained by patients after the appointment with the information that physicians gave patients during the appointment found that between 31% and 71% of information was forgotten *(6)*. Clinicians need specific techniques to reinforce important information for their patients that do not require large amounts of time and that help make the appointment more effective and efficient. Helpful techniques include:

1. People tend to remember those things that are presented first, thus state the most important points first.
2. Those things that are perceived as important are remembered better. Thus, a clinician who wants a person to remember a point could start by saying: "This is very important."
3. Simple instructions are remembered better than complex instructions.
4. Be specific and concrete rather than vague. For example, "Take off your socks and check your feet and between your toes every day" is more specific and easier to follow than "Be sure to check your feet."
5. Information, particularly key points or take home messages, written down in simple terms helps reinforce learning and information retention.
6. Ask patients to prepare for their medical appointment by writing down all questions that arise during the week prior to the appointment and bring that written list to the office with

them. This approach is a very efficient way to assess the patient and answer outstanding questions. People tend to remember information about issues that they have previously considered and that directly relates to them or their health.

Interview Techniques to Help with Patients who Struggle with their Self-Care

Motivational Interviewing *(88,89)* incorporates standard interviewing techniques in a process that is designed to help individuals who are struggling with health issues get back on track with their self-care. This technique, originally developed in the addictions field, provides a useful platform for busy clinicians to address barriers in an effective, simple manner.

Open-ended questions allow the patient to verbalize feelings and provide information in their own words thus preventing the clinician's preconceived ideas to dictate patient responses. *"Tell me about…" "How are you doing with taking your medications?" "What is it like to wear the orthotic?" "What problems are you having taking care of your diabetes?"* Although questions such as *"How are you doing?"* and *"How do you feel?"* appear open-ended, they are vague and have also taken on a social context that precludes more than a superficial response of "Fine."

Active listening entails consciously focusing on what the person means. This is not as easy as it sounds. Although everyone listens to some extent, busy clinicians may develop a preconceived idea of what the person means. Many people tend to think about what they will say next instead of focusing on what the patient is actually saying. Two useful tools for listening are reflection and summarizing:

1. Reflection. Repeat or paraphrase statements back to the person but using the tone of a question. *"You are having trouble with your exercise plan?" "You are frustrated with your treatment recommendations?"*
2. Summarizing. Summarizing the general idea of the patient's conversation shows that you have been listening and that you understand what the patient means. This technique also provides an opportunity to correct any misunderstandings. If the patient has outlined a plan or made other positive steps, summarizing can help reinforce their progress.

CONCLUSIONS

People with diabetes diagnosed with complications are at increased risk for diabetes-related distress and depression. Distress and depression impact the patient's ability to carry out self-care behaviors and follow through with treatment recommendations. This inability may limit success of regimens designed to prevent and treat foot ulceration. We offer some psychosocial, communication and education strategies that can be employed by physicians and other caregivers, and describe several and suggest a clinical assessment tools to identify patients who are having quality-of-life issues and who may benefit from referral to a mental health specialist for additional counseling and/or pharmacological intervention to help patients and family members obtain the most benefit from office visits.

ACKNOWLEDGMENTS

This work was supported by National Institutes of Health R01 DK60115 (KW) and National Institutes of Health Training Grant DK07260 (AS).

REFERENCES

1. Hamburg BA, Inoff GE. Coping with predictable crises of diabetes. *Diabetes Care* 1983;6(4): 409–416.
2. Jacobson AM, Weinger K. Psychosocial complications in diabetes, in *Medical Management of Diabetes* (Leahy J, Clark N, Cefalu W, eds.), Marcel Dekker, Inc., New York, 2000, pp. 559–572.
3. Weinger K, Welch G, Jacobson A. Psychological and psychiatric issues in diabetes mellitus, in *Principles of Diabetes Mellitus* (Poretsky L, ed.), Kluwer Academic Publishers, Norwell, MA, 2002, pp. 639–654.
4. Peyrot M, McMurry JF Jr, Kruger DF. A biopsychosocial model of glycemic control in diabetes: stress, coping and regimen adherence. *J Health Soc Behav* 1999;40(2):141–158.
5. Weinger K, McMurrich SJ. Behavioral strategies for improving self-management, in *Complete Nurse's Guide to Diabetes Care* (Childs B, Cypress M, Spollett G, eds.), American Diabetes Association, Alexandria, VA, 2005.
6. Ley P. Satisfaction, compliance and communication. *Br J Clin Psychol* 1982;21(Pt 4): 241–254.
7. Cohen SJ. Potential barriers to diabetes care. *Diabetes Care* 1983;6(5):499, 500.
8. Bailey TS, Yu HM, Rayfield EJ. Patterns of foot examination in a diabetes clinic. *Am J Med* 1985;78(3):371–374.
9. O'Brien KE, Chandramohan V, Nelson DA, Fischer JR Jr, Stevens G, Poremba JA. Effect of a physician-directed educational campaign on performance of proper diabetic foot exams in an outpatient setting. *J Gen Intern Med* 2003;18(4):258–265.
10. Malone JM, Snyder M, Anderson G, Bernhard VM, Holloway GA Jr, Bunt TJ. Prevention of amputation by diabetic education. *Am J Surg* 1989;158(6):520–523 (Discussion 523–524).
11. Barth R, Campbell LV, Allen S, Jupp JJ, Chisholm DJ. Intensive education improves knowledge, compliance, and foot problems in type 2 diabetes. *Diabet Med* 1991;8(2):111–117.
12. Apelqvist J, Larsson J. What is the most effective way to reduce incidence of amputation in the diabetic foot? *Diabetes Metab Res Rev* 2000;16(Suppl 1):S75–S83.
13. Thompson L, Nester C, Stuart L, Wiles P. Interclinician variation in diabetes foot assessment— a national lottery? *Diabet Med* 2005;22(2):196–199.
14. Boulton AJ. Why bother educating the multi-disciplinary team and the patient—the example of prevention of lower extremity amputation in diabetes. *Patient Educ Couns* 1995;26(1–3): 183–188.
15. Gregg EW, Sorlie P, Paulose-Ram R, et al. Prevalence of lower-extremity disease in the US adult population ≥40 years of age with and without diabetes: 1999–2000 national health and nutrition examination survey. *Diabetes Care* 2004;27(7):1591–1597.
16. Reiber GE, Vileikyte L, Boyko EJ, et al. Causal pathways for incident lower-extremity ulcers in patients with diabetes from two settings. *Diabetes Care* 1999;22(1):157–162.
17. American Diabetes Association. Economic consequences of diabetes mellitus in the US in 1997. *Diabetes Care* 1998;21(2):296–309.
18. Vileikyte L, Rubin RR, Leventhal H. Psychological aspects of diabetic neuropathic foot complications: an overview. *Diabetes Metab Res Rev* 2004;20(Suppl 1):S13–S18.
19. Litzelman DK, Slemenda CW, Langefeld CD, et al. Reduction of lower extremity clinical abnormalities in patients with non-insulin-dependent diabetes mellitus. A randomized, controlled trial. *Ann Intern Med* 1993;119(1):36–41.
20. Vileikyte L. Diabetic foot ulcers: a quality of life issue. *Diabetes Metab Res Rev* 2001;17(4):246–249.
21. Levin ME, Sicard GA, Baumann DS, Loechl B. Does crossing the legs decrease arterial pressure in diabetic patients with peripheral vascular disease? *Diabetes Care* 1993;16(10):1384–1386.
22. Kumar S, Ashe HA, Parnell LN, et al. The prevalence of foot ulceration and its correlates in type 2 diabetic patients: a population-based study. *Diabet Med* 1994;11(5):480–484.

23. Pecoraro RE, Reiber GE, Burgess EM. Pathways to diabetic limb amputation. Basis for prevention. *Diabetes Care* 1990;13(5):513–521.
24. Ebskov B, Josephsen P. Incidence of reamputation and death after gangrene of the lower extremity. *Prosthet Orthot Int* 1980;4(2):77–80.
25. Brod M. Quality of life issues in patients with diabetes and lower extremity ulcers: patients and care givers. *Qual Life Res* 1998;7(4):365–372.
26. Kinmond K, McGee P, Gough S, Ashford R. 'Loss of self': a psychosocial study of the quality of life of adults with diabetic foot ulceration. *J Tissue Viability* 2003;13(1):6–8, 10, 12 passim.
27. Carrington AL, Mawdsley SK, Morley M, Kincey J, Boulton AJ. Psychological status of diabetic people with or without lower limb disability. *Diabetes Res Clin Prac* 1996;32(1–2): 19–25.
28. Peyrot M, Rubin RR. Levels and risks of depression and anxiety symptomatology among diabetic adults. *Diabetes Care* 1997;20(4):585–590.
29. Phillips T, Stanton B, Provan A, Lew R. A study of the impact of leg ulcers on quality of life: financial, social, and psychologic implications. *J Am Acad Dermatol* 1994;31(1): 49–53.
30. Horgan O, MacLachlan M. Psychosocial adjustment to lower-limb amputation: a review. *Disabil Rehabil* 2004;26(14–15):837–850.
31. Hanley MA, Jensen MP, Ehde DM, Hoffman AJ, Patterson DR, Robinson LR. Psychosocial predictors of long-term adjustment to lower-limb amputation and phantom limb pain. *Disabil Rehabil* 2004;26(14–15):882–893.
32. Katz S, Gagliese L. Phantom pain: a continuing puzzle, in *Psychosocial Factors in Pain: Critical Perspectives* (Gatchel D, Turk D, eds.), The Guilford Press, New York, 1999, pp. 284–300.
33. Hill A. Phantom limb pain: a review of the literature on attributes and potential mechanisms. *J Pain Symptom Manage* 1999;17(2):125–142.
34. Gallagher P, Allen D, MacLachlan M. Phantom limb pain and residual limb pain following lower limb amputation: a descriptive analysis. *Disabil Rehabil* 2001;23(12):522–530.
35. Rybarczyk B, Edwards R, Behel J. Diversity in adjustment to a leg amputation: case illustrations of common themes. *Disabil Rehabil* 2004;26(14–15):944–953.
36. Rybarczyk B, Nyenhuis DL, Nicholas JJ, Cash SM. Body image, perceived social stigma, and the prediction of psychosocial adjustment to leg amputation. *Rehabil Psychol* 1995;40(2): 95–110.
37. Hogan P, Dall T, Nikolov P. Economic costs of diabetes in the US in 2002. *Diabetes Care* 2003; 26(3):917–932.
38. Pucher I, Kickinger W, Frischenschlager O. Coping with amputation and phantom limb pain. *J Psychosom Res* 1999;46(4):379–383.
39. Tennvall GR, Apelqvist J. Health-related quality of life in patients with diabetes mellitus and foot ulcers. *J Diabetes Complications* 2000;14:235–241.
40. Margolis DJ, Kantor J, Berlin JA. Healing of diabetic neuropathic foot ulcers receiving standard treatment. A meta-analysis. *Diabetes Care* 1999;22(5):692–695.
41. Margolis DJ, Allen-Taylor L, Hoffstad O, Berlin JA. Healing diabetic neuropathic foot ulcers: are we getting better? *Diabet Med* 2005;22(2):172–176.
42. Bradley C, Gamsu DS. Guidelines for encouraging psychological well-being: report of a Working Group of the World Health Organization Regional Office for Europe and International Diabetes Federation European Region St Vincent Declaration Action Programme for Diabetes. *Diabet Med* 1994;11(5):510–516.
43. Rubin R. Diabetes and quality of life. *Diabetes Spectr* 2000;13(1):21–23.
44. Snoek FJ. Quality of life: a closer look at measuring patients' well-being. *Diabetes Spectr* 2000; 13(1):24–28.
45. Reliability and validity of a diabetes quality-of-life measure for the diabetes control and complications trial (DCCT). The DCCT Research Group. *Diabetes Care* 1988;11(9):725–732.

46. Ingersoll GM, Marrero DG. A modified quality-of-life measure for youths: psychometric properties. *Diabetes Educ* 1991;17(2):114–118.
47. Influence of intensive diabetes treatment on quality-of-life outcomes in the diabetes control and complications trial. *Diabetes Care* 1996;19(3):195–203.
48. Bradley C. The well-being questionnaire, in *Handbook of Psychology and Diabetes* (Bradley C, ed.), Hardwood Academic Publishers, Chur, 1994, pp. 89–110.
49. Welch GW, Jacobson AM, Polonsky WH. The problem areas in diabetes scale. An evaluation of its clinical utility. *Diabetes Care* 1997;20(5):760–766.
50. Polonsky WH, Anderson BJ, Lohrer PA, et al. Assessment of diabetes-related distress. *Diabetes Care* 1995;18(6):754–760.
51. Weinger K, Jacobson AM. Psychosocial and quality of life correlates of glycemic control during intensive treatment of type 1 diabetes. *Patient Educ Couns* 2001;42(2):123–131.
52. Welch G, Weinger K, Anderson B, Polonsky WH. Responsiveness of the Problem Areas In Diabetes (PAID) questionnaire. *Diabet Med* 2003;20(1):69–72.
53. Ware J. *SF 36 Health Survey Manual and Interpretation Guide*, Health Institute New England Medical Center, Boston, MA, 1993.
54. Vileikyte L, Peyrot M, Bundy C, et al. The development and validation of a neuropathy- and foot ulcer-specific quality of life instrument. *Diabetes Care* 2003;26(9):2549–2555.
55. Coffey JT, Brandle M, Zhou H, et al. Valuing health-related quality of life in diabetes. *Diabetes Care* 2002;25(12):2238–2243.
56. Quality of life in type 2 diabetic patients is affected by complications but not by intensive policies to improve blood glucose or blood pressure control (UKPDS 37). UK Prospective Diabetes Study Group. *Diabetes Care* 1999;22(7):1125–1136.
57. Redekop WK, Koopmanschap MA, Stolk RP, Rutten GE, Wolffenbuttel BH, Niessen LW. Health-related quality of life and treatment satisfaction in Dutch patients with type 2 diabetes. *Diabetes Care* 2002;25(3):458–463.
58. Rubin RR, Peyrot M. Quality of life and diabetes. *Diabetes Metab Res Rev* 1999;15(3): 205–218.
59. Wikblad K, Leksell J, Wibell L. Health-related quality of life in relation to metabolic control and late complications in patients with insulin dependent diabetes mellitus. *Qual Life Res* 1996;5(1):123–130.
60. Price P. The diabetic foot: quality of life. *Clin Infect Dis* 2004;39(Suppl 2):S129–S131.
61. Ide M, Watanabe T, Toyonaga T. Sexuality in persons with limb amputation. *Prosthet Orthot Int* 2002;26(3):189–194.
62. Bodenheimer C, Kerrigan AJ, Garber SL, Monga TN. Sexuality in persons with lower extremity amputations. *Disabil Rehabil* 2000;22(9):409–415.
63. Ide M. Sexuality in persons with limb amputation: a meaningful discussion of re-integration. *Disabil Rehabil* 2004;26(14–15):939–943.
64. Kashani JH, Frank RG, Kashani SR, Wonderlich SA, Reid JC. Depression among amputees. *J Clin Psychiatry* 1983;44(7):256–258.
65. Lloyd CE, Dyer PH, Barnett AH. Prevalence of symptoms of depression and anxiety in a diabetes clinic population. *Diabet Med* 2000;17(3):198–202.
66. Anderson RJ, Freedland KE, Clouse RE, Lustman PJ. The prevalence of comorbid depression in adults with diabetes: a meta-analysis. *Diabetes Care* 2001;24(6):1069–1078.
67. Frank RG, Kashani JH, Kashani SR, Wonderlich SA, Umlauf RL, Ashkanazi GS. Psychological response to amputation as a function of age and time since amputation. *Br J Psychiatry* 1984;144:493–497.
68. Kovacs M, Mukerji P, Drash A, Iyengar S. Biomedical and psychiatric risk factors for retinopathy among children with IDDM. *Diabetes Care* 1995;18(12):1592–1599.
69. Roy A, Roy M. Depressive symptoms in African-American type 1 diabetics. *Depress Anxiety* 2001;13(1):28–31.

70. Black SA. Increased health burden associated with comorbid depression in older diabetic Mexican Americans. Results from the Hispanic Established Population for the Epidemiologic Study of the Elderly survey. *Diabetes Care* 1999;22(1):56–64.
71. Gary TL, Crum RM, Cooper-Patrick L, Ford D, Brancati FL. Depressive symptoms and metabolic control in African-Americans with type 2 diabetes. *Diabetes Care* 2000;23(1):23–29.
72. Ciechanowski PS, Katon WJ, Russo JE. Depression and diabetes: impact of depressive symptoms on adherence, function, and costs. *Arch Intern Med* 2000;160(21):3278–3285.
73. Sclar DA, Robison LM, Skaer TL, Galin RS. Depression in diabetes mellitus: a national survey of office-based encounters, 1990–1995. *Diabetes Educ* 1999;25(3):331–332, see also 335 and 340.
74. Jacobson AM, Weinger K. Treating depression in diabetic patients: is there an alternative to medications? *Ann Intern Med* 1998;129(8):656–657.
75. Kovacs M, Obrosky DS, Goldston D, Drash A. Major depressive disorder in youths with IDDM. A controlled prospective study of course and outcome. *Diabetes Care* 1997;20(1):45–51.
76. Perez-Stable EJ, Miranda J, Munoz RF, Ying YW. Depression in medical outpatients. Under recognition and misdiagnosis. *Arch Intern Med* 1990;150(5):1083–1088.
77. Lustman PJ, Griffith LS, Gavard JA, Clouse RE. Depression in adults with diabetes. *Diabetes Care* 1992;15(11):1631–1639.
78. Jacobson AM. The psychological care of patients with insulin-dependent diabetes mellitus. *N Engl J Med* 1996;334(19):1249–1253.
79. Cohen HW, Gibson G, Alderman MH. Excess risk of myocardial infarction in patients treated with antidepressant medications: association with use of tricyclic agents. *Am J Med* 2000;108(1):2–8.
80. de Groot M, Anderson R, Freedland KE, Clouse RE, Lustman PJ. Association of depression and diabetes complications: a meta-analysis. *Psychosom Med* 2001;63(4):619–630.
81. Beck AT, Steer RA. Internal consistencies of the original and revised Beck Depression Inventory. *J Clin Psychol* 1984;40(6):1365–1367.
82. Zigmond AS, Snaith RP. The hospital anxiety and depression scale. *Acta Psychiatr Scand* 1983;67(6):361–370.
83. Derogatis LR. *BSI 18: Brief Symptom Inventory. Administration, Scoring and Procedures Manual*, National Computer Systems, Inc., Minneapolis, MN, 2000.
84. Whooley MA, Avins AL, Miranda J, Browner WS. Case-finding instruments for depression. Two questions are as good as many. *J Gen Intern Med* 1997;12(7):439–445.
85. American Psychiatric Association. *Diagnostic and Statistical Manual of Mental Disorders*, (DSM-IV TFo, ed.), 4th ed. American Psychiatric Association, Washington, DC, 1994.
86. US Department of Health and Human Services DGP. Treatment of major depression (Clinical Practice Guidelines, No 5), in *Depression in Primary Care* (Research AfHCPa, ed.), US Government Printing Office, Washington, DC, 1993.
87. Gallagher P. Introduction to the special issue on psychosocial perspectives on amputation and prosthetics. *Disabil Rehabil* 2004;26(14–15):827–830.
88. Miller WR, Rollnick S. *Motivational Interviewing Preparing People for Change,* The Guilford Press, New York, 2002.
89. Rollnick S, Mason P, Butler C. *Health Behavior Change: A Guide for Practitioners*, Churchill Livingstone, Edinburgh, 1999.

25

The Role of Footwear in the Prevention
of Diabetic Foot Problems

Luigi Uccioli, MD

INTRODUCTION

Diabetes represents the primary cause of nontraumatic amputation in the Western World *(1)*. It is estimated that about 25% of subjects with diabetes will experience problems over the course of their lives with their feet and that one-third of these patients will undergo amputation *(2–4)*. Although these data highlight the extent of this problem in the diabetic population, they do not necessarily predicate inevitability: on the contrary, they serve to demonstrate that simple and relatively inexpensive measures may be able to reduce even up to 85% the number of amputations *(5–9)*. Some clinical conditions put the patient with diabetes "at risk of ulceration." An awareness of these conditions and the identification of subjects at risk may permit the introduction of suitable preventive strategies *(10–13)*.

Although peripheral vascular disease is only rarely a precipitating factor in ulcer formation *(3)*, neuropathy has a central role in the mechanisms underlying the lesion, representing a predisposing factor whereas other external factors may precipitate the situation and determine the appearance of ulcers *(14–16)*. Among the latter a decisive role is played by footwear: indeed, unsuitable footwear may not sufficiently protect the foot and in some cases may even be dangerous.

Given that the interaction between foot and footwear is crucial in the mechanism of ulceration, it is important that the health provider is not only aware of the importance of the selection of suitable footwear but that he or she is able to make a professional evaluation in this regard as correct footwear may represent a valid means of prevention.

Moreover, it is important to focus attention on the role of footwear and loading characteristics in repair mechanisms insofar as a neuropathic ulcer may heal spontaneously simply through an appropriate unloading at the site of the lesion.

Neuropathic complications may pose a risk of foot ulceration through two different mechanisms:

The first is related to sensory neuropathy *(17)*. The insensitivity of the feet to painful stimuli makes them particularly vulnerable in terms of external forces such as very high temperatures (water, sand, heaters, and so on) or to foreign bodies in the shoe (pebbles, coins, and so on) or even to very worn shoes or to those containing contusive particles

From: *The Diabetic Foot, Second Edition*
Edited by: A. Veves, J. M. Giurini, and F. W. LoGerfo © Humana Press Inc., Totowa, NJ

(e.g., tacks), or to unsuitable footwear in terms of size and/or shape. The footwear may be too tight or incorrectly sized, or unsuitable for deformed toes (with ensuing friction between the foot and shoe); in any case, painful symptoms are absent and are therefore unable to protect the foot from detrimental external factors (18). Numerous prospective studies demonstrate the relationship between neuropathy and ulceration. The determination of the vibratory perception threshold using biotesiometry or tactile sensitivity using monofilaments enables an evaluation of the degree of risk encountered by patients because of neuropathic complications (14,19–23).

The other mechanism through which neuropathy is responsible for foot lesions is related to the presence of both sensory and motor neuropathies (24). Motor neuropathy is responsible for a progressive atrophy of the intrinsic muscles of the foot. Foot shape is the result of an equilibrium between flexor and extensor muscles, therefore their atrophy induces foot deformities such as hammer or claw toes, hallux valgus, and prominent metatarsal heads. These changes are responsible for the development of areas of high plantar pressure (25,26). Although not exclusive to diabetic neuropathy, claw toe, hammer toe, and bunions are all conditions that when associated with peripheral neuropathy are particularly dangerous. On the one hand, they generate friction with footwear (e.g., claw toe not adequately accommodated in insufficient space in the frontal region with ensuing friction with the surface of the foot); on the other, they are associated with a lack of sense perception and consequently of sensitivity, and naturally a reduced defense capacity from the point of view of mechanical damage. Furthermore, these deformities result in areas of hyperpression, particularly at the level of the metatarsal heads, in which reactive hyperkeratosis first appears followed by ulceration (20,27,28).

In the presence of neuropathy foot deformities are responsible for the frontal shift of the submetatarsal adipose pads, following which the metatarsal heads come into direct contact with the ground (29). It is in this situation that the development of hyperkeratosis, that is a response mechanism to the overload, is in itself responsible for further hyperpression (indeed, it has been ascertained that the removal of a hyperkeratosis is able to reduce hyperpression up to 30%) (30). Some prospective studies have also demonstrated the relationship between areas of hyperpression and the subsequent development of ulceration (31). It should also be borne in mind that an increase in pressure associated with insensitivity represents an increased risk; indeed, subjects with rheumatoid arthritis with comparable hyperpression do not experience ulceration (32). Therefore, it is fairly evident that a reduction in hyperpression represents a means of reducing the risk of ulceration.

Limited joint mobility also seems to contribute in fact a reduction of the range of motion of the ankle joint has been associated with increased risk of ulceration. In addition patients with diabetes develop changes in plantar fascia and achilles tendon in terms of increased thickness. Plantar fascia might play a role in the pathogenesis of abnormal forefoot pressures in patients with diabetes; it has been hypothesized that its increased thickness might lead to the development of the cavus neuropathic foot.

In the neuropathic foot the horizontal forces of the intrinsic and extrinsic muscles are deficient and therefore their opposition to the flattening of the arch during gait is decreased. On the other hand, the horizontal forces coming from plantar fascia are increased because of its increased thickness and because of its sprain related to the displacement of the metatarsophalangeal joint resulting from development of the claw toes. Finally a rigid foot, thus less adaptable to the floor during the foot–floor interaction, develops; it remains rigid

Table 1
Risk Classes

Low	Patients with normal protective sensation
Medium	Loss of protective sensation, without foot deformities and without history of foot ulceration or previous amputation
High	Loss of protective sensation, with foot deformities but without history of foot ulceration and/or amputation
Very high	Loss of protective sensation, with foot deformities and with history of foot ulceration or amputation

during the whole walking cycle thus leading the appearance of the high plantar pressures. A relationship between plantar fascia thickness and forefoot increased vertical forces has been established thus supporting that soft tissue abnormalities may contribute to the development of a different pattern of pressure distribution under the foot *(33)*.

An important aspect to bear in mind is related to the role of footwear in the mechanisms associated with the pathogenesis and/or prevention of lesions. Several studies support the belief that inappropriate footwear causes ulceration *(18,34)*. It is fairly obvious that given their vulnerability, subjects with diabetes must select footwear that does not pose a further threat of risk and that ideally should serve as a form of protection. It is important that the physician, conscious of the importance of the role of footwear, be fully informed in order to make suitable recommendations. In turn, the patient must be made aware of the potential risk of lesion posed by unsuitable footwear, and must be encouraged to accept selecting a certain type of footwear that may not necessarily coincide with personal taste. In the discussion outlined later, we will first take a look at the various types of footwear most suitable for patients who do not present lesions, subdivided by category of risk. Subsequently we will discuss the options available for patients with active lesion with a view to releasing the pressure overload at the point of ulceration.

CATEGORIES OF RISK AND FOOTWEAR RECOMMENDATIONS

As outlined earlier, patients with diabetes are at risk of foot ulceration not merely because of diabetes but to diabetes complicated by neuropathy. It is clear that particular attention to footwear should be taken by these subjects at risk, insofar as suitable footwear is able to reduce abnormal pressure, to reduce the formation of callus and ulcers, and to protect from external trauma. Not all patients have the same level of risk, and a number of factors, including the presence/absence of protective sense perception, presence/absence of significant foot deformities and presence/absence of previous ulcers, should be evaluated in determining risk categories and planning corrective means of prevention *(35)*. Four risk categories have been identified on the basis of these criteria (Table 1) *(35)*.

Category 0: Patients Not at Risk of Ulceration

Patients Without Active or Previous Lesions

Diabetic patients without chronic complications and with a preserved protective sensation require adequate education, but no real change to footwear for daily use. In general terms, given their diabetic status, they should be simply encouraged to evaluate

Fig. 1. Shoes with soft sole and amply shaped soft upper available in different widths suitable for risk classes 0 and 1.

Table 2
Suggestions for the Right Selection of Footwear

Both feet should be measured with an appropriate measuring device
Both shoes should be fit while standing
The position at the first metatarso-phalangeal joint should be checked. It should be located in the widest portion of the shoe
The right length of the shoe should be checked; additional volume should be considered at the top of the toes. Allow 3/8 to 1/2 in. between the end of the shoe and the longest toe
The proper width should be tested; enough space should be present around the ball of the foot.
A soft and moldable upper with extra space should be selected in presence of foot deformities
A firm heel counter for rearfoot stability with a soft padded collar
Shoes with laces or straps should be selected because they allow a wider open and an easier entry into the shoes, and in addition they allow a better fitting with the foot shape

a number of factors when selecting footwear, such as whether the shoe is well-fitting and amply shaped with soft uppers and a sole able to absorb vertical forces, and therefore they should avoid tight-fitting footwear with narrow forefoot, tight toe box, or tight instep (Fig. 1). For every foot there is an ideal shape that avoids friction and the development of corns. It is important to consider not only shoe length but also width. Shoes made at least with different widths for each size should be preferred in order to better fit the natural shape of the foot without constriction. Education on selection of suitable footwear is very important (Table 2).

Category 1: Patients at Risk of Ulceration

The development of sensory neuropathy with an ensuing loss of protective sensation involves a subsequent risk of ulceration *(14,19–21)*. Education in patients with a loss of protective sensation assumes a very important role: moreover, a number of behavioral traits need to be inculcated such as never walking barefoot, avoiding mended socks, and learning to substitute the loss of sensation with alternative senses (e.g., eyesight or hand touch). These patients must learn to sample water temperature by hand before washing their feet in order to avoid burns, to detect foreign bodies such as pebbles before putting on their shoes, and to evaluate other dangerous signs (e.g., tacks or worn soles). Even if no studies have assessed the effectiveness of footwear in primary prevention, patients must be guided to an understanding that the selection of footwear cannot be based on the usual criteria, namely the immediate sensation of comfort. Indeed, in the presence of sensory neuropathy the patient perceives even tight shoes to be comfortable. Therefore, it is essential that the foot be measured in all its dimensions and that the footwear

Fig. 2. Oxford, soft flexible leather laced shoes of adequate size to accommodate pressure-dissipating accommodative insoles.

Fig. 3. Single layer, pressure-dissipating accommodative insole.

contain the foot without even the most minimal constriction. Education in the selection of the shoes is therefore very important in this category as well (Table 2). Oxford, soft leather laced shoes of adequate size to accommodate pressure-dissipating accommodative insoles or foot orthoses should be preferred (Figs. 2 and 3).

Category 2: Patients at High Risk of Ulceration

When the loss of protective sensation is complicated by foot deformities (e.g., bunion, claw toe, hammer toe) whether independent of diabetes (e.g., idiopathic bunion) or more frequently secondary to motor neuropathy, the risk of ulceration is considerably increased. Epidemiological studies examining risk factors in ulceration always take foot deformities into consideration as a condition that increases the risk of ulceration *(18,36)*.

In those cases in which foot deformities (e.g., of the toes) are accommodated in unsuitable footwear, the mechanism underlying the lesion involves friction caused by the upper part of the shoe, which in the first instance determines a superficial abrasion and later an outright ulcer. Ulcers associated with this sort of friction are usually localized on the top of the toes and on the lateral surfaces of the first and fifth toes. These cases necessitate a heightened awareness of the correct selection of footwear both in terms of shape, as the foot should not be constrained in any way, and from the point of view of materials used for the uppers. These materials should be soft and flexible, as well as adaptable to any surface irregularities in such a way as to guarantee perfect fitting and to avoid the threat of friction. Nonetheless, the increased risk associated with foot deformities is not exclusively because of the difficulty in accommodating deformed toes, but above all to the biomechanical changes in gait pattern provoked by such deformities. In patients with motor neuropathy together with toe deformities associated with atrophy of the lumbrical and interosseous muscles *(37)*, it is evident an alteration in the walking pattern which could be related to atrophy of the frontal and rear muscles of the leg *(38,39)* and to the modified control of the ankle joint; toe deformities involve a loss of walking function with a consequent appearance and persistence of overload at the metatarsal level in the propulsion and toe off phases *(40–43)*.

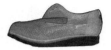

Fig. 4. Section of a shoe with "biomechanical properties:" the recessed heel allows a soft impact at heel strike; the point of rolling inserted immediately behind the metatarsal heads allows a smooth transition from midstance to propulsion; the presence of a wider angle between the sole and the ground at the most anterior part of the shoe further reduces the stress at the level of metatarsal heads during propulsion and toe off.

Table 3
Tovey Suggestions for Correct Selection of Shoes and Insoles in Diabetic Neuropathic Patients

Elastic insoles should ensure the right shock absorption
Insoles should allow the spreading of plantar pressure on a wider area
Shoes should be made with a rocker bottom
Extra space should be provided in the anterior portion of the shoe to accommodate
 deformed toes and to avoid undue hyperpressions from the shoe vamp

Therefore a further pathogenic mechanism of ulceration involves the development of areas of overload; indeed, because of motor neuropathy some areas become overloaded and bear the brunt of altered biomechanics, with ensuing hyperkeratosis in the first instance followed by ulceration *(44)*.

Patients in this category benefit greatly from the use of footwear that enables the correction or at least mitigation of these biomechanical defects *(45,46)*.

The aim underlying footwear recommendations in these patients is to offer an extra level of protection from mechanical stress involved in walking, in those cases in which there has been a loss of the capacity to perceive autonomously an excessive mechanical stress *(47,48)*. Shoes with "biomechanical properties" should allow the development of a protected walking pattern, with reduced plantar pressures. This may be guaranteed by the presence of a recessed heel that allows a soft impact at heel strike, by the presence of a point of rolling of the sole inserted immediately behind the metatarsal heads that allows a smooth transition from midstance to propulsion, and by the presence a wider angle between the sole and the ground at the most anterior part of the shoe that further reduces the stress at the level of metatarsal heads during propulsion and toe off (Fig. 4).

In 1984 Tovey outlined the fundamental requisites for footwear designed for subjects with diabetes (Table 3). These include the need for an appropriate unloading absorbed by total contact, custom-fabricated, pressure-dissipating accommodative foot orthoses (Fig. 5), inserted in deep lacing shoes manufactured in soft leather with a frontal region designed to suitably accommodate claw or hammer toes. Tovey also recommended the use of footwear designed with a rocker bottom in order to reduce the load in the execution of the step in the rolling phase *(49)*. However, since then there are no prospective data to demonstrate the role of footwear in the primary prevention of ulceration in patients with peripheral neuropathy. Data reported in the literature refer either to clinical experience in secondary prevention or to studies in which the parameters evaluated were plantar pressures measured instrumentally and unloaded using different aids *(45–47)*.

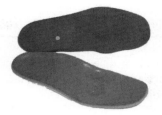

Fig. 5. Total contact, custom-fabricated, pressure-dissipating accommodative foot orthoses.

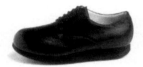

Fig. 6. Footwear with a rigid rocker sole. The rigid sole minimizes the metatarsal-phalangeal joint articulation tension and maximizes foot contact area during late stance phase.

Ashry and colleagues have used insole sensors to measure peak plantar pressures to evaluate the effectiveness of five footwear-insole strategies *(46)*. They found that comparing extra-depth shoes with and without insoles, peak pressures were significantly reduced with insoles, whereas there was no significant difference between the different insole modifications. Using the same measuring device Mueller and colleagues have evaluated *(50)* the peak plantar pressure in patients with diabetes and transmetatarsal amputation and they recorded that the full-length shoe with a total contact insert and a rigid rocker bottom sole was the most effective footwear combination in reducing peak plantar pressures on the distal residuum and the forefoot of the controlateral extremity in patients with diabetes and transmetatarsal amputation. Dalla Paola and colleagues have followed patients with diabetes after the first ray amputation and they found a lower reulceration and reamputation rate compared with that reported in the literature. They concluded that this finding could be attributed to the use of shoes with a rocker bottom sole and custom molded insoles *(51)*.

Kästenbauer and colleagues have shown that certain running shoe ("Adidas torsion equipment Cushion" running shoe) designed for maximal forefoot pressure relief are effective in decreasing plantar pressure, although the pressure relief obtained was not as great as that of the custom made soft insole in an in-depth shoe *(45)*.

Lavery and coworkers have compared the effectiveness of therapeutic, comfort and athletic shoes with and without viscoelastic insoles. They have concluded that when used in conjunction with a viscoelastic insole, both the comfort and athletic cross trainer shoes were as effective as the commonly described therapeutic shoes and therefore viable options to prevent the development or recurrence of foot ulcers.

The measurement of plantar pressure inside footwear has enabled to observe a significant differences in terms of the reduction of pressure between footwear with a rigid sole compared with a flexible sole *(48)*. An increased reduction in pressure is observed in the rigid model as this type of sole minimizes the metatarsal–phalangeal joint articulation tension and maximizes foot contact area during late stance phase (Fig. 6). This kind of shoe induces a modification in the walking pattern that is completely articulated at the ankle joint (the patient, particularly at the beginning of the use of this type of footwear,

Table 4
Characteristics of a Suitable Footwear

Soft leather upper without sewings preferably Oxford type with laces
Rigid rocker sole with a roller axis immediately behind the metatarsal heads
Extra depth to ensure enough space for the deformed toes and for the insertion of pressure-
    dissipating accommodative insoles or foot orthoses

Table 5
Characteristics of a Suitable Insert

Internal layer: soft material to relief areas of hyperpression
Intermediate layer: elastic material that helps in unloading and maximizes the contact area
External layer: less elastic material to support foot shape and function

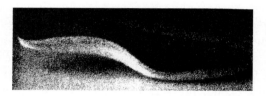

Fig. 7. Total contact inserts can reduce pressure peaks under the foot by maximizing the contact area and spreading the pressure over a larger plantar surface.

may complain about pain in the lower back muscles of the leg because of the fact that these muscles begin to bear a greater load). Indeed, it is important to consider the position of the axis of the roll of the step when designing this type of footwear. The characteristics of this type of footwear permit a significant reduction of the overload. Footwear with a point of the roll of the step placed immediately behind the metatarsal heads are able to guarantee a reduction of peak pressure up to 30% *(52,53)* (Table 4). A further reduction is acquired by the use of customized inserts; a reduction of a further 20% in peak pressure and peak time is possible depending on the materials used and the number of layers to realize the insert. Total contact inserts can reduce pressure peaks on the foot by maximizing contact area of the orthotic device to the foot, and spreading the plantar pressures over a larger plantar surface, clearly have a positive impact on the risk of ulceration (Table 5; Fig. 7) *(46,54–56)*.

Recently Bus, et al. have underlined that custom-made insoles are more effective than flat insoles in off-loading the first metatarsal head region. Nevertheless they observed a considerable variability between individuals and suggested that "because similar insole modifications apparently exert different effects in different patients, a comprehensive evaluation of custom designs using in-shoe pressure measurements should ideally be conducted before dispensing insoles to diabetic patients with neuropathy and foot deformity" *(57)*. However, in another study, therapeutic footwear with different

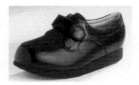

Fig. 8. Shoe with a rigid rocker sole and very high toe box to content deformed toes and multilayered customized insole.

types of footwear insoles (microcellular rubber, polyurethane foam or molded insoles) showed to significantly reduce foot pressures compared with patient's own footwear containing leather board insoles, they also proved effective in reducing the occurrence of new ulcers (4% vs 33%) *(58)*.

One of the most elementary rules of hygiene in these cases is simply never to use the same footwear for prolonged periods of time. Frequent change of footwear puts less stress on discrete areas of the skin and consequently reduces the risk of ulceration.

SECONDARY PREVENTION

Patients at Very High Risk of Ulceration

This category includes patients who have already had an ulcer that has healed. Diabetic patients with a history of relapsing plantar ulcers or patients with a previous minor amputation have abnormally elevated pressures under their feet during walking *(59)*. Peak pressures most often occur under the metatarsal heads and correlate with sites of ulceration *(60)*. The reduction of peak pressure through the use of appropriate footwear represents an important aspect in an effective program of treatment of the neuropathic foot *(61)*.

These patients present a very high risk of relapse. Statistical data demonstrate that this group of patients has a risk of up to 50% in a year *(62)*. In terms of recommendations for the selection of footwear for this group of patients, the principles outlined for patients with peripheral neuropathy hold true for this category as well. In particular, patients should be encouraged to select footwear with rigid rocker soles and molded insert, preferably multilayered insofar as this type is most beneficial in reducing peak pressures (Figs. 7 and 8) *(55,56)*.

In contrast to primary prevention, various studies have demonstrated the protective effect of footwear in secondary prevention, both in terms of made-to-measure solutions and prefabricated commercially designed models. Edmonds and Chanteleau have evaluated the protective effectiveness of made-to-measure footwear, comparing the rate of relapse between subjects either wearing or not wearing the recommended and supplied footwear. The use of suitable footwear represented a significantly lower rate of relapse *(63,64)*. Our experience using commercial models has also demonstrated a lower rate of relapse *(62)*. It was seen that the 1-year follow-up has been 27.7% in the treated group vs 58.3% in the control group. Striesow also, tested industrially produced special shoes realized according to Tovey guidelines and observed similar results *(65)*. More recently, Bush and Chantelau in a cohort study tested the efficacy of "off-the-shelf" therapeutic shoe with standardized insoles and they found that 15% of patients with shoes reulcerated at 1 year vs 60% of patients who did not wear the shoes *(66)*. The use of commercial footwear indeed offers a number of advantages. First of all it is possible to standardize the type of intervention. It is important to highlight that Edmonds in his review stresses the need to identify a single orthopedic procedure as a reference point in recommending corrective measures for the diabetic foot, given the general overall ignorance of the topic *(67)*. In the same way in the consensus development conference on diabetic foot wound care it is generically reported that "footwear should be prescribed, manufactured, and dispensed by individuals with experience in the care of diabetic foot" *(68)*. In addition the Medicare guidelines, related to the therapeutic shoe bill, do not clearly define qualifications of who furnish therapeutic footwear. The only requirement with respect to footwear expertise states "The footwear must be fitted and furnished by a podiatrist or other qualified individual such as a pedorthist, orthotist, or prosthetist." However, the guidelines do not specify standards for nonphysician entities. Suppliers do not have to submit any evidence of their expertise to Medicare *(69)*. It follows that there may be certain situations in which neither the physician is capable of making recommendations nor the orthopedic specialist is sufficiently aware of the problem, and in such cases the solutions offered may be ineffective in the least if not overtly damaging.

Clearly the availability of commercial models with proven success expands the number of patients who can take advantage of beneficial corrective procedures in response to their clinical needs. In addition other advantages may be related to the use of prefabricated models clinically tested, such as a general easier and faster availability of the shoes, the possibility of producing stylist models (Fig. 1) and the significant reduction of the costs related to the ownership of this kind of device with sure advantages for the general management of this complication.

Although general clinical recommendations for people with diabetes include provision of special footwear to individuals with diabetes and foot risk factors *(68,70)* the expert general agreement on the footwear benefits has been recently questioned by the results of a randomized controlled trial in which therapeutic shoes with custom insole or polyurethane insole did not show any difference in the reulceration rate in comparison with control groups *(71)*. The same group in a review article dealing with the effectiveness of diabetic therapeutic footwear in preventing reulceration report some concern when considering the appropriateness of therapeutic footwear recommendations for moderate-risk patients *(72)*. Some criticisms may be moved to the trial in the selection of the patients *(73–75)*, and indeed Maciejewski and colleagues underline the difficulties in conducting studies on the efficacy of the footwear in secondary prevention *(72)*. Therefore the question is still debatable and there is an urgent need for well-designed studies aimed to assess the cost-effectiveness of footwear in both primary and secondary prevention of neuropathic foot ulceration *(76)*.

INSERTS AND BIGGER SHOES

A problem that often arises is that of using inserts in normal shoes. In general, if the footwear is not designed to offer extra space for the insert, the use of a correctly sized shoe will increase pressure on the foot as the insert will naturally tighten the available space. The patient will try to resolve this problem by simply buying a bigger size. However, whereas this will ensure an extra length of 6.7 mm it will offer only an increase of 4 mm at the circumference of the first and fifth metatarsal heads. The ensuing instability of the foot provokes blisters on the surface of the skin, on the heel and on the surface of the back of the foot resulting from the action of transversal forces on the foot as it slips backward and forward. It is important to measure the diameter of the foot at the level of the metatarsal heads, add the thickness of the insert to this measurement, and to compare this with the diameter inside the footwear at that level. The suitability of the footwear depends on the availability of this extra space and not simply on shoe size. Ideally the footwear should have soft, preferably heat sensitive, uppers, which enable comfortable accommodation of the foot deformities, and the appropriately fitted insert.

FACTORS INVOLVED IN THE GENERAL RISK OF ULCERATION

When one considers the general risk of ulceration in a patient, several variables need to be borne in mind which may influence the risk quite considerably. Beyond the structural configuration of the foot, that is foot deformities, which we have seen represent a risk factor for increased plantar pressure (peak pressure) for example, at the level of the prominent metatarsal heads, it must be considered the function of the foot, that is the cumulative amount of time of loading of these peak areas (the risk of ulceration increases with the increase in the variable load peaks and overall time of overload). Another parameter to consider is the protective function of footwear and inserts. This protective function may be effective and may consequently annul the risk of ulceration owing to overload and the time of their application, which may be the case with suitable footwear and inserts. In other cases footwear may exercise no protective function whatsoever or may indeed be damaging. A final consideration involves the lifestyle of patients. The level of activity is understood to be the cumulative load during daily activity, which will naturally be quite different in those with a sedentary lifestyle compared with an active one. It is fairly clear that a neuropathic patient will not present ulcers if confined to bed all day, insofar as plantar overloads are not possible in such a situation *(77)*.

AIDS FOR PATIENTS WITH ACTIVE LESIONS

As we have already highlighted, patients with peripheral neuropathy tend to develop ulcers at the point of maximum load. Often patients are not able to, and they should not, stay in a bed for 4 or 6 weeks, which is ideally the time required to heal an ulcer in patients with normal arterial circulation and an absence of significant complications (e.g., overlapping infections). Often neuropathic ulcers do not heal because of the continued load placed on the ulcer during walking. It is fundamental in these cases to provide for an adequate unloading in order to favor healing *(78)*. Several options are available to ensure unloading in patients with active ulcers *(79)* (Table 6).

Total contact cast is the most extensively studied technique; it offers total unloading of the ulcer as well as the rapid mobilization of the patient who may resume normal activities immediately. As shown in several recent studies, total contact cast has become the gold standard for the treatment of diabetic foot ulcers *(80,81)*. It allows the immobilization of the tissues of the ulcer, it reduces the pressures through a distribution over a wide surface. However, the use of the total contact cast must follow specific indications (neuropathic lesions in the absolute absence of infections) and contraindications

Table 6
Options to Unload a Neuropathic Foot Ulcer

Total contact cast
Other casts/boots (air cast or walking cast)
Temporary shoes
Sandals
Felted foam dressings

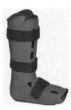

Fig. 9. Aircast: this device allows a good control of high pressures at the ulcer site by means of subpatellar unloading.

(ischemic lesions and infected lesions; furthermore, their use is contra indicated in blind patients and in those with pathological obesity or ataxia) *(82)*.

These plaster casts cover the lesion and are removed and substituted weekly in order to ensure a better fit as the edema withdraws and to inspect the wound.

Alternatively, one may use the scotch cast, a sort of removable boot made of stiff, light material padded with wadding in order to reduce pressure. This procedure is suitable for elderly persons who do not tolerate the plaster cast or in those cases in which ulcers are situated in difficult areas. Indeed, the scotch cast is a sort of compromise between the plaster cast and other aids, as they are made-to-measure and easily removable *(79,83)*.

Other commercial techniques involve the use of stirrups or other pneumatic means of subpatellar unloading (air cast and walking cast) (Fig. 9). The high cost of these aids has prohibited their widespread use; moreover, their results do not seem to be more beneficial than those reported for the plaster cast *(48,84)*. One of the limitations to use these walking casts is the low patients' compliance. In fact the easy removability may allow patients to wear it only in certain occasions. On the other hand, this special feature makes their use possible also in clinical conditions in which it is necessary to follow strictly the lesion. To solve this problem, Armstrong et al. have proposed the use of the "instant" total contact cast that is a walker rendered nonremovable by wrapping it with cast material *(85)*. This solution can have all the advantages of the walker without the disadvantages related to a poor compliance.

Nonetheless, the plaster cast is unsuitable in some conditions. Other aids must be used in these cases, namely temporary shoes as talus shoes that enable an unloading of the lesion in the forefoot because of the absence of a sole in the front part of the shoe (Fig.10). Using this healing device the patients walk by loading only the rearfoot. This type of footwear is particularly indicated in young persons who do not present problems

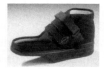

Fig. 10. Talus shoe: it enables the unloading of a forefoot ulcer, because the patients walk by loading only the rearfoot.

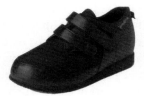

Fig. 11. Temporary footwear with extra volume and rigid rocker sole.

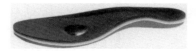

Fig. 12. Foot orthoses for temporary footwear.

of equilibrium. Other aids include temporary footwears with extra volume (extra deep 1/2 in. or super deep 3/4 in.) and rigid rocker sole (Fig. 11). The extra space it is necessary to content a bigger foot because of the edema and of the infection that can be present, an insert that can be grossly molded to form a depression in which the ulcerated area can be accommodated and unloaded (Fig. 12), and bandages that can be different in volume according to the needs of the ulcer. The rigid sole guarantees the immobilization of the metatarsal-phalangeal joint and a reduced load at the level of metatarsal heads *(50)*. The foot ulcer unloading given by temporary footwear is not equivalent to that of total contact cast or walking casts *(79)*, however this kind of device may have other advantages such as its wider usability because of the absence of adverse effects, a better acceptance and therefore better compliance by the patients because of their feeling of a quite normal lifestyle with the possibility of having little walks, of driving the car, although taking care of their foot ulcers.

FOOTWEAR IN CHARCOT'S FOOT

Charcot's foot is characterized by complications of bones and joints of the foot in patients with diabetes and peripheral neuropathy. However, this is not always the case as the condition may occur in other forms of neuropathy such as siringomielia, tabe dorsalis, and so on. A clear case of Charcot's foot is characterized by a complete involvement of the bones and joints structures and the loss of the structural organization of the foot. In its most typical form involving the tarsal bones there is a collapse of the plantar roof, the foot becoming short and squat and the plantar surface assuming a rocking profile and the appearance of high pressures at midfoot, an area that becomes at risk of ulceration *(86)*. Corrective intervention in these patients involves diverse phase-related options. In the less dramatic case in which the bone involvement is detected before bone collapse, the use of a plaster cast, followed by a corrective strategy involving the use of a plantar support of the arch which enables the stabilization of the lesion, it is able to prevent the structural damage to the foot. In other cases a diagnosis is made when the bone structure has already deteriorated and the tarsal bones have lost their articulation. The use of a plaster case is necessary in this case as well at least until the lesion has been stabilized *(87)*. It should be borne in mind that the time frames involved in the use of a plaster cast are fairly long (in some cases up to 6 months), and that its use is based on empirical observations of the skin temperature as there is no supporting scientific data. Subsequent corrective strategies will largely depend on the ensuing structural deformity, insofar as if the patient is able to wear shoes, albeit customized footwear, surgical intervention may not be necessary whereas surgery is usually indicated otherwise. Corrective strategies aim at reducing plantar high plantar pressures and subsequently the risk of ulceration *(88)*. However, in a recent survey, Pinzur has reported that, using commercially available therapeutic footwear and custom foot orthoses, more than 50% patients with Charcot arthropathy at the midfoot level can be successfully managed without surgery *(89)*.

THE PRESCRIPTION AND USE OF SUITABLE FOOTWEAR

One problem in prescribing and wearing protective shoes is that most individuals with diabetes and their physicians are aware of potential diabetic foot morbidity, and very few take advantage of prophylactic footwear *(90)*. Considerable barriers exist to the ownership and use of these shoes. First of all some of these barriers are related to the steps needed to obtain reimbursement for shoes and inserts, that indeed do not allow the furniture, in many instances, of more than one pair of shoes every 12 months.

Second reason is related to the appearance of shoe and patients with foot problems are looking for footwear that is presentable and fashionable as well as protective *(91)*. The third point is the empowerment of the patients in using the protective footwear, because they avoid using the prescribed footwear in many occasions during the day life, and Knowles found that only 22% of the subjects used to wear their prescribed footwear all day *(72)*. It is well-known that diabetic footwear to be effective must be worn at least 60% of the time, and the only way to get this result is to increase patient's perception of the diabetic foot. Macfarlane and Jensen have shown that the use of diabetic shoes is related to the perceived value of the shoe and not to the patient's previous history of foot complications or to the aesthetics of diabetic footwear *(92)*. Many strategies need to be applied to increase the ownership and use of the protective shoes.

In May 1993, the US Congress passed legislation to add coverage of therapeutic shoe for diabetic Medicare beneficiaries of risk of foot disease as a benefit of Medicare Port B coverage. This was done after a 3-year demonstration project that found no evidence that such a benefit had increased overall Medicare costs *(93)*.

However, the number of footwear beneficiaries in respect to the potential number has been reported in less than 1 in 50 Medicare-aged patients with diabetes receiving shoes in 1996 according to therapeutic shoe bill *(94)*. This means that it is necessary to increase awareness of the benefit among eligible beneficiaries. In a recent experience the mailing of motivational brochures has been followed by an increase in the number of persons with diabetes making therapeutic footwear claims *(95)*. Another direction to increase the ownership is to simplify the documentation and shorten the time necessary to obtain shoes and insoles. Finally push the factories in making shoes protective as well as fashionable.

CONCLUSION

The above discussion clearly outlines the important role of footwear in prevention of the foot lesions and their relapse. The health providers should be aware of these important aspects and be able to make precise recommendations regarding the use of suitable footwear.

REFERENCES

1. Reiber GE, Boyko EJ, Smith DG. Lower extremity foot ulcers and amputations in diabetes, in *Diabetes in America*. (Harris MI, Cowie CC, Stern MP, Boyko EJ, Reiber GE, Bennett PH, eds.), 2nd ed., US Govt. Printing Office, 1995 (NIH publ. No. 95-1468), Washington, DC.
2. Centers for Disease Control. *Diabetes Surveillance*, 1993. U.S. Department of Health and Human Services, Atlanta, GA, 1993.
3. Pecoraro RE, Reiber GE, Burgess EM. Pathways to diabetic limb amputation: basis for prevention. *Diabetes Care* 1990;13:513–521.
4. Moss SE, Klein BEK. The prevalence and incidence of lower extremity amputation in diabetic population. *Arch Intern Med* 1992;152:610–616.
5. Litzelman DK, Slemenda CW, Langefeld CD, et al. Reduction of lower extremity clinical abnormalities in patients with non-insulin-dependent diabetes mellitus. *Ann Intern Med* 1993; 119:36–41.
6. Edmonds ME, Foster A, Watkins PJ. Can careful foot care in the diabetic patient prevent major amputation? in *Limb Salvage and Amputation for Vascular Disease*. (Greenhalgh RM, Jamieson CW, Nicolaides AN, eds.), WB Sauders, Philadelphia, 1988, pp. 407–417.
7. Davidson JK, Alogna M, Goldsmith M, Borden J. Assessment of program effectiveness at Grady Memorial Hospital—Atlanta. in *Educating Diabetic Patients*. (Steiner G, Lawrence PA, eds.), Springer, New York, 1981, pp. 329–348.
8. Runyan JW Jr, Vander Zwaag R, Joiner MB, Miller ST. The Memphis Diabetes Continuing Care Program. *Diabetes Care* 1980;3:382–386.
9. Assal JP, Muhlhauser I, Pernet A, Gfeller R, Jorgens V, Berger M. Patient education as the basis for diabetes care in clinical practice and research. *Diabetologia* 1985;28:602–613.
10. Boulton AJM, Kubrusly DB, Bowker JH, et al. Impaired vibratory perception and diabetic foot ulceration. *Diabet Med* 1986;3:335–337.
11. Sims DS Jr, Cavanagh PR, Ulbrecht JS. Risk factors in the diabetic foot. *J Am Phys Ther Assoc* 1988;68:1887–1902.
12. Lavery LA, Armstrong DG, Vela SA, Quebedeaux JL, Fleischli J. Practical criteria for screening patients at high risk for diabetic foot ulcerations. *Arch Intern Med* 1998;158: 157–162.
13. McCabe CJ, Stevenson RC, Dolan AM. Evaluation of a diabetic foot screening and education program. *Diabet Med* 1998;15:80–84.
14. Young MJ, Breddly JL, Veves A, Boulton AJM. The prediction of diabetic neuropathic foot ulceration using vibration perception thresholds: a prospective study. *Diabetes Care* 1994; 17:557–560.
15. McNeely MJ, Boyko EJ, Ahroni Jh, et al. The independent contributions of diabetic neuropathy and vasculopathy in foot ulceration. *Diabetes Care* 1995;18:216–219.

16. Reiber GE, Vileikyte L, Boyko EJ, et al. Causal pathways for incident lower-extremity ulcers in patients with diabetes from two setting. *Diabetes Care* 1999;22:157–162.
17. Harris M, Eastman R, Cowie C. Symptoms of sensory neuropathy in adults with NIDDM in the U.S. population. *Diabetes Care* 1982;16:1446–1452.
18. Apelqvist J, Larsson J, Agardh CD. The influence of external precipitating factors and peripheral neuropathy on the development and outcome of diabetic foot ulcers. *J Diabetes Complications* 1990;4:21–25.
19. Litzelman DK, Marriott DJ, Vinicor F. Independent physiological predictors of foot lesions in patients with NIDDM. *Diabetes Care* 1997;20:1273–1278.
20. Birke JA, Sims DS. Plantar sensory threshold in ulcerative foot. *Lepr Rev* 1986;57:216–267.
21. Sosenko JM, Kato M, Soto R, Bild DE. Comparison of quantitative sensory-threshold measures for their association with foot ulceration in diabetic patients. *Diabetes Care* 1990;13: 1057–1061.
22. Kumar S, Fernando DJS, Veves A, Knowles EA, Young MJ, Boulton AJM. Semmes Weinstein monofilaments: a simple, effective and inexpensive screening device for identifying diabetic patients at risk of foot ulceration. *Diabetes Care* 1991;13:63–68.
23. Rith-Najarian SJ, Stolusky T, Gohdes DM. Identifying diabetic patients at high risk for lower-extremity amputation in a primary health care setting. *Diabetes Care* 1992;15: 1386–1389.
24. Cavanagh PR, Simoneau GG, Ulbrecht JS. Ulceration, unsteadiness, and uncertainity the biomechanical consequences of diabetes mellitus. *J Biomechanics* 1993;26:23–40.
25. Coughlin MS. Mallet toes, hammer toes, claw toes, and corns: causes and treatments of lesser toe deformities. *Postgrad Med* 1984;75:191–198.
26. Habershaw G, Donovan JC. Biomechanical considerations of the diabetic foot. in *Management of Diabetic Foot Problems.* (Kozak GP, Hoar CS, Rowbotham JL, Wheelock FC, Gibbons GW, Campbell D, eds.), WB Saunders, Philadelphia, 1984, pp. 32–44.
27. Ctercteko GC, Dhanendran M, Hutton WC, Lequesne LP. Vertical forces acting on the feet of diabetic patients with neuropathic ulceration. *Br J Surg* 1981;68:608–614.
28. Boulton AJM, Betts RP, Franks CI, Ward JD, Duckworth T. The natural history of foot pressure abnormalities in neuropathic diabetic subjects. *Diabetic Res* 1987;5:73–77.
29. Gooding GAW, Stess RM, Graf PM. Sonography of the sole of the foot: evidence for loss of foot pad thickness in diabetes and its relationship to ulceration of the foot. *Invest Radiol* 1986;21:45–48.
30. Young MJ, Cavanagh PR, Thomas G, Johnson MM, Murray H, Boulton AJM. The effect of callus removal on dynamic plantar foot pressures in diabetic patients. *Diabetes Med Supp* 1992;9:55–57.
31. Veves A, Murray HJ, Young MJ, Boulton AJM. The risk of foot ulceration in diabetic patients with high foot pressure: a prospective study. *Diabetologia* 1992;35:660–663.
32. Masson EA, Hay EM, Stockley I, Veves A, Betts RP, Boulton AJM. Abnormal foot pressures alone may not cause ulceration. *Diabet Med* 1989;6:426–428.
33. D'Ambrogi E, Giurato L, D'Agostino MA, et al. Contribution of plantar fascia to the increased forefoot pressures in diabetic patients. *Diabetes Care* 2003;26:1525–1529.
34. MacFarlane RM, Jeffcoate WJ. Factors contributing to the presentation of diabetic foot ulcers. *Diabetic Med* 1997;16:867–870.
35. Lavery LA, Armstrong DG, Vela SA, Quebedeax TL, Fleischli JC. Practical criteria for screening patients at high risk for diabetic foot ulceration. *Arch Intern Med* 1998;158:157–162.
36. Faglia E, Favales F, Morabito A. New ulceration, new major amputation, and survival rates in diabetic subjects hospitalized for foot ulceration from 1990 to 1993: a 6.5-year follow-up. *Diabetes Care* 2001;24:78–83.
37. Mayfield JA, Reiber GE, Sanders LJ, Janisse D, Pogach LM. Preventive foot care in people with diabetes. *Diabetes Care* 1999;21:2161–2177.

38. Andersen H, Gadeberg PC, Brock B, Jakobsen J. Muscular atrophy in diabetic neuropathy: a stereological magnetic resonance imaging study. *Diabetologia* 1997;40:1062–1069.
39. Andersen H, Poulsen PL, Mogensen CE, Jakobsen J. Isokinetic muscle strength in long-term IDDM patients in relation to diabetic complications. *Diabetes* 1996;45:440–445.
40. Payne CB. Biomechanics of the foot in diabetes mellitus. Some theoretical considerations. *J Am Podiatr Med Assoc* 1998;88(6):285–289.
41. Payne CB. Relief of plantar pressure in diabetic patients. *Diabet Med* 1998;15(6):518–522.
42. Uccioli L, Caselli A, Giacomozzi C, et al. Pattern of abnormal tangential forces in the diabetic neuropathic foot. *Clin Biom* 2001;16:446–454.
43. Giacomozzi C, Caselli A, Macellari V, Giurato L, Lardieri L, Uccioli L. Walking strategy in diabetic patients with peripheral neuropathy. *Diabetes Care* 2002;25(8):1451–1457.
44. Delbrid L, Appleberg M, Reeve TS. Factors associated with development of foot lesions in the diabetic. *Surgery* 1983;93(1):78–82.
45. Kastenbauer T, Sokol G, Auinger M, Irsigler. Running shoes for relief of plantar pressure in diabetic patients. *Diabet Med* 1998;15(6):518–522.
46. Ashry HR, Lavery LA, Murdoch DP, Frolich M, Lavery DC. Effectiveness of diabetic insoles to reduce foot pressures. *J Foot Ankle Surg* 1997;36(4):268–271.
47. Mueller MJ. Therapeutic footwear helps protect the diabetic foot. *J Am Podiatr Med Assoc* 1997;87(8):360–364.
48. Lavery LA, Vela SA, Fleischli JG, Armstrong DG, Lavery DC. Reducing plantar pressure in the neuropathic foot. A comparison of footwear. *Diabetes Care* 1997;20(11):1706–1710.
49. Tovey FI. The manufacture of diabetic footwear. *Diabet Med* 1984;1:69–71.
50. Mueller MJ, Strube MJ, Allen BT. Therapeutic footwear can reduce plantar pressure in patients with diabetes and transmetatarsal amputation. *Diabetes Care* 1997;20(4):637–641.
51. Dalla Paola L, Faglia E, Caminiti M, Clerici G, Ninkovic S, Deanesi V. Ulcer recurrence following first ray amputation in diabetic patients: a cohort prospective study. *Diabetes Care* 2003;26:1874–1878.
52. Van Schie C, Ulbrecht JS, Becker MB, Cavanagh PR. Design criteria for rigid rocker shoes. *Foot Ankle Int* 2001;22:184–185.
53. Cavanagh PR, Ulbrecht JS, Caput GM. Biomechanical aspects of diabetic foot disease: aetiology, treatment and prevention. *Diabet Med* 1996;13(1):517–522.
54. Lord M, Riad H. Pressure redistribution by holded inserts in diabetic footwear: a pilot study. *J Rehabil Res Dev* 1994;31(3):214–221.
55. Mueller MJ. Application of plantar pressure assessment in footwear and insert design. *J Orthop Sports Phys Ther* 1999;29:745–755.
56. Foto JG, Birke J. Evaluation of multidensity orthotic materials used in footwear for patients with diabetes. *Foot Ankle Int* 1998;19(12):836–841.
57. Bus SA, Ulbrecht JS, Cavanagh PR. Pressure relief and load redistribution by custom-made insoles in diabetic patients with neuropathy and foot deformity. *Clin Biomech* 2004;19: 629–638.
58. Viswanathan V, Madhavan S, Gnanasundaram S, et al. Effectiveness of different types of footwear insoles for the diabetic neuropathic foot: a follow-up study. *Diabetes Care* 2004;27:474–477.
59. Brand PW. Repetitive stress in the development of diabetic foot ulcers. in *The Diabetic Foot*. (Levin ME, Davidson JK, eds.), 4th ed., Mosby, St. Louis, MO, 1988, pp. 83–90.
60. Veves A, Murray HJ, Young MJ, Boulton AJM. The risk of foot ulceration in diabetic patients with high foot pressure: a prospective study. *Diabetologia* 1992;35:660–663.
61. Litzelman DK, Marriot DJ, Vinicor F. The role of footwear in the prevention of foot lesion in patients with NIDDH. *Diabetes Care* 1997;20(2):156–162.
62. Uccioli L, Faglia E, Monticone G, et al. Manufactured shoes in the prevention of diabetic foot ulcers. *Diabetes Care* 1995;18:1376–1378.

63. Edmonds ME, Blundell MP, Morris ME, Thomas EM, Cotton LT, Watkins PJ. Improved survival of the diabetic foot: the role of a specialized foot clinic. *Q J Med* 1986;60:763–771.
64. Chantelau E, Haage P. An audit of cushioned diabetic footwear: relation to patient compliance. *Diabet Med* 1994;11:114–116.
65. Striesow F. Special manufactured shoes for prevention of recurrent ulcer in diabetic foot syndrome. *Med Klin* 1998;93(12):695–700.
66. Bush K, Chantelau E. Effectiveness of a new brand of stock "diabetic" shoes to protect against diabetic foot ulcer relapse: a prospective cohort study. *Diabet Med* 2003;20:665–669.
67. Edmonds ME. Experience in a multidisciplinary diabetic foot clinic. in The foot in diabetes: proceedings of the First National Conference on the Diabetic Foot, Malvern, England, May 1986. (Connor H, Boulton AJM, Ward JD, eds.), John Wiley, Chichester, England, 1987, pp. 121–134.
68. American Diabetes Association. Preventive foot care in people with diabetes. *Diabetes Care* 2003;26(Suppl 1):S78–S79.
69. Department of Health and Human Services. Medicare payments for therapeutic shoes. August 1998 OEI-03-97-00300.
70. Apelquist J, Bakker K, van Houtum WH, Nabuurs-Franssen MH, Schaper NC. International consensus and practical guidelines on the management and prevention of the diabetic foot. *Diabetes Metab Res Rev* 2000;16:S84–S92.
71. Reiber GE, Smith DG, Wallace C, et al. Effect of therapeutic footwear on foot reulceration in patients with diabetes: a randomized clinical trial. *JAMA* 2002;287:2552–2558.
72. Maciejewski ML, Reiber GE, Smith DG, Wallace C, Hayes S, Boyko EJ. Effectiveness of diabetic therapeutic footwear in preventing re-ulceration. *Diabetes Care* 2004;27:1774–1782.
73. Cavanagh PR, Boulton AJM, Sheehan P, Ulbrecht JS, Caputo GM, Armstrong DG. Therapeutic footwear in patients with diabetes (Letter). *JAMA* 2002;288:1231.
74. Chantelau E. Therapeutic footwear in patients with diabetes (Letter). *JAMA* 2002;288: 1231, 1232.
75. Reiber GE, Smith DG, Wallace C, et al. Therapeutic footwear in patients with diabetes (Letter). *JAMA* 2002;288:1232.
76. Boulton AJM, Jude EB. Therapeutic footwear in diabetes. *Diabetes Care* 2004;27:1832, 1833.
77. Cavanagh PR, Ulbrecht JS. Biomechanical aspects of foot problems in diabetes. in *The Foot in Diabetes* (Boulton AJM, Connor H, Cavanagh PR, eds.), 2nd ed., John Wiley, New York, 1994, pp. 25–35.
78. Stess RM, Jensen SR, Mirmiran R. The role of dynamic plantar pressure in diabetic foot ulcers. *Diabetes Care* 1997;20(5):855–858.
79. Armstrong DG, Lavery LA. Evidence-based options for off-loading diabetic wounds. *Clin Podiatr Med Surg* 1998;15(1):95–104.
80. Caravaggi C, Faglia E, De Giglio R, et al. Effectiveness and safety of a nonremovable fiberglass off-bearing cast versus a therapeutic shoe in the treatment of neuropathic foot ulcers: a randomized study. *Diabetes Care* 2000;23:1746–1751.
81. Armstrong DG, Nguyen HC, Lavery LA, van Schie CH, Boulton AJ, Harkless LB. Off-loading the diabetic foot wound: a randomized clinical trial. *Diabetes Care* 2001;24:1019–1022.
82. Borssen B, Lithner F. Plaster casts in the management of advanced ischaemic and neuropathic diabetic foot lesions. *Diabet Med* 1989;6(8):720–723.
83. Knowles EA, Armstrong DG, Hayat SA, Khawaja KI, Malik RA, Boulton AJ. Offloading diabetic foot wounds using the scotchcast boot: a retrospective study. *Ostomy Wound Manage* 2002;48:50–53.
84. Baumhauer JF, Wervey R, McWilliams J, Harris GF, Shereff MJ. A comparison study of plantar foot pressure in a standardized shoe, total contact cast, and prefabricated pneumatic walking brace. *Foot Ankle Int* 1997;18(1):26–33.
85. Armstrong DG, Short B, Espensen EH, Abu-Rumman PL, Nixon BP, Boulton AJ. Technique for fabrication of an "instant total-contact cast" for treatment of neuropathic diabetic foot ulcers. *J Am Podiatr Med Assoc* 2002;92(7):405–408.

86. Armstrong DG, Todd WF, Lavery LA, Harkless LB, Bushman TR. The natural history of acute Charcot's arthropathy in a diabetic foot specialty clinic. *Diabet Med* 1997;14(5):357–363.
87. Armstrong DG, Lavery LA. Elevated peak plantar pressures in patients who have Charcot arthropathy. *J Bone Joint Surg Am* 1998;80(3):365–369.
88. Lavery LA, Armstrong DG, Walker SC. Healing rates of diabetic foot ulcers associated with midfoot fracture due to Charcot's arthropathy. *Diabet Med* 1997;14:46–49.
89. Pinzur M. Surgical versus accommodative treatment for Charcot arthropathy of the midfoot. *Foot Ankle Int* 2004;25:545–549.
90. Pinzur MS, Shields NN, Goelitz B, et al. American Orthopaedic Foot and Ankle Society shoe survey of diabetic patients. *Foot Ankle Int* 1999;20:703–707.
91. Knowles EA, Boulton AJ. Do people with diabetes wear their prescribed footwear? *Diabet Med* 1996;13:1064–1068.
92. Macfarlane DJ, Jensen JL. Factors in diabetic footwear compliance. *J Am Podiatr Med Assoc* 2003;93:485–491.
93. Woolridge J, Moreno L. Evaluation of the costs to medicare of covering therapeutic shoes for diabetic patients. *Diabetes Care* 1994;17:541–547.
94. Sugarman JR, Reiber GE, Baumgrdner G, Prela CM, Lowery J. Use of the therapeutic footwear benefit among diabetic medicare beneficiaries in three states, 1995. *Diabetes Care* 1998;21:777–781.
95. LeMaster JW, Sugarman JR, Baumgardner G, Reiber GE. Motivational brochures increase the number of medicare-eligible persons with diabetes making therapeutic footwear claims. *Diabetes Care* 2003;26:1679–1684.

INDEX